ORTHODONTIC TREATMENT
OF THE CLASS II NONCOMPLIANT PATIENT

Commissioning Editor: Michael Parkinson
Development Editor: Hannah Kenner
Project Manager: Jane Dingwall
Design: Stewart Larking
Illustration Manager: Bruce Hogarth

ORTHODONTIC TREATMENT OF THE CLASS II NONCOMPLIANT PATIENT

CURRENT PRINCIPLES AND TECHNIQUES

EDITED BY

MOSCHOS A. PAPADOPOULOS DDS, Dr Med Dent

Associate Professor
Department of Orthodontics
School of Dentistry
Aristotle University of Thessaloniki
Thessaloniki, Greece

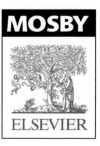

Edinburgh London New York Oxford Philadelphia St Louis Sydney Toronto 2006

MOSBY
ELSEVIER

First published 2006

ISBN-13: 978-0-7234-3391-0
ISBN-10: 0-7234-3391-7

British Library Cataloguing in Publication Data
A catalogue record for this book is available from the British Library

Library of Congress Cataloging in Publication Data
A catalog record for this book is available from the Library of Congress

Note
Knowledge and best practice in this field are constantly changing. As new research and experience broaden our knowledge, changes in practice, treatment and drug therapy may become necessary or appropriate. Readers are advised to check the most current information provided (i) on procedures featured or (ii) by the manufacturer of each product to be administered, to verify the recommended dose or formula, the method and duration of administration, and contraindications. It is the responsibility of the practitioner, relying on their own experience and knowledge of the patient, to make diagnoses, to determine dosages and the best treatment for each individual patient, and to take all appropriate safety precautions. To the fullest extent of the law, neither the Publisher nor the Editor assumes any liability for any injury and/or damage to persons or property arising out or related to any use of the material contained in this book.

The Publisher

ELSEVIER your source for books, journals and multimedia in the health sciences
www.elsevierhealth.com

The publisher's policy is to use paper manufactured from sustainable forests

Working together to grow libraries in developing countries

www.elsevier.com | www.bookaid.org | www.sabre.org

ELSEVIER   BOOK AID International   Sabre Foundation

Printed in China

Preface

During orthodontic treatment, cooperation or compliance of the patients is a major factor for a successful treatment outcome. In order to achieve successful treatment results, patients are expected to follow the recommended regimens suggested by their orthodontists. Unfortunately, lack of patient compliance is one of the major problems in orthodontic treatment and often the clinicians have to deal with this issue almost daily. Orthodontic treatment in patients with limited compliance can, among other things, result in a longer treatment time, destruction of the teeth and periodontium, extraction of additional teeth, frustration for the patient and additional stress for the orthodontist and staff. This is the reason why a lot of effort has been directed over the years to developing noncompliance techniques.

Noncompliance approaches are a very important option for the orthodontic treatment of patients with Class II malocclusion who present with minimal or no cooperation, especially when nonextraction treatment protocols have to be utilized. Conventional orthodontic procedures usually require patient cooperation, which very often is a significant problem to overcome in order to achieve successful treatment outcomes. During the last decades a great variety of noncompliance appliances and techniques have been proposed in order to correct Class II malocclusion, either by advancing the mandible to a more forward position or by distalizing the maxillary molars into a Class I relationship.

The aim of this book is to cover the subject of noncompliance Class II orthodontic treatment in a comprehensive and critical way, presenting the principles and techniques of the most important currently available noncompliance appliances used for the treatment of Class II malocclusion, while focusing on their clinical management and effectiveness.

The book is divided into five sections, starting from the problem of compliance (Section I), describing several intermaxillary appliances (Section II), intramaxillary distalization appliances (Section III), and intramaxillary appliances with absolute anchorage (Section IV), and closing with the evidence-based knowledge on the efficacy of these appliances (Section V).

In detail, the book contains information regarding the following subjects, chapter by chapter. In Section I, Chapter 1 introduces the reader to the main aspects of the noncompliance treatment in orthodontics, and Chapter 2 provides a classification of the noncompliance appliances used for the treatment of Class II malocclusion. In Section II, Chapter 3 presents an overview of the various currently available noncompliance intermaxillary appliances used in Class II orthodontic treatment, while Chapters 4–14 discuss in detail the current principles and the clinical management of these appliances, including the Herbst appliance, the Cantilever Bite Jumper (CBJ), the Ritto Appliance, the Mandibular Protraction Appliance, the Mandibular Anterior Repositioning Appliance (MARA), the Jasper Jumper, the Flex Developer, the Eureka Spring, the Twin Force Bite Corrector, and the Sabbagh Universal Spring (SUS). In Section III, Chapter 15 presents an overview of the various intramaxillary distalization appliances utilized for the management of Class II malocclusion, while Chapters 16–23 discuss thoroughly the current principles and the clinical management of these appliances, such as the Pendulum appliance, the Penguin Pendulum, the Distal Jet, the Keles Slider, the Jones Jig and modifications, magnets, the First Class Appliance and the Keles TPA. Section IV focuses on the intramaxillary appliances with absolute anchorage: Chapter 24 presents an overview of these appliances, Chapter 25 describes the use of implants as absolute anchorage for Class II correction, and Chapter 26 provides information concerning the use of onplants for maxillary molar distalization. The final chapter, Chapter 27 (Section IV), provides the reader with all currently available evidence concerning the clinical efficacy of the noncompliance appliances used for Class II correction.

Effort was made by the editor to invite orthodontists who are expert in each specific subject to contribute chapters to this book. Almost all the authors have either developed or introduced sophisticated appliances, or they have been actively involved in their clinical evaluation.

It is the hope of the editor that this book will provide all the background needed for the better understanding and more efficient use of the currently available noncompliance appliances and that students, faculty, and practitioners will find this book useful for the clinical management of noncompliant patients presenting with Class II malocclusion.

Moschos A. Papadopoulos
Thessaloniki, Greece

List of contributors

Claudio Arcuri, MD, DDS
Associate Professor, Fatebenefratelli Hospital,
Department of Oral Pathology,
University of Rome "Tor Vergata",
Rome, Italy

Lars Bondemark, DDS, Odont Dr
Associate Professor, Head of the Department
of Orthodontics,
Faculty of Odontology,
Malmö University, Malmö, Sweden

Steven Jay Bowman, DDS
Adjunct Professor, Department of
Orthodontics,
University of Saint Louis, St Louis, MO, USA

Friedrich K. Byloff, DDS, MD, Dip Orth
Private Practice, Graz, Austria

†Aldo Carano, Dr Odont, MS, Spec Orthod
Adjunct Professor, Department of
Orthodontics,
University of Ferrara, Ferrara, Italy *and*
Adjunct Professor, Department of
Orthodontics,
University of Saint Louis, St Louis, MO, USA

Fabio Oliveira Coelho, DDS
Graduate Student of Orthodontics, Uniararas
University *and*
MS candidate, São Paulo, São Luis, Maranhão,
Brazil

M. Ali Darendeliler, BDS, Dip Orth, Cert Orth, PhD
Professor and Chair, Discipline of Orthodontics,
Faculty of Dentistry, Sydney Dental Hospital,
University of Sydney,
Sydney, Australia

† = deceased

John P. DeVincenzo, DDS, MS
Adjunct Associate Professor, Department of
Orthodontics,
School of Dentistry, Loma Linda University,
Loma Linda, CA, USA

James E. Eckhart, DDS
Private Practice, Torrance, CA, USA

Carlos Martins Coelho Filho, DDS, MSD
Former Professor of Orthodontics,
Federal University of Maranhão *and*
Private Practice, São Luis, Maranhão, Brazil

Arturo Fortini, MD, DDS
Private Practice, Florence, Italy

Lorenzo Franchi, DDS, PhD
Research Associate, Department of
Orthodontics,
University of Florence, Florence, Italy *and*
Thomas M. Graber Visiting Scholar,
Department of Orthodontics and Pediatric
Dentistry,
School of Dentistry, University of Michigan,
Ann Arbor, MI, USA

Aldo Giancotti, DDS, MS
Assistant Professor, Fatebenefratelli Hospital,
Department of Orthodontics,
University of Rome "Tor Vergata",
Rome, Italy

James J. Jasper, DDS
Private Practice, Santa Barbara, CA, USA

Ahmet Keles, DDS, DMSc
Associate Research Investigator,
The Forsyth Institute, Boston, MA, USA *and*
Private Practice, Istanbul, Turkey

Joe H. Mayes, DDS, MSD
Clinical Assistant Professor, Department of
Orthodontics,
Baylor College of Dentistry *and*
Consultant to the Craniofacial Virtual Reality
Lab,
University of California (USC) *and*
Private Practice, Lubbock, TX, USA

Alfred Peter Muchitsch, MD, DDS
Assistant Professor, Clinical Department of
Orthodontics,
School of Dentistry, Medical University of Graz,
Graz, Austria

Ravindra Nanda, BDS, M Dent Sc, PhD
Professor and Head, Department of
Orthodontics,
Oral Surgery, Pediatric Dentistry and AEGD,
School of Dental Medicine, University of
Connecticut,
Farmington, CT, USA

Hans U. Paulsen, DDS, Odont Dr
Visiting Professor, Karolinska Institutet,
Stockholm, Sweden *and*
Former Associate Professor, Department of
Orthodontics,
University of Aarhus, Aarhus *and*
Department of Orthodontics, Copenhagen
Municipal Dental Health Service, Copenhagen,
Denmark

António Korrodi Ritto, DDS, PhD
Private Practice, Leiria, Portugal

Jeff Rothenberg, DDS
Private Practice, Miami, FL, USA

Aladin Sabbagh, DDS
Private Practice, Nuremberg, Germany

Gang Shen, BDS, MDS, PhD
Associate Professor, Discipline of Orthodontics,
Faculty of Dentistry, Sydney Dental Hospital,
University of Sydney,
Sydney, Australia

Flavio Uribe, DSS, MDS
Assistant Professor, Division of Orthodontics,
School of Dental Medicine, University of
Connecticut,
Farmington, CT, USA

Frank J. Weiland, DMD, PhD
Former Associate Professor, Department of
Orthodontics,
University Dental School, Graz *and*
Private Practice, Graz, Austria

Heinz Winsauer, DDS
Private Practice, Bregenz, Austria

Andrej Zentner, BDS, PhD, Dr habil, FDS RCS
Professor and Chairman, Department of
Orthodontics and Social Dentistry, Academic
Center for Dentistry Amsterdam (ACTA),
Amsterdam, The Netherlands

Acknowledgments

The editor is most grateful to all colleagues involved in the preparation of the chapters included in this book for their valuable contributions, and especially to Dr A. Carano, who recently passed away. He was a very decent person and a great scientist who, although seriously ill, succeeded in contributing a chapter concerning his innovation, the Distal Jet appliance. The editor wishes also to express his sincere appreciation to his mentor, Professor T. Rakosi, for his inspiration and guidance during the very first years of his postgraduate studies in orthodontics, and to Professor A. E. Athanasiou for his friendship and his continuing support over the years. Dr A. Mavropoulos, Dr A. Karamouzos, and Professor S. Kiliaridis are also acknowledged for their significant contribution in the preparation of the two published papers concerning the sectional jig assembly. Further, the journals *American Journal of Orthodontics and Dentofacial Orthopedics, Clinical Orthodontics and Research, European Journal of Orthodontics, Hellenic Orthodontic Review, Journal of Orofacial Orthopedics, The Angle Orthodontist* and *World Journal of Orthodontics* are acknowledged for granting permission to use in Chapters 4, 10, 19, 20, 22, 23 and 26, certain texts, figures, and diagrams which were previously published by their journals, as well as Mr I. Gkiaouris for his assistance during the preparation of the literature reviews used for Chapters 3, 15, and 27. Finally, Mr M. Parkinson, Senior Commissioning Editor, Ms H. Kenner, Development Editor, and Ms J. Dingwall, Project Manager, are also acknowledged for their excellent cooperation during the preparation and publication procedures of this book, as well as Elsevier Health Sciences for the high quality of the published work.

Dedication

To my family for their love,
understanding and their full
support over the years

Contents

SECTION III

INTRAMAXILLARY DISTALIZATION APPLIANCES USED FOR THE MANAGEMENT OF CLASS II NONCOMPLIANT PATIENTS

SECTION IV

INTRAMAXILLARY APPLIANCES WITH ABSOLUTE ANCHORAGE USED FOR THE MANAGEMENT OF CLASS II MALOCCLUSION

SECTION V

CLINICAL EFFICACY OF THE NONCOMPLIANCE APPLIANCES

SECTION ONE

CLASS II ORTHODONTIC TREATMENT AND COMPLIANCE

This section includes chapters on the following:

1   The problem of compliance in orthodontics
2   Classification of the noncompliance appliances used for Class II correction

CHAPTER 1

The problem of compliance in orthodontics

Andrej Zentner

Background and Definitions

In recent decades biologic understanding and technologic advancement have substantially improved the efficiency of conventional orthodontic treatment. However, its outcome is still to a large extent dependent on the patient's compliance. Whilst there is no consistent definition of this term, "compliance" contains elements relating to patients' self-care responsibilities, their role in the treatment process and collaboration with the care providers. Alternative terms such as adherence, cooperation, mutuality, and therapeutic alliance are also used. "Therapeutic alliance" is applied to the process of patient–provider interactions, "compliance" and "adherence" refer to the outcome of such interactions while "adherence" also stresses the responsibility of the clinician to form a therapeutic relationship with the patient and enhance the outcome.[1]

Compliance is a very important healthcare issue and has been studied since the 1950s from a wide range of perspectives, including medical care and nursing, psychology, and health economics. Several theories have been adopted from behavioral psychology and various intervention approaches applied to compliance and health behavior modification. The interested reader is referred to relevant literature for more background reading on these topics.[2–8] Compliance with orthodontic treatment has also attracted considerable research attention and the current knowledge on various aspects of this issue is summarized in recently published comprehensive reviews.[9,10]

Orthodontic treatment may cause unpleasant sensations and impede speech while appliance wear may interfere with daily life, is difficult to control, and may be easily forgotten. From the life perspective of a child or adolescent, treatments lasting over 2 years may appear extremely long and most orthodontic treatments are provided in adolescence which is a time of life abundant in complex social and developmental issues. Furthermore, orthodontic correction is an elective treatment and, in contrast to serious diseases, non-compliance has no vital consequences. Incidentally, preventive health behaviors, which, subjectively, are more closely comparable to compliance in orthodontics than management of serious chronic diseases, are generally rather difficult to achieve. For instance, long-term adherence to preventive moderate physical exercise is disappointing[11] and maintenance of successful health behavior changes seems also quite difficult, as shown by the report that 43% of individuals who had quit tobacco smoking returned to regular smoking after 12 months of continuous abstinence.[12]

It is recognized that compliance is a problem with a considerable challenge in orthodontic patient management.[9,10] For a better understanding of this problem, two issues require thorough consideration: the factors influencing compliance, and its assessment and prediction.

Factors Related to Compliance

The factors associated with adherence to treatment occur in the following key areas:

- the psychosocial characteristics of the patient
- the nature of the treatment regimen
- the relationship between the clinicians and the patient and their parents.

Patient Characteristics

These encompass personality characteristics, demographic parameters, social support, knowledge of the treatment regimen, and health-related behaviors such as health value, motivation, and locus of control.

Personality Characteristics

It is assumed that the patient's personality characteristics and performance at school are closely associated with orthodontic compliance.[13–15] Cooperative orthodontic patients tend to have better grades, show less deviant behavior, are considered academically brighter and more sociable by their teachers, and reveal higher levels of self-perceived cognitive competence.[15] Psychologic assessment of orthodontic patients[16–18] has outlined the following profiles of uncooperative and cooperative patients. Irrespective of gender, patients who tend to be uncooperative are inclined to attitudinal preferences conventionally regarded as masculine, which are expressed as active, aggressive, and realistic behaviors and self-images, rather than sensitive, esthetic, and idealistic ones. Impulsiveness, need for egoassertion, individualism, impatience, intolerance, and negligence are also characteristic psychologic traits of noncompliant patient.[16,17,19] The patients who are more likely to show higher levels of treatment compliance tend to be enthusiastic, outgoing, energetic, self-controlled, responsible, trusting, diligent, and obliging individuals.[16]

Demographic Aspects

With regard to patients' age, it is known from behavioral medicine that the level of adherence of children and adolescents is lower than that of adults, and that adolescents are less compliant than younger children.[5] In addition, the young child's adherence to the treatment regimen depends on both his/her own adherence and that of the parents, and there is often confusion in the families of adolescents over allocation of responsibility for adherence to the treatment regimen.[5]

In orthodontics, age is not considered to be a factor explicitly influencing the adherence to treatment.[15,20] This is probably attributable to the elective nature of orthodontic treatment and children's and adolescents' individual psychologic maturation. For instance, even adolescent development might have different effects on individual patients, leading either to adoption of a healthy lifestyle and enhancement of self-responsibility or, in contrast, to establishment of health-risking behavioral patterns.[19,21,22] The potential influence of other demographic parameters such as gender, socioeconomic status and private versus third-party treatment financing is also very inconsistent.[15] Normal events of everyday life, such as daily routine, sports, social activities, transient emotional disposition and persons with whom the patients spend their time, also influence the degree of compliance.[23]

Social Support

The aspects of social support which are relevant to compliance comprise:

- the supportive behavior of the patient's family and friends
- the individual's perception of the support provided by their family and friends
- the nature of the social network around the patient.[5]

The patients who perceive their families and friends to be supportive are more adherent to medical care and this effect is more evident with children and individuals with an external locus of control.[5]

Orthodontic studies of the significance of parents' attitudes toward child rearing and the influence of child–parent relationship or parents' attitude to treatment on compliance of children and adolescents have, however, provided no conclusive evidence.[13,16,17,24] It has been suggested that parental beliefs are important for compliance of children and that assessment of the child–parent relationship might help predict the level of cooperation.[24] However, it appears from other studies that the personal psychologic characteristics of the child may be more decisive in determining the level of compliance.[13,17,21] Nevertheless, parents seem to play a prominent role in influencing children's decision to seek orthodontic treatment[25] and parental beliefs in many cases influence compliance which, however, tends to be limited to the earlier stages of treatment.[20,21,26] The significance of peer group relationships for individual development, especially during adolescence, is well known.[22] Whilst the influence of the peer group on health-related behavior of adolescents is recognized,[27] there is currently little information regarding its role in compliance with orthodontic treatment.

Knowledge of the Treatment Regimen

Whilst it appears obvious that patients are unlikely to adhere to treatment regimens about which their knowledge is limited or inaccurate, the possession of this knowledge on its own does not guarantee their adherence. This is in line with the long-recognized finding that knowledge, attitudes, and behavior are not causally linked.[5] It has been suggested that in order to enhance compliance, at the start of treatment both the patients and their parents should be sufficiently informed about the treatment regimens and expected level of compliance.[20] However, it is important to be aware of the limits of information retention after orthodontic consultations.[28]

Health-Related Behavior

Health motivation, health value, and health locus of control have a strong influence on compliance with medical care[5] and orthodontic treatment.[20,27] Recent studies suggest a beneficial influence of excellent dental appearance and of past orthodontic treatment on oral health attitudes and oral health-related quality of life of young adults.[29,30] It is believed that health-related behavior in general and patients' attitude to orthodontic treatment in particular might considerably influence orthodontic compliance. Health behaviors comprise personal efforts aimed at reducing behavioral pathogens or health-compromising behaviors, as well as increasing the practice of behaviors which act as behavioral immunogens or health-promoting behaviors.[27]

Of particular relevance in this respect are patients' attitudes toward dental esthetics, perceived severity of malocclusion, desire for orthodontic correction and expectations from orthodontic treatment in the sense of an anticipated self-efficacy.[25,31,32] The latter may be defined as the individual's belief in their ability to function competently.[32] Favorable compliance seems to be related to perceived severity of malocclusion[13,20,33,34] and to internal control orientation.[21,26,35] According to the locus of control theory, internal control orientation implies that patients attribute treatment outcomes to their personal efforts without relying primarily on chance or endeavors of others.[36] It is likely that those orthodontic patients who make fewer external attributions will retain some sense of responsibility, and possibly control, over treatment outcomes and believe that their participation and cooperation can facilitate treatment progress.[21]

Treatment Characteristics

Attributes of a treatment regimen considered to be important for compliance are:

- the complexity of the regimen
- its duration
- the degree of discomfort and unwanted side effects
- the necessity for lifestyle changes
- its financial costs.[5]

It is known from behavioral medicine that adherence to simplified short-term regimens is better than that to more complex and prolonged ones.[5] Regimens that involve substantial lifestyle changes or are otherwise inconvenient to the patients or their families are also less likely to be adhered to than regimens that can be readily absorbed into daily routine.[5] There is no conclusive evidence with regard to the potential importance of the financial costs of treatment as a barrier to compliance. Both in medical care and orthodontics, research has failed to establish a clear relationship between adherence and socioeconomic status of the patient.[5,15] There is an interesting, albeit untested assumption that more expensive treatments might require a greater health motivation. This aspect is of particular interest when considering great differences in costs of orthodontic treatment, such as, for instance, the variation observed across European countries with comparable general standards of living.[37]

There is surprisingly little evidence on the influence of the complexity and duration of orthodontic treatment on compliance. It has been found that cooperative behavior of both adolescent[21,38] and adult patients[39] declines about 18 and 10–12 months into treatment, respectively.

In general, patients tend to be less adherent to a treatment regimen that is painful or has side effects.[5] As orthodontic patients may experience a considerable amount of discomfort from treatment, it is reasonable to expect that their initial experience with orthodontic treatment, adaptation to it and its acceptance at an early stage might strongly influence the degree of compliance at subsequent stages. General personality variables and specific attitudes to orthodontics once more seem to play an important role. The results of some investigations suggest that the patient's attitude to orthodontics at the beginning of treatment may predict their capability to accommodate to initial discomfort associated with an orthodontic appliance, which in turn may predict their acceptance of appliance and treatment on the whole and the degree of subsequent compliance.[40,41] Appliance adaptation and treatment acceptance or denial are short-term events occurring within a few days after the start of treatment.[40,41] This evidence implies that the treating clinician should consider patients' adaptation at the earliest treatment stages, with regard to both realistic expectations of future compliance and prevention of long-lasting establishment of a stereotype denial of orthodontics.

Some appliance designs may diminish cooperation by causing unpleasant tactile sensations, feelings of constraint in the mouth, stretching of the soft tissues, pressure on the mucosa, displacement of the tongue, soreness of the teeth, and even pain.[17,42–45] Removable appliances such as headgear, plates, and functional appliances may be rejected by the patient because of pain, discomfort, problems with speech or simple annoyance.[23] Pain, functional and esthetic impairment, and associated complaints are the principal reasons for patients' wish to discontinue treatment[42] and for early treatment termination by the patient.[46] Patients' self-confidence might be affected by speech impairment and visibility of the appliance, especially during social interactions when attention is focused on the face, eyes, and mouth.[23,34] Effects of appliance type on oral complaints, such as higher degree of pain or speech impairment during wearing of bionator and headgear,[44] increased incidence of perceived pain, tension, sensitivity and pressure under treatment with functional and fixed appliances[40] or differences in initial acceptance of various designs of functional appliances[45] have been described.

It seems likely, therefore, that because of different experiences, the type of appliance will have a substantial effect on initial adaptation to treatment. Appliances which are more easily accepted by the patients and those designed to minimize dependence on patient wear offer a promising solution to some compliance problems encountered in conventional orthodontic treatment.

Clinician–Patient Relationship

It is known from both medical and orthodontic literature that the quality of this relationship, including factors such as communication, openness and warmth, has a substantial influence on compliance. Patients who perceive their treating clinician to be friendly and attentive are more likely to adhere to their treatment.[5,14] There is great potential for a beneficial influence of the doctor's verbal and nonverbal communication skills on compliance.[14,20,47]

Assessment and Prediction of Compliance

Although the data on the degree of compliance with orthodontic treatment regimens are rather limited, they suggest that there are appreciable problems in adherence to removable appliance wear. Microelectronic monitoring showed an average of 7.65 hours per day of functional appliance wear which was only a 50–60% fulfillment of the wearing instructions, decreasing to below 35% at the sixth appointment.[48] This rather low degree of adherence to functional appliance wear was almost mirrored by the compliance with headgear wear assessed in other investigations. As estimated by means of a headgear timer, adherence to headgear regimens was 55.8%[31] and 54.2%[49] of the recommended hours of wear. Patients were inclined to overrate their own adherence and objectively measured appliance wear was about 55–66% of the reported wearing time.[50] The correlation coefficient Cohen's kappa between the patients' estimates and the actual degree of compliance was 0.13.[50] In the same investigation, treating clinicians were only able to score a 43.5% accordance rate with the objectively measured appliance wear, and produced 33.2% overestimates and 23.3% underestimates of the actual compliance.

Various aspects of compliance prediction are discussed in detail in a recently published review.[15] It appears that demographic parameters, such as age, gender, cultural and socioeconomic characteristics, are unreliable as compliance predictors. It is known that the meshing of patients' personality characteristics, their relationships with family, peers and orthodontist, as well as performance at school, are closely linked with compliance and might serve as valuable sources of additional information for the management of compliance. However, no single parameter or a clearly defined parameter group has so far been identified as a reliable predictor.[13,15,51]

As stated above, health-related behaviors are important factors influencing compliance and, theoretically, if assessed at the start of treatment, might be useful for predicting compliance. The results of recent studies support the view that the patient's desire for orthodontic correction,[24] their appreciation of dental esthetics and attitude to orthodontic treatment at its start[41] may serve as useful predictors of the level of compliance to be expected. On these grounds, it may be recommended that the initial attitude of the patient toward orthodontics is thoroughly considered and carefully discussed with the patient, ensuring that their expectations are realistic. Assessment of the patient's initial level of oral hygiene and the extent of its improvement after detailed oral hygiene instructions has been used as an indicator of the previous oral health-related behavior[24] and may serve as a useful adjunct for compliance prediction.

It must be stressed, however, that these parameters may be used subjectively in addition to the clinician's personal impression of the patient, and that at present there are no reliable structured tests of compliance prediction. Although detailed psychologic testing of health-related behaviors at the start of treatment would provide valuable additional information, the practicability of anything beyond a subjective general impression gained by the clinician appears very limited.

Concluding Remarks

The problem of compliance is complex. Its understanding involves constant exploration of the cognitive and affective processes which determine social behavior, lifestyle, health values, and attitudes of individual patients and their parents. Various tactics have been suggested to improve compliance.[20,52] However, in the absence of research-based, structured, practical methods of compliance management, these tactics tend to be subjective and are based predominantly on common sense and general experience of the clinician.

When discussing compliance, it is important to avoid the clinician-centered assumption that patients are passive recipients of treatment. In a patient-centered healthcare approach, patients are free to participate in clinical decision making, discuss requirements on compliance, choose between alternatives, and assume responsibility for their own care. In orthodontics, this approach would stipulate that alternative treatment strategies are presented to and discussed with the patient. Considering that conventional orthodontic mechanotherapy relies on patient cooperation, regimens or appliances which appear more acceptable to patients and are designed to minimize dependence on patient cooperation offer a promising potential solution to some compliance problems encountered in orthodontic treatment.

References

1. Fawcett J. Compliance: definitions and key issues. J Clin Psychiatry 1995;56:4–10.

2. Stuart RB, ed. Adherence, compliance and generalization in behavioral medicine. New York: Brunner/Mazel; 1982.

3. Bruhn JG. The application of theory in childhood asthma self-help programs. J Allergy Clin Immunol 1983;72:561–577.

4. McGrath PJ, Firestone P, eds. Pediatric and adolescent behavioural medicine: issues in treatment. New York: Springer; 1983.

5. Fotheringham MJ, Sawyer MG. Adherence to recommended medical regimens in childhood and adolescence. J Paediatr Child Health 1995;31:72–78.

6. Prochaska JO, Velicer WF. The transtheoretical model of health behavior change. Am J Health Promot 1997;12:38–48.

7. Elder JP, Ayala GX, Harris S. Theories and intervention approaches to health-behavior change in primary care. Am J Prev Med 1999;17:275–384.

8. Schou L. The relevance of behavioral sciences in dental practice. Int Dent J 2000;50:324–332.

9. McNamara JA, Trotman C-A, eds. Creating the compliant patient. Craniofacial Growth Series, Vol 33. Ann Arbor: Center for Human Growth and Development; 1997.

10. Sinha PK, Nanda RS, Fillingim RB (guest eds). Psychologic issues related to orthodontics. Semin Orthod 2000;6(4).

11. Adams J, White M. Are activity promotion interventions based on the transtheoretical model effective? A critical review. Br J Sports Med 2003;37:106–114.

12. US Department of Health and Human Services. The health benefits of smoking cessation: a report of the Surgeon General. DHHS Publication No. CDC 90-8416. Washington, DC: US Government Printing Office, 1990.

13. Nanda RS, Kierl MJ. Prediction of cooperation in orthodontic treatment. Am J Orthod Dentofacial Orthop 1992;102:15–21.

14. Jay MS. Compliance: the adolescent/provider partnership. In: McNamara JA, Trotman C-A, eds. Creating the compliant patient. Craniofacial Growth

Series, Vol 33. Ann Arbor: Center for Human Growth and Development; 1997: 47–58.

15. Sergl HG, Zentner A. Predicting patient compliance in orthodontics. Semin Orthod 2000;6:231–236.

16. Allan TK, Hodgson EW. The use of personality measurements as a discrimination of patient cooperation in an orthodontic practice. Am J Orthod 1968;54:433–440.

17. Sergl HG, Klages U, Rauh C, Rupp I. Psychische Determinanten der Mitarbeit kieferorthopädischer Patienten – ein Beitrag zur Frage der Kooperationsprognose. Fortschr Kieferorthop 1987;48:117–122.

18. Southard KA, Tolley EA, Arheart KL, Hackett-Renner CA, Southard TE. Application of the Millon Adolescent Personality Inventory in evaluating orthodontic compliance. Am J Orthod Dentofacial Orthop 1991;100:553–561.

19. Sergl HG, Klages U, Pempera J. On the prediction of dentist-evaluated patient compliance in orthodontics. Eur J Orthod 1992;14:463–468.

20. Albino J, Lawrence S, Lopes C, Nash L, Tedesco L. Cooperation of adolescents in orthodontic treatment. J Behavior Med 1991;14:53–70.

21. Albino J. Factors influencing adolescent cooperation in orthodontic treatment. Semin Orthod 2000;6:214–223.

22. Petersen AC, Kuipers KS. Understanding adolescence: adolescent development and implications for the adolescent as a patient. In: McNamara JA, Trotman C-A, eds. Creating the compliant patient. Craniofacial Growth Series, Vol 33. Ann Arbor: Center for Human Growth and Development; 1997: 1–24.

23. Zentner A, Stelte V, Sergl HG. Patients' attitudes and non-compliance in orthodontic treatment. Eur J Orthod 1996;18:429 (abstract).

24. Mehra T, Nanda RS, Sinha PK. Orthodontists' assessment and management of compliance. Angle Orthod 1998;68:115–122.

25. Fox RM, Albino JE, Green LJ, Tedesco LA. Development and validation of a measure of attitudes toward malocclusion. J Dent Res 1982; 61:1039–1043.

26. Bartsch A, Witt E, Sahm G, Schneider S. Correlates of objective patient compliance with removable appliance wear. Am J Orthod Dentofacial Orthop 1993;104:378–386.

27. Cooper ML, Shapiro CM. Motivations for health behaviors among adolescents. In: McNamara JA, Trotman C-A, eds. Creating the compliant patient. Craniofacial Growth Series, Vol 33. Ann Arbor: Center for Human Growth and Development; 1997: 25–46.

28. Thomson AM, Cunningham SJ, Hunt NP. A comparison of information retention at an initial orthodontic consultation. Eur J Orthod 2001; 23:169–178.

29. Klages U, Bruckner A, Zentner A. Dental aesthetics, self-awareness, and oral health-related quality of life in young adults. Eur J Orthod 2004;26: 507–514.

30. Klages U, Bruckner A, Guld Y, Zentner A. Dental esthetics, orthodontic treatment and oral health attitudes in young adults. Am J Orthod Dentofacial Orthop 2005;128:442–449.

31. Clemmer EJ, Hayes EW. Patient cooperation in wearing orthodontic headgear. Am J Orthod 1979;75:517–524.

32. Albino J, Tedesco LA. Esthetic need for orthodontic treatment. In: Melsen B, ed. Current controversies in orthodontics. Berlin: Quintessence; 1991: 11–24.

33. Lewit DW, Virolainen K. Conformity and independence in adolescents' motivation for orthodontic treatment. Child Develop 1968; 38:1189–1200.

34. Lewis HG, Brown WA. The attitude of patients to the wearing of removable orthodontic appliance. Br Dent J 1973;134:87–90.

35. El-Mangoury NH. Orthodontic cooperation. Am J Orthod 1981;80:604–622.

36. Rotter JB. Generalized expectancies for internal versus external control of reinforcement. Psychol Monogr 1966;80:1–28.

37. van der Linden FPGM, Schmiedel WJ, Bijlstra RJ. Het specialisme orthodontie in Europees perspectief. Ned Tijdschr Tandheelkd 2003;110:14–19.

38. Gabriel HF. Motivation of the headgear patient. Angle Orthod 1968;38:129–135.

39. Vanarsdall RL, Musich DR. Adult orthodontics: diagnosis and treatment. In: Graber TM, Vanarsdall RL, eds. Orthodontics: current principles and techniques. St. Louis: Mosby; 1994: 750–836.

40. Sergl HG, Klages U, Zentner A. Pain and discomfort during orthodontic treatment: causative factors and effects on compliance. Am J Orthod Dentofacial Orthop 1998;114:684–691.

41. Sergl HG, Klages U, Zentner A. Functional and social discomfort during orthodontic treatment – effects on compliance and prediction of patients' adaptation by personality variables. Eur J Orthod 2000;22:307–315.

42. Oliver RG, Knappman YM. Attitudes to orthodontic treatment. Br J Orthod 1985;12:179–188.

43. Egolf RJ, BeGole EA, Upshaw HS. Factors associated with orthodontic patient compliance with intraoral elastic and headgear wear. Am J Orthod Dentofacial Orthop 1990;97:336–348.

44. Johnson PD, Cohen DA, Aiosa L, McGorray S, Wheeler T. Attitudes and compliance of pre-adolescent children during early treatment of Class II malocclusion. Clin Orthod Res 1998;1:20–28.

45. Sergl HG, Zentner A. A comparative assessment of acceptance of different types of functional appliances. Eur J Orthod 1998;20:517–524.

46. Brattström V, Ingersson M, Aberg E. Treatment cooperation in orthodontic patients. Br J Orthod 1991;18:37–42.

47. Klages U, Sergl HG, Burucker J. Relations between verbal behavior of the orthodontist and communicative cooperation of the patient in regular orthodontic visits. Am J Orthod Dentofacial Orthop 1992;102:265–269.

48. Sahm G, Bartsch A, Witt E. Micro-electronic monitoring of functional appliance wear. Eur J Orthod 1990;12:297–301.

49. Cureton SL, Regennitter FJ, Yancey JM. Clinical versus quantitative assessment of headgear compliance. Am J Orthod Dentofacial Orthop 1993;104:277–284.

50. Sahm G, Bartsch A, Witt E. Reliability of patient reports on compliance. Eur J Orthod 1990;12:438–446.

51. Bos A, Hoogstraten J, Prahl-Andersen B. On the use of personality characteristics in predicting compliance in orthodontic practice. Am J Orthod Dentofacial Orthop 2003;123:568–570.

52. Rosen DS. Creating the successful adolescent patient: a practical patient-oriented approach. In: McNamara JA, Trotman C-A, eds. Creating the compliant patient. Craniofacial Growth Series, Vol 33. Ann Arbor: Center for Human Growth and Development; 1997: 59–72.

CHAPTER 2

Classification of the noncompliance appliances used for Class II correction

Moschos A. Papadopoulos

CONTENTS

Introduction

During orthodontic treatment, the cooperation or compliance of the patient is a major factor for a successful treatment outcome. According to Haynes, compliance, as it relates to healthcare, is the "extent to which a person's behavior (in terms of taking medications, following diets, or executing lifestyle changes) coincides with medical or health advice."[1] This means that in order to achieve successful treatment results, patients are expected to follow the recommended regimens suggested by their orthodontists. Unfortunately, noncompliance of the patient is a serious and common problem and orthodontists have to deal with this issue almost daily. Orthodontic treatment in patients with limited compliance can result in, among other things, a longer treatment time, destruction of the teeth and periodontium, extraction of additional teeth, frustration for the patient, and additional stress for the orthodontist and staff.[2]

During the last decades, many appliances and techniques that reduce or minimize the need for patient compliance have been introduced in order to correct Class II malocclusion. It should be noted, however, that these noncompliance treatment modalities are not solely indicated in patients with minimal compliance but can also be applied to compliant patients. They can be used, for example, in patients with almost completed prepubertal growth, at the early phase of permanent dentition, and when second maxillary molars have already erupted. Using these modalities, the treatment procedures are better controlled by the orthodontist and therefore more predictable results can be expected.

The noncompliance appliances used in Class II correction present some common characteristics.

- The forces applied in order either to advance the mandible or to move molars distally are produced by means of fixed auxiliaries, either intra- or intermaxillary.[3–8]
- Almost always, they require the use of dental and/or palatal anchorage such as multibanded fixed appliances, lingual or transpalatal arches, and modified palatal buttons.[6,8,9–18]
- In the majority of these appliances, and especially those used for molar distalization, much use is made of resilient wires, such as super-elastic nickel-titanium (NiTi) and titanium-molybdenum alloys (TMA).[6–10,12,14,15,19,20] However, anchorage loss often occurs during molar distalization with these modalities and represents a major negative aspect of their application.[12–18,21,22]

Depending on their mode of action and type of anchorage, all these appliances can be classified into two categories. Intermaxillary noncompliance appliances, which derive their anchorage in an intermaxillary manner, act in both maxillary and mandibular arches in order to advance the mandible, e.g. the Herbst appliance (Dentaurum Inc., Ispringen, Germany),[3,23] the Jasper Jumper (American Orthodontics, Sheboygan, WI),[4] the Adjustable Bite Corrector (OrthoPlus Inc., Santa Rosa, CA),[24] and the Eureka Spring (Eureka Orthodontics, San Louis Obispo, CA, USA).[5] Intramaxillary noncompliance appliances, which derive their anchorage in an intramaxillary or absolute anchorage manner, act only in the maxillary arch in order to move molars distally, e.g. the Pendulum Appliance,[6] the Distal Jet (American Orthodontics, Sheboygan, WI),[7] repelling magnets,[21,25,26] the Jones Jig (American Orthodontics, Sheboygan, WI),[8] and palatal implants. A detailed presentation of the currently available appliances, including the author who introduced them and/or the manufacturer, is shown in Tables 2.1, 2.2 and 2.3.

Intermaxillary Noncompliance Appliances

A feasible way to further classify the intermaxillary noncompliance appliances is to categorize them according to the features of the

Table 2.1. Classification of the noncompliance appliances. I. Intermaxillary appliances.

Appliance	Author	Manufacturer*
a. Rigid intermaxillary appliances (RIMA)		
Herbst Appliance		
Banded Herbst Design	Pancherz (1979)[3]	Dentaurum Inc.
Cast Splint Herbst Design	Pancherz (1997)[27]	
Stainless Steel Crown Herbst Design	Langford (1982),[28] Dischinger (1989)[29]	
Acrylic Splint Herbst Design *(cemented or bonded)*	Howe (1982)[30]	Specialty Appliance Works
(removable)	Howe (1987)[31]	
(upper bonded and lower removable)	McNamara et al (2001)[32]	
Modifications		
Goodman's Modified Herbst	Goodman & McKenna (1985)[33]	
Upper Stainless Steel Crowns & Lower Acrylic	Valant (1989)[34]	Dentaurum Inc.
Mandibular Advancement Locking Unit (MALU)	Schiavoni et al (1996),[35] Haegglund & Segerdal (1997)[36]	Saga Dental Supply AS
Magnetic Telescopic Device	Ritto (1997)[37]	
Flip-Lock Herbst Appliance	Miller (1996)[38]	TP Orthodontics Inc.
Hanks Telescoping Herbst Appliance	Hanks (2003)[39]	American Orthodontics
Ventral Telescope		Professional Positioners Inc.
Universal Bite Jumper (UBJ)	Calvez (1998)[40]	
Open-Bite Intrusion Herbst	Dischinger (2001)[41]	AOA/Pro Orthodontic Appliances
IST (Intraoral Snoring Therapy) Appliance		Scheu-Dental GmbH
Acrylic Splint with Hinge System accord. to Dr. Amoric		Scheu-Dental GmbH
Cantilever Bite Jumper (CBJ)	Mayes (1996)[42]	AOA/Pro Orthodontic Appliances/ Ormco Corporation
Molar-Moving Bite Jumper (MMBJ)	Mayes (1998)[43]	AOA/Pro Orthodontic Appliances/ Ormco Corporation
Mandibular Advancing Repositioning Splint (MARS)	Clements & Jacobson (1982)[44]	Dentaurum Inc. & Rocky Mountain Orthodontics
Mandibular Corrector Appliance (MCA)	Jones (1985)[45]	Cormar Inc.
Biopedic Appliance		GAC International Inc.
Ritto Appliance	Ritto Orthod Cyber-J Archives[46]	
Mandibular Protraction Appliance (MPA)		
Type I	Coelho Filho (1995)[47]	
Type II	Coelho Filho (1997)[48]	
Type III	Coelho Filho (1998)[49]	
Type IV	Coelho Filho (2001)[50]	
Mandibular Anterior Repositioning Appliance (MARA)	Eckhart (1998)[51]	AOA/Pro Orthodontic Appliances/ Ormco Corporation
Functional Mandibular Advancer (FMA)	Kinzinger et al (2002)[52]	
b. Flexible intermaxillary appliances (FIMA)		
Jasper Jumper	Jasper (1987)[53]	American Orthodontics
Scandee Tubular Jumper		Saga Dental Supply AS
Flex Developer (FD)	Winsauer (2002)[54]	LPI Ormco
Amoric Torsion Coils	Amoric (1994)[55]	

Table 2.1. Classification of the noncompliance appliances. I. Intermaxillary appliances (*cont'd*).

Appliance	Author	Manufacturer*
Adjustable Bite Corrector (ABC)	West (1995)[24]	OrthoPlus Inc.
Bite Fixer	Awbrey (1999)[56]	Ormco Corporation
Gentle Jumper		American Orthodontics
Klapper SUPERspring II	Klapper (1999)[57]	ORTHOdesign
Churro Jumper	Castanon et al (1998)[58]	
Forsus Nitinol Flat Spring	Heinig & Goz (2001)[59]	3M Unitek Orthodontic Products
Ribbon Jumper		American Orthodontics
c. Hybrid appliances (combination of RIMA and FIMA)		
Eureka Spring	DeVincenzo (1997)[5]	Eureka Orthodontics
Sabbagh Universal Spring (SUS)		Dentaurum Inc.
Forsus Fatigue Resistant Device		3M Unitek Orthodontic Products
Forsus Fatigue Resistant Device with Direct Push Rod		3M Unitek Orthodontic Products
Twin Force Bite Corrector	Corbett & Molina (2001)[60]	Ortho Organizers Inc.
Twin Force Bite Corrector – Double Lock		Ortho Organizers Inc.
d. Appliances acting as substitute for elastics		
The Calibrated Force Module		Cormar Inc.
Alpern Class II Closers		GAC International Inc.
Saif Springs	Starnes (1998)[61]	Pacific Coast Manufacturing Inc.

* Complete manufacturer information is provided in Table 2.4

Table 2.2. Classification of the noncompliance appliances. II. Distalization appliances deriving their anchorage in an intramaxillary manner.

Appliance	Author	Manufacturer
a. Flexible palatally positioned distalization force system		
Pendulum Appliance	Hilgers (1992)[6]	
Modifications		
Hilgers Palatal Expander	Hilgers (1991)[62]	AOA/Pro Orthodontic Appliances/Ormco Corporation
Pend-X (Pendex) Appliance	Hilgers (1992)[6]	AOA/Pro Orthodontic Appliances/Ormco Corporation
Mayes' Penguin Design	Mayes (1999)[63]	AOA/Pro Orthodontic Appliances/Ormco Corporation
Hilgers PhD Appliance	Hilgers (1998)[64]	AOA/Pro Orthodontic Appliances/Ormco Corporation
GrumRax Appliance	Grummons (1999)[65]	AOA/Pro Orthodontic Appliances/Ormco Corporation
T-Rex Appliance	Snodgrass (1996)[66]	AOA/Pro Orthodontic Appliances/Ormco Corporation
Tracey/Hilgers MDA Expander (Mini-Distalizing Appliance)		AOA/Pro Orthodontic Appliances/Ormco Corporation
M-Pendulum Appliance	Scuzzo et al (1999)[67]	
K-Pendulum Appliance	Kinzinger et al (2000)[68]	
Bipendulum and Quad Pendulum Appliance	Kinzinger et al (2002)[69]	Ormco Corporation
Intraoral Bodily Molar Distalizer (IBMD)	Keles & Sayinsu (2000)[70]	
Simplified Molar Distalizer	Walde (2003)[71]	TP Orthodontics Inc.
Distal Jet Appliance	Carano & Testa (1996)[7]	American Orthodontics
Modifications		
Modified Distal Jet Appliance	Quick & Harris (2000)[72]	

Table 2.2. Classification of the noncompliance appliances. II. Distalization appliances deriving their anchorage in an intramaxillary manner (*cont'd*).

Appliance	Author	Manufacturer
Keles Slider	Keles (2001)[73]	(patent pending)
Nance Appliance with NiTi Coil Springs		
(Open-Coil Springs)	Reiner (1992)[74]	3M Unitek Orthodontic Products
(Neosentalloy Coils)	Bondemark (2000)[75]	GAC International Inc.
Fast Back Appliance	Lanteri et al (2002)[76]	Leone SpA
b. Flexible buccally positioned distalization force system		
Jones Jig	Jones & White (1992)[8]	American Orthodontics
Modifications		
Lokar Molar Distalizing Appliance	Scott (1996)[77]	Ormco Corporation
Modified Sectional Jig Assembly	Papadopoulos (1998)[78]	
NiTi Coil Springs	Gianelly et al (1991)[9]	
NiTi Coil Springs	Erverdi et al (1997)[79]	Ortho Organizers Inc.
Sentalloy Coil Springs and Edgewise Appliance	Pieringer et al (1997)[80]	GAC International Inc.
Repelling Magnets		
Samarium-Cobalt Magnets	Blechman (1985)[81]	
Repelling Magnets	Gianelly et al (1988, 1989)[21,82]	Medical Magnetics Inc.
Magneforce	Blechman & Alexander (1995)[83]	Ormco Corporation
Repelling Samarium-Cobalt Magnets	Bondemark (2000)[75]	Modular Magnetic Inc.
Magnet Force System		Ortho Organizers Inc.
NiTi Wires		
Neosentalloy Wires	Locatelli et al (1992)[10]	GAC International Inc.
Nickel Titanium Double Loop System (neosentalloy wires)	Giancotti & Cozza (1998)[84]	GAC International Inc.
K-Loop	Kalra (1995)[20]	Ormco Corporation
U-Shaped Vertical Loop	Vlock (1998)[85]	
Distalizing Arches		
Bimetric Distalizing Arch	Wilson (1978)[86]	Rocky Mountain Orthodontics
Multi-Distalizing Arch (MDA)		Ortho Organizers Inc.
Molar Distalization Bow	Jeckel & Rakosi (1991)[19]	
Korn Lip Bumper		American Orthodontics
Acrylic Distalization Splints		
Acrylic Splint with NiTi Coils (Sentalloy Coils)	Manhartsberger (1994)[87]	GAC International Inc.
Removable Molar Distalization Splint	Ritto (1997)[88]	Eureka Orthodontics/Great Lakes Orthodontics Ltd.
Carriere Distalizer	Carriere (Syllabus)[89]	ClassOne Orthodontics
c. Flexible palatally and buccally positioned distalization force system		
Piston Appliance (Greenfield Molar Distalizer)	Greenfield (1995)[90]	nX Orthodontic Services Ltd.
Nance Appliance with NiTi Coil Springs (Open-Coil Springs and Edgewise Appliance)	Puente (1997)[91]	GAC International Inc.
d. Rigid palatally positioned distalization force system		
Veltri's Distalizer	Veltri & Baldini (2001)[92]	Leone SpA
New Distalizer	Baccetti & Franchi (2000)[93]	Leone SpA
P-Rax Molar Distalizer	Paz (2001)[94]	AOA/Pro Orthodontic Appliances/Ormco Corporation
e. Hybrid appliances (combination of rigid buccally and flexible palatally positioned distalization force system)		
First Class Appliance	Fortini et al (1999)[95]	Leone SpA

Table 2.2. Classification of the noncompliance appliances. II. Distalization appliances deriving their anchorage in an intramaxillary manner (*cont'd*).

Appliance	Author	Manufacturer
f. Transpalatal arches for molar rotation and/or distalization		
Stainless Steel Transpalatal Arches	Celtin & Ten Hoeve (1983)[96]	
Prefabricated (Stainless Steel) Transpalatal Arches	Dahlquist et al (1996)[97]	GAC International Inc.
Zachrisson-type Transpalatal Bar (ZTPB)		Rocky Mountain Orthodontics
Palatal Rotation Arch	Cooke & Wreakes (1978)[98]	
Nitanium Molar Rotator2	Corbett (1996)[99]	Ortho Organizers Inc.
Nitanium Palatal Expander2	Corbett (1997)[100]	Ortho Organizers Inc.
3D (Wilson) Palatal Appliance		Rocky Mountain Orthodontics
TMA Transpalatal Arch	Mandurino & Balducci (2001)[101]	Ormco Corporation
Keles TPA	Keles & Impram (2003)[102]	Ormco Corporation
Distalix	Langlade (2003)[103]	Rocky Mountain Orthodontics

Table 2.3. Classification of the noncompliance appliances. III. Intramaxillary appliances deriving their anchorage in an absolute anchorage manner.

Implant	Author	Manufacturer
a. Palatally positioned implants used as anchorage for molar distalization		
Graz Implant-Supported Pendulum (GISP)	Byloff et al (2000)[104]	Mondeal Medical Systems GmbH
Palatal Implant with Pendulum Appliance (Indirect Loading)	Karcher et al (2002)[105]	Mondeal Medical Systems GmbH
Straumann Orthosystem	Giancotti et al (2002)[106]	Straumann AG
with Coil Springs and NiTi Wires (Indirect Loading)		
with Distal Jet (Direct Loading)		
with Modified Acrylic Nance Button (Direct Loading)		
with Modified Pendulum Appliance (Direct Loading)		
Frialit-2 Implant System (Synchro Screw Implants)	Keles et al (2003)[107]	Friadent GmbH
Midplant System (Core Implant with Orthodontic Implant	Maino et al (2002)[108]	HDC
Connection Easy Application)		
with Neosentalloy Coil and Sentalloy Wires (Indirect Loading)		
with Modified Pendulum Appliance (Direct Loading)		
with Distal Jet (Direct Loading)		
Bioresorbable Implant Anchor for Orthodontics System (BIOS)	Glatzmaier et al (1995, 1996)[109,110]	Biovision GmbH
Short Epithetic Implants	Bernhart et al (2001)[111]	Nobel Biocare AB
Distalization of First Molars, Cantilever Mechanics		
Anchorage Screw	Karaman et al (2002)[112]	Stryker Leibinger GmbH & Co. KG
with Distal Jet (Direct Loading)		
Mini-Screws	Kyung et al (2003)[113]	
with Transpalatal Arch (Indirect Loading)		
Onplant System	Bondemark et al (2002)[114]	Nobel Biocare AB
with Coil Springs and NiTi Wires (Indirect Loading)		
b. Palatally positioned implants used as posterior anchorage for anterior teeth retraction		
Straumann Orthosystem		
Canine, Anterior Teeth Retraction	Wehrbein et al (1996)[115,116]	Straumann AG
Canine Retraction	Bantleon et al (2002)[117]	Straumann AG
Premolar, Canine, Anterior Teeth Retraction	Giancotti et al (2002)[106,118]	Straumann AG

Table 2.3. Classification of the noncompliance appliances. III. Intramaxillary appliances deriving their anchorage in an absolute anchorage manner (*cont'd*).

Implant	Author	Manufacturer
Midplant System (Core Implant with Orthodontic Implant Connection Easy Application) *Premolar, Canine, Anterior Teeth Retraction*	Maino et al (2002)[108]	HDC
Mini-Implants *Orthosystem-Titanium-Mini-Implants* *Premolar Distalization and Intrusion (Animal Study)*	Fritz et al (2003)[119]	Straumann AG
Short Epithetic Implants *Intrusion, Retraction of Anterior Teeth* *Retraction of Anterior Segment, Cantilever Mechanics*	Bernhart et al (2001)[111]	Nobel Biocare AB
Mini-Screws *Retraction of Anterior Teeth* *Miniscrew No. 204-1210, Retraction of Anterior Teeth*	Costa et al (1998)[120] Lee et al (2001)[121]	OsteoMed Corp.
Onplants *OnPlant, Retraction of Anterior Teeth (Animal Study)* *OrthoImplant, Retraction of Anterior Teeth*	Block & Hoffman (1995)[122] Celenza & Hochman (2000)[123]	Straumann AG
c. Buccally positioned implants used as posterior anchorage for anterior teeth retraction		
Mini-Screws *Micro Plus Titanium Plating System, Canine Retraction (suggested)* *Intrusion, Retraction of Anterior Teeth* *Micro Screw No. 59-12106, Retraction of Anterior Teeth* *Spider Screw for Skeletal Anchorage*	Kanomi (1997)[124] Costa et al (1998)[120] Park et al (2001)[125] Maino et al (2003)[126]	Stryker Leibinger GmbH & Co. KG Stryker Leibinger GmbH & Co. KG HDC
Mini-Plates (Zygomatic Anchorage) *L-Shaped Titanium Mini-Plates for Canine Distalization* *Zygoma Anchor, Retraction of Anterior Teeth*	Erverdi et al (2002)[127] De Clerck et al (2002)[128]	Stryker Leibinger GmbH & Co. KG Surgi-Tec

force system which is used to advance the mandible. In this way, they can be classified into four main categories (Table 2.1):

- rigid intermaxillary appliances (RIMA)
- flexible intermaxillary appliances (FIMA)
- hybrid appliances (combination of RIMA and FIMA)
- appliances acting as substitute for elastics.

Intramaxillary Noncompliance Distalization Appliances

The noncompliance distalization appliances, which derive their anchorage in an intramaxillary manner, can be classified according to the characteristics and the localization of the force system which is used to distalize the maxillary molars. In this way six categories can be formed (Table 2.2):

- appliances with a flexible distalization force system palatally positioned
- appliances with a flexible distalization force system buccally positioned

- appliances with a double flexible distalization force system positioned both palatally and buccally
- appliances with a rigid distalization force system palatally positioned
- hybrid appliances with a combination of a rigid distalization force system buccally positioned and a flexible one palatally positioned
- transpalatal arches that can be used for molar rotation and/or distalization.

Intramaxillary Noncompliance Appliances with Absolute Anchorage

Osseointegrated implants can be combined with various appliances or orthodontic modalities to provide a stable anchorage for the treatment of Class II malocclusion in terms of posterior teeth distalization and/or anterior teeth retraction and intrusion. Taking into consideration the different locations of their insertion as well as

Table 2.4. List of companies with trademarks and registrations.

Company	Postal address	Website
3M Unitek Orthodontic Products	2724 South Peck Road, Monrovia, CA	www.3m.com/unitek
American Orthodontics	1714 Cambridge Ave., Sheboygan, WI 53082	www.americanortho.com
AOA/Pro Orthodontic Appliances	P.O. Box 725, Sturtevant, WI 53177	www.ormco.com/aoa
Biovision GmbH	Merzhauser Str. 112, D-79100 Freiburg, Germany	www.biovision-biomaterial.de
ClassOne Orthodontics	5064 - 50th Street, Lubbock, TX 79414	www.classoneorthodontics.com
Cormar Inc.	Box 115C, Salisbury, MD 21801	
Dentaurum Inc.	Turnstraße 31, D-75228 Ispringen, Germany	www.dentaurum.com
Eureka Orthodontics	1312 Garden Street, San Louis Obispo, CA 93401	www.eurekaortho.com
Friadent GmbH	Postfach 710111, D-68221 Mannheim, Germany	www.friadent.de
GAC International Inc.	185 Oval Drive, Islandia, NY 11749	www.gacintl.com
Great Lakes Orthodontics Ltd	200 Cooper Avenue, PO Box 5111, Tonawanda, NY	www.greatlakesortho.com
HDC, Health Development Company	Via dell' Industria 19, I-36030 Sarcedo, Italy	www.hdc-italy.com
Leone SpA	Via P. a Quaracchi 50, I-50019 Sesto Fiorentino, Firenze, Italy	www.leone.it
LPI Ormco, Ludwig Pittermann GesmbH	Unter Oberndorf 50, A-3034 Maria Anzbach, Austria	www.flexdeveloper.com
Medical Magnetics Inc.	79 N. Franklin Turnpike, Ramsey, NJ 07446	
Modular Magnetic Inc.	New City, NY	
Mondeal Medical Systems GmbH	Moltkestrasse 39, D-78532 Tuttlingen, Germany	www.mondeal.de
Nobel Biocare AB	Box 5190, 40226 Gothenburg, Sweden	www.nobelbiocare.com
nX Orthodontic Services Ltd	9381 West Sample Road, Coral Springs, FL 33065	www.nxortho.com
Ormco Corporation	1717 West Collins Ave., Orange, CA 92867	www.ormco.com
Ortho Organizers Inc.	1619 S. Rancho Santa Fe Road, San Marcos, CA 92069	www.orthoorganizers.com
ORTHOdesign	744 Falls Circle, Lake Forest, IL 60045	
OrthoPlus Inc.	1275 Fourth St., Suite 381, Santa Rosa, CA 95404	
OsteoMed Corp.	3885 Arapaho Road, Addison, TX 75001	www.osteomedcorp.com
Pacific Coast Manufacturing Inc.	18506 142nd Ave. NE, Woodinville, WA 98072	
Professional Positioners Inc.	2525 Three Mile Road, Racine, WI 53404-1328	
Rocky Mountain Orthodontics	PO Box 17085, Denver, CO	www.rmortho.com
Saga Dental Supply AS	Pb.216, N-2202 Kongsvinger, Norway	
Scheu-Dental GmbH	Am Burgberg 20, D-58642 Iserlohn, Germany	www.scheu-dental.com
Specialty Appliance Works	1415 W. Argyle St., Jackson, MI 49202	
Straumann AG	Hauptstrasse 26d, CH-4437 Waldenburg, Switzerland	www.straumann.com
Stryker Leibinger GmbH & Co. KG	Bötzinger Straße 37-41, 79111 Freiburg, Germany	www.strykerleibingereurope.com
Surgi-Tec	Industriepark Waggelwater, Lieven Bauwensstraat 20, B-8200 Brugge, Belgium	www.surgi-tec.com
TP Orthodontics Inc.	100 Center Plaza, LaPorte, IN 46350-962	www.tportho.com

the goals of their use, they can be classified in three main categories (Table 2.3):

- palatally positioned implants used as anchorage for molar distalization
- palatally positioned implants used as posterior anchorage for anterior teeth retraction
- buccally positioned implants used as posterior anchorage for anterior teeth retraction.

References

1. Haynes RB. Compliance in health care. Baltimore: Johns Hopkins University Press; 1979.

2. Southard KA, Tolley EA, Arheart KL, Hackett-Renner CA, Southard TE. Application of the Millon Adolescent Personality Inventory in evaluating orthodontic compliance. Am J Orthod Dentofacial Orthop 1991;100:553–561.

3. Pancherz H. Treatment of Class II malocclusions by jumping the bite with the Herbst appliance. A cephalometric investigation. Am J Orthod 1979;76:423–442.

4. Jasper JJ, McNamara JA Jr. The correction of interarch malocclusions using a fixed force module. Am J Orthod Dentofacial Orthop 1995;108:641–650.

5. DeVincenzo JP. The Eureka Spring: a new interarch force delivery system. J Clin Orthod 1997;31:454–467.

6. Hilgers JJ. The pendulum appliance for Class II noncompliance therapy. J Clin Orthod 1992; 26:706–714.

7. Carano A, Testa M. The distal jet for upper molar distalization. J Clin Orthod 1996;30:374–380.

8. Jones RD, White MJ. Rapid Class II molar correction with an open-coil jig. J Clin Orthod 1992;26:661–664.

9. Gianelly AA, Bednar J, Dietz VS. Japanese NiTi coils used to move molars distally. Am J Orthod Dentofacial Orthop 1991;99:564–566.

10. Locatelli R, Bednar J, Dietz VS, Gianelly AA. Molar distalization with superelastic NiTi wire. J Clin Orthod 1992;26:277–279.

11. Bondemark L, Kurol J, Bernhold M. Repelling magnets versus superelastic nickel-titanium coils in simultaneous distal movement of maxillary first and second molars. Angle Orthod 1994; 64:189–198.

12. Ghosh J, Nanda RS. Evaluation of an intraoral maxillary molar distalization technique. Am J Orthod Dentofacial Orthop 1996;110:639–646.

13. Byloff FK, Darendeliler MA. Distal molar movement using the pendulum appliance. Part 1: Clinical and radiological evaluation. Angle Orthod 1997;67:249–260.

14. Gulati S, Kharbanda OP, Parkash H. Dental and skeletal changes after intraoral molar distalization with sectional jig assembly. Am J Orthod Dentofacial Orthop 1998;114:319–327.

15. Runge ME, Martin JT, Bukai F. Analysis of rapid maxillary molar distal movement without patient cooperation. Am J Orthod Dentofacial Orthop 1999;115:153–157.

16. Brickman CD, Sinha PK, Nanda RS. Evaluation of the Jones jig appliance for distal molar movement. Am J Orthod Dentofacial Orthop 2000; 118:526–534.

17. Bussick TJ, McNamara JA Jr. Dentoalveolar and skeletal changes associated with the pendulum appliance. Am J Orthod Dentofacial Orthop 2000;117:333–343.

18. Haydar S, Uner O. Comparison of Jones jig molar distalization appliance with extraoral traction. Am J Orthod Dentofacial Orthop 2000; 117:49–53.

19. Jeckel N, Rakosi T. Molar distalization by intra-oral force application. Eur J Orthod 1991;3:43–46.

20. Kalra V. The K-loop molar distalizing appliance. J Clin Orthod 1995;29:298–301.

21. Gianelly AA, Vaitas AS, Thomas WM. The use of magnets to move molars distally. Am J Orthod Dentofacial Orthop 1989;96:161–167.

22. Bondemark L, Kurol J. Distalization of maxillary first and second molars simultaneously with repelling magnets. Eur J Orthod 1992; 14:264–272.

23. Herbst E. Atlas und Grundriss der Zahnärztlichen Orthopädie. Munich: JF Lehmann Verlag; 1910.

24. West RP. The Adjustable Bite Corrector. J Clin Orthod 1995;10:269–275.

25. Papadopoulos MA. Clinical applications of magnets in orthodontics. Hell Orthod Rev 1999;1:31–42.

26. Papadopoulos MA. A study of the biomechanical characteristics of magnetic force systems used in orthodontics. Hell Orthod Rev 1999;2:89–97.

27. Pancherz H. The modern Herbst appliance. In: Graber TM, Rakosi T, Petrovic AG, eds. Dentofacial orthopedics with functional appliances, 2nd edn. St Louis: Mosby-Year Book; 1997; 336–366.

28. Langford NM Jr. Updating fabrication of the Herbst appliance. J Clin Orthod 1982;16:173–174.

29. Dischinger TG. Edgewise bioprogressive Herbst appliance. J Clin Orthod 1989;23:608–617.

30. Howe RP. The bonded Herbst appliance. J Clin Orthod 1982;16:663–667.

31. Howe RP. Removable plastic Herbst retainer. J Clin Orthod 1987;21:533–537.

32. McNamara JA Jr, Brudon WL, Buckhardt DR, Huge SA. The Herbst appliance. In: McNamara JA Jr, Brudon WL, eds. Orthodontics and dentofacial orthopedics. Ann Arbor: Needham Press; 2001: 285–318.

33. Goodman P, McKenna P. Modified Herbst appliance for the mixed dentition. J Clin Orthod 1985;19:811–814.

34. Valant JR. Increasing maxillary arch length with a modified Herbst appliance. J Clin Orthod 1989;23:810–814.

35. Schiavoni R, Bonapace C, Grenga V. Modified edgewise-Herbst appliance. J Clin Orthod 1996; 30:681–687.

36. Haegglund P, Segerdal S. The Swedish-style integrated Herbst appliance. J Clin Orthod 1997;31:378–390.

37. Ritto AK. Tratamento das Classes II divisão 1 com a Biela Magnética. Dissertation thesis; 1997.

38. Miller RA. The flip-lock Herbst appliance. J Clin Orthod 1996;30:552–558.

39. Hanks SD. Herbst therapy: trying to get out of the 20th century. Good Practice Newsletter of American Orthodontics 2003;4:2–4. Available online at: www.americanortho.com/clinical/images/Vol%204_1.pdf

40. Calvez X. The universal bite jumper. J Clin Orthod 1998;32:493–499.

41. Dischinger TG. Open-bite intrusion Herbst. AOA Orthodont Appl 2001;5:1–4. Available online at: www.aoalab.com/learning/publications/aoaVol/aoaVol5No2.pdf

42. Mayes JH. The cantilever bite-jumper system: exploring the possibilities. Orthodontic CYBER-journal 1996. Available online at: www.oc-j.com/issue3/p0000077.htm

43. Mayes JH. The molar-moving bite jumper (MMBJ). Clin Impressions 1998;7:16–19.

44. Clements RM Jr, Jacobson A. The MARS appliance. Report of a case. Am J Orthod 1982;82:445–455.

45. Jones M. Mandibular corrector. J Clin Orthod 1985;19:362–368.

46. Ritto AK. The Ritto Appliance – a new fixed functional appliance. Orthodontic CYBERjournal, archives. Available online at: www.oc-j.com/ritto/ritto.htm and www.oc-j.com/GARY/ritto.htm

47. Coelho Filho CM. Mandibular protraction appliances for Class II treatment. J Clin Orthod 1995;29:319–336.

48. Coelho Filho CM. Clinical applications of the mandibular protraction appliance. J Clin Orthod 1997;31:92–102.

49. Coelho Filho CM. The Mandibular Protraction Appliance No. 3. J Clin Orthod 1998;32:379–384.

50. Coelho Filho CM. Mandibular protraction appliance IV. J Clin Orthod 2001;35:18–24.

51. Eckhart JE. Introducing the MARA. Clin Impressions 1998;7:2–5, 24–27.

52. Kinzinger G, Ostheimer J, Forster F, Kwandt PB, Reul H, Diedrich P. Development of a new fixed functional appliance for treatment of skeletal class II malocclusion first report. J Orofac Orthop 2002;63:384–399.

53. Jasper JJ. The Jasper Jumper – a fixed functional appliance. Sheybogan: American Orthodontics; 1987.

54. Winsauer H. Flex Developer. Adjustable power developer – variable length and force. Maria Anzbach: LPI-Ormco, 2002. Available online at: www.flexdeveloper.com

55. Amoric M. Les ressorts intermaxillaires en torsion. Rev Orthop Dentofacial 1994;28:115–117.

56. Awbrey JJ. The bite fixer. Clin Impressions 1999;8:10–17, 31.

57. Klapper L. The SUPERspring II: a new appliance for noncompliant Class II patients. J Clin Orthod 1999;33:50–54.

58. Castanon R, Valdes MS, White LW. Clinical use of the Churro jumper. J Clin Orthod 1998; 32:731–745.

59. Heinig N, Goz G. Clinical application and effects of the Forsus spring. A study of a new Herbst hybrid. J Orofac Orthop 2001;62: 436–450.

60. Corbett MC, Molina FG. Twin Force Bite Corrector. Light force and patient friendly. Syllabus, Ortho Organizers, 2001.

61. Starnes LO. Comprehensive phase I treatment in the middle mixed dentition. J Clin Orthod 1998;32:98–110.

62. Hilgers JJ. A palatal expansion appliance for noncompliance therapy. J Clin Orthod 1991; 25:491–497.

63. Mayes JH. The Texas Penguin... a new approach to pendulum therapy. AOA Orthodont Appl 1999;3:1–2. Available online at: www.aoalab.com/learning/publications/aoaVol/aoaVol3N1.pdf

64. Hilgers JJ. The Hilgers PhD. AOA Orthodont Appl 1998;2:5. Available online at: www.aoalab.com/learning/publications/aoaVol/aoaVol2N1.pdf

65. Grummons D. Maxillary asymmetry and frontal analysis. Clin Impressions 1999;8:2–16, 23.

66. Snodgrass DJ. A fixed appliance for maxillary expansion, molar rotation, and molar distalization. J Clin Orthod 1996;30:156–159.

67. Scuzzo G, Pisani F, Takemoto K. Maxillary molar distalization with a modified pendulum appliance. J Clin Orthod 1999;33:645–650.

68. Kinzinger G, Fuhrmann R, Gross U, Diedrich P. Modified pendulum appliance including distal screw and uprighting activation for noncompliance therapy of Class II malocclusion in children and adolescents. J Orofac Orthop 2000;61:175–190.

69. Kinzinger G, Fritz U, Diedrich P. Bipendulum and quad pendulum for noncompliance molar distalization in adult patients. J Orofac Orthop 2002;63:154–162.

70. Keles A, Sayinsu K. A new approach in maxillary molar distalization: intraoral bodily molar distalizer. Am J Orthod Dentofacial Orthop 2000;117:39–48.

71. Walde KC. The simplified molar distalizer. J Clin Orthod 2003;37:616–619.

72. Quick AN, Harris AM. Molar distalization with a modified distal jet appliance. J Clin Orthod 2000;34:419–423.

73. Keles A. Maxillary unilateral molar distalization with sliding mechanics: a preliminary investigation. Eur J Orthod 2001;23:507–515.

74. Reiner TJ. Modified Nance appliance for unilateral molar distalization. J Clin Orthod 1992;26:402–404.

75. Bondemark L. A comparative analysis of distal maxillary molar movement produced by a new lingual intra-arch Ni-Ti coil appliance and a magnetic appliance. Eur J Orthod 2000; 22:683–695.

76. Lanteri C, Francolini F, Lanteri V. Distalization using the Fast Back. Leone News Int 2002;Feb:1–3.

77. Scott MW. Molar distalization: more ammunition for your operatory. Clin Impressions 1996; 5:16–27.

78. Papadopoulos MA. Simultaneous distalization of maxillary first and second molars by means of superelastic NiTi coils. Hell Orthod Rev 1998; 1:71–76.

79. Erverdi N, Koyuturk O, Kucukkeles N. Nickel-titanium coil springs and repelling magnets: a comparison of two different intra-oral molar distalization techniques. Br J Orthod 1997; 24:47–53.

80. Pieringer M, Droschl H, Permann R. Distalization with a Nance appliance and coil springs. J Clin Orthod 1997;31:321–326.

81. Blechman AM. Magnetic force systems in orthodontics: clinical results of a pilot study. Am J Orthod 1985;87:201–210.

82. Gianelly AA, Vaitas AS, Thomas WM, Berger DG. Distalization of molars with repelling magnets. J Clin Orthod 1988;22:40–44.

83. Blechman AM, Alexander C. New miniaturized magnets for molar distalization. Clin Impressions 1995;4:14–19.

84. Giancotti A, Cozza P. Nickel titanium double-loop system for simultaneous distalization of first and second molars. J Clin Orthod 1998; 32:255–260.

85. Vlock R. A fixed appliance for rapid distalization of upper molars. Orthodontic CYBERjournal 1998;3. Available online at: www.oc-j.com/issue7/vlock.htm

86. Wilson WL. Modular orthodontic systems. Part 2. J Clin Orthod 1978;12:358–375.

87. Manhartsberger C. [Headgear-free molar distalization.] Fortschr Kieferorthop 1994; 55:330–336.

88. Ritto AK. Removable distalization splint. Orthodontic CYBERjournal 1997;2. Available online at: www.oc-j.com/issue6/ritto.htm & http://www.oc-j.com/issue2/ritto.htm

89. Carriere L. Syllabus on the Carriere distalizer and its use. ClassOne Orthodontics. Available online at: www.classoneorthodontics.com/customer_files/Class_One_Carriere.pdf

90. Greenfield RL. Fixed piston appliance for rapid Class II correction. J Clin Orthod 1995; 29:174–183.

91. Puente M. Class II correction with an edgewise-modified Nance appliance. J Clin Orthod 1997;31:178–182.

92. Veltri N, Baldini A. Slow sagittal and bilateral palatal expansion for the treatment of class II malocclusions. Leone Bollettino Int 2001; 3:5–9.

93. Baccetti T, Franchi L. A new appliance for molar distalization. Leone Bollettino Int 2000;2:3–7.

94. Paz ME. Nonextraction therapy benefits from small expansion appliance. Clin Impressions 2001;10:12–15.

95. Fortini A, Lupoli M, Parri M. The First Class Appliance for rapid molar distalization. J Clin Orthod 1999;33:322–328.

96. Cetlin NM, Ten Hoeve A. Nonextraction treatment. J Clin Orthod 1983;17:396–413.

97. Dahlquist A, Gebauer U, Ingervall B. The effect of a transpalatal arch for the correction of first molar rotation. Eur J Orthod 1996;18: 257–267.

98. Cooke MS, Wreakes G. Molar derotation with a modified palatal arch: an improved technique. Br J Orthod 1978;5:201–203.

99. Corbett MC. Molar rotation and beyond. J Clin Orthod 1996;30:272–275.

100. Corbett MC. Slow and continuous maxillary expansion, molar rotation, and molar distalization. J Clin Orthod 1997;31:253–263.

101. Mandurino M, Balducci L. Asymmetric distalization with a TMA transpalatal arch. J Clin Orthod 2001;35:174–178.

102. Keles A, Impram S. An effective and precise method for rapid molar derotation: Keles TPA. World J Orthod 2003;4:229–236.

103. Langlade M. Clinical distalization with the Distalix. World J Orthod 2003;4:215–228.

104. Byloff FK, Karcher H, Clar E, Stoff F. An implant to eliminate anchorage loss during molar distalization: a case report involving the Graz implant-supported pendulum. Int J Adult Orthod Orthognath Surg 2000;15:129–137.

105. Karcher H, Byloff FK, Clar E. The Graz implant supported pendulum, a technical note. J Craniomaxillofac Surg 2002;30:87–90.

106. Giancotti A, Muzzi F, Greco M, Arcuri C. Palatal implant-supported distalizing devices: clinical application of the Straumann Orthosystem. World J Orthod 2002;3:135–139.

107. Keles A, Erverdi N, Sezen S. Bodily distalization of molars with absolute anchorage. Angle Orthod 2003;73:471–482.

108. Maino BG, Mura P, Gianelly AA. A Retrievable palatal implant for absolute anchorage in orthodontics. World J Orthod 2002;3: 125–134.

109. Glatzmaier J, Wehrbein H, Diedrich P. Die Entwicklung eines resorbierbaren Implantatsystems zur orthodontischen Verankerung. Fortschr Kieferorthop 1995;56:175–181.

110. Glatzmaier J, Wehrbein H, Diedrich P. Biodegradable implants for orthodontic anchorage. A preliminary biomechanical study. Eur J Orthod 1996;18:465–469.

111. Bernhart T, Freudenthaler J, Dortbudak O, Bantleon HP, Watzek G. Short epithetic implants for orthodontic anchorage in the paramedian region of the palate. A clinical study. Clin Oral Implants Res 2001;12:624–631.

112. Karaman AI, Basciftci FA, Polat O. Unilateral distal molar movement with an implant-supported distal jet appliance. Angle Orthod 2002;72: 167–174.

113. Kyung SH, Hong SG, Park YC. Distalization of maxillary molars with a midpalatal miniscrew. J Clin Orthod 2003;37:22–26.

114. Bondemark L, Feldmann I, Feldmann H. Distal molar movement with an intra-arch device provided with the onplant system for absolute anchorage. World J Orthod 2002;3:117–124.

115. Wehrbein H, Glatzmaier J, Mundwiller U, Diedrich P. The orthosystem: a new implant system for orthodontic anchorage in the palate. J Orofac Orthop 1996;57:142–153.

116. Wehrbein H, Merz BR, Diedrich P, Glatzmaier J. The use of palatal implants for orthodontic anchorage. Design and clinical application of the orthosystem. Clin Oral Implants Res 1996; 7:410–416.

117. Bantleon HP, Bernhart T, Crismani AG, Zachrisson BU. Stable orthodontic anchorage with palatal osseointegrated implants. World J Orthod 2002;3:109–116.

118. Giancotti A, Muzzi F, Santini F, Arcuri C. Straumann Orthosystem method for orthodontic anchorage step-by-step procedure. World J Orthod 2002;3:140–146.

119. Fritz U, Diedrich P, Kinzinger G, Al-Said M. The anchorage quality of mini-implants towards translatory and extrusive forces. J Orofac Orthop 2003;64:293–304.

120. Costa A, Raffaini M, Melsen B. Miniscrews as orthodontic anchorage: a preliminary report. Int J Adult Orthodont Orthognath Surg 1998; 13:201–209.

121. Lee JS, Park HS, Kyung HM. Micro-implant anchorage for lingual treatment of a skeletal Class II malocclusion. J Clin Orthod 2001;35: 643–647.

122. Block MS, Hoffman DR. A new device for absolute anchorage for orthodontics. Am J Orthod Dentofacial Orthop 1995;107:251–258.

123. Celenza F, Hochman MN. Absolute anchorage in orthodontics: direct and indirect implant-assisted modalities. J Clin Orthod 2000;34:397–402.

124. Kanomi R. Mini-implant for orthodontic anchorage. J Clin Orthod 1997;31:763–767.

125. Park HS, Bae SM, Kyung HM, Sung JH. Micro-implant anchorage for treatment of skeletal Class I bialveolar protrusion. J Clin Orthod 2001; 35:417–422.

126. Maino BG, Bednar J, Pagin P, Mura P. The spider screw for skeletal anchorage. J Clin Orthod 2003;27:90–97.

127. Erverdi N, Tosun T, Keles A. A new anchorage site for the treatment of anterior open bite: zygomatic anchorage. A case report. World J Orthod 2002;3:147–153.

128. De Clerck H, Geerinckx V, Siciliano S. The Zygoma Anchorage System. J Clin Orthod 2002;36:455–459.

SECTION TWO

INTERMAXILLARY APPLIANCES USED FOR THE MANAGEMENT OF CLASS II NONCOMPLIANT PATIENTS

This section includes chapters on the following:

CHAPTER 3

Overview of the intermaxillary noncompliance appliances

Moschos A. Papadopoulos

Rigid Intermaxillary Appliances (RIMA)

There are several types of intermaxillary noncompliance appliances used for the correction of Class II malocclusion. The Herbst appliance (Dentaurum, Ispringen, Germany) is a rigid intermaxillary appliance known to be an effective device for this purpose. Following its re-introduction by Pancherz,[1] several modifications as well as new appliances based on the principles of the Herbst appliance have been proposed by various authors (see Table 2.1).

Herbst Appliance

Usually, the Herbst appliance is attached to bands (banded Herbst design) (see Figs 4.1 and 4.2)[1,2] or cast splints (cast splint Herbst design) (see Figs 4.7, 4.8 and 4.9).[3,4] The appliance can also be attached to stainless steel crowns (stainless steel crown Herbst design)[5–7] and to acrylic splints (acrylic splint Herbst design) (see Fig. 4.12).[8,9] These are the four basic designs of the Herbst appliance. Other Herbst variations include space-closing Herbst designs, cantilevered Herbst designs, and expansion designs.[10–12]

The Herbst appliance is a fixed appliance which functions like an artificial joint between the maxilla and the mandible.[1,2] The original design (banded Herbst design) consists of a bilateral telescopic mechanism attached to orthodontic bands on maxillary first permanent molars and on mandibular first premolars, which maintains the mandible in a continuous protruded position or, in other words, in a continuous anterior jumped position. Bands can also be placed on first maxillary premolars and first mandibular permanent molars, while a lingual bar is used to connect the maxillary or mandibular premolars with the molars.[13,14] When the mandibular first premolars have not erupted, the permanent canines can be banded but in this case there is an increased possibility of buccal mucosa ulceration at the corner of the mouth.[15]

A more recent version of the Herbst appliance was developed by Pancherz,[3] in which the bands are replaced by cast splints (cast splint Herbst design), which fit precisely and cover the teeth in their lateral segments, fabricated from cobalt-chromium alloy and cemented with glass ionomer cement to the teeth.[3,4] Usually, the maxillary and mandibular anterior teeth are incorporated into the anchorage with brackets and the use of sectional archwires.

Each of the telescopic mechanisms consists of a tube and a plunger which fit together, two pivots and two locking screws.[1,3,15] The pivot for the tube is soldered to the maxillary first molar band and the pivot for the plunger to the mandibular first premolar band. The tubes and plungers are attached to the pivots with the locking screws and can easily rotate around their point of attachment. A large interpivot distance prevents the disengagement of the telescopic mechanism due to the plunger slipping out of the tube. Consequently, the upper pivots should be positioned distally on the molar bands and the lower pivots mesially on the premolar bands. In addition, the plunger should be as long as possible to prevent its slippage out of the tube and to avoid damage of the appliance in case the plunger is jammed on the tube opening. If the plunger is much longer than the tube, it extends behind the tube distally to the maxillary first molar and may wound the buccal mucosa.[1,10,16] In contrast, if the plunger is too short it may slip out of the tube when the patient opens the mouth wide.[1,10]

The bands on which the tube and the plunger are attached should be fabricated from at least 0.15 mm or 0.010″ thick orthodontic material, which prevents any breakage during treatment with the Herbst appliance and also allows increased extension in the occlusocervical direction to achieve adequate retention of the bands on the teeth.[13–15]

The appliance permits the mandible to perform opening movements and also small lateral movements, mainly because of the loose fit of the tube and plunger at their sites of attachment. These lateral movements can be increased by widening the pivot openings of the tubes and plungers (see Fig. 4.6).[1,13,15,17] If larger lateral movements are desired, the Herbst telescope with balls will give greater freedom (see Figs 4.7 and 4.8).

For stabilization of the anchorage teeth, two main systems can be used: partial anchorage and total anchorage.[15] For *partial anchorage*, in the maxillary dental arch the bands of the first permanent molars and first premolars are connected with a half-round (1.5 × 0.75 mm) lingual or buccal sectional archwire on each side. In the mandibular dental arch the bands of the first premolars are connected with a half-round (1.5 × 0.75 mm) or a round (1 mm) lingual archwire touching the lingual surfaces of the anterior teeth.[2,3,15] When partial anchorage is considered to be inadequate, the incorporation of supplementary dental units is advised, thus transforming partial anchorage into *total anchorage*.[3,15] In this type of anchorage, a labial archwire is ligated to brackets on the first premolars, cuspids, and incisors in the maxillary dental arch (see Fig. 4.5). In addition, a transpalatal arch can be attached on the first molar bands.[16] In the mandibular dental arch, bands are cemented on the first molars and connected to the lingual archwire which is extended distally. Additionally, a premolar-to-premolar labial rectangular archwire attached to brackets on the anterior teeth can be used.[18]

When maxillary expansion is also required, a rapid palatal expansion screw can be soldered to the premolar and molar bands or to the cast splint[3,15] (see Fig. 4.3d). The maxillary expansion can be accomplished simultaneously[12,14,15,19,20] or prior to Herbst appliance treatment.[20,21] The Herbst appliance can also be used in combination with headgear when banded[22,23] or when splinted.[24]

The telescopic mechanism of the Herbst appliance exerts a posteriorly directed force on the maxilla and its dentition and an anterior force on the mandible and its dentition.[17,25–27] Thus, the mandibular length is increased due to the stimulation of condylar growth and the remodeling process in the articular fossa, which can be attributed to the anterior jumped position of the mandible.[1,2,25] The amount of mandibular protrusion is determined by the length of the tube, to which the length of the plunger is adjusted. In most cases the mandible is advanced to an initial incisal edge-to-edge position at the start of the treatment, and the dental arches are placed in a Class I or overcorrected Class I relationship[1–4,14,15,17,19,20,28–34] while in some cases a step-by-step advancement procedure is followed (usually by adding shims over the mandibular plungers) until an edge-to-edge incisal relationship is established[14,17,23,24] (see Fig. 4.9).

Prior to the mandibular advancement procedure and before starting treatment with the Herbst appliance, a proper transverse relationship should be achieved,[9] the maxillary and mandibular teeth should be well aligned and the dental arches should fit each other in the normal sagittal position.[1,14,15] After the Herbst appliance has been inserted, a small adjustment period of 7–10 days is required, during which the patient may experience some chewing difficulties and therefore a soft diet is recommended.[1,13,15,17,28]

Treatment with the banded Herbst appliance usually lasts 6–8 months.[1,2,15,19,29,35] However, a longer treatment period of 9–15 months is also recommended for better treatment outcomes.[10] When the desired effects have been obtained and a Class I or overcorrected Class I relationship has been achieved, the appliance is removed.

Following Herbst treatment, a retention phase is required in order to avoid any relapse of the dental relationships, due to undesirable growth patterns or because of lip–tongue dysfunction habits.[15,35] In patients with mixed dentition and unstable cuspal interdigitation,[1,15,25] this phase can last 1–2 years[35–38] or until stable occlusal relationships are established when the permanent teeth have erupted.[15,39] This is accomplished by means of activators, such as the Andresen activator[4,15,18,35] or positioners.[33] When a second phase with fixed appliances follows, retention is required for 8–12 months to maintain stable occlusal relationships[1,15,19,25,35] while Class II elastics can also be used.[16]

Many authors have proposed the use of stainless steel crowns as anchor units instead of bands.[5,6,40–45] The stainless steel crown Herbst design was first introduced by Langford[5] to avoid breakages of the bands. According to the author, crowns are placed on the maxillary first molars and the mandibular first premolars (or canines). The advantages of the stainless steel crown Herbst appliance include resistance to the stresses placed on the appliance, elimination of loose crowns or breakage during treatment, and avoidance of excessive protrusion of the mandibular incisors.[5] Dischinger proposed the edgewise bioprogressive Herbst appliance to minimize limitations of the Herbst design and to incorporate edgewise brackets and mechanics in the correction of Class II malocclusions.[6] Similar stainless steel crown Herbst designs were also introduced by Smith (type II)[43,44] and by Hilgers.[45] Another stainless steel crown Herbst design is the cantilever Herbst, which includes mandibular extension arms attached to stainless steel crowns on the mandibular first molars and can be used in mixed and early permanent dentition.[21,43,44] The arms extend anteriorly from the mandibular first molar lateral to the dentition and end in the premolar area. The Herbst pivots are soldered to the cantilever arms close to the buccal surface of the mandibular first premolars and support wires are used in the shape of occlusal rests to the mandibular deciduous second molars or permanent second molars for additional stabilization.

The Acrylic Splint Herbst Appliance consists of the telescopic mechanism which is attached to acrylic splints cemented or bonded on the maxillary and mandibular dentition. For the attachment of the bite-jumping mechanism, a wire framework is used, over which 2.5–3 mm acrylic is adapted.[8,21,46,47] A transpalatal arch or, more usually, a rapid palatal expansion screw attached to the wire framework connects the left and right parts of the splint together. The acrylic maxillary and mandibular splints can also be removable. The appliance can be worn on a full-time basis and removed only for oral hygiene, or on a part-time basis.[9,48,49] Mainly due to the fact that bonding of the acrylic splints increases the risk of decalcification,[9,47] McNamara et al[21] recommend that the Acrylic Splint Herbst Appliance should be removable in most cases. However, bonding of the maxillary splint may be necessary, for example in cases involving rapid palatal expansion, in patients whose teeth shape does not provide adequate retention during jaw movements, or when additional anchorage is required. In these cases, the upper splint can be bonded while the lower one can be removable.[9,21,47,50]

The acrylic maxillary splint can accommodate various auxiliaries, such as rectangular buccal tubes to allow the use of utility archwires for incisor proclination and intrusion,[46] rapid palatal expanders in case of posterior crossbites,[8,9,46] transpalatal bars to minimize rotation and displacement of the maxillary posterior teeth,[8] headgear tubes, and posterior bite blocks,[9,51,52] while in the mandibular splint buccal tubes can be used to add removable Frankel-type labial pads to interrupt hyperactive mentalis activity or to engage lip bumpers.[8,21,46]

Modifications of the Herbst Appliance

Goodman's Modified Herbst Appliance
This appliance consists of stainless steel crowns placed on the maxillary first permanent molars[53] and, if additional anchorage is required on maxillary first deciduous molars, a transpalatal arch fabricated from 0.045″ round wire connecting the crowns, bands on the mandibular first molars, frameworks for both mandibular and maxillary arches made of 14-gauge half-round wire, and the Herbst telescopic mechanism. The maxillary pivots are soldered to the most distobuccal points of the crowns, parallel to the distal and the occlusal surfaces, while the mandibular pivots are soldered to the wire framework on a level with the mesial surface of the first deciduous molars. A wax-bite in an edge-to-edge incisal position is taken and the cementation of the appliance follows after a trial procedure. The appliance is placed for 7–8 months after which any additional advancement could take place for 3–4 more months, while the patient is recalled every 6 weeks, for a total period of 9–11 months.

Upper Stainless Steel Crowns and Lower Acrylic
Another modification of the Herbst appliance was developed by Larry White and introduced by Valant & Sinclair.[54] It consists of stainless steel crowns placed on the maxillary first permanent molars and a removable mandibular acrylic splint with occlusal coverage including a wire framework.[54,55] The lower part is removed for oral hygiene, while patient compliance is maintained, since the removal of the mandibular component leaves the telescoping mechanism impinging on the buccal vestibular mucosa of the mandible. The appliance is indicated in skeletal Class II and dental Class II, division 1 malocclusion in adolescents and the treatment lasts about 10 months.[54]

A similar design, the Emden Herbst (Dentaurum, Ispringen, Germany; Great Lakes Orthodontics, Tonawanda, NY), was introduced by Zreik.[56] This incorporates additionally double buccal tubes on the maxillary crowns which can be used for the insertion of utility, sectional or continuous archwires, allowing the placement of full fixed appliances 6 weeks after Herbst placement. Further, the Magnusson system (Dentaurum, Ispringen, Germany) is very similar to the modification introduced by Valant & Sinclair,[54] with the difference that the crowns on the maxillary first molars are connected with a transpalatal arch.[57]

Mandibular Advancement Locking Unit (MALU)
The Mandibular Advancement Locking Unit (MALU) (Saga Dental Supply AS, Kongsvinger, Norway) was introduced by Schiavoni et al[58] and consists of two tubes, two plungers, two upper "Mobee" hinges with ball-pins, and two lower key hinges with brass pins. Bands are placed on the maxillary first molars with 0.051″ headgear tubes, while a palatal arch can be used in cases of overexpansion. Regarding the mandible, bands are placed on the mandibular first molars, while the anterior teeth are bonded from canine to canine with 0.022″ brackets, and a 0.021 × 0.025″ stainless steel archwire with labial root torque in the anterior section is used, bent back at the distal ends. The Mobee hinge is inserted into the hole at end of the MALU tube and secured to the first molar headgear with the ball-pin, while the lower key hinge is inserted into the hole at the end of the plunger and locked to the mandibular base arch with the brass pin. The length of the tube–plunger assembly is specified by the amount of mandibular advancement required, and further advancements of 1–5 mm can be performed using spacers. According to Haegglund & Segerdal,[59] the MALU attachment can also be used by connecting the pistons to an auxiliary archwire, thus integrating the Herbst telescopic mechanism to fixed appliances.

Magnetic Telescopic Device
According to Ritto,[60] the Magnetic Telescopic Device consists of two tubes and two plungers with a semicircular section and with NdFeB magnets, which are positioned to exert a repelling force, while fitting is achieved using the MALU system. Its main advantages include the linking of a magnetic field on a functional appliance, while its disadvantages involve its thickness, the laboratory work necessary to prepare it, and the covering of the magnets.[61]

Flip-Lock Herbst Appliance
The Flip-Lock Herbst Appliance (TP Orthodontics, LaPorte, IN) reduces the number of moving parts that can lead to breakage or failure. It uses ball-joint connectors instead of screw attachments, and it needs no retaining springs.[62] The ball-joint connectors are attached to stainless steel crowns on maxillary first molars and mandibular first premolars. Further, bands are placed on mandibular first molars and a lingual arch connects them with the crowns on first premolars. The rods have forked ends to be crimped onto the mandibular balls. According to Miller,[62] molar tubes can be soldered on maxillary first molar crowns to combine Herbst treatment with fixed appliances, while simultaneous maxillary expansion can be accomplished with a jackscrew appliance, if needed. The advantages of the Flip-Lock Herbst Appliance include patient comfort and tolerance and the fact that it improves lateral movements of the mandible.

Hanks Telescoping Herbst Appliance
The Hanks Telescoping Herbst Appliance (American Orthodontics, Sheboygan, WI) consists of two tubes, a ball and socket joint, and a

rod attached to the mandibular premolars or cantilever arms, and functions like a free-sliding radio antenna.[63] The outer tube of the axle captures the middle tube and the middle tube slides inside the outer tube stopped at the mesial end of the outer tube. The rod is captured by the middle tube and slides inside the middle tube until it is stopped at the mesial end of the middle tube. This way, the assembly will not disengage due to the stops built into the free-sliding rod and tubes. The advantages of the Hanks Telescoping Herbst include one-piece design, which prevents disengagement, reduced ulcerations, greater lateral movements of the mandible because of the ball and socket joints, fewer emergency appointments, patient comfort and user-friendly components.[63]

Ventral Telescope

The Ventral Telescope (Professional Positioners, Racine, WI) is, according to Ritto,[61] the first intermaxillary appliance fabricated as a single unit and is fixed via ball attachments. The Ventral Telescope is available in two sizes and is activated by unscrewing the tube, thereby causing approximately 3 mm of activation. Its advantages include elimination of the risk of the appliance disassembling when maximum opening occurs, and easy and simple operation, while its disadvantages include thickness and fractures of the brake which stabilizes the joint.[61]

Universal Bite Jumper

The Universal Bite Jumper was introduced by Calvez[64] and is similar to the Herbst appliance but smaller and more adaptable, while an active coil spring can be added when needed. The jumper is fitted in the mouth and cut to the proper length depending on the amount of mandibular advancement. The activation is achieved by crimping 2–4 mm crimping bushes onto the rods, whereas when coil springs are used, no activation is required.

Open-Bite Intrusion Herbst

The Open-Bite Intrusion Herbst (AOA/Pro Orthodontic Appliances, Sturtevant, WI) for mixed dentition consists of a maxillary and a mandibular part.[65] The maxillary part consists of crowns cemented on the maxillary second deciduous molars and permanent first molars, stops which extend from the deciduous second molars to the deciduous first molars, 0.036″ stainless steel intrusion wires with helix loops soldered to the deciduous second molars to intrude the maxillary permanent first molars, cantilever extensions with 0.022″ archwire tubes soldered to the deciduous second molar crowns, and positioning axles distal to the deciduous second molar crowns and just mesial to the permanent first molar crowns. The telescopic axles are initially soldered to the axles to maintain the position of the primary second molars while intruding the permanent first molars, while axles positioned to the first molar crowns are used to connect the Herbst mechanism and maintain the intruded molars during Class II correction.

The mandibular portion of the appliance consists of crowns placed on the deciduous second molars, cantilever arms which are counteracted inferiorly and gingivally to produce increased vertical force, with stops extending to the primary first molars, while additional stops extend from the mandibular second molar crowns to the deciduous and permanent first molars to stabilize the mandibular cantilevers and prevent their tipping down or towards the teeth. Brackets are also placed on both the mandibular and maxillary incisors to increase anchorage during molar intrusion.

After intrusion of the maxillary permanent molars, the deciduous second molars are in occlusion, thereby maintaining the bite open. When intrusion is completed, the Herbst rods and tubes are attached to the intruded maxillary first molars, while extraction of the maxillary deciduous first and second molars should follow. Thus, the mandible autorotates and the maxillary molar position is maintained. After stabilization of the molar position, the Herbst appliance is used to correct Class II malocclusion.

Regarding the permanent dentition, there are maxillary appliances designed for first molar intrusion with first premolar and first molar crowns or for second molar intrusion including first premolar and second molar crowns, while the mandibular appliance is designed with first molar crowns.

The Open-Bite Intrusion Herbst is indicated in high-angle openbite Class II patients with mixed and permanent dentition. The intrusion procedure is completed first and then the Class II correction follows.[65]

IST (Intraoral Snoring Therapy) Appliance

The IST Appliance (Scheu-Dental GmbH, Iserlohn, Germany) was developed by Hinz, consists of removable acrylic splints and a telescopic mechanism, and is indicated in patients suffering from breathing problems during sleep, such as obstructive sleep apnea. The appliance reduces snoring by protruding the mandible, thus reducing the obstruction in the pharyngeal area. Its advantages include a construction that allows change in the amount of protrusion separately on each side, up to 8 mm, and an end stop for prevention of disengagement.[61]

Acrylic Splint with Hinge System

The Hinge System (Scheu-Dental GmbH, Iserlohn, Germany) consists of hinges, profile wires and fastening parts and is used in Class II cases with removable splints. The fastening parts are anchored on a profile wire and polymerized in a splint.

Cantilever Bite Jumper (CBJ)

The Cantilever Bite Jumper (AOA/Pro Orthodontic Appliances, Sturtevant, WI) can be regarded as another modification of the Herbst appliance. It was developed in the mid-1980s by Mayes[66] and works like an artificial joint. It consists of stainless steel crowns placed on the mandibular and maxillary first permanent molars, cantilever arms,

Herbst pivots, a 0.045″ lingual bar, and a transpalatal arch when palatal expansion is required (see Fig. 5.6).

The mandibular cantilevers are extended anteriorly from the mandibular first molars lateral to the dentition and end mesial to the first premolar area or approximately to the middle or to the anterior part of the deciduous mandibular first molar.[41,66] The Herbst pivot is soldered to the mandibular cantilever arm close to the buccal surface of the mandibular first premolar. The lingual bar is attached on the mandibular first molar crowns and is kept in touch with the lingual surfaces of the mandibular anterior teeth.

After appliance placement, the mandible is advanced in an edge-to-edge incisal position when greater orthopedic response is required, and this position is maintained for about 12 months to avoid serious relapse. When more dental changes are needed, the mandibular advancement can be performed in gradual increments, 3 mm every 2 months, until an edge-to-edge incisal relationship is achieved, which is maintained for about 9 months.[66] The CBJ can be combined with expansion of the upper and lower arch.[41] The maxillary expansion can be achieved by selecting between rapid palatal expander, quad helix, Goshgarian transpalatal arch, U-shaped arch or W-arch. The mandibular arch can be expanded with lingual bars, Frozat or labial expanders.

Molar-Moving Bite Jumper (MMBJ)

The Molar-Moving Bite Jumper (AOA/Pro Orthodontic Appliances, Sturtevant, WI) was developed by Mayes[42] to correct Class II malocclusion and to simultaneously close the spaces when the lower second premolars are missing. There are two types of MMBJ, which use common components in the maxilla. In particular, both types use CBJ maxillary molar crowns with preattached axles. The first type uses stainless steel crowns on mandibular first premolars bilaterally, bands on the first permanent molars, and 9 mm NiTi coil springs attached on the molar band hooks and on hooks welded on the premolar bands. A 0.045″ lingual bar inserted in the 0.045″ lingual molar tubes and welded to the premolar crowns prevents mesial crown tipping during the molar mesial movement. The NiTi coil springs exert a mesial force of 150 g on the mandibular first molar, which can be restricted by placing a stop on the lingual bar.

The second type can be used with unilaterally missing second premolars. It consists of a similar lingual bar, bands on the mandibular first premolars and the first molar on the missing premolar's side, a CBJ crown placed on the first molar of the other side, and a 9 mm NiTi coil spring attached on the molar band hook and on a hook welded on the premolar band. The mandibular CBJ molar crown with preattached cantilever results in a slight opening of the bite, thus allowing more rapid mesial movement of the other first mandibular molar.[42]

Prior to appliance placement, second deciduous molars should be extracted in order to achieve mesial molar movement, and if maxillary expansion is required, it should also take place before inserting the appliance. According to Mayes,[42] the MMBJ is indicated for the correction of Class II malocclusions when the second premolars are missing, both unilaterally and bilaterally.

Mandibular Advancing Repositioning Splint (MARS)

The Mandibular Advancing Repositioning Splint (Dentaurum Inc., Ispringen, Germany; Rocky Mountain Orthodontics, Denver, CO) was introduced by Clements & Jacobson.[67] The MARS appliance consists of bilaterally telescopic units, the struts, maxillary and mandibular multibanded appliances, and locking devices consisting of a slot and setscrew. Each telescopic unit is composed of a plunger and a cylinder or hollow tube and their free ends are attached to the upper and lower archwires with the use of the locking devices, which secure their position on the archwire. The MARS appliance tube is attached mesially to the most distal maxillary molar incorporated into the fixed appliance, and the plunger is attached distal to the mandibular canines. The locking device is attached to both plunger and tube with a loose-fitting screw to provide rotational movement of the telescopic mechanism around the point of attachment, allowing the mandible to perform lateral movements.

The MARS appliance should be placed in position only after initial rotations, space closure, and alignment procedures have been completed. A heavy rectangular archwire which fits completely in the bracket slots should be used for the fixed appliance. The dental arches should be brought into an incisal edge-to-edge relationship. A less protrusive mandibular position should be selected if the patient cannot tolerate muscular discomfort, and with subsequent advancements the mandible should be brought into a more forward position. The MARS appliance should be removed when a super Class I relationship and a stable cuspal interdigitation have been achieved.[67]

Mandibular Corrector Appliance (MCA)

The Mandibular Corrector Appliance (Cormar Inc., Salisbury, MD) was introduced by Jones.[68] The appliance consists of bilateral repositioning arms, multibanded appliances with almost full-size edgewise archwires and connectors. The archwire dimensions should be 0.0175 × 0.025″ when 0.018″ bracket-slots are used or 0.021 × 0.025″ when 0.022″ bracket-slots are used.[68] The repositioning arms are attached to the archwire with connectors distal on the mandibular canine brackets and mesial to the tubes of the terminal maxillary molars. The length of the repositioning arms is determined after advancing the mandible for about 3–4 mm. After this initial advancement, additional reactivations of 2–4 mm can take place every 4 weeks until the incisors are brought into an edge-to-edge position. In cases of midline deviations, the correction can be performed by advancing the mandible more on one side.

Treatment with the MCA lasts 6 months if an overjet correction of 3–4 mm is required, whereas when 7–8 mm correction is needed the treatment time may be increased up to 12–14 months. After a super Class I molar relationship has been achieved and the mandible is kept in a stable position without being retracted, the MCA can be removed and short Class II elastics can be placed to bring the posterior teeth into tight intercuspation.

Biopedic Appliance

The Biopedic (GAC International Inc., Islandia, NY), designed by Collins, was introduced in 1997 and consists of buccal attachments soldered to mandibular and maxillary first molar crowns.[61,69] The attachments contain a standard edgewise tube and a 0.070″ molar tube, while large rods pass through the tubes. The maxillary rod, which is inserted from the distal, is fixed by a screw clamp mesial to the maxillary first molar, while the mandibular rod is inserted from the mesial of the molar tube and is fixed at the distal by a similar screw.[69] The rods are connected via a rigid shaft, while two pivots on their ends allow the appliance to be rotated when the patient opens his mouth. The Biopedic appliance is activated by moving the mandibular rod mesially and fixing the screw.[61,69]

Ritto Appliance®

The Ritto Appliance was developed by Ritto and is described as a miniaturized telescopic device with simplified intraoral application and activation[70] (see Figs 6.1 and 6.7). It is a one-piece device with telescopic action, which is fabricated in a single format able to be used bilaterally, attached to upper and lower archwires. A steel ball-pin and a lock-controlled sliding brake are used as fixing components. In addition, two maxillary and two mandibular bands and brackets on the mandibular arch can support the appliance adequately. The appliance is activated by sliding the lock around the lower arch distally and fixing it against the appliance. The activation is performed in two steps, an initial adjustment activation of 2–3 mm and a subsequent activation of 1–2 mm 1 week later, while further activations of 4–5 mm can be performed after 3 weeks.

Mandibular Protraction Appliance (MPA)

The Mandibular Protraction Appliance was introduced by Coelho Filho[71] for the correction of Class II malocclusion. It has been continuously developed since its initial introduction and four different types have been proposed, all by Coelho Filho.

The first type (MPA I) consists of one-piece bilateral telescopic parts attached to mandibular and maxillary archwires (see Fig. 7.1a). Each part is fabricated from 0.032″ stainless steel wire with circular loops at a right angle to the ends of the wire. These two loops are in a reverse direction. The mandibular archwire incorporates stops distal to the canines, such as circles, crimpable hooks or loops, to prevent direct contact between the telescopic part and the brackets, and enough lingual torque in the anterior segment to resist the mandibular incisor proclination caused by the mesial forces of the appliance. Premolar brackets should be avoided to provide adequate space for sliding along the mandibular tube.[71] The length of the telescopic device is determined by the distance between the mesial of the upper molar tube and the stop made in the mandibular archwire distal to the canine when the mandible is brought forward with the dental arches in a Class I relationship. During mouth opening, the MPA I slides along the mandibular archwire in a distal direction and mesially along the maxillary archwire; during closing it rests against the mandibular archwire stop and maxillary buccal tube.

Despite the effectiveness of the appliance in carefully selected patients, difficulties such as omitting the mandibular premolar brackets, the limited mouth opening, and the dislodgment of the molar bands led the author to develop a second design. The MPA II consists of bilateral telescopic parts in two pieces and a small rigid stainless steel coil or tubing[70,72] (see Fig. 7.1b). Each telescopic device is fabricated from two pieces of 0.032″ or 0.036″ stainless steel wire with circular loops in one of their ends. The coil or tubing is placed over one of the wires and one end of the wire is inserted through the other wire's loop in such a way that each of the wires can slide through the other up to the limit of the wire coil. Then, circular loops are formed at the other ends of the wire. The coils prevent interfering of the wires and ensure their correct relationship.

To overcome breakage and problems, restricted opening and patient intolerance connected with the use of the MPA I, and difficulties in the fabrication of the MPA II, Coelho Filho[73] introduced a third MPA design (see Fig. 7.1c). The main difference between the MPA III and previous designs is the incorporation of telescopic tubes and mandibular rods. These rods rotate within the circular loops placed in the mandibular archwires distally to the canines, while the longer section of the mandibular rods slides within the telescopic tubes. Several adaptations have been made to this design, such as the use of nickel titanium open-coil springs over the mandibular rods, thus exerting continuous and light Class II forces. The appliance can also be used in a reversed way for the correction of Class III malocclusions and anterior crossbites.[73]

The latest version of the MPA (MPA IV) consists of a T-tube, a maxillary molar locking pin, a mandibular rod, and a rigid mandibular stainless steel archwire with two circular loops distal to the canine[74] (see Fig. 7.1d). The mandibular rod is inserted into the longer section of the T-tube and the molar locking pin is inserted into the smaller section of the T-tube. To place the appliance, the mandibular rod is inserted into the circular loop of the mandibular archwire, the mandible is protruded to an edge-to-edge position, and the molar locking pin is inserted into the maxillary molar tube from the distal and bent mesial for stabilization. Thus, the maxillary extremity of the appliance can slide around the pin wire (see Fig. 7.3). The appliance can also be inserted from the mesial. If activation is necessary, this can be performed by inserting a piece of nickel titanium open-coil spring between the mandibular rod and the telescopic tube.[74,75]

Mandibular Anterior Repositioning Appliance (MARA™)

The MARA (AOA/Pro Orthodontic Appliances, Sturtevant, WI) is an intermaxillary appliance which keeps the mandible in a continuous protruded position. It was first developed by Douglas Toll in 1991 and redesigned in 1995.[76] It can be considered as a fixed twin block due to the fact that it incorporates two opposing vertical surfaces placed in such a way as to keep the mandible in a forward position (see Fig. 8.13).

The MARA consists of four stainless steel crowns (or rigid bands) attached to the first permanent molars. Each lower molar crown incorporates a double tube soldered on it, consisting of a 0.045″ tube and a 0.022 × 0.028″ tube for the maxillary and mandibular arch-wires. A 0.059″ arm is also soldered to each lower crown, projecting perpendicular to its buccal surface, which engages the elbows of the upper molar. For stabilization, the lower crowns can be connected to each other through a soldered lingual arch, especially if no braces are used. A lingual arch is also recommended to prevent crowding of the second premolars and mesiolingual rotation of the mandibular first molars.[77,78]

Each upper molar crown also incorporates the same double tube as the lower crown. In addition, 0.062″ square tubes are soldered to each of the upper crowns, into which slide the corresponding 0.060″ square upper elbows.[76–79] These upper elbows are inserted in the upper square tubes while guiding the patient into an advanced forward position, and are hung vertically. The elbows are tied in by ligatures or elastics after placement of the MARA.[76,77,80] The buccal position of the upper elbows is controlled by torquing them with a simple tool, while their anteroposterior position is controlled by shims.[76] In addition, Simon & Haerian added a buccal shield to the lower arm to increase patient comfort.[81]

Occlusal rests can also be used on the maxillary and mandibular second molars or premolars.[78] According to Eckhart,[80] the upper occlusal rests on the second molars are used to prevent intrusion and tip-back of the maxillary first molars and extrusion of the maxillary second molars. Brackets on the maxillary second premolars should not be used to avoid interfering with the elbow during its insertion and removal.[77,78] The MARA can be combined with maxillary and mandibular expanders, transpalatal arches, adjustments loops, fixed orthodontic appliances, and maxillary molar distalization appliances.[78,79,81]

Before appliance placement, the maxillary incisors should be aligned, properly torqued, and intruded if required, so as not to interfere with the mandibular advancement, while the maxillary arch should be wide enough to allow the elbows to hang buccally to the lower crowns.[77,78] The mandible is usually advanced, either in one step or in gradual increments, into an overcorrected Class I relationship to counteract the expected small relapse usually observed during the posttreatment period.[76–79] When 4–5 mm of mandibular advancement is required, the mandible is advanced to an edge-to-edge incisor position. When 8–9 mm correction is needed, the advancement is performed in two steps to avoid excessive strain on the temporo-mandibular joint or appliance breakage.[78] In the first step, the mandible is advanced initially 4–5 mm, maintained in that position for about 6 months, and then advanced in an edge-to-edge position for an additional period of 6 months.[78] Alternatively, the advance-ment can be performed in gradual increments of 2–3 mm every 8–12 weeks, by adding shims on the elbows.[77–79]

After insertion of the MARA, the patient should be informed that it will take 4–10 days to be comfortable with the new, advanced mandibular position, during which period some chewing difficulties may occur.[78,79] If the patient is a mouth breather or suffers from bruxism, vertical elastics can be placed during sleeping to keep the mouth closed.[78] The posterior open bite which may be observed after appliance placement is reduced, while the posterior teeth erupt normally without interference with the appliance.[77]

Treatment duration with the MARA depends on the severity of the Class II malocclusion and the patient's age but usually lasts about 12–15 months.[76,78,79] The patient is monitored at 12–16 week intervals for further adjustments or reactivations.[78,79]

After treatment with the MARA is completed and the dental arches are brought into a Class I relationship, the appliance is removed and fixed multibanded appliances can be used to further adjust the occlusion.[78,79] If the mandible is not advanced in an overcorrected position, Class II elastics can be used for approximately 6 months after appliance removal.[78] If the molars are in open bite due to the occlusal coverage when crowns are used, vertical elastics should be used to close the space.[77]

Functional Mandibular Advancer (FMA)

The FMA, which was developed by Kinzinger et al[82] as an alternative to the Herbst appliance for the correction of Class II malocclusions, is a rigid intermaxillary appliance based on the principle of the inclined plane. It is similar to the MARA but with some fundamental differences. It consists of cast splints, crowns or bands on which the main parts of the appliance, the guide pins and inclined planes, are laser welded buccally. The bite-jumping appliance of the FMA is attached at a 60° angle to the horizontal, thus actively guiding the mandible in a forward position while closing, which provides unrestricted mandibular motion and increases patient adaptation. According to Kinzinger et al,[82] the anterior shape of the bite-jumping device and the active components of the abutments were designed to allow mandibular guidance even in partial jaw closure, thus ensuring its effectiveness even in patients with habitual open mouth posture. The appliance is reactivated by adjusting the threaded insert supports over a length of 2 mm, using guide pins of different width or by fitting the sliding surfaces of the inclined planes with spacers of different thicknesses. Therefore, the mandibular advancement can be accomplished following a step-by-step procedure which provides better patient adaptation, especially for adult patients.[82]

Flexible Intermaxillary Appliances (FIMA)

The main representative of the flexible intermaxillary appliances (FIMA) is the Jasper Jumper[83] (see Table 2.1). Other appliances of the same category include the Flex Developer,[84] the Amoric Torsion Coils,[85] the Adjustable Bite Corrector,[86] the Bite Fixer,[87] the Klapper

SUPERspring II,[88] the Churro Jumper,[89] and the Forsus Nitinol Flat Spring.[90]

Jasper Jumper™

The Jasper Jumper (American Orthodontics, Sheboygan, WI) is a flexible intermaxillary appliance first introduced by Jasper in 1987 in an attempt to address the restriction of the mandibular lateral movements that occurs with Herbst appliance use.[83,91,92] It consists of a flexible force module constructed of a stainless steel coil spring enclosed in a polyurethane covering attached at both ends to stainless steel endcaps with holes to facilitate the anchoring of the appliance (see Fig. 10.2).[91,92] The modules are different for the right and left sides and they are supplied in seven lengths, ranging from 26 to 38 mm in 2 mm increments. Ball-pins, small plastic Teflon friction balls or Lexan beads and auxiliary sectional archwires are the anchor parts of the appliance, which are used to attach the appliance on the maxillary and mandibular fixed appliances.

The appropriate size of the Jasper Jumper is determined by guiding the mandible in centric relation and measuring the distance between the mesial of the maxillary first molar headgear tube and the point of insertion to the mandibular arch at the distal of the small plastic beads, adding 12 mm (see Fig. 10.3).[91,93]

Several methods are available to anchor the Jasper Jumper force module to the permanent or mixed dentition.[92,94] The appliance is usually attached to previously placed fixed appliances.[91,92,94] The force module is anchored to the upper headgear tube with a ball-pin passing through the upper hole of the jumper and through the distal end of the headgear tube. Then, the mesial extension of the pin is bent back over the tube to keep it in position.[89,93,95]

The attachment of the force module to the mandibular archwire can be performed in two different ways.[93] In the first, described originally by Dr Jasper, offsets are placed in the full engaged mandibular archwires distal to the canine brackets and the first (or the first and second) premolar bracket is removed. A small plastic bead is slid onto the archwire to provide an anterior stop, followed by the lower end of the jumper, and then the arch is ligated in place (see Fig. 10.6).[91,92,94]

However, the most effective method uses an auxiliary tube on the mandibular first molar and $0.017 \times 0.025''$ sectional archwires. The distal end of the sectional archwire, which incorporates an out-set bayonet bent mesial to the mandibular molar's auxiliary tube, is inserted into this tube, while the mesial end is looped over the main archwire between the first premolar and the canine (see Fig. 10.8). Thus there is no need to remove the premolar brackets and the patient has a greater range of jaw movement.[90–94,96]

In patients with mixed dentition, the maxillary attachment is similar to that described above, while the mandibular attachment is achieved through an archwire extending between the mandibular first molar bands and lateral incisor brackets, thus avoiding the deciduous canine and molar areas (see Fig. 10.5).[92,94] However, in these patients a transpalatal arch and a fixed lingual arch should always be used to prevent undesirable treatment effects.[92,94]

The Jasper Jumper exerts a light, continuous force and can deliver functional, bite jumping, headgear-like forces, activator-like forces, elastic-like forces or a combination of these.[93,96] When the force module is straight, it is in passive condition and is activated when the teeth come into occlusion, thus compressing the spring. Four millimeters of compression can deliver about 250 g of force.[91] The appliance delivers sagittally directed forces with a posterior direction to the maxilla and the maxillary dentition and reciprocal anteriorly directed forces on the mandible and its dentition, intrusive forces on the maxillary posterior teeth and the mandibular anterior teeth, and buccal forces which tend to expand the maxillary arch.[91,97,98]

Prior to appliance placement, heavy rectangular archwires should be placed in the maxillary and mandibular arches.[93] In addition, a lingual arch can be used in the mandibular arch in order to increase lower anchorage, except in extraction cases, and brackets with −5° lingual torque should be bonded to the lower anterior teeth for the same reason.[93] In the maxillary arch, a transpalatal bar should be used to enhance lateral anchorage. However, when maxillary molar distalization is needed, the use of transpalatal bars and cinching or tying back the maxillary archwire should be avoided.[91]

Reactivation of the appliance can take place 2–3 months after the initial activation by shortening the ball-pin attached to the maxillary first molar bands or by adding crimpable stops mesial to the ball on the mandibular archwire.[91] Treatment with the Jasper Jumper usually lasts 3–9 months, after which the appliance can be left passively in place for 3–4 months for retention, and then finishing procedures can follow for about 12 months.[93,96] The Jasper Jumper can also be combined with rapid palatal expanders.[99]

A removable version of the Jasper Jumper has been presented by Sari et al,[100] which consists of two separate acrylic plates covering the occlusal and lingual surfaces of the teeth. The anchorage has been increased by incorporating clasps, while the jumpers are placed diagonally on each side between the upper and lower plates. In addition, a facebow has been attached to the upper plate from between the first and second premolars to enable the application of extraoral forces.[100]

Scandee Tubular Jumper

The Scandee Tubular Jumper (Saga Dental AS, Kongsvinger, Norway) is a very similar device to the Jasper Jumper, although it is not prefabricated. It is offered as a kit including all the individual components and can be assembled by the clinician. The appliance is a coated intermaxillary torsion spring which consists of the spring, the connectors, the covering, and the ball-pins.[61] The spring is cut to the appropriate length by the clinician and there is no distinction between left and right sides. In cases of appliance fracture, it is only necessary to replace the individual components. The Scandee Tubular Jumper's thickness is considered as its main disadvantage.

Flex Developer (FD)

The Flex Developer (LPI Ormco, Ludwig Pittermann GesmbH, Maria Anzbach, Austria) was introduced by Winsauer[84] and is supplied as a kit to be assembled by the clinician. The force module is an elastic minirod made of polyamide, while additional components include an anterior hooklet module, a posterior attachment module, a preformed auxiliary bypass arch, a securing mini-disk, and a ball-pin. The anterior locking module is relockable, thus permitting easy insertion and removal (see Figs 11.1 and 11.2). The appliance is used in combination with full multibanded appliances and is attached to the headgear tubes of maxillary first molar bands and to the mandibular bypass arch (see Fig. 11.10).

The length of the bypass arch is determined by measuring the distance between the distal edge of the mandibular molar tube and the back edge of the mandibular canine bracket, adding 5 mm. The distal end of the bypass arch is inserted into the archwire tube of the mandibular first molar band, while its mesial end is placed between the premolar and canine brackets.

The length of the elastic minirod is determined by measuring the distance between the entrance of the maxillary headgear tube and the labial end of the bypass arch, using a specially designed gauge.

The FD delivers a continuous force of 50–1000 g between the maxilla and the mandible, which is derived from the elastic minirod. The force delivered by the FD can be adjusted by thinning the minirod's diameter, while its length can also be reduced to allow proper fit of the appliance.[84]

After the necessary preparations are made, such as the length adjustment, ensuring that the posterior attachment module and the anterior hooklet are parallel, and the placement of the ball-pin into the headgear tube from the distal, the patient protrudes the mandible in the desired position and the anterior hooklet is secured on the bypass archwire.[84] To reactivate the FD, the ball-pin can be shortened to the mesial or the bypass arch can be shortened toward distal, thus pushing back the sliding arch and bending its end upwards. Alternatively, the sliding section of the arch can be shortened by adding an acrylic ball at its mesial end. Lip bumpers, headgears or reversed headgears can also be used in combination with the FD.

Amoric Torsion Coils

This bilateral flexible intermaxillary appliance, developed by Amoric,[85] consists of two uncovered springs with rings on their ends, which slide into each other.[61,85] The rings are fixed to the maxillary and mandibular archwires using double ligatures. The appliance's force depends on the distance between the fixing points on the arch.

Adjustable Bite Corrector (ABC)

The ABC (OrthoPlus Inc., Santa Rosa, CA) is another flexible intermaxillary appliance, which functions similarly to the Herbst appliance and Jasper Jumper, and is also assembled by the orthodontist. It consists of a 0.018″ stainless steel universal stretchable closed-coil spring, an internally threaded end-cap, a nickel titanium wire in the center lumen of the spring, molar clips, and eyelet pins.[86]

The appliance is attached to full bracketed upper and lower arches and can be used on either side of the mouth with a simple 180° rotation of the lower end-cap to change its orientation. The molar clips or the eyelet pins allow easy removal and replacement of the endpiece at the maxillary molar headgear tube, for quick repair or adjustment during treatment. The appliance is attached to the mandibular arch by means of a sectional arch ("starter jig") with an eyelet at its distal end, which is large enough for attaching the jig to the molar hook.

The forward-directed force of the appliance is produced by the nickel titanium wire located in the center lumen of the spring, which keeps the mandible in a continuous protruded position during functional movements. If the patient opens the mouth widely, the closed-coil spring is able to stretch about 25% beyond its initial length without permanent deformation, thus minimizing the possibility of appliance breakage or accidentally changing its length.[86] The length of the closed-coil spring is determined by advancing the mandible in a corrected position with ideal overbite and overjet and then measuring the distance between the mesial opening of the headgear tube on the maxillary first molar band and a point 3 mm below the contact between the mandibular canine and first premolar. An additional 4 mm increase in the length is possible, beyond which there is a risk of pulling the spring out of the end-cap when the patient opens wide and pulls on the spring.

To avoid proclination of the mandibular incisors, a full-size rectangular archwire should be used in the lower incisor area, while a transpalatal arch should be applied in order to avoid undesired expansion of the maxillary first molars. The appliance can also be combined with maxillary expanders.[86]

Bite Fixer

The Bite Fixer (Ormco, Orange, CA) is a prefabricated intermaxillary coil spring, attached and crimped to the end fitting to prevent breakage between the spring and the end fitting. Plastic tubing is inserted in the spring to prevent it from becoming a food trap.[87] The Bite Fixer is supplied in a kit with various sizes for both left and right sides. The appliance can be used only in combination with full bracketed upper and lower arches. The spring is attached to the headgear tubes of the maxillary first molars by means of ball-pins. Attachment of the spring to the mandibular arch can be accomplished in three different ways:[87]

- by attaching the force module directly to the mandibular archwire between the brackets of the first premolar and the canine
- by attaching the force module directly to the mandibular archwire and performing step-out bends distal to the canines after removing either or both premolar brackets
- by using a sectional archwire attached to the lower first molar band and the mandibular archwire between the premolar and canine bracket.

In all cases an acrylic bead should also be used, acting as a stop to prevent the force module from sliding mesially.

Of the three different ways of attachment, the use of sectional wires is strongly recommended because it presents many advantages.[87]

- Sectional archwires can be pre-bent, saving time.
- The premolar brackets do not have to be removed.
- The force module is allowed to slide freely along the sectional wire, and therefore the patient's range of motion is increased, thus decreasing the possibility of breakage.
- If breakage does occur, it is usually the auxiliary wire, which can be easily replaced.
- Anchorage is increased, which helps to prevent the lower incisors from proclining.

To attach the appliance, the ball-pin is placed through the distal end of the Bite Fixer's end-cap, is pulled anteriorly through the distal end of the headgear tube of the maxillary first molar band, and then an additional loop is made to the distal to anchor it in that position. Activation at a second appointment is recommended, after the placement of the appliance, to reduce the possibility for appliance breakage and allow patient adaptation, and is accomplished by pulling the ball-pin more anteriorly.[87] The patient should be instructed not to open the mandible too widely due to the increased risk for appliance breakage. The appliance can be reactivated when the posterior segments move distally and the spring becomes passive.[87]

Before alignment of the appliance, leveling and decompensation of the upper and lower arch should be completed, while brackets with fully engaged stainless steel archwires in both arches should be used to increase anchorage.

Treatment with the Bite Fixer usually lasts about 8–10 months to achieve orthopedic effects, and when the dental arches are in an overcorrected Class I relationship the appliance is removed. When only dentoalveolar changes are required, treatment duration is approximately 4–6 months until the molars have been distalized, after which the force module can stay in place to increase anchorage during retraction of the premolars and the anterior teeth.[87] After appliance removal, elastics can be placed for 6–8 months to further correct the occlusion.

Higgins incorporated the Bite Fixer springs in the "Class II spring appliance" designed for unilateral or bilateral use.[101] The Class II spring appliance consists of a maxillary expansion appliance (Ormco Compact Screw; Ormco, Orange, CA) attached to bands placed on the maxillary first permanent molars and first or second permanent or deciduous premolars, a triple L-arch (lower labial lingual arch) fabricated from 0.045″ Elgiloy wire, and the Bite Fixer springs. The appliance can be used in mixed dentition, since no brackets and archwires are required. To prevent the bite fixer from sliding to the mesial, Gurin locks (3M Unitek, Monrovia, CA) are used on the lower labial lingual arch, which also allow easy activation of the springs. A solder stop should be used at the distal aspect of the labial bow to prevent distortion of the spring. Higgins recommends the use of longer springs to provide maximum opening and minimum breakage risk, to keep the spring active in a wider range of mandibular motion and the force in a more horizontal direction.[101] The mandible should be advanced in an edge-to-edge position, while the appliance is removed when an overcorrected Class I relationship has been achieved.

Gentle Jumper

The Gentle Jumper (American Orthodontics, Sheboygan, WI) is a very similar device to the Bite Fixer. When activated 4 mm, the Gentle Jumper exerts just 75 g of force, in comparison to the 360 g of force of the Jasper Jumper. The appliance is better suited to mixed dentition cases.

Klapper SUPERspring II

The SUPERspring II (ORTHOdesign, Lake Forest, IL) is a flexible intermaxillary device based on a spring which was developed by Klapper.[88] It rests in the vestibule and is attached to the maxillary first molar band and to the mandibular archwire distal to the mandibular canine. The anterior open helical loop of the spring is tied in the mandibular archwire like a J-hook distal to the canines, while the maxillary end of the spring is attached to the maxillary first molar through a special oval tube instead of a headgear tube and is secured with a stainless steel ligature. The springs are available in two sizes. The SUPERspring II exerts a continuous distalizing force on the maxillary molars and an intruding force on the mandibular anterior teeth and the maxillary first molars. The anteroposterior force can be modified by extending the anterior attachment wire and/or by changing the angulation of the posterior attachment wire.[88]

Churro Jumper

The Churro Jumper was developed as an improvement of the mandibular protraction appliance and was introduced by Castanon et al.[89] It consists of a jumper fabricated by the clinician from a 0.028 × 0.032″ stainless steel wire, containing 15–20 symmetrical and closely placed circles, and two circles in each end. The appliance is attached to the maxillary molar band by means of a 0.036″ pin passing through the circle on the distal end of the jumper and through the distal end of the headgear tube, and is secured by bending the pin downward on the mesial end of the tube. The mesial end, which is an open circle, is positioned over the mandibular archwire distal to the canine bracket. The mandibular premolar brackets should not be bonded and a buccal offset should be placed to allow unrestricted sliding of the jumper along the archwire.[89] The length of the Churro Jumper is determined by measuring the distance between the mesial of the headgear tube and the distal of the mandibular canine bracket, adding 10–12 mm.

After placement, the Churro Jumper is in a passive state and is activated only after the pin is pulled forward, causing the jumper to bow outward to the cheek. Thus, the appliance delivers a distally directed and intrusive force on the maxillary molar and a forward and intrusive force on the mandibular incisors.[89] The appliance is reactivated by pulling the headgear pin mesially. Treatment with the

Churro Jumper usually takes 4–6 months when correcting Class II malocclusions. The appliance should be left in place until a stable Class I cuspal interdigitation is observed in the posterior area.[89]

Forsus Nitinol Flat Spring

The Forsus Nitinol Flat Spring (3M Unitek, Monrovia, CA) is another flexible intermaxillary appliance which keeps the mandible in a continuous protruded position. It consists of a 0.5×3.0 mm spring bar (45% nickel, 55% titanium) covered with a transparent plastic coating and with its bent ends attaching to bands and archwires.[90]

The Forsus Spring is attached to the headgear tubes of the maxillary first molar bands and to the mandibular archwire distal to the canine bracket using a bayonet bend. Moreover, a stainless steel ball stop can be placed on the archwire to create a mesial stop for the Forsus Spring.[90] The spring slides along the archwire when the mandibular first premolar bracket is omitted or along a bypass sectional archwire if the bracket has been bonded.[90]

The length of the spring is determined by the distance between the mesial surface of the maxillary first molar headgear tube and the distal surface of the mandibular canine bracket plus 10–12 mm, when the patient has closed in habitual occlusion (4 mm for play, 4 mm for the headgear tube and 4–5 mm for the activation).[90] The appliance is reactivated by adding crimpable stops on the bypass archwire 5 mm mesial to the spring or distal to the stainless steel ball stop.

The Ribbon Jumper

The nickel titanium Ribbon Jumper (American Orthodontics, Sheboygan, WI) is a very similar device to the Forsus Nitinol Flat Spring, which offers light continuous forces in order to advance the mandible and to distalize molars. The appliance applies an intraoral force that is slightly less than the Jasper Jumper, but exceeds the forces delivered by the Gentle Jumper.

Hybrid Appliances (Combination of RIMA and FIMA)

Among the hybrid intermaxillary appliances that use a combination of rigid and flexible force systems, the Eureka Spring[102] is one of the most commonly used in noncompliance Class II orthodontic treatment (see Table 2.1). The Sabbagh Universal Spring (SUS), the Forsus Fatigue-Resistant Device, and the Twin Force Bite Corrector[101] also belong to this category of appliances.

Eureka Spring™

The Eureka Spring (Eureka Orthodontics, San Luis Obispo, CA) is a hybrid appliance which was developed by DeVincenzo[102] and consists of an open coil spring encased in a plunger, flexible ball-and-socket attachments, and a shaft for guiding the spring (see Fig. 12.1).

The open coil spring is attached directly to the upper or lower archwire with a closed or open ring clamp. The plunger has a 0.002″ tolerance in the cylinder, and a triple telescopic action allows mouth opening to 60 mm, beyond which the appliance is disengaged, but it can be easily reassembled by the patient. The cylinder is connected to the molar tube with a 0.032″ wire annealed at its anterior end and a 0.036″ ball at the posterior end functioning like a universal joint, thus allowing lateral and vertical movements of the cylinder.[102]

The advantages of the Eureka Spring include lack of reliance on patient compliance, esthetic appearance, resistance to breakage, maintenance of good oral hygiene, prevention of tissue irritation, rapid tooth movement, optimal force direction, 24-hour continuous force application even when the mouth is opened to 20 mm, functional acceptability, easy installation, low cost, and minimal inventory requirements.[102]

Sabbagh Universal Spring (SUS)

The Sabbagh Universal Spring (Dentaurum Inc., Ispringen, Germany) is another hybrid appliance which consists of a SUS telescopic element, a U-loop anteriorly and a telescope rod with a U-loop posteriorly positioned. The telescopic unit consists of an inner spring over an inner tube, a guide tube and a middle telescopic tube (see Fig. 14.1).

The SUS is attached to the maxillary molar headgear tube and to the mandibular archwire (see Fig. 14.2). To fit the appliance, a 1 mm ball retainer clasp is placed from the distal through the loop in the headgear tube and is bent mesially on the tube. After bending of the tube inwards, the telescopic rod with U-loop is inserted into the maxillary fixed SUS telescopic element, and the U-loop is attached to the lower stainless steel archwire, which should be at least $0.016 \times 0.022″$, between the first premolar and the canine bracket.

The size of the spring can be adjusted by inserting or unscrewing the inner telescopic tube or by presetting the length of the inner tube with an activation key. When skeletal effect is required, the spring force should be minimized, whereas when dentoalveolar effect is mostly needed, the spring force should be maximized. The spring can be activated by inserting or unscrewing the inner telescope tube manually or with an activation key, by extending or shortening the distal distance of the ball-pin in the headgear tube, by inserting activation springs or by placing the U-loop between the mandibular incisor and canine bracket.

Forsus™ Fatigue-Resistant Device

The Forsus Fatigue-Resistant Device (3M Unitek, Monrovia, CA) is a hybrid appliance designed to address the problem of fatigue failure and consists of a three-piece telescopic spring device. The appliance is attached to the maxillary first molar headgear tube with an L-shaped ball-pin and to the mandibular archwire through a bypass archwire. The appropriate length of the rod is selected to allow full spring compression without advancing the mandible, when advancement is not required. To simplify the insertion, a direct push rod is incorporated in the device, which permits direct attachment to the mandibular archwire. According to Dionne,[104] ligating of the mandibular canine-to-first molar brackets as a group is advised to avoid creating space distal to the canine.

To reactivate the spring, ring bushings can be added distal on the stop of the distal rod, thus compressing the spring 2–3 mm, or a longer rod can be used to maintain engagement. Patients should be informed not to open their mouth widely due to the risk of disengagement.

The Forsus Fatigue-Resistant Device has also been used instead of the Bite Fixer springs in the Class II spring appliance, described above. This version is known as the crossbow appliance.

Twin Force Bite Corrector (TFBC)

The Twin Force Bite Corrector (Ortho Organizers Inc., San Marcos, CA) is also a hybrid appliance which consists of dual plungers containing nickel titanium springs with ball-and-socket joints in their ends, an anchor wire, and an archwire clamp.[103] To eliminate the need for a headgear tube, the TFBC with a double lock was developed (see Figs 13.1–13.3). The appliance is attached to the lower archwire between the canine and the first premolar with a ball-and-socket wire clamp and to the maxillary molar headgear tube with the anchor wire which has a ball-and-socket adjustable joint.

Before appliance placement, palatal expansion and alignment of the maxillary and mandibular dental arches should be completed.[103] Bands with double buccal tubes should also be placed on the maxillary first molars, and lingual sheaths in order to facilitate the use of transpalatal arches. In addition, the mandibular arch should be leveled, the overbite should be opened, and mandibular and maxillary $0.017 \times 0.025''$ or $0.018 \times 0.025''$ archwires should be engaged. A lingual lower arch can also be used to enhance anchorage.[103]

The TFBC exerts a continuous light force of 100–200 g and does not require activation. The appliance permits lateral movements and a wide range of motion due to the ball joints. To avoid mandibular incisor proclination, an elastic chain or a figure-eight wire tie can be used bracket-to-bracket from molar to molar, and cinch back bends at the distal ends of the archwire.[103]

After appliance placement, the patient should be seen in a week and then monitored once a month.[103] After the desired occlusion has been achieved, the appliance is maintained in place for 2–3 months, then it is removed and Class II elastics are used to stabilize the cuspal interdigitation. Retention appliances can be used to maintain the mandibular position.[103]

Appliances Acting as Substitutes for Elastics

Three devices are included in the category of noncompliance appliances acting as substitutes for elastics (see Table 2.1). These are the Calibrated Force Module, the Alpern Class II Closers and the Saif Springs.[105]

Calibrated Force Module

The Calibrated Force Module is a device originally designed to substitute for Class II elastics. It was developed in 1988 by Cormar Inc. (Salisbury, MD) and is available in three sizes.[61] It is attached to the lower archwire distal of the mandibular molars and fixed by a screw, and to the upper archwire distal or mesial to the maxillary canines. Constant forces of about 150–200 g can be delivered due to the spring coil incorporated in the appliance.

Alpern Class II Closers

The Alpern Class II Closers (or Alpern Sentalloy Interarch Coil Springs) (GAC International Inc., Islandia, NY) are used for the correction of Class II malocclusions instead of elastics in patients with compliance problems.[61] They consist of a small telescopic device which encloses in its interior Sentalloy coil springs and two hooks for fixing. The coil springs are used to reduce breakage and provide a near-constant 250 g pull for predictable results. The appliance is fixed to the mandibular molar and to the maxillary canine bracket, and its telescopic action provides a satisfactory mouth opening. The appliance is available in four different sizes.

Saif Springs

The Saif Springs (Pacific Coast Manufacturing Inc., Woodinville, WA) is a fixed force system which can be used to replace headgear or elastics in the correction of interarch deficiencies.[105] The device is available in two sizes (7 mm and 10 mm). Prior to appliance placement, the overbite should be corrected, bands should be placed on molars with hooks for spring attachment, and full engaged rectangular archwires should be placed in both arches.[105] The eyelet end of the spring is attached to the mandibular first molar hook, which is then closed to avoid slipping of the eyelet. The appliance is placed on the maxillary archwire by crimping a hook on the vertical leg of the wire and making an offset bend between the canine and lateral incisor, where the hook will be placed, to prevent sliding of the crimpable hook on the archwire and opening spaces. Then, the spring should be activated by 2–3 mm. Starnes suggests that the force should be directed as horizontally as possible.[105] After the springs are placed, the patient should be monitored every 2 weeks. A Class II malocclusion can be corrected in 1–3 months. Usually, an overcorrection and stabilization is suggested to compensate for possible relapse after appliance removal.

References

1. Pancherz H. Treatment of Class II malocclusions by jumping the bite with the Herbst appliance. A cephalometric investigation. Am J Orthod 1979;76:423–442.

2. Pancherz H. The mechanism of Class II correction in Herbst appliance treatment. A cephalometric investigation. Am J Orthod 1982;82:104–113.

3. Pancherz H. The modern Herbst appliance. In: Graber TM, Rakosi T, Petrovic AG, eds. Dentofacial orthopedics with functional appliances, 2nd edn. St Louis: Mosby-Year Book; 1997: 336–366.

4. Ruf S, Pancherz H. Does bite-jumping damage the TMJ? A prospective longitudinal clinical and MRI study of Herbst patients. Angle Orthod 2000;70:183–199.

5. Langford NM Jr. Updating fabrication of the Herbst appliance. J Clin Orthod 1982; 16:173–174.

6. Dischinger TG. Edgewise bioprogressive Herbst appliance. J Clin Orthod 1989;23:608–617.

7. Burkhardt DR, McNamara JA Jr, Baccetti T. Maxillary molar distalization or mandibular enhancement: a cephalometric comparison of comprehensive orthodontic treatment including the pendulum and the Herbst appliances. Am J Orthod Dentofacial Orthop 2003;123:108–116.

8. Howe RP. The bonded Herbst appliance. J Clin Orthod 1982;16:663–667.

9. McNamara JA, Howe RP. Clinical management of the acrylic splint Herbst appliance. Am J Orthod Dentofacial Orthop 1988;94:142–149.

10. White LW. Current Herbst appliance therapy. J Clin Orthod 1994;28:296–309.

11. Snodgrass D. A modified, lingually supported cantilevered Herbst appliance. Funct Orthod 1996;13:20–26, 28.

12. Rogers MB. Herbst appliance variations. J Clin Orthod 2003;37:156–159.

13. Langford NM Jr. The Herbst appliance. J Clin Orthod 1981;15:558–561.

14. Rogers MB. The banded Herbst appliance. J Clin Orthod 2001;35:494–499.

15. Pancherz H. The Herbst appliance – its biologic effects and clinical use. Am J Orthod 1985; 87:1–20.

16. Eberhard H, Hirschfelder U. Treatment of Class II, Division 2 in the late growth period. J Orofac Orthop 1998;59:352–361.

17. Allen-Noble P. Clinical management of crown/banded Herbst appliances. Allesee Orthodontic Appliances/Pro Lab, 2002. Available online at: www.ormco.com/pubs/AOA/Manuals/Herbst 2002.pdf

18. Pancherz H, Hansen K. Mandibular anchorage in Herbst treatment. Eur J Orthod 1988;10:149–164.

19. Pancherz H, Ruf S. The Herbst appliance: research-based updated clinical possibilities. World J Orthod 2000;1:17–31.

20. Sinha P. Clinical applications of the Herbst appliance. Good Practice Newsletter of American Orthodontics 2002;3:2–3. Available online at: www.americanortho.com

21. McNamara JA Jr, Brudon WL, Buckhardt DR, Huge SA. The Herbst appliance. In: McNamara JA Jr, Brudon WL, eds. Orthodontics and dentofacial orthopedics. Ann Arbor: Needham Press; 2001: 285–318.

22. Wieslander L. Intensive treatment of severe Class II malocclusions with a headgear-Herbst appliance in the early mixed dentition. Am J Orthod 1984;86:1–13.

23. Du X, Hagg U, Rabie AB. Effects of headgear Herbst and mandibular step-by-step advancement versus conventional Herbst appliance and maximal jumping of the mandible. Eur J Orthod 2002;24:167–174.

24. Hagg U, Du X, Rabie AB. Initial and late treatment effects of headgear-Herbst appliance with mandibular step-by-step advancement. Am J Orthod Dentofacial Orthop 2002;122:477–485.

25. Pancherz H, Hansen K. Occlusal changes during and after Herbst treatment: a cephalometric investigation. Eur J Orthod 1986;8:215–228.

26. Konik M, Pancherz H, Hansen K. The mechanism of Class II correction in late Herbst treatment. Am J Orthod Dentofacial Orthop 1997;112:87–91.

27. Wong GW, So LL, Hagg U. A comparative study of sagittal correction with the Herbst appliance in two different ethnic groups. Eur J Orthod 1997;19:195–204.

28. Pancherz H, Anehus-Pancherz M. The effect of continuous bite jumping with the Herbst appliance on the masticatory system: a functional analysis of treated Class II malocclusions. Eur J Orthod 1982;4:37–44.

29. Pancherz H, Fackel U. The skeletofacial growth pattern pre- and post-dentofacial orthopaedics. A long-term study of Class II malocclusions treated with the Herbst appliance. Eur J Orthod 1990;12:209–218.

30. Pancherz H, Ruf S, Thomalske-Faubert C. Mandibular articular disk position changes during Herbst treatment: a prospective longitudinal MRI study. Am J Orthod Dentofacial Orthop 1999;116:207–214.

31. Ruf S, Pancherz H. Dentoskeletal effects and facial profile changes in young adults treated with the Herbst appliance. Angle Orthod 1999; 69:239–246.

32. Ruf S, Pancherz H. Temporomandibular joint remodeling in adolescents and young adults during Herbst treatment: a prospective longitudinal magnetic resonance imaging and cephalometric radiographic investigation. Am J Orthod Dentofacial Orthop 1999;115:607–618.

33. Paulsen HU, Karle A. Computer tomographic and radiographic changes in the temporomandibular joints of two young adults with occlusal asymmetry, treated with the Herbst appliance. Eur J Orthod 2000;22:649–656.

34. O'Brien K, Wright J, Conboy F, et al. Effectiveness of treatment for Class II malocclusion with the Herbst or twin-block appliances: a randomized, controlled trial. Am J Orthod Dentofacial Orthop 2003;124:128–137.

35. Pancherz H. The nature of Class II relapse after Herbst appliance treatment: a cephalometric long-term investigation. Am J Orthod Dentofacial Orthop 1991;100:220–233.

36. Pancherz H, Anehus-Pancherz M. The headgear effect of the Herbst appliance: a cephalometric long-term study. Am J Orthod Dentofacial Orthop 1993;103:510–520.

37. Pancherz H, Anehus-Pancherz M. Facial profile changes during and after Herbst appliance treatment. Eur J Orthod 1994;16:275–286.

38. Hansen K, Iemamnueisuk P, Pancherz H. Long-term effects of the Herbst appliance on the dental arches and arch relationships: a biometric study. Br J Orthod 1995;22:123–134.

39. Pancherz H. The effects, limitations, and long-term dentofacial adaptations to treatment with the Herbst appliance. Semin Orthod 1997;3:232–243.

40. Mayes JH. Improving appliance efficiency with the cantilever Herbst – a new answer to old problems. Clin Impressions 1994;3:2–5,17–19.

41. Mayes J. The cantilever bite-jumper system, Exploring the possibilities. Orthodontic CYBER-journal 1996. Available online at: www.oc-j.com/issue3/p0000077.htm

42. Mayes JH. The molar-moving bite jumper (MMBJ). Clin Impressions 1998;7:16–19.

43. Smith JR. Matching the Herbst to the malocclusion. Clin Impressions 1998;7:6–12, 20–23.

44. Smith JR. Matching the Herbst to the malocclusion: Part II. Clin Impressions 1999; 8:14–23.

45. Hilgers JJ. Hyper efficient orthodontic treatment using tandem mechanics. Semin Orthod 1998;4:17–25.

46. Howe RP. Updating the bonded Herbst appliance. J Clin Orthod 1983;17:122–124.

47. McNamara JA. Fabrication of the acrylic splint Herbst appliance. Am J Orthod Dentofacial Orthop 1988;94:10–18.

48. Howe RP. Removable plastic Herbst retainer. J Clin Orthod 1987;21:533–537.

49. Howe RP. Lower premolar extraction/removable plastic Herbst treatment for mandibular retrognathia. Am J Orthod Dentofacial Orthop 1987;92:275–285.

50. Kucukkeles N, Arun T. Bio-thermal Herbst application during the mixed dentition period. J Clin Pediatr Dent 1994;18:253–258.

51. Schiavoni R, Grenga V, Macri V. Treatment of Class II high angle malocclusions with the Herbst appliance: a cephalometric investigation. Am J Orthod Dentofacial Orthop 1992; 102:393–409.

52. Schiavoni R, Grenga V. Nonextraction treatment of a high-angle Class II case with a modified Herbst appliance. J Clin Orthod 1994;28:453–457.

53. Goodman P, McKenna P. Modified Herbst appliance for the mixed dentition. J Clin Orthod 1985;19:811–814.

54. Valant JR, Sinclair PM. Treatment effects of the Herbst appliance. Am J Orthod Dentofacial Orthop 1989;95:138–147.

55. Valant JR. Increasing maxillary arch length with a modified Herbst appliance. J Clin Orthod 1989;23:810–814.

56. Zreik T. A fixed-removable Herbst appliance. J Clin Orthod 1994;28:246–248.

57. Dentaurum. The Herbst bite jumping hinge. Instructions for use. Ispringen, Germany: Dentaurum; 2003. Available online at: www. dentaurum.com/eng/Orthodontie/pdf/989-518-20_Herbst-Scharnier.pdf

58. Schiavoni R, Bonapace C, Grenga V. Modified edgewise-Herbst appliance. J Clin Orthod 1996;30:681–687.

59. Haegglund P, Segerdal S. The Swedish-style integrated Herbst appliance. J Clin Orthod 1997;31:378–390.

60. Ritto AK. Tratamento das Classes II divisão 1 com a Biela Magnética. Dissertation thesis, 1997.

61. Ritto AK. Fixed functional appliances – an updated classification. Orthodontic CYBER-journal. Available online at: www.oc-j.com/june01/rittoffa.htm

62. Miller RA. The flip-lock Herbst appliance. J Clin Orthod 1996;30:552–558.

63. Hanks SD. Herbst therapy: trying to get out of the 20th century. Good Practice Newsletter of American Orthodontics 2003;4:2–4. Available online at: www.americanortho.com/clinical/images/Vol%204_1.pdf

64. Calvez X. The universal bite jumper. J Clin Orthod 1998;32:493–499.

65. Dischinger TG. Open-bite intrusion Herbst. AOA Orthodontic Appliances 2001;5:1–4. Available online at: www.aoalab.com/learning/publications/aoaVol/aoaVol5No2.pdf

66. Faulkner J. An interview with Dr. Joe Mayes on the Cantilever Bite Jumper. Orthodontic CYBERjournal 1997. Available online at: www.oc-j.com/issue5/mayes.htm

67. Clements RM Jr, Jacobson A. The MARS appliance. Report of a case. Am J Orthod 1982;82:445–455.

68. Jones M. Mandibular corrector. J Clin Orthod 1985;19:362–368.

69. DeVincenzo DJ. Treatment options for sagittal corrections in noncompliant patients. In: Graber TM, Vanarsdall RL Jr, eds. Orthodontics. Current principles and techniques. St Louis: Mosby; 2000: 779–800.

70. Ritto AK. The Ritto Appliance – a new fixed functional appliance. Orthodontic CYBERjournal, Archives. Available online at: www.oc-j.com/ritto/ritto.htm and www.oc-j.com/GARY/ritto.htm

71. Coelho Filho CM. Mandibular protraction appliances for Class II treatment. J Clin Orthod 1995;29:319–336.

72. Coelho Filho CM. Alternative uses for the mandibular protraction appliance. Syllabus. Presented at the 97th Annual Session of the AAO, Philadelphia, 1997.

73. Coelho Filho CM. The Mandibular Protraction Appliance No. 3. J Clin Orthod 1998;32:379–384.

74. Coelho Filho CM. Mandibular protraction appliance IV. J Clin Orthod 2001;35:18–24.

75. Coelho Filho CM, White L. Treating adults with the mandibular protraction appliance. Orthodontic CYBERjournal, Archives. Available online at: www.oc-j.com/jan03/MPA2.htm

76. Eckhart JE. The MARA Appliance. AOA Orthodontic Appliances 1997;1:1–2. Available online at: www.aoalab.com/learning/publications/aoaVol/aoaVol1N1.pdf

77. Eckhart JE. Introducing the MARA. Clin Impressions 1998;7:2–5, 24–27.

78. Allen-Noble PS. Clinical management of the MARA. A manual for orthodontists and staff. Allesee Orthodontic Appliances/Pro Lab, 2002. Available online at: www.ormco.com/pubs/AOA/Manuals/MARA2002.pdf

79. Eckhart JE, White LW. Class II therapy with the Mandibular Anterior Repositioning Appliance. World J Orthod 2003;4:135–144.

80. Eckhart JE. MARA provides effective adult treatment. Clin Impressions 2001;10:16–17.

81. Simon E, Haerian A. Efficient treatment by design: using the MARA for Class IIs. AOA Orthodontic Appliances 2001;5:1,3. Available online at: www.aoalab.com/learning/publications/aoaVol/aoaVol5N1.pdf

82. Kinzinger G, Ostheimer J, Forster F, Kwandt PB, Reul H, Diedrich P. Development of a new fixed functional appliance for treatment of skeletal class II malocclusion first report. J Orofac Orthop 2002;63:384–399.

83. Jasper JJ. The Jasper Jumper – a fixed functional appliance. Sheybogan: American Orthodontics; 1987.

84. Winsauer H. Flex Developer. Adjustable power developer – variable length and force. Maria Anzbach, Austria: LPI-Ormco; 2002. Available online at: www.flexdeveloper.com

85. Amoric M. Les ressorts intermaxillaires en torsion. Rev Orthop Dentofacial 1994;28:115–117.

86. West RP. The adjustable bite corrector. J Clin Orthod 1995;29:650–657.

87. Awbrey JJ. The bite fixer. Clin Impressions 1999;8:10–17, 31.

88. Klapper L. The SUPERspring II: a new appliance for non-compliant Class II patients. J Clin Orthod 1999;33:50–54.

89. Castanon R, Valdes MS, White LW. Clinical use of the Churro jumper. J Clin Orthod 1998;32:731–745.

90. Heinig N, Goz G. Clinical application and effects of the Forsus spring. A study of a new Herbst hybrid. J Orofac Orthop 2001;62:436–450.

91. Jasper JJ, McNamara JA Jr. The correction of interarch malocclusions using a fixed force module. Am J Orthod Dentofacial Orthop 1995;108:641–650.

92. McNamara JA Jr, Brudon WL. The Jasper Jumper. In: McNamara JA Jr, Brudon WL, eds. Orthodontics and dentofacial orthopedics. Ann Arbor: Needham Press; 2001: 333–342.

93. Blackwood HO 3rd. Clinical management of the Jasper Jumper. J Clin Orthod 1991;25:755–760.

94. Jasper JJ, McNamara JA Jr, Mollenhauer B. The Modified Herbst Appliance (Jasper Jumper). In: Graber TM, Rakosi T, Petrovic AG, eds. Dentofacial orthopedics with functional appliances, 2nd edn. St Louis: Mosby-Year Book; 1997: 366–378.

95. Bowman SJ. Class II combination therapy (distal jet and Jasper Jumpers): a case report. J Orthod 2000;27:213–218.

96. Cope JB, Buschang PH, Cope DD, Parker J, Blackwood HO 3rd. Quantitative evaluation of craniofacial changes with Jasper Jumper therapy. Angle Orthod 1994;64:113–122.

97. Covell DA Jr, Trammell DW, Boero RP, West R. A cephalometric study of class II Division 1 malocclusions treated with the Jasper Jumper appliance. Angle Orthod 1999;69:311–320.

98. Stucki N, Ingervall B. The use of the Jasper Jumper for the correction of Class II malocclusion in the young permanent dentition. Eur J Orthod 1998;20:271–281.

99. Mills CM, McCulloch KJ. Case report: modified use of the Jasper Jumper appliance in a skeletal Class II mixed dentition case requiring palatal expansion. Angle Orthod 1997;67:277–282.

100. Sari Z, Goyenc Y, Doruk C, Usumez S. Comparative evaluation of a new removable Jasper Jumper functional appliance vs an activator-headgear combination. Angle Orthod 2003;73:286–293.

101. Higgins DW. Using bite-jumping springs in phase 1 treatment. AOA Orthodontic Appliances 2001;5:4–5. Available online at: www.aoalab.com/learning/publications/aoaVol/aoaVol5N1.pdf

102. DeVincenzo J. The Eureka Spring: a new interarch force delivery system. J Clin Orthod 1997;31:454–467.

103. Corbett MC, Molina FG. Twin Force Bite Corrector. Light force and patient friendly. Syllabus. San Marcos: Ortho Organizers; 2001.

104. Dionne DG. Clinical Trial Report: Forsus™Fatigue Resistant Device. Orthodontic Perspectives Volume IX No.1:11–12. Available online at: www.3m.com/us/healthcare/unitek/pdf/OPVol9No1.PDF

105. Starnes LO. Comprehensive phase I treatment in the middle mixed dentition. J Clin Orthod 1998;32:98–110.

CHAPTER 4

The Herbst appliance

Hans U. Paulsen, Moschos A. Papadopoulos

Introduction

There are several types of intermaxillary appliances used for the correction of Class II malocclusion. The Herbst appliance (Dentaurum, Ispringen, Germany) is a fixed intermaxillary appliance known to be an effective device for this purpose. Emil Herbst developed his appliance in the early 1900s[1] based on the idea of "jumping the bite," which was introduced by Kingsley in 1880,[2] and published his results in 1934.[3] Interest in Herbst appliance treatment was renewed after its reintroduction by H. Pancherz, mainly due to his initial favorable reports.[4]

Perhaps more than any other type of intermaxillary appliance, whether fixed or removable, the treatment effects produced by the Herbst appliance have been well documented, especially by Pancherz and colleagues.[4–25] During the last decades this treatment method has become increasingly popular because of its favorable results as well as its reduced need for patient compliance.

Herbst Designs

Usually, the Herbst appliance is attached to bands (banded Herbst design)[4,6] or cast splints (cast splint Herbst design).[26,27] The appliance can also be attached to stainless steel crowns (stainless steel crown Herbst design)[28–30] and to acrylic splints (acrylic splint Herbst design)[31,32] which, in addition to the banded and cast splint designs, form the four basic designs of the Herbst appliance. Other Herbst variations include space-closing Herbst designs, cantilevered Herbst designs, and expansion designs.[33–35]

Banded and Cast Splint Herbst Design

The Herbst appliance is a fixed appliance which functions like an artificial joint between the maxilla and the mandible.[1,3,4,6] The original design (banded Herbst design) consists of a bilateral telescopic mechanism attached to orthodontic bands on the maxillary first permanent molars and mandibular first premolars, which maintains the mandible in a continuous protruded position or, in other words, in a continuous anterior jumped position (Figs 4.1–4.3). Bands can also be placed on the first maxillary premolars and first mandibular permanent molars, while a lingual bar is used to connect the maxillary or mandibular premolars with the molars (see Fig. 4.3e).[36,37] If the mandibular first premolars have not erupted, the permanent canines can be banded, but in this case there is an increased possibility of buccal mucosa ulceration at the corner of the mouth.[8]

A more recent version of the Herbst appliance was developed by Pancherz, in which the bands are replaced by cast splints (cast splint Herbst design), which fit precisely and cover the teeth in their lateral segments, fabricated from chromium-cobalt and cemented with glass ionomer cement to the teeth.[26,27] Usually, the maxillary and mandibular anterior teeth are incorporated into the anchorage with brackets and the use of sectional archwires (Fig. 4.4).

According to Hägg et al, both appliances produce similar effects on the dentofacial structures.[38] However, the splinted Herbst appliances are preferable to the banded Herbst appliances because more clinical and laboratory time is required to service and/or replace fractured or dislodged banded appliances.

Each telescopic mechanism consists of a tube and a plunger which fit together, two pivots, and two locking screws.[4,8,26] The pivot for the tube is soldered to the maxillary first molar band and the pivot for the plunger to the mandibular first premolar band (Fig. 4.5). The tubes and plungers are attached to the pivots with locking screws and can freely rotate around their point of attachment (Fig. 4.6); locking balls (Dentaurum no. 4) can also be used which allow more freedom

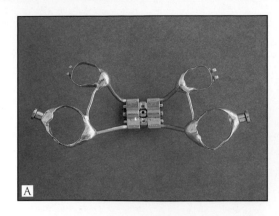
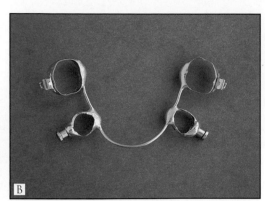

Figure 4.1 The banded Herbst appliance. **A)** The upper framework. **B)** The lower framework.

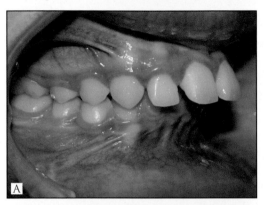
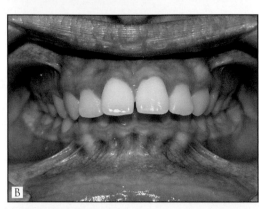
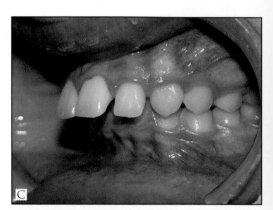

Figure 4.2 Intraoral photographs of a patient before insertion of the Herbst appliance.

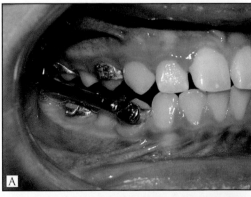
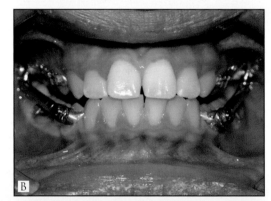
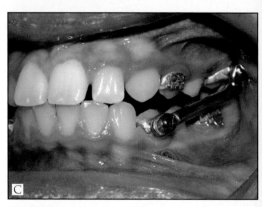

Figure 4.3 Intraoral photographs of a patient immediately after insertion of the Herbst appliance.

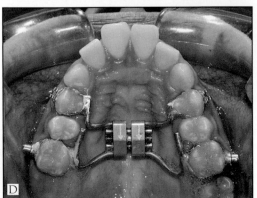
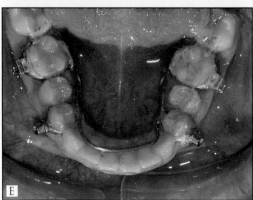

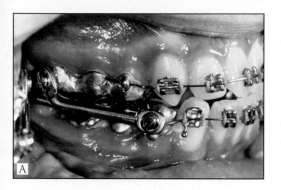
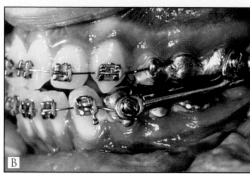

Figure 4.4 The chrome-cobalt casted Herbst appliance with screws.

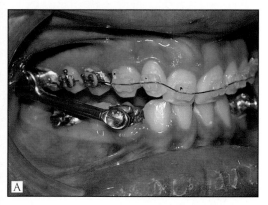
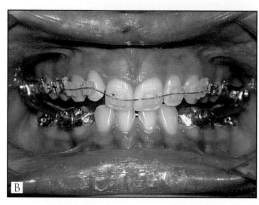
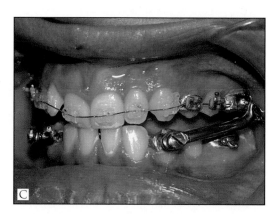

Figure 4.5 Intraoral photographs of a patient immediately after insertion of the Herbst appliance with total anchorage.

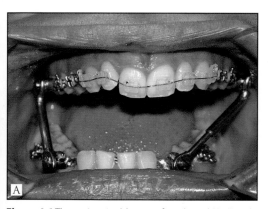
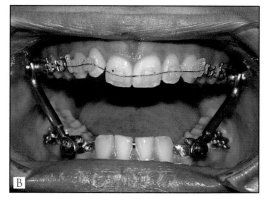
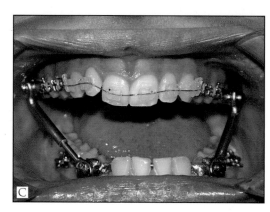

Figure 4.6 The patient is able to perform lateral (**A,C**) and opening movements (**B**).

for lateral jaw movements (Figs 4.7 and 4.8). A large interpivot distance prevents the disengagement of the telescopic mechanism due to the plunger slipping out of the tube.[8,26] Consequently, the upper pivots should be positioned distally on the molar bands and the lower pivots mesially on the premolar bands. In addition, the plunger should be as long as possible to prevent its slippage out of the tube and to avoid damage of the appliance if the plunger gets jammed on the tube opening.[8,26] If the plunger is much longer than the tube, it extends behind the tube distally to the maxillary first molar and may wound the buccal mucosa.[4,33,39] In contrast, if the plunger is too short it may slip out of the tube when patients open their mouth wide.[4,33] The telescope can be extended using small tubes or rings sized from 1.0 to 7.0 mm (Dentaurum) to move the mandible forward step by step, to reduce the maxillary overjet, ending up with a little overcorrection. The bands on which the tube and the plunger are attached should be fabricated from at least 0.15 mm or 0.010″ thick orthodontic material, which prevents any breakage during the treatment and also allows increased extension in the occlusocervical direction to achieve adequate retention of the bands on the teeth.[8,36,37]

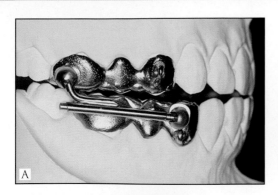
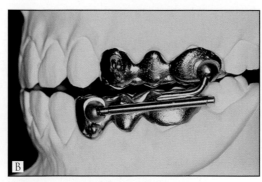

Figure 4.7 The chrome-cobalt casted Herbst appliance with ball joints (Dentaurum 4). (*Courtesy of Roskilde Orto-teknik, Roskilde, Denmark*)

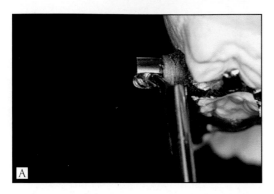
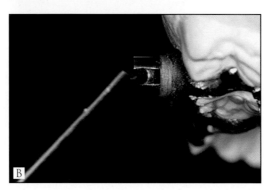

Figure 4.8 Ball joints allow better mobility function for patient comfort. (*Courtesy of Roskilde Orto-teknik, Roskilde, Denmark*)

The appliance permits the mandible to perform not only opening movements but also small lateral movements, mainly because of the loose fit of the tube and plunger at their sites of attachment. These lateral movements can be increased by widening the pivot openings of the tubes and plungers[4,8,36,40] (see Fig. 4.6); if larger lateral movements are desired, the Herbst telescope with balls will allow wider freedom (see Figs 4.7 and 4.8).

For stabilization of the anchorage teeth, two main systems can be used: partial anchorage and total anchorage.[8] For *partial anchorage*, in the maxillary dental arch the bands of the first permanent molars and first premolars are connected with a half-round (1.5 × 0.75 mm) lingual or buccal sectional archwire on each side.[6,8,26] In the mandibular dental arch the bands of the first premolars are connected with a half-round (1.5 × 0.75 mm) or a round (1 mm) lingual archwire touching the lingual surfaces of the anterior teeth.[6,8,26] When partial anchorage is considered to be inadequate, the incorporation of supplementary dental units is advised, thus transforming partial anchorage into *total anchorage*.[8,26] In this type of anchorage, a labial archwire is ligated to brackets on the first premolars, cuspids, and incisors in the maxillary dental arch (see Fig. 4.5). In addition, a transpalatal arch can be attached on the first molar bands.[39] In the mandibular dental arch, bands are cemented on the first molars and connected to the lingual archwire which is extended distally.[8,26] Additionally, a premolar-to-premolar labial rectangular archwire attached to brackets on the anterior teeth can be used (see Fig. 4.9).[15] A cast Herbst appliance in chromium-cobalt can be created in four separated pieces with tubes for fixed appliances to the front regions. If the archwire in the front section

has a dimension of 0.016 × 0.022″, the lingual wire in the mandibular front is not needed. This architecture will make it easier for the clinician to insert and remove the appliance sections.

When maxillary expansion is also required, a rapid palatal expansion screw can be soldered to the premolar and molar bands or to the cast splint (see Fig. 4.3d).[8,26] The maxillary expansion can be accomplished simultaneously[8,35,37,41,42] or prior to Herbst appliance treatment.[42,43] The Herbst appliance can also be used in combination with headgear when banded[44,45] or splinted.[46]

The telescopic mechanism of the Herbst appliance exerts a posteriorly directed force on the maxilla and its dentition and an anterior force on the mandible and its dentition.[14,40,47,48] Thus, the mandibular length is increased due to the stimulation of condylar growth and the remodeling process in the articular fossa, which can be attributed to the anterior jumped position of the mandible.[4,6,14,19,21,22,25] The amount of mandibular protrusion is determined by the length of the tube, to which the length of the plunger is adjusted. In most cases the mandible is advanced to an initial incisal edge-to-edge position at the start of the treatment, and the dental arches are placed in a Class I or overcorrected Class I relationship,[4,6,8,12,18,25–27,37,40–42,49–52] while in some cases a step-by-step advancement procedure is followed (usually by adding shims over the mandibular plungers) until an edge-to-edge incisal relationship is established (Fig. 4.9).[37,40,45,46]

Prior to the mandibular advancement procedure and before starting treatment with the Herbst appliance, a proper transverse relationship should be achieved,[32] the maxillary and mandibular teeth should be well aligned and the dental arches should fit each other in the normal sagittal position.[4,8,37] Further, in cases of skeletal

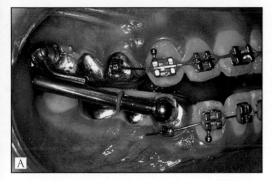 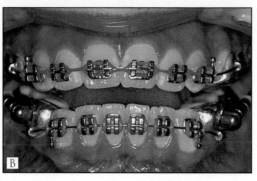 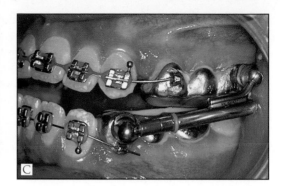

Figure 4.9 Step-by-step advancement by means of rings in different millimeters inserted through the telescopes.

midline discrepancies the patient should be encouraged to align the midlines when taking the wax-bite registration, while the correction of dental midline discrepancies can be accomplished during Herbst treatment with selective growth stimulation of the adaptive growth in the condyles[25] or after Herbst removal when fixed appliances are placed.[8,37] After the Herbst appliance has been inserted, a small adjustment period of 7–10 days is required, during which the patient may experience some chewing difficulties and therefore a soft diet is recommended.[4,8,12,36,40] Treatment with the banded Herbst appliance usually lasts 6–8 months.[4,6,8,10,18,41] However, a longer treatment period of 9–15 months is also recommended for better treatment outcomes.[33] When the desired effects have been obtained and a Class I or overcorrected Class I relationship has been achieved, the appliance is removed.

Herbst treatment alone does not usually completely correct Class II cases.[8] The desired result is achieved by subsequent use of multibracket appliances, as a second phase of treatment,[8,32,41] or overcorrecting to a slight Class III malocclusion by inserting tubes or rings to 2–3 mm negative overjet and, after the active treatment, using a tooth positioner in black rubber to finally correct and maintain the dental and skeletal interrelationships (Figs 4.10 and 4.11). In Class II, division 2 patients, a three-phase procedure can be followed which includes a first orthodontic phase to align the anterior maxillary teeth with multibracket appliances, a subsequent orthopedic phase to normalize the Class II malocclusion using the Herbst appliance, and a final orthodontic phase during which tooth irregularities and arch discrepancy problems are resolved with fixed appliances, with or without teeth extractions.[8] Another way is to change the Class II, division 2 malocclusion to a Class II, division 1 during the Herbst phase of treatment with a sectional fixed appliance in the front.

Following Herbst treatment, a retention phase is required in order to avoid any relapse of the dental relationships, due to the undesirable normal growth pattern or because of lip–tongue dysfunction habits.[8,10] In patients with mixed dentition and unstable cuspal interdigitation,[4,8,14] this phase can last 1–2 years[10,53–55] or until stable occlusal relationships are established when the permanent teeth have erupted.[8,56] It is accomplished by means of activators, such as the

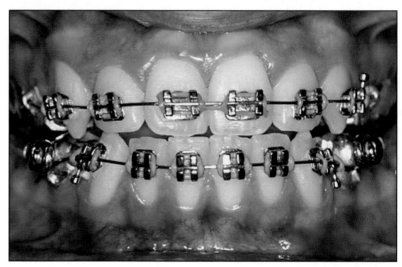

Figure 4.10 Casted Herbst appliance with fixed sectional archwires.

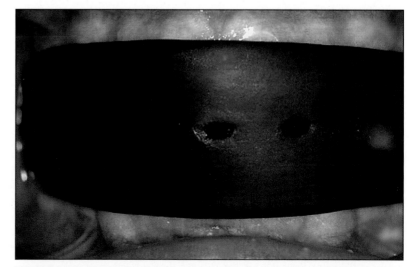

Figure 4.11 Tooth positioner to finally correct and maintain the dental and skeletal interrelationships.

Andresen Activator[8,10,15,27] or positioners[25] until normal growth has ceased. When a second phase with fixed appliances follows, retention is required for 8–12 months to maintain stable occlusal relationships[4,8,10,14,41] while Class II elastics can also be used.[39] The key concept for retention is: occlusal stabilization until growth has ceased.

Stainless Steel Crown Herbst Design

Many authors have proposed the use of stainless steel crowns as anchor units instead of bands.[28,29,57–62] The stainless steel crown Herbst design was first introduced by Langford to avoid breakages of the bands.[28] According to the author, crowns are placed on the maxillary first molars and the mandibular first premolars (or canines). The advantages of the Stainless Steel Crown Herbst Appliance include resistance to the stresses placed on the appliance, elimination of loose crowns or breakage during treatment, and avoidance of excessive protrusion of the mandibular incisors.[28]

Dischinger proposed the Edgewise Bioprogressive Herbst Appliance to minimize limitations of the Herbst design and to incorporate edgewise brackets and mechanics in the correction of Class II malocclusions.[29] This design includes stainless steel crowns which are attached on the maxillary first permanent molars and usually on the mandibular first premolars, while the mandibular first permanent molars are banded. A 0.040″ lingual wire connects the mandibular crowns and bands. The maxillary arch and the mandibular incisors are bracketed. Double buccal tubes are placed on the maxillary crowns through which an archwire can be placed to intrude the maxillary incisors. Tubes are also attached on the mandibular stainless steel crowns to accommodate an archwire. No transpalatal arches are used in the maxilla so that the first permanent molars can rotate as the Class II relationship is corrected during Herbst treatment. However, according to McNamara et al,[43] the incorporation of a Hyrax-type expansion screw or a transpalatal arch in the maxillary appliance adds rigidity to the appliance and minimizes the possibility of loosening. Similar stainless steel crown Herbst designs were also introduced by Smith (type II)[60,61] and Hilgers.[62]

Another stainless steel crown Herbst design is the Cantilever Herbst, which includes mandibular extension arms attached to stainless steel crowns on the mandibular first molars and can be used in the mixed and early permanent dentition.[43,60,61] The arms extend anteriorly from the mandibular first molar lateral to the dentition and end in the premolar area. The Herbst pivots are soldered to the cantilever arms close to the buccal surface of the mandibular first premolars, and support wires are used in the shape of occlusal rests to the mandibular deciduous second molars or permanent second molars for additional stabilization.

A similar design was also introduced by Sinha,[42] while Dischinger[63] proposed the Edgewise Herbst Appliance. According to this design, stainless steel crowns are cemented on the maxillary and mandibular permanent first molars or on the second deciduous lower molars if the first molars are covered by an operculum. In the permanent dentition,

brackets are placed on the six maxillary anterior teeth and on the mandibular incisors, which provide −10° torque to prevent proclination. In the mixed dentition, brackets are placed only on the incisors. Double buccal tubes on the molar crowns permit the use of archwires to intrude the maxillary incisors. In the mandibular arch, a 2 mm half-round cantilever is positioned between the first molar and the interproximal area between the first premolar and the canine. The axle is placed at the mesial end of the cantilever and a 0.022 × 0.028″ archwire tube is placed above and below the axle. Furthermore, no lingual arch is used to prevent incisor tipping and to allow easier placement of the appliance, and again no transpalatal arch is used to permit molar rotation during treatment. The main advantages of this design include the minimal need for patient cooperation and the ability to perform orthodontic and orthopedic therapy simultaneously.[63] Mayes[57,58] has further developed the Cantilever Herbst by introducing the Cantilever Bite Jumper System (Ormco, Orange, CA), which is described thoroughly in Chapter 5.

Acrylic Splint Herbst Design

The Acrylic Splint Herbst Appliance consists of the telescopic mechanism which is attached to acrylic splints cemented or bonded on the maxillary and mandibular dentition (Fig. 4.12). For the attachment of the bite-jumping mechanism, a wire framework is used, over which 2.5–3 mm acrylic is adapted.[31,43,64,65] The maxillary splint covers all the maxillary teeth except the incisors and the acrylic coverage extends from the free gingival margin of the buccal surfaces over the occlusal ending to the free gingival margin on the lingual surfaces.[64] A transpalatal arch or, more usually, a rapid palatal expansion screw attached to the wire framework connects the left and right parts of the splint together. Regarding the mandibular splint, the incisal one-third of the mandibular canine and incisor crowns is covered with acrylic, which can reduce incisor proclination, the posterior teeth are fully covered, while occlusal rests are placed on the second molars when erupted.[43,64] To facilitate removal of the appliance, Howe recommended the maintenance of openings over the cusps of the posterior teeth in both upper and lower splints.[64] The advantages of the bonded acrylic splint include attachment of the mandibular and maxillary dental arch without the use of bands, which enables use of the appliance in patients at any dental development stage,[31] minimal tooth movement during treatment, prevention of tooth impingement and reduction of breakage incidents.[31,66] However, the inhibition of normal tooth eruption, the difficulty of maintaining good oral hygiene, as well as the problem of removing the bonding material, particularly on the proximal tooth surfaces, can be regarded as disadvantages.[8]

The acrylic maxillary and mandibular splints can also be removable, with some differences in comparison to the bonded type, such as full coverage of all teeth including the maxillary incisors[67] or full coverage of the maxillary canines (without the incisors) and half coverage of the labial surfaces of the mandibular incisors.[43,65] The pivots of the Herbst bite-jumping mechanism are soldered to the base archwire at the mesial surface of the mandibular first premolar, and ball clasps

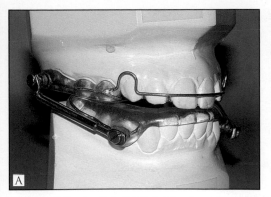 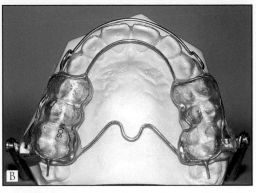 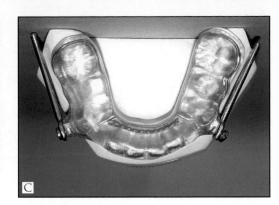

Figure 4.12 The Acrylic Splint Herbst Appliance. *(Courtesy of Metaxas Brothers, Orthodontic Laboratory, Thessaloniki, Greece)*

can be added to increase retention.[43,68] The appliance can be worn on a full-time basis and removed only for oral hygiene, or on a part-time basis.[32,67,68]

Mainly due to the fact that bonding of the acrylic splints increases the risk of decalcification,[32,43,65] McNamara et al[43] recommend that the Acrylic Splint Herbst Appliance should be removable in most cases. However, bonding of the maxillary splint may be necessary, for example in cases involving rapid palatal expansion, in patients whose teeth shape does not provide adequate retention during jaw movements, or when additional anchorage is required. In these patients, the upper splint can be bonded while the lower one can be removable.[32,43,65,69]

Mandibular advancement with the Acrylic Herbst Appliance takes place in a similar way as with the banded or stainless steel crown design. Some authors propose a mandibular advancement into an edge-to-edge position,[70] while others recommend an initial advancement of 2–4 mm followed by subsequent advancements at 2–3 month intervals.[32,65,67,68,71] However, a vertical advancement of 3 mm in the incisor region should always be performed to allow space for fabrication of the acrylic splints. In addition, during bite registration a proper alignment of the skeletal midlines should be achieved first, using the dental midlines as reference points.[32]

After placement of the appliance, instructions should be given for restriction of sugar intake and maintenance of good oral hygiene with brushing and fluoride rinsing. Furthermore, the patient should be informed about chewing difficulties, muscular pain and discomfort which may occur but are of a temporary nature.[31,32,43,71] The Acrylic Herbst Appliance is usually removed after 9–12 months of treatment, when a Class I relationship has been achieved.[32,70,72,73]

The acrylic maxillary splint can accommodate various auxiliaries, such as rectangular buccal tubes to allow the use of utility archwires for incisor proclination and intrusion,[64] rapid palatal expanders in case of posterior crossbites,[31,32,64] transpalatal bars to minimize rotation and displacement of the maxillary posterior teeth,[31] headgear tubes, and posterior bite blocks,[32,70,73] while in the mandibular splint buccal tubes can be used to add removable Frankel-type labial pads to interrupt the hyperactive mentalis activity or to engage lip bumpers.[31,43,64]

Indications for the Herbst Appliance

The Herbst appliance is indicated for the noncompliance treatment of Class II skeletal discrepancies, mainly in young patients, to influence the growth efficiently,[4,8,17,26,33,36,40–42,51,74,75] in high angle patients due to the increase in sagittal condylar growth,[33,41,76] in patients with deep anterior overbite,[7,40] in cases of mandibular midline deviation,[25,33] in mouth breathers due to the lack of interference while breathing,[8] and in patients with anterior disk displacement.[49] Further, the Herbst appliance is most suitable for the treatment of Class II malocclusion in patients with retrognathic mandibles and retroclined maxillary incisors.[4,8,33,41] The removable Acrylic Herbst Appliance can also be used in patients suffering from obstructive sleep apnea, in order to improve the clinical symptoms.[77–82]

Herbst treatment is also indicated in postadolescent patients who have passed their maximum pubertal growth, due to the fact that the appliance can take advantage of the residual growth and treatment lasts only 6–8 months.[8,26,33,41,42,47,50,51,74,75] Furthermore, Herbst treatment can also be performed during the postpubertal period in young adults[24,25,27,39] as an alternative to orthognathic surgery due to the favorable results in the intermaxillary jaw base relationships and skeletal profile convexity, the lower cost and risk for the patient.[41,50,51]

The appropriate somatic maturation period to initiate Herbst treatment is considered as a critical parameter for successful results. Herbst treatment before the pubertal peak of growth can lead to a normal skeletal and soft tissue morphology at a young age, which could be the foundation for a normal growth of these structures,[44] and was initially suggested as more suitable.[8] However, this early approach requires retention of the treatment outcomes until the eruption of all the permanent teeth into a stable cuspal interdigitation and the possibility of occlusal relapse is expected to increase.[13,41] By initiating treatment in the permanent dentition at or just after the pubertal growth peak, the increase in the condylar growth and the shorter retention phase required could lead to a more stable occlusion and reduced posttreatment relapse.[10,13,19,41,83] However, Konik et al[47] found that Herbst treatment was equally efficient in prepubertal and postpubertal patients although greater anchorage loss (proclination of the lower incisors) should be anticipated in postpubertal patients.

Contraindications to the Herbst Appliance

The prognosis of Herbst treatment is best in subjects with a brachyfacial growth pattern. Unfavorable growth, unstable occlusal conditions, and oral habits that persist after treatment are potential risk factors for occlusal relapse.[8] According to Rogers,[84] the appliance is contraindicated in autistic children and in patients with severe bruxism.

Advantages of the Herbst Appliance

Compared to other removable functional appliances, the Herbst appliance is fixed to the teeth and thereby is able to work 24 hours a day.[13,16–18,33,36,40] In addition, the duration of treatment is relatively short (6–8 months), while the removable functional appliances usually require 2–4 years, thus making the Herbst appliance suitable for postpubertal patients[13] and young adults.[24,25]

The main advantages of the Herbst appliance include the short and standardized treatment duration,[4,8,13,16,18,40] the lack of reliance on patient compliance to attain the desired treatment effects,[4,13,17,18,28,33,36,37,52] the easy acceptance,[8,12,16,28] and patient tolerance.[4,8] In addition, the distalizing effect on the maxillary first molars contributes to the avoidance of extractions in Class II malocclusions with maxillary crowding.[53] Other advantages include the improvement in the patient's profile immediately after placement, the absence of removable parts, the maintenance of good oral hygiene, the simultaneous use of fixed appliances, and the ability to modify the appliance for various clinical applications.[37,40]

Disadvantages of the Herbst Appliance

The main disadvantages of the Herbst appliance include anchorage loss of the upper (diastemas between the upper canines and first premolars) and lower teeth (proclination of the lower incisors during treatment),[6,10,14,15,17,28,69,85] chewing problems during the first week of the treatment,[4,12,36] soft tissue impingement, breakage or distortion of the appliance, bent rods, loose or broken bands (Fig. 4.13), and in some cases broken or loose screws.[4,33,36,38,52,84]

Case Studies

Figures 4.14–4.28 show a 14-year-old girl treated during the adolescent period, before and after 7 months' treatment, 1.5 years after treatment, and at 5 years' control. They also show an evaluation of the treatment outcome, based on cephalometric tracings orientated on "stable" structures before and directly after treatment and 1.5 years

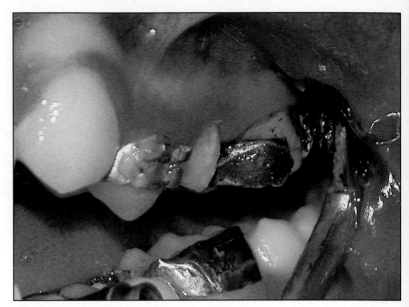

Figure 4.13 Broken band of the left maxillary first molar.

after treatment. During treatment, the alveolar processes have been tipped with the teeth from incisors to molars, backward in the maxilla and forward in the mandible. Condylar growth can easily be seen on the mandibular sketch and the radiographs of the condyles. The condylar growth amount is normally fitting with the forward inclination of the alveolar process of the mandible. Transforming the mandibular sketch to the face profile shows an anterior rotation of the mandible and a tipping of the occlusal plane forward. One and a half years after treatment, the elastic effect of the Herbst treatment upon the alveolar process with teeth has been adjusted. The lower incisors are parallel with the original lower incisor inclination.

Figures 4.29–4.41 show a 13-year-old girl treated during the adolescent period, before and after treatment, and 1 year after treatment. They also show an evaluation of the treatment outcome, based on cephalometric tracings oriented on "stable" structures before and after treatment and 1 year after treatment. During treatment the alveolar processes have been tipped with teeth, backward in the maxilla and forward in the mandible. Condylar growth in an upward and backward direction can easily be seen on the mandibular sketch. The condylar growth amount is fitting with the forward inclination of the alveolar process of the mandible. Transforming the mandibular sketch to the face profile shows an anterior rotation of the mandible and a tipping forward of the occlusal plane. One year after treatment, the elastic effect of the Herbst treatment upon the alveolar process with teeth has been adjusted to some degree. The occlusal plane has changed from the original plane. The lower incisors are parallel with the original lower incisor inclination. The ongoing condylar growth after treatment has changed to the original, more vertical direction. If extreme growth is ongoing, the mandible will rotate anteriorly and a crowding of lower incisors will appear during development of a deep bite. The treatment

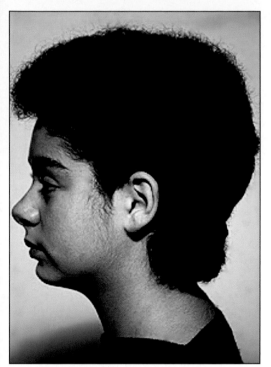

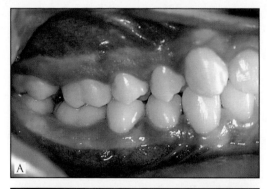

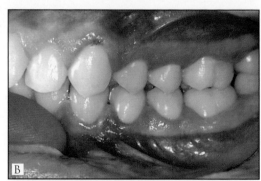

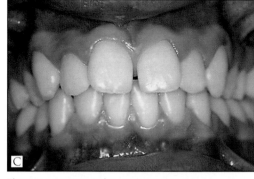

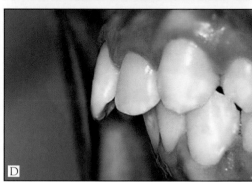

Figures 4.14–4.28 Herbst treatment of a 14-year-old girl.   **Figures 4.15, 4.16** Before Herbst treatment.

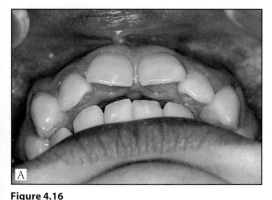

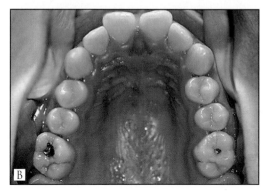

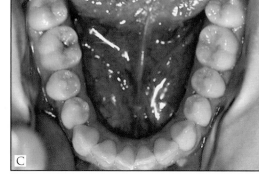

Figure 4.16

result was therefore occlusal retained with a positioner until growth had permanently ceased.

Clinical Efficacy of the Herbst Appliance

According to most investigators, the Herbst appliance is an effective and reliable method of correcting Class II malocclusion without relying on patient compliance. Herbst treatment affects not only the dentition but also the craniofacial skeleton, the associated soft tissues, and the temporomandibular joint. The following section discusses the effects of the Herbst appliance during treatment, in the short-term posttreatment period (6–12 months after Herbst

removal), and in the long-term posttreatment period (more than 6–12 months post treatment).

Sagittal Changes

Use of the Herbst appliance in Class II patients appears to have a restraining effect on the maxillary growth, as shown by the 0.4–1.2° decrease in the SNA angle during treatment.[4,6,8,14,15,17,18,30,46,48,83,85–91] In contrast, Pancherz found a slight increase in the SNA angle during Herbst treatment.[10] After the end of Herbst treatment, the SNA relapsed to almost pretreatment values in a short period,[14,15,85] while Pancherz[10] found an additional increase between 0.4° and 0.7°. In the long-term posttreatment period the SNA angle

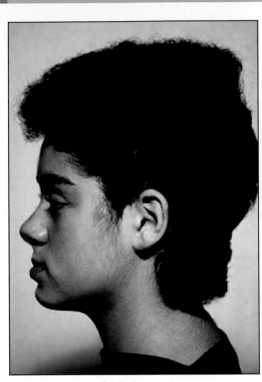

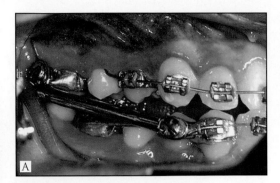

Figure 4.18

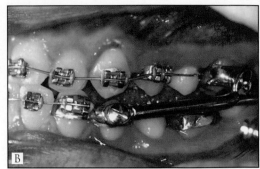

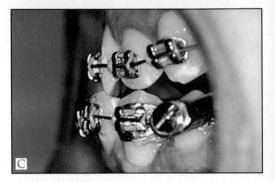

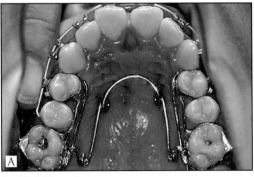

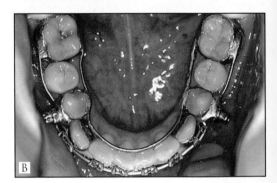

Figure 4.19

Figures 4.17–4.19 After Herbst insertion.
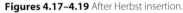

increased between 0.2° and 4°,[10,83,87] whereas other investigators observed a decrease of 0.6–0.8° for the same period.[85,90]

The restraining effect on the maxilla was also evident by the reduction in forward movement of the maxillary base (A-point). In particular, the maxillary base moved forward 0.1–1.2 mm during treatment,[8,21,45,47,50,52,76,85,87,89,90–93] which was found to be 0.2–1.2 mm less than the forward movement observed in the normal population or in the control group[87,91,92] whereas in some studies it moved backward 0.5–1.0 mm.[8,30,44–46] During treatment, the Herbst appliance exerts a posterior and upward force on the maxilla and the maxillary dentition, which can be compared to the effect of the high-pull headgear.[39,53,56,86,91] This headgear effect is enhanced by using the headgear-Herbst appliance, and remains stable when using the headgear-activator for retention.[46] The restraining effect on the maxilla was diminished in the short- and long-term posttreatment periods as the maxillary base moved forward 0.8–1.4 mm[14,21,46,85] and 1.3–5.1 mm[18,53,83,85,87,90,94] respectively, thus showing that maxillary growth inhibition by the Herbst appliance was of a temporary nature.

The increase in sagittal mandibular growth was evident by the increase in the SNB angle which was found to be between 0.2° and 2.6° during Herbst treatment,[4,7,8,10,14,15,17,21,30,39,48,66,85–91] while an increase of up to 3.1° was also observed in severe Class II, division 1 patients.[66] During the short-term posttreatment period the SNB angle remained substantially unchanged[39,85] or slightly increased by 0.3–0.5°.[10,14] In the long-term posttreatment period, the SNB angle was found to be unchanged by Hansen et al[85] whereas in some studies an increase of 0.3–2.6° was evident.[10,83,87,90]

The sagittal intermaxillary jaw relationships were also improved after Herbst appliance treatment. In particular, the ANB angle was

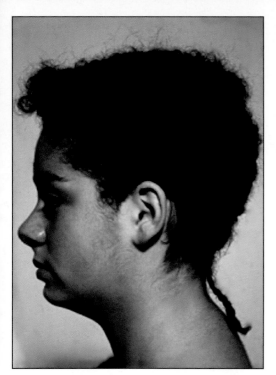

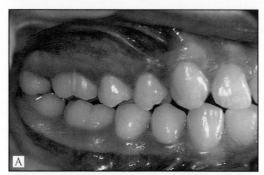

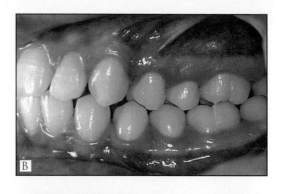

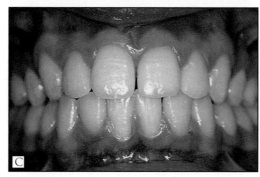

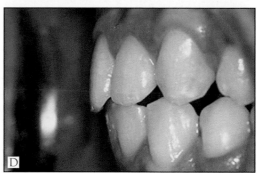

Figures 4.20-4.23 After 7 months' treatment with 1.5-year follow-up (2 year total).

Figure 4.21

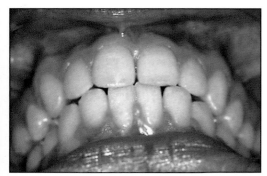

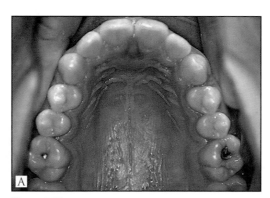

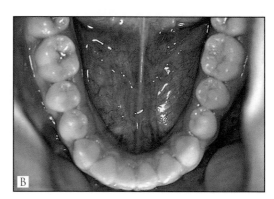

Figure 4.22

Figure 4.23

decreased between 1.1° and 3.9° as a result of the changes observed in the SNA and SNB angles, which could be attributed to the skeletal changes produced by the treatment.[4,7,8,14,15,17,18,30,39,44,48,66,85-91,94,95] After Herbst removal, the ANB angle was slightly increased 0.1–0.4° during the short-term posttreatment period.[10,14,15,21,39] However, a decrease of between 0.4° and 4.0° was observed during the long-term posttreatment period,[83,85,90,94] while Pancherz[10] found an increase between 0.2° and 1.0°. The Wits appraisal was also affected during Herbst treatment, and a decrease between 2.4 and 3.0 mm was found.[14,15,39,88,89] In Class II, division 2 patients this decrease was greater (3.0–5.1 mm).[89,96] In the short-term posttreatment period, the Wits appraisal remained substantially unchanged.[14,15,39,96]

The increase in mandibular length produced by the Herbst appliance during treatment was also confirmed by various variables. The Co-Pg distance increased between 3.0 and 7.5 mm during treatment, whereas in the control group the increase in the mandibular length did not exceed 0.5–1 mm;[4,6,52,66,91,92] the Co-Gn distance increased between 3.4 and 6.4 mm[30,44,88,95] while the control group presented only an increase of 2 mm.[95] The Ar-Pg distance was increased between 1.5 and 5 mm.[18,48,50,76] Finally, the S-Pg distance was also increased by 4.2 mm.[18] On a long-term posttreatment basis, the mandibular length was also increased significantly as shown by the 5.6 mm increase of the S-Pg and the 5.7 mm increase of the Ar-Pg distance.[18]

In addition, a 0.9–5.0 mm forward movement of the mandibular jaw base (as measured by Pg-point) was

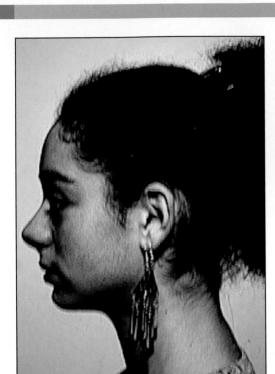

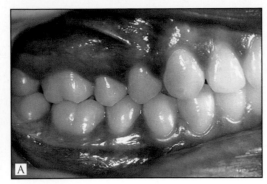

Figure 4.25

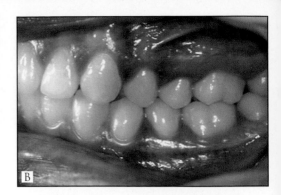

Figure 4.26

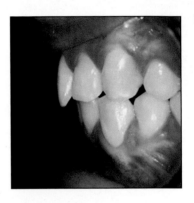

Figures 4.24–4.26 Five-year follow-up after treatment.

found.[6,8,14,17,30,45–48,50,52,66,76,83,85,87–93,97] Further, the mandibular base was moved forward 1.7 mm during the short-term posttreatment period[14] and 2.6–7.6 mm during the long-term posttreatment period.[83,85,87,90,98] In contrast to the previous findings, Wieslander found no significant long-term effect of Herbst treatment on the mandibular structures and in the mandibular position in comparison with the changes in the control group.[94]

The Herbst appliance also had a significant effect on sagittal condylar growth,[19,21] which was increased 1.8–3.8 mm during treatment, about 1.0–1.5 mm greater than that observed in control group patients before maximum pubertal growth.[13,46] The maximum sagittal condylar growth was observed in subjects around the maximum pubertal growth period.[13] In contrast, other investigators observed that the sagittal condylar growth was minimal.[70,88,91,92] Regarding the effective condylar growth, as demonstrated by the change in the position of the Co-point, an upward movement between 1.5 and 3.1 mm and a 2.1–4.0 mm backward movement were observed during Herbst treatment,[51,75,97,98] which were greater than the Bolton group for both adolescents and young adults.[51,75,98] Furthermore, the changes in the adolescents were approximately twice those observed in the young adults group.[51] This change in the Co-point could be attributed to the sagittal condylar growth stimulation,[13,98] the glenoid fossa remodeling,[4,98] and the repositioning of the condyle in the fossa.[98] The effective condylar growth changes were followed by similar Pg position changes during treatment (1.1–3.9 mm downward and 0.9–2.2 mm forward),[97,98]

with the exception of the posterior mandibular autorotation (0.4°) which, when observed, resulted in a more downward movement of the Pg-point.[98]

The dental changes observed in both the maxilla and the mandible can be attributed to the fact that the Herbst appliance exerts a posteriorly directed force on the maxillary dentition and an anteriorly directed force on the mandibular dentition,[4,6,10,13,17,47,89] which results in distalization of the maxillary molars, retroclination of the maxillary incisors, mesial movement of the mandibular molars, and proclination of the mandibular incisors.[6,13,17,66,95] The latter is undesirable, especially in patients with initial incisor proclination and can be considered as anchorage loss along with the spaces between maxillary canines and first premolars (headgear effect), which are often observed after Herbst treatment.[6] However, the mandibular incisors showed a tendency to return to their former position after Herbst removal, without causing anterior crowding.[14,15] According to Pancherz,[6] dental changes during Herbst treatment are generally undesirable, with the exception of cases presenting anterior maxillary crowding, in which the distal movement of the posterior teeth is favorable.

Regarding the influence of the Herbst appliance on the maxillary molars, a distal molar movement between 0.6 and 3.0 mm and a distal tipping of 5.6–6.4° were observed during treatment.[6,8,10,14,17,39,45–48,50,53,83,86–88,90,92,95] In contrast, Croft et al,[91] O'Brien et al[52] and Burkhardt et al[30] found a 0.2–0.6 mm mesial movement. After Herbst removal, the maxillary first molars

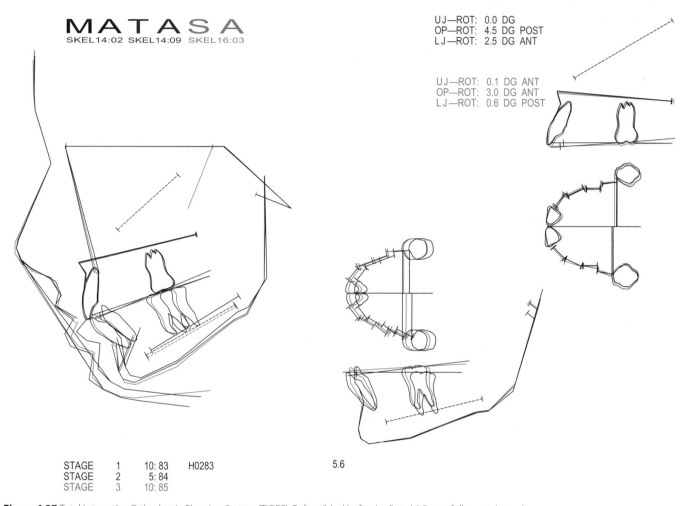

MATASA
SKEL14:02 SKEL14:09 SKEL16:03

UJ—ROT: 0.0 DG
OP—ROT: 4.5 DG POST
LJ—ROT: 2.5 DG ANT

UJ—ROT: 0.1 DG ANT
OP—ROT: 3.0 DG ANT
LJ—ROT: 0.6 DG POST

STAGE 1 10: 83 H0283
STAGE 2 5: 84
STAGE 3 10: 85

5.6

Figure 4.27 Total Interactive Orthodontic Planning System (TIOPS). Before (black), after (red) and 1.5-year follow-up (green).

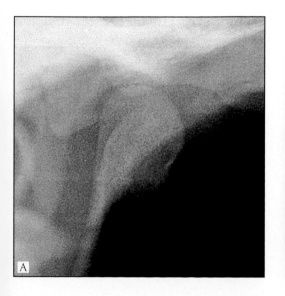

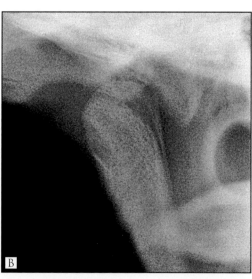

A

B

Figure 4.28 Condylar bone modeling at both condyles. Radiographic evaluation in open position during 6 months' treatment.

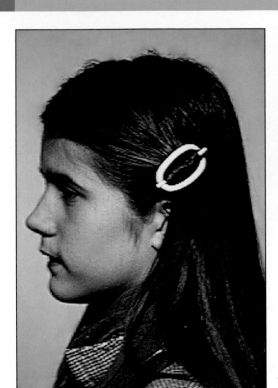

Figure 4.29–4.41 Herbst treatment of a 13-year-old girl.

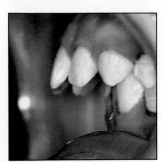

Figures 4.30–4.32 Before Herbst treatment.

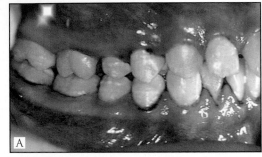

Figure 4.31

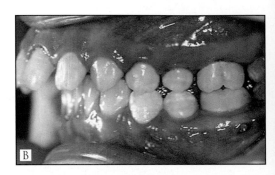

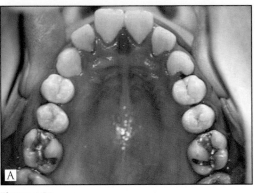

Figure 4.32

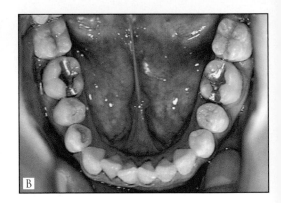

moved mesially 0.7–1.4 mm during the short-term posttreatment period[10,14,46,53,87] and 1.6–1.9 mm during the long-term posttreatment period.[10,83,87,92]

The mandibular first molars were moved mesially between 0.9 and 5.5 mm as a result of the anteriorly directed force of the Herbst appliance.[6,8,13–15,17,21,30,45–48,50,52,66,76,83,86,88–92,95] The mandibular molars moved distally 0.4–0.8 during the short-term posttreatment period[10,14,46,66,83,92] and a further 0.4–0.8 mm during the long-term posttreatment period.[10,83,87]

According to most investigators, both dental (mesial movement of the mandibular molars and distal movement of the maxillary molars) and skeletal changes (increased mandibular growth) contributed to the molar correction observed during Herbst treatment. In particular, the molar relationship was corrected between

3.0 and 9.3 mm,[6,8,13,14,17,30,47,48,52,87,89–93] while Hagg et al[46] and Du et al[45] found an even greater molar relationship correction, with a maximum of 10.9 mm. The molar relationship relapsed 1.1–1.7 mm during the short-term posttreatment period[14,46,92] and 0.4–2.6 mm during the long-term posttreatment period.[83,87,90]

Regarding the effect of the Herbst appliance on the maxillary incisors, a distal movement between 0.5 and 3.6 mm and a retroclination between 3.2° and 8.2° were evident at the end of the treatment phase,[10,14,17,21,30,39,45–48,50,52,76,83,88–90,95] which can be attributed to the pull of the transseptal fibers due to molar distalization or the altered position of the lower lip.[6] In contrast, other investigators found no significant differences in the incisor position[4,6,8,86] or a mesial movement of 0.8 mm.[91] In Class II, division 2 patients the maxillary incisors moved forward 3.0 mm and

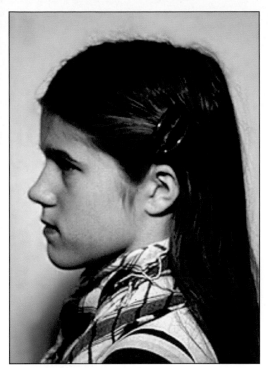

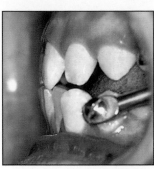

Figure 4.34

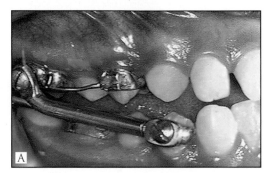

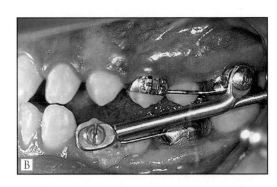

Figure 4.35

Figures 4.33–4.36 During Herbst treatment (1.5 years).

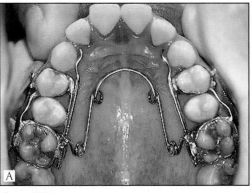

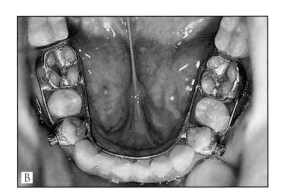

Figure 4.36

proclined 15.3°, which can be considered as favorable in treating this type of malocclusion.[89,96] During the short-term posttreatment period the maxillary incisor position remained unaffected,[10,14,46,92] while a retroclination of 0.6° was observed in Class II, division 2 patients.[96] Finally, during the long-term posttreatment period the maxillary incisors relapsed by moving mesially 0.4–2.1 mm;[10,87,90] however, other investigators did not observe a significant change in the incisor position during the same period.[83]

The mandibular incisors were also affected by the Herbst treatment, mainly because of the mesial forces exerted on the mandibular dentition, which resulted in a proclination between 5.4° and 10.8° and a mesial movement between 0.2 and 4.0 mm.[4,6,8,10,13–15,17,21,30,39,45–48,50,52,66,74,83,85–87,89,90,92,95,96,99] In contrast, Eberhard & Hirschfelder[39] and Hansen et al[83] found no

significant influence of the Herbst appliance on mandibular incisor position. The mandibular incisor proclination observed during Herbst treatment did not have an effect on the preexisting gingival recession or did not cause gingival recession.[99] Regarding the mandibular incisors' posttreatment changes, a distal movement between 0.9 and 3.3 mm was observed in the short-term period,[14,15,46,85,92] thus returning approximately to their initial position.[14,15] Furthermore, the mandibular incisor proclination was reduced between 6° and 7.9° during the first year of the posttreatment period[10,15,46,85] and 2.3° in Class II, division 2 patients.[96] During the long-term posttreatment period the mandibular incisors moved distally between 1.6 mm and 3.8 mm,[10,83,85,87,90] while a retroclination of 1.9–2.5° in relation to the sella–nasion line was evident,[85,90] which can be attributed to mandibular growth

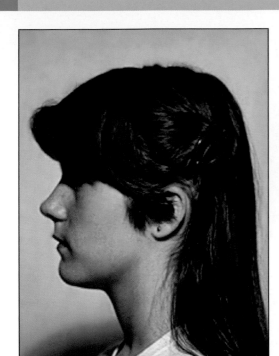

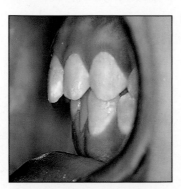

Figure 4.38

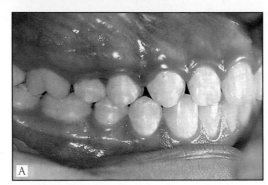

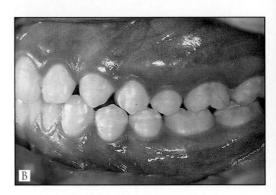

Figure 4.39

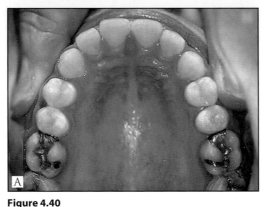

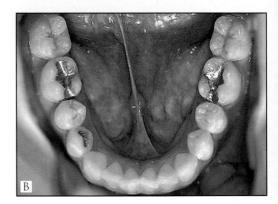

Figure 4.40

Figures 4.37–4.40 Follow-up 1 year after treatment.

rotational changes[85] or to the greater SNB angle in the Herbst group at the start of treatment.[90]

The overjet was corrected as a result of the dental and skeletal changes produced by the Herbst treatment. In particular, a reduction between 3.3 and 9.8 mm was evident at the end of the treatment.[4,6,8,10,13–15,17,21,30,44,47,48,50,52,55,66,76,83,87,90–93] This reduction was even more pronounced (approx. 10.5 mm) when the headgear Herbst and a step-by-step mandibular advancement were used.[44–46] In Class II, division 2 patients the overjet was reduced 3.1 mm.[89] After Herbst removal, the overjet relapsed between 1.7 and 3.0 mm during the short-term posttreatment period,[10,14,15,46,55] which can be attributed to the relapse in the mandibular incisor inclination[8] or to

the recovery of the upper and lower teeth movements.[10] In contrast, Franchi et al[92] found that the overjet remained almost unaffected. On a long-term posttreatment basis, a relapse in the overjet between 0.3 and 2.4 mm was observed.[10,83,87,90,94] In total, the Herbst appliance caused an overjet correction between 3.3 and 5.7 mm from the pretreatment to the long-term posttreatment period.[10,55,83,87,90]

Finally, when considering the effect of the Herbst appliance in relation to the age of the patients, it was found that skeletal changes were more marked in early adolescent subjects, while dental changes were more pronounced in late adolescent or young adult patients.[13,41,50,51]

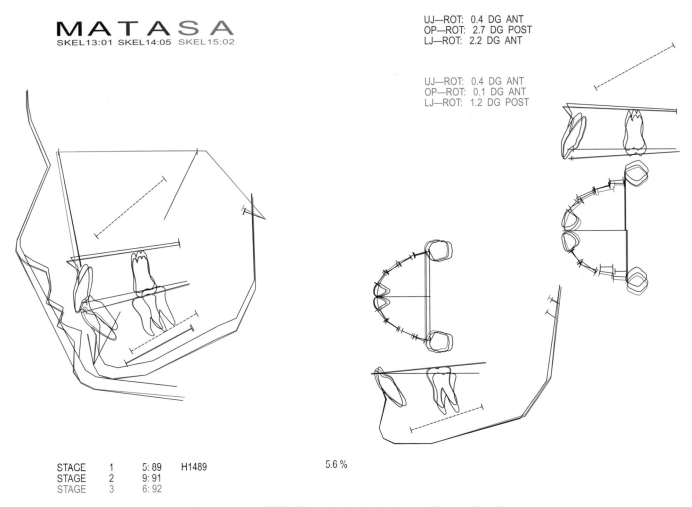

Figure 4.41 Total Interactive Orthodontic Planning System (TIOPS). Before (black), after (red) and at follow-up (green).

Vertical Changes

According to most investigators, the Herbst appliance affected the skeletal and dental structures vertically, in both the mandible and the maxilla. The use of the Herbst appliance in Class II patients appeared to affect the maxillary growth by causing its redirection,[18,46,88] while mandibular growth was also affected, as it became more sagittally directed.[91,100]

Regarding the effect of the Herbst appliance on the maxilla, it was found that the palatal plane inclination (NL/NSL angle) was changed during the treatment and posttreatment period, showing a rotational effect of the Herbst telescopic mechanism on the maxillary skeleton. In particular, the palatal plane tipped downwards 0.2–1.0°.[4,6,10,18,48,53,83,85–88,90] In patients treated after the maximum pubertal growth the NL/NSL angle was decreased 0.4°.[83] During the short-term posttreatment period the palatal plane angle did not present significant changes, which was similar to what happened during treatment.[10,18,53,85] However, during the long-term posttreatment period a significant increase of 1.0° was observed.[53,90] This was in contrast with the 0.5–0.6° decrease[10,83] or nonsignificant changes[85] observed in other studies. On average, Pancherz & Anehus-Pancherz[53] found that the palatal plane tipped significantly downward by 1.1° during the whole examination period and this was about twice what was seen in the Bolton control group.

The occlusal plane tipped clockwise during treatment (as was shown by the increase of the OL/NSL angle) between 1.1° and 5.1°, which was significantly different from the control group mainly because of the distalization and intrusion of the maxillary first molars.[6,8,10,14,17,21,39,48,53,88–90,95] However, it tipped counterclockwise 1.3–2.8° in the short-term posttreatment period[10,14,53] and further counterclockwise during the long-term posttreatment period.[10,21,90]

Regarding the effect of the Herbst appliance on the mandibular plane angle (ML/NSL), the majority of the investigators found an increase of 0.1–2.0° during Herbst treatment.[4,6,8,10,14,15,17,18,21,39,45,48,85,86,89,90,101] However, others observed that the ML/NSL angle was decreased 0.1–1.5°,[30,45,46,83,95,101] whereas some investigators found that it remained unaffected.[4,87,93]

After Herbst removal, the mandibular plane angle decreased between 0.5° and 0.7° during the short-term posttreatment period,[10,15,46] whereas Pancherz & Hansen[14] observed that it remained approximately unchanged. During the long-term posttreatment period the mandibular plane angle further decreased 1.6–5.8°,[10,18,21,83,85,87,90,101] which can be attributed to the marked forward rotation of the mandible[90] or to normal growth.[101] In the long term, Ruf & Pancherz found that the Herbst appliance did not have a significant effect on the ML/NSL angle, although a wide range of treatment responses was observed, and concluded that Herbst treatment does not seem to result in an undesired backward rotation of the mandible.[101]

According to the findings of Valant & Sinclair,[86] the initial opening observed after Herbst insertion was compensated for during the active treatment and settling periods. The 0.8° increase of the mandibular plane angle at the start of the treatment, due to the incisal edge-to-edge construction bite, leads to a posterior rotation of the mandible,[101] while the decrease observed after Herbst removal can be attributed to the vertical effects during the late treatment and retention periods, which permitted an anterior rotation of the mandible,[18,46] and the headgear effect, which intruded the maxillary molars[7,53].

Regarding the vertical jaw relationships, the maxillomandibular plane angle (ML/NL) was decreased by 0.2–1.1° at the end of the Herbst treatment,[4,6,10,21,39,83,87,92,93] while other investigators found an increase of 0.1–2.6°.[39,48] The same angle decreased by 0.2–1.3° in the short term and between 1.6° and 4.2° in the long-term posttreatment periods.[6,10,39,83,85]

The anterior lower facial height (ANS-Me) was increased 0.4 to 4.1 mm[4,8,30,45,66,70,88,95] but according to Pancherz,[8] no difference was evident between the treatment and the control groups in the 12-month posttreatment period. Further, Hagg et al[46] observed an increase of 2.7 mm of the anterior lower facial height during treatment, which remained unchanged during the retention period. However, when measuring the net treatment effect, the same investigators observed a decrease of 0.9 mm during treatment and a further decrease of 1.8 mm during the retention period. According to Nelson et al,[93] the anterior lower facial height increased 3.2 mm during Herbst treatment and the 6-month retention period. Finally, Paulsen et al[21] and Sidhu et al[66] found that both the anterior and posterior facial heights increased during treatment. This increase resulted in a mandibular translation without causing unfavorable rotation.

Regarding changes in the mandibular morphology, the gonion angle (RL/ML) was found approximately unchanged at the end of treatment.[4,17] However, Pancherz & Fackel[18] and Paulsen et al[21] observed that the gonion angle was increased 2.0–5.0° although it was reduced by the same amount in the posttreatment period and therefore no significant differences were found comparing the pre- and posttreatment changes. One year after Herbst removal the gonion angle was decreased by 1.0°,[96] while during the long-term observation period it was further decreased between 2.1° and 7.7°.[18,83] When examining the treatment outcomes in relation to the vertical jaw base relationship, it was found that the dental and skeletal treatment changes resulting in a Class II correction were not dependent on the pretreatment severity, meaning that favorable treatment changes can also be expected in hyperdivergent patients.[76,88] According to Ruf & Pancherz,[76] the increased skeletal reaction in hyperdivergent patients, the bone apposition in the posterior condylar pole and the inherited horizontal condylar growth direction contributed to the unexpected favorable skeletal effect observed in those patients, in comparison with the hypodivergent group. Further, Schiavoni et al[70] found that the banded Herbst appliance did not cause a modification of the vertical growth pattern in normohypodivergent patients, while in hyperdivergent patients the high-pull headgear and the acrylic Herbst splints allowed better control of the vertical dimension.

The Herbst appliance also affected the dental components of both maxilla and mandible. Regarding maxillary dental changes, it was observed that the maxillary first molars were intruded between 0.5 and 1.1 mm during the treatment period.[8,46,53,95,96] In contrast, an extrusion of 1.4–1.5 mm was evident in other studies.[30,96] The maxillary first molars were extruded between 1.1 and 1.4 mm during the short-term posttreatment period and 3.5 mm during the long-term follow-up.[46,53] Pancherz & Anehus-Pancherz[53] found that after a 7-year observation period, including the treatment and the short- and long-term posttreatment periods, the maxillary first molars were extruded by 3.9 mm. The maxillary second premolars also extruded during Herbst treatment.[8] Regarding the maxillary incisors, an extrusion between 0.2 and 2.2 mm was observed at the end of treatment[30,45,46] while no significant changes were found during the retention period.[46]

With regard to the mandibular dental changes, the incisors were intruded by 0.4–2.4 mm, which can be partially attributed to the proclination of these teeth, and the molars extruded 1.3–2.8 mm.[8,45,46,66,95,96] However, Burkhardt et al[30] observed an incisor extrusion of 0.1–1.4 mm. During the 6-month retention period, the mandibular molars and incisors extruded equally by 0.6 mm.[46] Regarding the mandibular first premolars, an intrusion was found at the end of the treatment, due to the fact that these teeth served as anchors to the appliance.[39] Finally, the mandibular second premolars were extruded after treatment.[8]

The incisal edge-to-edge relationship leaves the buccal segment out of occlusion, which contributes to the allowance of normal vertical tooth eruption and growth in the posterior segments.[4,6,17,18] Thus, a reduction in the overbite should be anticipated.[4] After Herbst treatment the overbite was reduced between 1.9 and 5.6 mm.[4,7,8,10,21,30,55,66,87,93,96] A relapse of 1.7–1.8 mm during the short-term posttreatment period was evident, mainly because of the relapse in the inclination of the mandibular incisors to the mandibular line.[8,83] In addition, an increase of 0.5–1.1 mm was observed during long-term follow-up.[10,55,87] In fact, these measured effects are caused by an elastic rocking reaction of the alveolar process, forward during treatment and backward after treatment.[21] Thus, the total overbite reduction during the total observation period was between 1.0 and 2.6 mm.[10,55]

Transverse Changes

During Herbst treatment, maxillary arch length, intercanine width, and intermolar width were increased significantly, while the mandibular arch displayed minimal change.[86]

Similarly, Hansen et al found an increase of the upper and lower arch perimeters after Herbst treatment, which relapsed during the short-term observation period.[55] According to these investigators, the same effects were observed in the mandibular and mandibular intercanine arch width and the upper intermolar width, while the lower intermolar width appeared to be unaffected by treatment. In the long-term observation period, the arch perimeters showed a normal dental developmental pattern.

Soft Tissue Changes

At the end of Herbst treatment the soft tissue profile was improved.[4,54,102] The upper lip was retruded during treatment[30,54] while the lower lip remained unchanged[54] or retruded less than the upper lip.[30] During the short-term posttreatment period the upper and lower lips retruded nonsignificantly, while in the same period the facial profile showed a relapse.[54] Regarding the long-term posttreatment effects on the soft tissues, a retrusion of 4.4–4.5 mm of the upper lip was observed, while the lower lip showed a retrusion of 2.9–3.4 mm.[54] The soft tissue profile changes of the upper and lower lip retrusion can be at least partially attributed to the increase in nasal growth, which affected the position of the lips in relation to the E-line[54] and to the tendency of the lower incisors to relapse.[14,54]

Finally, according to Schweitzer & Pancherz,[96] Herbst treatment in Class II, division 2 patients resulted in a reduction of the lower lip overlap on the maxillary incisors by 1.8 mm, which remained stable during the 12-month posttreatment period, despite the minor relapse observed in the incisor tooth positions and its relationships.

Effects on Temporomandibular Joint

The placement of the Herbst appliance caused an anterior and downward movement of the condyle which induced adaptive growth, modeling and remodeling of the condyle, the glenoid fossa, and the articular tubercle.[4,19,21] Condylar adaptive growth, modeling and remodeling were observed at the posterior–superior border of the condyle, and glenoid fossa remodeling at the anterior surface of the postglenoid spine,[51] while it was also observed that fossa remodeling followed that of the condyle and both contributed to the mandibular forward growth.[21,51,75] The newly formed bone remained unchanged after Herbst treatment in adult patients, where normal growth had ceased (Fig. 4.42).[19]

Human condylar cartilage and bone were examined in autopsy material from 20 individuals aged 18–31 years by Paulsen et al.[24] Histomorphometry, scanning electron microscopy, and cartilage histology were used to analyze the tissue. Correlation analyses between ages and all parameters were conducted. There was a statistically significant correlation between age and the hypertropic chondrocytes ($r = -0.50$, $p<0.05$), and age and the hypertropic chondrocytes in bone ($r = -0.48$, $p<0.05$) (Fig. 4.43). Quantitative and qualitative investigations of the turnover activity in the fibrocartilage and the bone tissue, describing the activity of hypertropic chondrocytes and the trabecular bone tissue, demonstrated condylar growth potential in the group up to 30 years of age. Growth activity seemed to decline with age.[24]

The mechanism of the condylar and glenoid fossa modifications was proposed by Voudouris & Kuftinec[103] and tested by Voudouris et al.[104,105] The growth relativity hypothesis involved mandibular displacement, viscoelastic tissue extension forces to the condyle through several different attachments and transduction of forces radiating beneath the fibrocartilage of the glenoid fossa and condyle, which resulted in redirected and enhanced condylar-glenoid fossa growth,[103] mainly due to significant bone modeling (Fig. 4.44).[21] Thus, significant bone formation was observed in the glenoid fossa which showed a downward and forward direction.[105]

The articular disk, which retruded at the start of the treatment as an adaptive response to the incisal edge-to-edge position, returned to approximately its initial position after appliance removal, and a slightly retruded position remained in only a few patients.[49] Further, the temporomandibular joint (TMJ) was not affected during Herbst treatment,[4,6,8,41,74] as the condyles returned to their normal fossa position after removal of the appliance,[14] mainly due to the increase of the sagittal condylar growth,[4,75,106] and the remodeling of the glenoid fossa.[4,75] For these reasons, the condyle–fossa relationship was unaffected at the end of the therapy.[75,107]

Some undesirable functional disturbances were observed during Herbst treatment, such as TMJ sounds,[108] masticatory muscle tenderness,[8,108] and TMJ tenderness on palpation, which can be attributed to the lack of occlusal buffer during the first months of treatment.[8,12] The distortion of the TMJ during mastication could be attributed to the changes in the sensory information from the mechanoreceptors of the periodontal membranes and the TMJs.[12] According to Ruf & Pancherz,[27] bite jumping with the Herbst appliance did not cause muscular temporomandibular disorders (TMD), decreased the prevalence of capsulitis and structural condylar bone changes, and did not cause disk displacement in patients with normal pretreatment disk position. Furthermore, the frequency of condylar displacement, TMJ sound findings or TMDs in patients treated with the Herbst appliance was not significantly greater than that of the normal population, both for the short-term and long-term periods.[74,109] In addition, anamnesis, clinical, and radiographic findings were similar to those observed in untreated groups.[108]

Thus, the functional disturbances observed were characterized by their temporary nature. Herbst treatment did not seem to have any adverse effects on the TMJ function or cause TMDs or unfavorable structural changes on a short- or long-term basis.[8,27,74,108,109] Also, TMJ sounds, muscle tenderness, and symptoms which were observed before the initiation of treatment were resolved mainly due to the normal occlusal conditions

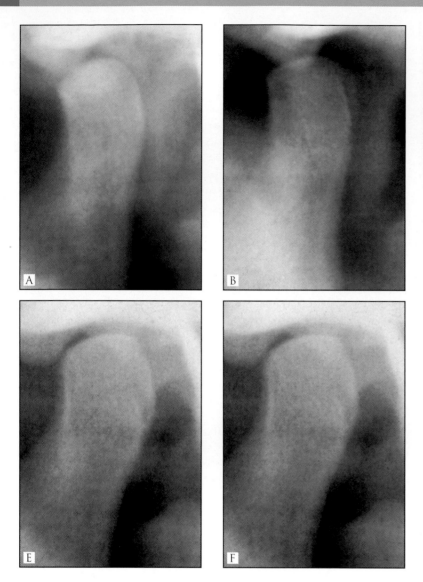

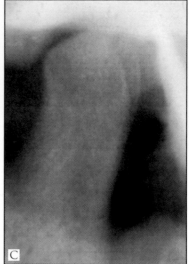

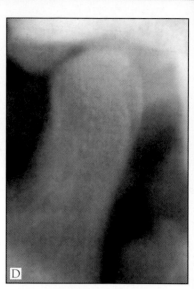

Figure 4.42 Radiographs showing bone modeling in a female at adulthood. **A)** Before treatment. **B)** Three months' treatment. **C)** Six months' treatment. **D)** One year after treatment. **E)** Two years after treatment. **F)** Three years after treatment. *(From Paulsen 1997,[19] with kind permission of Oxford University Press)*

established, and possibly because of the repositioning of the displaced disk caused by the jumped position of the condyle during treatment.[4,6,8]

Effects on Muscles

Regarding the effects of the Herbst appliance on the masticatory muscles, the incisal edge-to-edge relationship caused a noticeable reduction in the electromyographic (EMG) activity of both the masseter and temporal muscles during maximal biting in an intercuspal position, which recovered noticeably almost to pretreatment values 3–6 months after placement of the Herbst appliance.[11,12,110] Regarding the lateral pterygoid muscle activity, an increase in the EMG pattern was observed after wearing the appliance which was reduced markedly in a 6-month period,[111,112] which led to the conclusion that muscular adaptation takes place

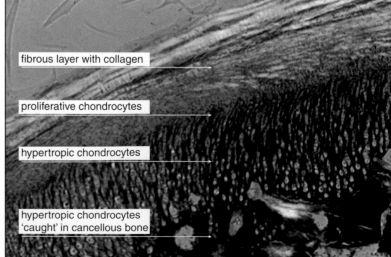

Figure 4.43 Histologic histomorphology of an autopsy condyle of a 22-year-old male. Vertical sections stained with Masson Trichrome and viewed under polarized light with lambda filter. Fibrous cartilage shows active, bone-forming tissue: fibrous layer with collagen, proliferative chondrocytes, hypertropic chondrocytes in columns, and hypertropic chondrocytes "caught" in cancellous bone. *(From Paulsen et al,[24] with kind permission of Blackwell Muustaard)*

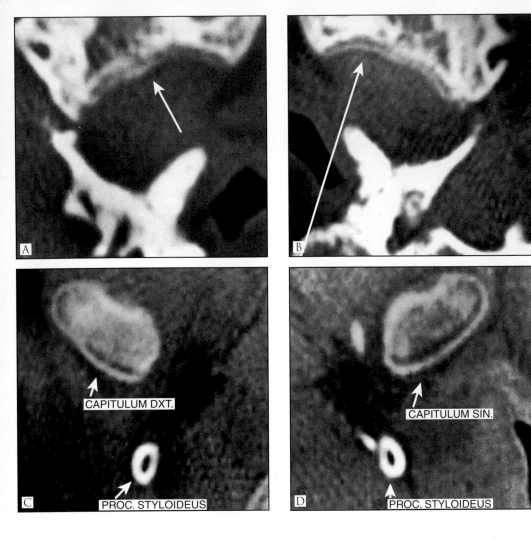

Figure 4.44 CT scanning of the TMJ after 3 months' Herbst treatment. Bone modeling of the distal part of the condyles and mesial part of the fossae can be seen, shown by double contours. *(From Paulsen et al 1995,[21] with kind permission of Oxford University Press)*

soon after Herbst placement, and before the appearance of morphologic changes due to functional treatment.[112]

When the Herbst appliance was removed, the EMG activity of the masseter and temporal muscles was found to be increased in comparison to pretreatment values,[11] although this increase was greater for the masseter than for the temporal muscle. Twelve months post treatment, when the occlusion was stabilized, the contraction pattern in the two muscles was similar to that observed in subjects with normal occlusion.[8]

In a study of Herbst treatment effect in a hypodivergent patient in late adolescence, Bakke & Paulsen[20] found a reduction of the powerful masseter muscle strength by about 40% and an increase of the minimal pterygoideus muscle strength after achievement of a normodivergent jaw relation with a more equal strength of these muscles, in accordance with findings by Moeller.[113] In addition, the moment arms of the masseter muscle increased, mainly due to the mandibular protrusion which caused changes in the muscle and jaw geometry.[114] In contrast, the moment arms of the temporal muscle presented no significant changes, possibly because the temporal muscle application vector is far from the area where the geometric changes occurred. Moreover, the mechanical advantages of masseter and temporal muscles related to the occlusal bite force on the mandibular and occlusal planes, as well as the number and intensity of occlusal contacts, were reduced after treatment.[114]

References

1. Herbst E. Atlas und Grundriss der Zahnärztlichen Orthopädie. Munich: JF Lehmann Verlag; 1910.
2. Kingsley NW. A treatise on oral deformities as a branch of mechanical surgery. New York: D Appleton; 1880.
3. Herbst E. Dreissigjährige Erfahrungen mit dem Retentions-Scharnier. Zahnärztl Rundschau 1934;43:1515–1524, 1563–1568, 1611–1616.
4. Pancherz H. Treatment of Class II malocclusions by jumping the bite with the Herbst appliance. A cephalometric investigation. Am J Orthod 1979; 76:423–442.
5. Pancherz H. The effect of continuous bite jumping on the dentofacial complex: a follow-up study after Herbst appliance treatment of

Class II malocclusions. Eur J Orthod 1981; 3:49–60.

6. Pancherz H. The mechanism of Class II correction in Herbst appliance treatment. A cephalometric investigation. Am J Orthod 1982;82:104–113.

7. Pancherz H. Vertical dentofacial changes during Herbst appliance treatment: a cephalometric investigation. Swed Dent J Supp 1982; 15:189–196.

8. Pancherz H. The Herbst appliance – its biologic effects and clinical use. Am J Orthod 1985; 87:1–20.

9. Pancherz H, Stickel A. [Position changes of mandibular condyle in Herbst treatment. Radiographic study.] Inf Orthod Kieferorthop 1989;21:515–527.

10. Pancherz H. The nature of Class II relapse after Herbst appliance treatment: a cephalometric long-term investigation. Am J Orthod Dentofacial Orthop 1991;100:220–233.

11. Pancherz H, Anehus-Pancherz M. Muscle activity in Class II, division 1 malocclusions treated by bite jumping with the Herbst appliance. An electromyographic study. Am J Orthod 1980;78:321–329.

12. Pancherz H, Anehus-Pancherz M. The effect of continuous bite jumping with the Herbst appliance on the masticatory system: a functional analysis of treated Class II malocclusions. Eur J Orthod 1982;4:37–44.

13. Pancherz H, Hagg U. Dentofacial orthopedics in relation to somatic maturation. An analysis of 70 consecutive cases treated with the Herbst appliance. Am J Orthod 1985;88:273–287.

14. Pancherz H, Hansen K. Occlusal changes during and after Herbst treatment: a cephalometric investigation. Eur J Orthod 1986;8:215–228.

15. Pancherz H, Hansen K. Mandibular anchorage in Herbst treatment. Eur J Orthod 1988; 10:149–164.

16. Hagg U, Pancherz H. Dentofacial orthopaedics in relation to chronological age, growth period and skeletal development. An analysis of 72 male patients with Class II division 1 malocclusion treated with the Herbst appliance. Eur J Orthod 1988;10:169–176.

17. Pancherz H, Malmgren O, Hagg U, Omblus J, Hansen K. Class II correction in Herbst and Bass therapy. Eur J Orthod 1989;11:17–30.

18. Pancherz H, Fackel U. The skeletofacial growth pattern pre- and post-dentofacial orthopaedics. A long-term study of Class II malocclusions treated with the Herbst appliance. Eur J Orthod 1990;12:209–218.

19. Paulsen HU. Morphological changes of the TMJ condyles of 100 patients treated with the Herbst appliance in the period of puberty to adulthood: a long-term radiographic study. Eur J Orthod 1997;19:657–668.

20. Bakke M, Paulsen HU. Herbst treatment in late adolescence: clinical, electromyographic, kinesiographic, and radiographic analysis of one case. Eur J Orthod 1989;11:397–407.

21. Paulsen HU, Karle A, Bakke M, Herskind A. CT-scanning and radiographic analysis of temporoandibular joints and cephalometric analysis in a case of Herbst treatment in late puberty. Eur J Orthod 1995;17:167–175.

22. Paulsen HU. [Herbst apparatus and Jasper jumper.] Tandlaegernes Tidsskr 1990;5: 362–365.

23. Paulsen HU, Rabol A, Sørensen SS. Bone scintigraphy of human temporomandibular joints during Herbst treatment: a case report. Eur J Orthod 1998;20:369–374.

24. Paulsen HU, Thomsen JS, Hougen HP, Mosekilde L. A histomorphometric and scanning electron microscopy study of human condylar cartilage and bone tissue changes in relation to age. Clin Orthod Res 1999;2:67–78.

25. Paulsen HU, Karle A. Computer tomographic and radiographic changes in the temporomandibular joints of two young adults with occlusal asymmetry, treated with the Herbst appliance. Eur J Orthod 2000;22:649–656.

26. Pancherz H. The modern Herbst appliance. In: Graber TM, Rakosi T, Petrovic AG, eds. Dentofacial orthopedics with functional appliances, 2nd edn. St Louis: Mosby-Year Book; 1997: 336–366.

27. Ruf S, Pancherz H. Does bite-jumping damage the TMJ? A prospective longitudinal clinical and MRI study of Herbst patients. Angle Orthod 2000;70:183–199.

28. Langford NM Jr. Updating fabrication of the Herbst appliance. J Clin Orthod 1982;16:173–174.

29. Dischinger TG. Edgewise bioprogressive Herbst appliance. J Clin Orthod 1989;23:608–617.

30. Burkhardt DR, McNamara JA Jr, Baccetti T. Maxillary molar distalization or mandibular enhancement: a cephalometric comparison of comprehensive orthodontic treatment including the pendulum and the Herbst appliances. Am J Orthod Dentofacial Orthop 2003; 123:108–116.

31. Howe RP. The bonded Herbst appliance. J Clin Orthod 1982;16:663–667.

32. McNamara JA, Howe RP. Clinical management of the acrylic splint Herbst appliance. Am J Orthod Dentofacial Orthop 1988;94:142–149.

33. White LW. Current Herbst appliance therapy. J Clin Orthod 1994;28:296–309.

34. Snodgrass D. A modified, lingually supported cantilevered Herbst appliance. Funct Orthod 1996;13:20–26, 28.

35. Rogers MB. Herbst appliance variations. J Clin Orthod 2003;37:156–159.

36. Langford NM Jr. The Herbst appliance. J Clin Orthod 1981;15:558–561.

37. Rogers MB. The banded Herbst appliance. J Clin Orthod 2001;35:494–499.

38. Hägg U, Tse EL, Rabie AB, Robinson W. A comparison of splinted and banded Herbst appliances: treatment changes and complications. Aust J Orthod 2002;18:76–81.

39. Eberhard H, Hirschfelder U. Treatment of Class II, Division 2 in the late growth period. J Orofac Orthop 1998;59:352–361.

40. Allen-Noble P. Clinical management of crown/banded Herbst appliances. Allesee Orthodontic Appliances/Pro Lab, 2002. Available online at: www.ormco.com/pubs/AOA/Manuals/Herbst2002.pdf

41. Pancherz H, Ruf S. The Herbst appliance: research-based updated clinical possibilities. World J Orthod 2000;1:17–31.

42. Sinha P. Clinical applications of the Herbst appliance. Good Practice Newsletter of American Orthodontics 2002;3:2–3. Available online at: www.americanortho.com

43. McNamara JA Jr, Brudon WL, Buckhardt DR, Huge SA. The Herbst appliance. In: McNamara JA Jr, Brudon WL, eds. Orthodontics and dentofacial orthopedics. Ann Arbor: Needham Press; 2001: 285–318.

44. Wieslander L. Intensive treatment of severe Class II malocclusions with a headgear-Herbst appliance in the early mixed dentition. Am J Orthod 1984; 86:1–13.

45. Du X, Hagg U, Rabie AB. Effects of headgear Herbst and mandibular step-by-step advancement versus conventional Herbst appliance and maximal jumping of the mandible. Eur J Orthod 2002;24:167–174.

46. Hagg U, Du X, Rabie AB. Initial and late treatment effects of headgear-Herbst appliance with mandibular step-by-step advancement. Am J Orthod Dentofacial Orthop 2002;122:477–485.

47. Konik M, Pancherz H, Hansen K. The mechanism of Class II correction in late Herbst treatment. Am J Orthod Dentofacial Orthop 1997;112:87–91.

48. Wong GW, So LL, Hagg U. A comparative study of sagittal correction with the Herbst appliance in two different ethnic groups. Eur J Orthod 1997;19:195–204.

49. Pancherz H, Ruf S, Thomalske-Faubert C. Mandibular articular disk position changes during Herbst treatment: a prospective longitudinal MRI study. Am J Orthod Dentofacial Orthop 1999;116:207–214.

50. Ruf S, Pancherz H. Dentoskeletal effects and facial profile changes in young adults treated with the Herbst appliance. Angle Orthod 1999;69:239–246.

51. Ruf S, Pancherz H. Temporomandibular joint remodeling in adolescents and young adults during Herbst treatment: a prospective longitudinal magnetic resonance imaging and cephalometric radiographic investigation. Am J Orthod Dentofacial Orthop 1999;115:607–618.

52. O'Brien K, Wright J, Conboy F, et al. Effectiveness of treatment for Class II malocclusion with the Herbst or twin-block appliances: a randomized, controlled trial. Am J Orthod Dentofacial Orthop 2003;124:128–137.

53. Pancherz H, Anehus-Pancherz M. The headgear effect of the Herbst appliance: a cephalometric long-term study. Am J Orthod Dentofacial Orthop 1993;103:510–520.

54. Pancherz H, Anehus-Pancherz M. Facial profile changes during and after Herbst appliance treatment. Eur J Orthod 1994;16:275–286.

55. Hansen K, Iemamnueisuk P, Pancherz H. Long-term effects of the Herbst appliance on the dental arches and arch relationships: a biometric study. Br J Orthod 1995;22:123–134.

56. Pancherz H. The effects, limitations, and long-term dentofacial adaptations to treatment with the Herbst appliance. Semin Orthod 1997;3:232–243.

57. Mayes JH. Improving appliance efficiency with the cantilever Herbst – a new answer to old problems. Clin Impressions 1994;3:2–5,17–19.

58. Mayes JH. The cantilever bite-jumper system, Exploring the possibilities. Orthodontic CYBER-journal 1996. Available online at: www.oc-j.com/issue3/p0000077.htm

59. Mayes JH. The molar-moving bite jumper (MMBJ). Clin Impressions 1998;7:16–19.

60. Smith JR. Matching the Herbst to the mal-occlusion. Clin Impressions 1998;7:6–12, 20–23.

61. Smith JR. Matching the Herbst to the malocclusion: Part II. Clin Impressions 1999;8:14–23.

62. Hilgers JJ. Hyper efficient orthodontic treatment using tandem mechanics. Semin Orthod 1998; 4:17–25.

63. Dischinger T. Edgewise Herbst appliance. J Clin Orthod 1995;29:738–742.

64. Howe RP. Updating the bonded Herbst appliance. J Clin Orthod 1983;17:122–124.

65. McNamara JA. Fabrication of the acrylic splint Herbst appliance. Am J Orthod Dentofacial Orthop 1988;94:10–18.

66. Sidhu MS, Kharbanda OP, Sidhu SS. Cephalometric analysis of changes produced by a modified Herbst appliance in the treatment of Class II division 1 malocclusion. Br J Orthod 1995;22:1–12.

67. Howe RP. Removable plastic Herbst retainer. J Clin Orthod 1987;21:533–537.

68. Howe RP. Lower premolar extraction/removable plastic Herbst treatment for mandibular retrognathia. Am J Orthod Dentofacial Orthop 1987;92:275–285.

69. Kucukkeles N, Arun T. Bio-thermal Herbst application during the mixed dentition period. J Clin Pediatr Dent 1994;18:253–258.

70. Schiavoni R, Grenga V, Macri V. Treatment of Class II high angle malocclusions with the Herbst appliance: a cephalometric investigation. Am J Orthod Dentofacial Orthop 1992;102:393–409.

71. Howe RP, McNamara JA Jr. Clinical management of the bonded Herbst appliance. J Clin Orthod 1983;17:456–463.

72. Howe RP. The acrylic-splint Herbst. Problem solving. J Clin Orthod 1984;18:497–501.

73. Schiavoni R, Grenga V. Nonextraction treatment of a high-angle Class II case with a modified Herbst appliance. J Clin Orthod 1994;28:453–457.

74. Ruf S, Pancherz H. Long-term TMJ effects of Herbst treatment: a clinical and MRI study. Am J Orthod Dentofacial Orthop 1998;114:475–483.

75. Ruf S, Pancherz H. Temporomandibular joint growth adaptation in Herbst treatment: a prospective magnetic resonance imaging and cephalometric roentgenographic study. Eur J Orthod 1998;20:375–388.

76. Ruf S, Pancherz H. The mechanism of Class II correction during Herbst therapy in relation to the vertical jaw base relationship: a cephalometric roentgenographic study. Angle Orthod 1997; 67:271–276.

77. Rider EA. Removable Herbst appliance for treatment of obstructive sleep apnea. J Clin Orthod 1988;22:256–257.

78. Sjoholm TT, Polo OJ, Rauhala ER, Vuoriluoto J, Helenius HY. Mandibular advancement with dental appliances in obstructive sleep apnoea. J Oral Rehabil 1994;21:595–603.

79. Millman RP, Rosenberg CL, Carlisle CC, Kramer NR, Kahn DM, Bonitati AE. The efficacy of oral appliances in the treatment of persistent sleep apnea after uvulopalatopharyngoplasty. Chest 1998;113:992–996.

80. Johal A, Battagel JM. An investigation into the changes in airway dimension and the efficacy of mandibular advancement appliances in subjects with obstructive sleep apnoea. Br J Orthod 1999; 26:205–210.

81. Bloch KE, Iseli A, Zhang JN, et al. A randomized, controlled crossover trial of two oral appliances for sleep apnea treatment. Am J Respir Crit Care Med 2000;162:246–251.

82. Shadaba A, Battagel JM, Owa A, Croft CB, Kotecha BT. Evaluation of the Herbst Mandibular Advancement Splint in the management of patients with sleep-related breathing disorders. Clin Otolaryngol 2000;25:404–412.

83. Hansen K, Pancherz H, Hagg U. Long-term effects of the Herbst appliance in relation to the treatment growth period: a cephalometric study. Eur J Orthod 1991;13:471–481.

84. Rogers MB. Troubleshooting the Herbst appliance. J Clin Orthod 2002;36:268–274.

85. Hansen K, Koutsonas TG, Pancherz H. Long-term effects of Herbst treatment on the mandibular incisor segment: a cephalometric and biometric investigation. Am J Orthod Dentofacial Orthop 1997;112:92–103.

86. Valant JR, Sinclair PM. Treatment effects of the Herbst appliance. Am J Orthod Dentofacial Orthop 1989;95:138–147.

87. Hansen K, Pancherz H. Long-term effects of Herbst treatment in relation to normal growth development: a cephalometric study. Eur J Orthod 1992;14:285–295.

88. Windmiller EC. The acrylic-splint Herbst appliance: a cephalometric evaluation. Am J Orthod Dentofacial Orthop 1993;104:73–84.

89. Obijou C, Pancherz H. Herbst appliance treatment of Class II, division 2 malocclusions. Am J Orthod Dentofacial Orthop 1997;112:287–291.

90. Omblus J, Malmgren O, Pancherz H, Hagg U, Hansen K. Long-term effects of Class II correction in Herbst and Bass therapy. Eur J Orthod 1997;19:185–193.

91. Croft RS, Buschang PH, English JD, Meyer R. A cephalometric and tomographic evaluation of Herbst treatment in the mixed dentition. Am J Orthod Dentofacial Orthop 1999;116:435–443.

92. Franchi L, Baccetti T, McNamara JA Jr. Treatment and post-treatment effects of acrylic splint Herbst appliance therapy. Am J Orthod Dentofacial Orthop 1999;115:429–438.

93. Nelson B, Hansen K, Hagg U. Class II correction in patients treated with class II elastics and with fixed functional appliances: a comparative study. Am J Orthod Dentofacial Orthop 2000; 118:142–149.

94. Wieslander L. Long-term effect of treatment with the headgear-Herbst appliance in the early mixed dentition. Stability or relapse? Am J Orthod Dentofacial Orthop 1993;104:319–329.

95. McNamara JA Jr, Howe RP, Dischinger TG. A comparison of the Herbst and Frankel appliances in the treatment of Class II malocclusion. Am J Orthod Dentofacial Orthop 1990;98:134–144.

96. Schweitzer M, Pancherz H. The incisor-lip relationship in Herbst/multibracket appliance treatment of Class II, Division 2 malocclusions. Angle Orthod 2001;71:358–363.

97. Baltromejus S, Ruf S, Pancherz H. Effective temporomandibular joint growth and chin position changes: activator versus Herbst treatment. A cephalometric roentgenographic study. Eur J Orthod 2002;24:627–637.

98. Pancherz H, Ruf S, Kohlhas P. "Effective condylar growth" and chin position changes in Herbst treatment: a cephalometric roentgenographic long-term study. Am J Orthod Dentofacial Orthop 1998;114:437–446.

99. Ruf S, Hansen K, Pancherz H. Does orthodontic proclination of lower incisors in children and adolescents cause gingival recession? Am J Orthod Dentofacial Orthop 1998;114:100–106.

100. Hagg U. Change in mandibular growth direction by means of a Herbst appliance? A case report. Am J Orthod Dentofacial Orthop 1992;102: 456–463.

101. Ruf S, Pancherz H. The effect of Herbst appliance treatment on the mandibular plane angle: a cephalometric roentgenographic study. Am J Orthod Dentofacial Orthop 1996;110:225–229.

102. Eicke C, Wieslander L. [Soft-tissue profile changes through therapy with the Herbst hinge appliance.] Schweiz Monatsschr Zahnmed 1990; 100:149–153.

103. Voudouris JC, Kuftinec MM. Improved clinical use of Twin-block and Herbst as a result of radiating viscoelastic tissue forces on the condyle and fossa in treatment and long-term retention: growth relativity. Am J Orthod Dentofacial Orthop 2000;117:247–266.

104. Voudouris JC, Woodside DG, Altuna G, et al. Condyle-fossa modifications and muscle interactions during Herbst treatment, part 2. Results and conclusions. Am J Orthod Dentofacial Orthop 2003;124:13–29.

105. Voudouris JC, Woodside DG, Altuna G, Kuftinec MM, Angelopoulos G, Bourque PJ. Condyle-fossa modifications and muscle interactions during Herbst treatment, part 1. New technological methods. Am J Orthod Dentofacial Orthop 2003;123:604–613.

106. Pancherz H, Littmann C. [Morphology and position of mandible in Herbst treatment. Cephalometric analysis of changes to end of growth period.] Inf Orthod Kieferorthop 1989; 21:493–513.

107. Popowich K, Nebbe B, Major PW. Effect of Herbst treatment on temporomandibular joint morphology: a systematic literature review. Am J Orthod Dentofacial Orthop 2003;123: 388–394.

108. Hansen K, Pancherz H, Petersson A. Long-term effects of the Herbst appliance on the craniomandibular system with special reference to the TMJ. Eur J Orthod 1990;12:244–253.

109. Hansen K. Post-treatment effects of the Herbst appliance. A radiographic, clinical and biometric investigation. Swed Dent J Suppl 1992;88: 1–49.

110. Leung DK, Hagg U. An electromyographic investigation of the first six months of progressive mandibular advancement of the Herbst appliance in adolescents. Angle Orthod 2001;71:177–184.

111. Hiyama S. [An electromyographic study on functional adaptations – associated with herbst appliance.] Kokubyo Gakkai Zasshi 1996; 63:18–30.

112. Hiyama S, Ono PT, Ishiwata Y, Kuroda T, McNamara JA Jr. Neuromuscular and skeletal adaptations following mandibular forward positioning induced by the Herbst appliance. Angle Orthod 2000;70:442–453.

113. Moeller E. The chewing apparatus. An electromyographic study of the action of the muscles of mastication and its correlation to facial morphology. Acta Physiol Scand 1966;69:sup 280.

114. Athanasiou AE, Papadopoulos MA, Nasiopoulos AT, Ioannidou I, Kolokithas G. Changes in the mechanical advantages of the masseter and temporal muscles and the number and intensity of occlusal contacts following Herbst appliance treatment of Class II, division 1 malocclusion: an early evaluation. J Marmara University Dental Faculty 2004;5:435–444.

The Cantilever Bite Jumper (CBJ)

Joe H. Mayes

Introduction

In 1981 I was privileged to hear Dr Pancherz speak about the Herbst appliance used to correct Class II relationships. The appliance not only corrected a dental Class II to a dental Class I but also offered a marked improvement of the classic Class II facial profile.[1] The facial changes achieved were amazing and predictable once compliance was removed from the treatment plan. I had just placed the last Frankel I was to ever use on my son. I was in the process of giving up on finding removable appliances that would be worn as prescribed.[2] Now I had been introduced to an appliance that was not removable and offered very noticeable profile enhancements.

Throughout the history of orthodontics, headgears, Class II elastics, and surgery have been the most common forms of Class II correction. Other than surgery, all methods of correction involved patient cooperation. Using headgears on normally positioned upper jaws tends to move a normal upper jaw distal to try to match with a retrusive lower jaw. Using Class II elastics to correct Class II relationships only moves teeth and has little, if any, effect on the supporting bone. Their use may also flair the lower incisors beyond desirable esthetic and periodontal ideals.

Surgery, on the other hand, offers a skeletal correction of a mostly skeletal problem.[3]

Careful evaluation of Class II patients will show that 80% or more will have facial esthetic improvement with an advanced lower jaw. I always have the Class II patient slide their lower jaw into a Class I relationship and evaluate the face with the jaw protruded. If the patient has a more balanced profile, they will wear a CBJ. If the face looks Class III, the problem is a dental one and the patient will be corrected using a pendulum device to distalize the upper molars.[4] If the face looks very flat, all efforts will be made to fill the lips after the Class II correction and this is probably a surgery case involving both jaw advancements.

If the Class II patient has a skeletal component and the face is more attractive with the lower jaw forward, a bite-jumping appliance will be used to enhance mandibular growth as much as possible.[5] The most important key to mandibular growth enhancement is timing of the treatment. The later in the growth cycle, the less growth is left to create relapse of the correction. In other words, the ideal treatment time for me to start the case is when I can band or bond the second molars when it becomes time for bracket placement after Class II correction.

If a cemented bite-jumping appliance is used, compliance is eliminated. The appliance cannot be removed and will be worn as requested. Once patient compliance problems were overcome, expected results of controlling growth direction followed (and, to a large extent, the amount of growth in that direction). More recent research indicates that bite-jumping appliances have the ability to inhibit maxillary growth as well as enhancing mandibular growth. It has also been shown that bite-jumping appliances push maxillary molars distal and advance mandibular molars and incisors.[6]

The original bite-jumping appliance (Herbst appliance) was designed by Dr Emil Herbst and reintroduced by Dr Pancherz using maxillary and mandibular first molars and first bicuspids. The bands were connected with heavy wire soldered to each band and carried a tube and piston assembly that allowed mandibular movement but permanently postured the mandible forward.

Multiple designs of this appliance have since been developed and the Cantilever Bite Jumper (CBJ) is one of the most recent. The Cantilever Bite Jumper uses four stainless steel crowns attached to the maxillary and mandibular molars (Fig. 5.1). This is the simplest of

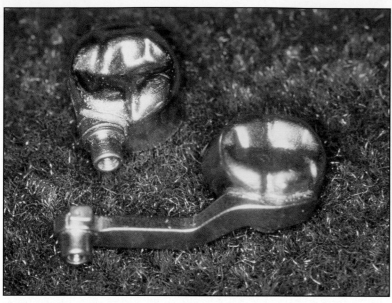

Figure 5.1 Close-up of upper crowns with axles gold braised and lower crowns with cantilever arms gold braised.

attachments as there are only four attachment points, two in each arch. The axles are soldered to the maxillary crowns and the axles are cast with the cantilever arm that is soldered to and extends mesially from the mandibular first molars (Fig. 5.2). A 0.022 × 0.028″ tube is attached to the occlusal part of the cantilever arm just above the axle. This facilitates placement of auxiliary appliances.

Advantages of Using the CBJ

- It is a fixed appliance and eliminates compliance problems.
- There is minimal breakage or loosening of the appliance.
- Stainless steel crowns are less expensive than bands, easier to fit and stay on better than bands.
- The appliance is comfortable and easy to clean.
- Class II corrections more predictable and controlled.
- The patient and parents notice an immediate improvement in facial appearance.
- Because of the auxiliary tube, bonded appliances may be used with the CBJ.

When to Use a CBJ

- If the maxilla has good A/P position (expansion will still be generally required) and a recessive lower jaw is present. If an obtuse nasolabial angle is present and would increase with use of headgear, Class II elastics, upper molar distalization and upper bicuspid extractions or surgery are not an option.
- When early treatment of a skeletal Class II with an anterior open bite is present. After the Class II correction has occurred, the stainless steel crowns are removed and the upper deciduous molars and canines are removed *that day*. The combination of

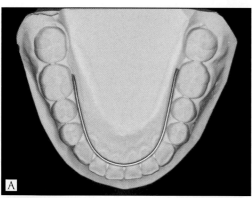

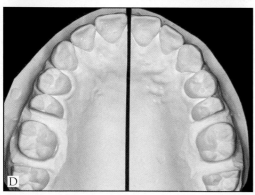

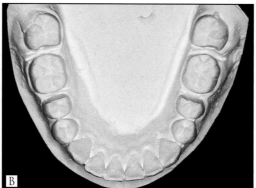

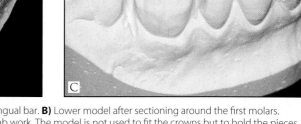

Figure 5.2 A) Model with prefabricated 0.045″ lingual bar. **B)** Lower model after sectioning around the first molars. **C)** Amount of model needed to be removed for lab work. The model is not used to fit the crowns but to hold the pieces in correct relationship and absorb the heat of soldering the lingual bar. **D)** Upper model with sectioning around the first molars and a die saw cut down the midpalatal suture.

Class II correction and deciduous tooth removal accounts for 5–6° of facial axis closure (the molars will be 2–4 mm out of occlusion due to being intruded during treatment).

- With adult patients in whom surgery is not an option and mostly dentoalveolar changes will give an adequate result.

The CBJ works well with my treatment philosophy of only treating Class I uncrowded cases. This is a three-part treatment:

- correct the width
- correct any A/P discrepancies
- place braces on Class I uncrowded cases for as short a time as possible.

It also fits in very well with my treatment efficiency requirements. They fall into four groups and form the acronym PACE.

- Proper diagnosis is the first step.
- Appropriate treatment timing prevents treatment going on too long.
- Compliance-free appliances remove a lot of the variance and quality in treatment.
- Exact bracket placement allows the use of two archwires per arch and an average 9.5–10 months of bracket wearing. Remember, from the patient's perspective there is only one good thing about brackets: their removal when treatment is finished. Everything else is bad: loose brackets, pokey archwires, loose bands, etc. All these things indicate a practice that is not operated at maximum efficiency.

What Occurs During Bite Jumper Therapy?

Clinical and radiographic evidence from my office and research indicates that the following occur with bite jumper therapy.

- Maxillary molars move distally and expand (very slightly).
- Mandibular molars and incisors move mesially.
- Condylar growth and slight remodeling of the fossae occur in growing patients.
- In nongrowing patients (adults), the fossae migrate forward, there is a distal tipping of the head of the condyle and dentoalveolar changes that occur to correct the malocclusion.[7]

An In-Office Clinical Study of 125 Consecutively Treated Cases

In 1986 I started a clinical case study of bite jumper patients to get a better grasp of what was occurring with their treatment. I divided 125 consecutively treated CBJ patients into five groups of 25 each. Each group contained 25 consecutively treated and similar cases.[8]

In the first group, the mandibles were advanced in 3 mm increments. The advancements were done at 8-week intervals until a super Class I occlusion was achieved. This position was held for

9 months. The second group consisted of 25 consecutively treated patients with their mandibles brought to a super Class I and held there for 12 months. In the third group of 25, the mandibles were advanced to a super Class I as in the second group; the difference was that full maxillary braces were placed with tiebacks for more maxillary anchorage. The fourth group was the same as the third group with the addition of a mandibular lip bumper attached to the mandibular cantilever arms. The fifth and final group consisted of adults to measure their orthodontic and orthopedic results.

Results of the Study

When the mandible was advanced 3 mm in the first group, the mandibular incisors advanced 1.6–3.1 mm, with an average advancement of 2.3 mm. The maxillary molars moved distally 2.1–5.4 mm, with an average distal movement of 3.8 mm. Mandibular growth of this group was 1.1–3.0 mm more than growth forecasting predicted, with an average of 1.9 mm more growth than predicted.

In the second group, when the mandible was advanced immediately to a super Class I, the mandibular incisors advanced 0.5–1.3 mm with an average of 0.9 mm. The maxillary molars were distalized 0.9–3.8 mm with an average of 1.7 mm distalization. Mandibular growth was 1.9–4.1 mm more than growth forecasts predicted, with an average of 2.8 mm more growth.

The third group consisted of immediate advancements to super Class I in conjunction with maxillary braces for anchorage. In this group the mandibular incisors advanced 0.4–1.2 mm with an average advancement of 0.8 mm. Maxillary molars moved distal 0.0–0.3 mm with an average distal movement of 0.2 mm. Mandibular growth exceeded the predicted amount by 2.6–6.1 mm, with an average of 3.9 mm.

The fourth group was the same as the third group with the exception of a fixed mandibular lip bumper. In this group, mandibular incisors moved forward 0.6–1.4 mm and advanced an average of 0.7 mm. The maxillary molars moved distally 0.0–0.4 mm with an average of 0.2 mm distalization. Mandibular growth exceeded forecasting by 2.4–6 mm, with an average of 3.9 mm.

In the adult group (average age 22+ years), the mandibular incisors advanced 0.9–2.5 mm and averaged 2.1 mm of advancement. Maxillary molars were moved distally 2.1–6.2 mm and averaged 3.7 mm. This group's mandibles showed an average forward growth/movement of 2.1 mm. Also, it was noted that the fossae migrated mesially an average of 0.8 mm.

Conclusions from the Study

This in-office study of 125 consecutively treated cases suggests several things. First, if more dental change is needed, the appliance should be advanced in smaller increments. Second, if more skeletal change is desired, the appliance should be advanced immediately to a super Class I and maintained. With a large forward jump of the mandible, the appliance seems to become a muscle-driven system.

This is due in large part to the teeth becoming extremely sore if the pressure from the rod stop resting on the end of the tube transmits large forces to the teeth. Third, it was noted that lip bumpers have little or no effect on treatment outcomes when using bite jumpers. Finally, it appeared that there is a small component of skeletal change in adults. As a general rule, adults will not tolerate advances beyond 3 mm, but both skeletal and dental changes occur to correct the Class II relationship (most of the time a Nance is placed to maintain the maxillary molar distalization).

In-Office Delivery of the CBJ

Most Class II malocclusions will require maxillary expansion when the mandible is postured forward into a super Class I occlusion. This may be checked by having the patient slide the lower jaw forward to edge-to-edge incisors. If separators and upper impression are done at this visit, a maxillary expander can be delivered at the next visit. The RPE screw is prebent and the 0.060″ wires are cut to length and the anterior tip rounded.[9]

At the next or delivery appointment, bands are fit on the maxillary molars and a new impression is made with the bands in place. The bands are placed in the impression and held in place with 0.016″ wires. The impression is poured in plaster with slurry water. At this time separators are placed for the mandibular molars and a mandibular impression is made to premake the CBJ lingual bar. In a few minutes the model with the bands on it is ready to solder the premade upper expander. After soldering and polishing, the appliance is trial fit in the mouth. The RPE (rapid palatal expander) is cemented with glass ionomer cement and the parents are shown how to make the necessary turns for the desired expansion. The patient is scheduled to return in 3 weeks for delivery of the CBJ.

The maxillary model used to premake the upper expander and the mandibular model are relieved around the first molars and a 0.045″ lingual bar is bent to fit the mandibular model (see Fig. 5.2). The maxillary model is then sectioned with a die saw through the midpalatal suture. This cut will allow separation of the two halves of the maxilla to duplicate what happens with the RPE. The two halves of the model will facilitate making the transpalatal bar that will maintain the expansion and is removed in 3 months.

The RPE is removed when the patient returns for delivery of the CBJ and cleaned in preparation for its use in the lab. Stainless steel crowns from the CBJ kit are fit in the mouth and any adjustments to the cantilever arms are made at this time. Measure the distance from the mesial of the axle on the maxillary molar to the distal of the axle on the cantilever with the lower jaw postured forward the desired amount. These measurements will allow the correct selection of the precut rod and tube assemblies and posture the mandible in the desired position when the appliance is delivered (Fig. 5.3).

The maxillary model halves are placed on a soldering tile. The removed RPE is placed on the two halves and each half held to the tile with sticky wax. The RPE is carefully removed and the stainless steel crowns with axles already attached to them are placed on the first molars. As the stainless steel crowns fit looser than bands, the

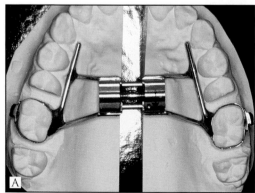
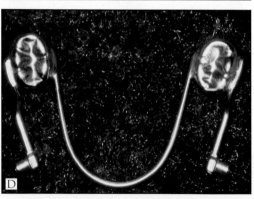
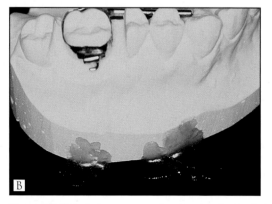
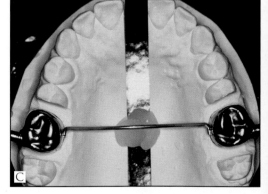

Figure 5.3 A) Typical upper expander placed on the two halves of the upper model to simulate expansion. **B)** Sticky wax is used to attach the model to the soldering tile to hold the two halves of the upper model at the correct expansion. **C)** 0.045″ palatal bar ready for soldering to the upper crowns fit in the mouth. **D)** Soldered and polished lower part of the appliance.

resultant play allows this technique to work very well. A 0.045″ transpalatal bar is bent and soldered to the lingual of the maxillary crowns (see Fig. 5.3).

The prebent 0.045″ lingual bar and lower stainless steel crowns are placed on the mandibular model and any adjustments made. The crowns and lingual bar are then held in place with sticky wax. The mandibular part of the CBJ is soldered and both upper and lower parts of the appliance are polished. Select the premeasured rod and tube assemblies. These have been previously cut to length and the rod ends rounded. The attachment to the axles have been routed and beveled to allow as much lateral excursive movement as possible (Fig. 5.4). The tubes are attached to the maxillary crowns using Ceka-Bond on the screw threads. At this time the appliance is ready for trial fit in the mouth.

Once the CBJ has been correctly fit in the mouth, it is removed and the final steps (Fig. 5.5) completed before cementing with glass ionomer cement (gold Protech is my favorite). The crowns are notched on the mesiobuccal of the mandibular crowns and the maxillary crowns are notched on the mesiopalatal. These notches will facilitate crown removal when therapy is completed. The final preparation is to crimp the crowns for a better fit. Once the appliance is ready for cementation and the crowns are approximately half full of cement, dry the molars and with a Q-tip place a thin layer of Chapstick in the occlusal anatomy. This will make clean-up easier when the appliance is removed. Do not use Vaseline as its viscosity

may allow it to flow over the side of the teeth and affect the strength of cementation.[9]

The rods are placed in the tubes and guided over the axles on the cantilever arms. Check to make sure the position of the mandible is correct. Positioning can be adjusted with shims on the rod which force advancement of that side's mandibular axle. When the mandible is in the desired position and posterior separators have been placed over the axles on the cantilever arms, attach the rods using Ceka-Bond on the screw threads (Figs 5.6 and 5.7). The appliance may be adjusted at any time in the future in the same way. However, the Ceka-Bond does not allow the screws to become loose. Therefore, use a pair of pliers to twist the screw a quarter turn before using the hex head, to prevent stripping of the inside of the screw head.

CBJ Removal

The Chapstick that was placed in the occlusal grooves and the notching of the crowns will make CBJ removal much easier. The crowns are divided with a #557 bur in a high-speed handpiece. The cut is started at the notch and continued up the side of the crown and along the central groove. The mandibular crown is grasped with the cantilever arm and twisted to remove the crown. The maxillary crown is easily removed by placing a small screwdriver in the cut in the central groove and twisting to break the cement

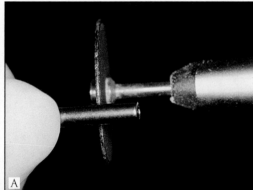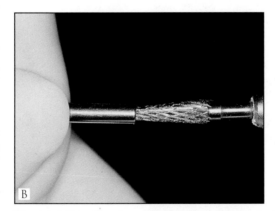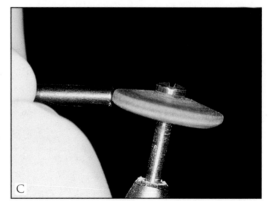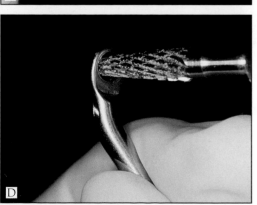

Figure 5.4 A) Cutting tubes to length. **B)** Removing burs in the tube. **C)** Rounding and smoothing the cut tube. **D)** Opening the part of the tube that slides over the upper axle to increase lateral range of motion.

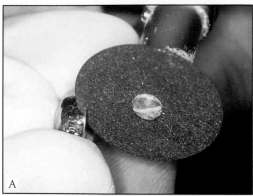

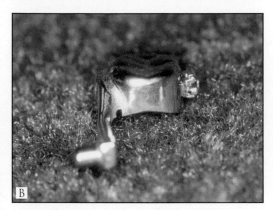

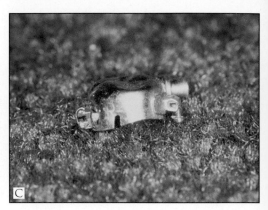

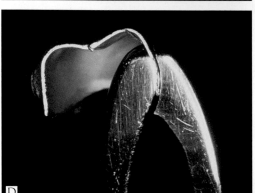

Figure 5.5 A) Separating disk used to notch the crowns before cementation. Note direction of rotation of the disk. **B)** Notched lower crowns on the mesiobuccal. **C)** Notched upper crowns on the mesiopalatal. **D)** Cutaway of crown showing effectiveness of the crown crimping plier.

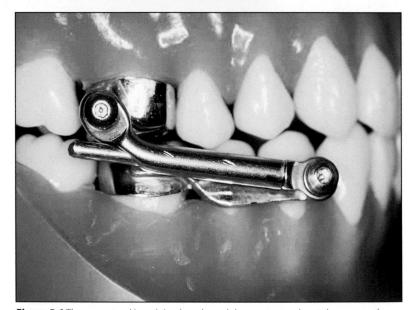

Figure 5.6 The correct rod length is when the rod does not extend past the upper axle.

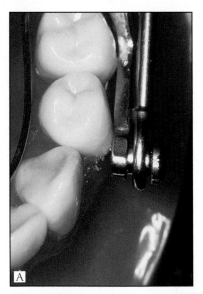

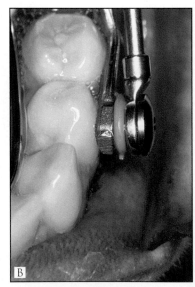

Figure 5.7 A shows original straight rod, **B** shows new offset rod with separator on axle and large head screw.

seal. Normally a large chip of cement will be removed as there was no attachment to the occlusal anatomy. The remaining cement may be removed by scraping or bond removing burs. The first molars will have been intruded as a result of the crowns opening the bite, but the molars will be extruded to normal position with the first archwire.

Instructions and Information

Patients and parents should be advised of difficulties in chewing during the first 3–7 days. Once the patient adjusts, they will forget that the appliance is in place for the most part. Patients are instructed to eat a soft diet and chew small bites. Offer them encouragement and

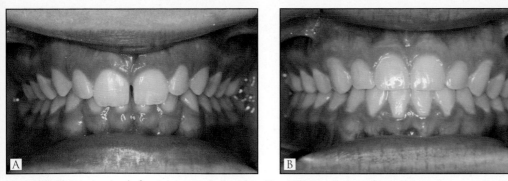

Figure 5.8 A) Anterior view before treatment of a deep bite Class II. **B)** Anterior view after treatment.

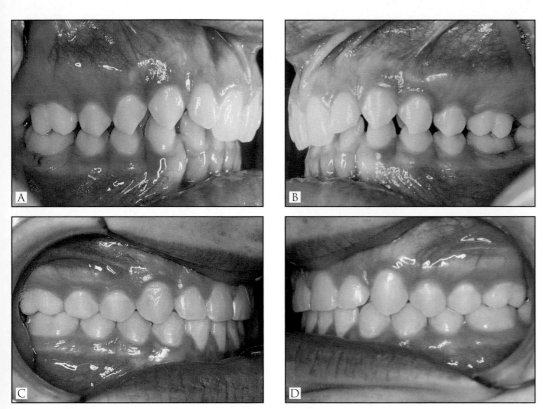

Figure 5.9 A,B) Buccal views of before treatment of a deep bite Class II. **C,D)** Buccal views after treatment.

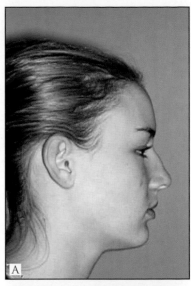

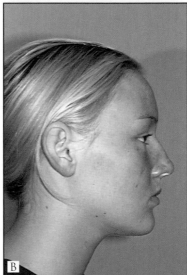

Figure 5.10 Profile views (**A**) before and (**B**) after CBJ treatment.

have them look at their new profile using a double mirror technique. Make patients and parents aware of potential problems such as the appliance coming apart on opening wide, loose screws, breakage, etc. Information leaflets can be helpful for patients.

Case Studies

Patient 1 presented with a dental and skeletal Class II malocclusion. A deep bite with lingually tipped upper anteriors and no crowding was noted. The treatment plan called for an upper expander followed by CBJ therapy to correct the dental and skeletal problem followed by full corrective appliances. Treatment time was 23 months and involved 13 total visits from new patient exam to retainer delivery (Figs 5.8–5.10).

Patient 2 presented with a unilateral Class II malocclusion of his left side and fairly good Class I occlusion on his right side. He also had a mandibular shift to the left of the middle of his face. Nonextraction treatment was chosen, using an upper expander followed by unilateral CBJ correction of the midline and Class II on his left. Unilateral cases

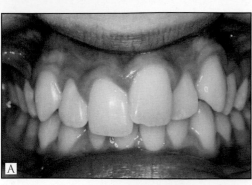
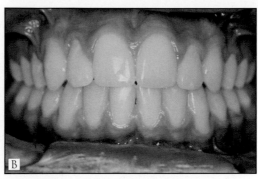

Figure 5.11 A) Anterior view before treatment of a unilateral Class II case. **B)** Anterior view after treatment.

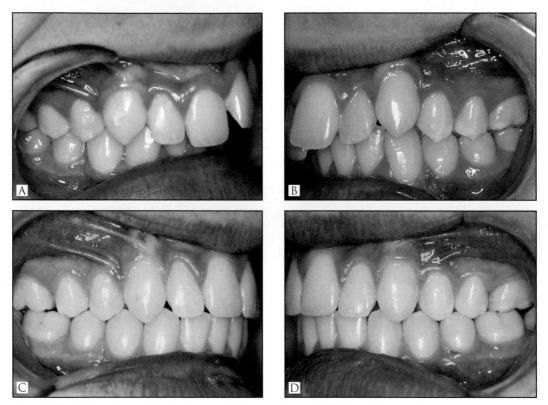

Figure 5.12 A,B) Buccal views of before treatment of a unilateral Class II. **C,D)** Buccal views after treatment.

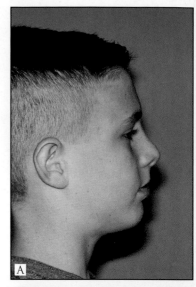
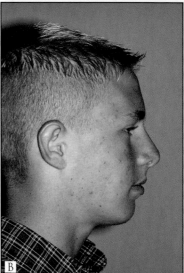

Figure 5.13 Profile views of before (**A**) and after (**B**) treatment of a unilateral Class II case. Note the slight profile improvement characteristic of unilateral cases.

do not achieve the same profile improvements that bilateral corrections do. His treatment involved 21 months of active treatment and 14 visits from new patient exam to retainer delivery (Figs 5.11–5.13).

Patient 3 presented with a Class II malocclusion with severe crowding and a retrognathic mandible. Due to the amount of crowding in the arches, extraction therapy was instigated followed by upper expansion and CBJ therapy. Full appliances were placed for space closure and final detailing of the occlusion.

Treatment time was 24 months with 15 visits from new patient exam to retainer delivery. Note the marked profile improvement (Figs 5.14–5.16).

Conclusion

My overall treatment philosophy is to correct any width problems first. Next, correct any anterior–posterior problems. Third, and

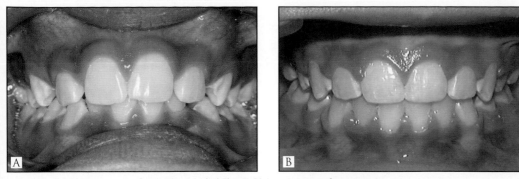

Figure 5.14 A) Anterior view of severely crowded Class II. **B)** Anterior view after treatment.

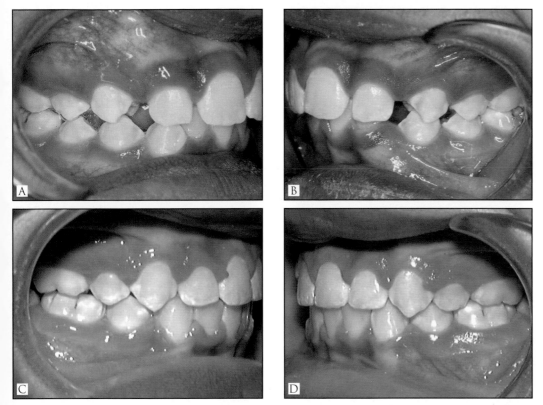

Figure 5.15 A,B) Buccal views before treatment of a severely crowded Class II case. **C,D)** Buccal views after treatment.

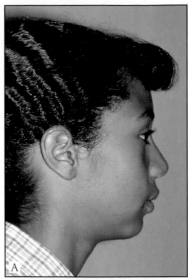

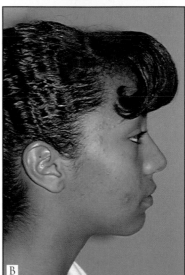

Figure 5.16 Profile views before (**A**) and after (**B**) treatment of a severely crowded Class II.

finally, place brackets on Class I uncrowded cases for the shortest time possible. The CBJ works well with my treatment philosophy. The appliance may be adjusted to offer more or less skeletal correction. When a CBJ is used for skeletal Class II corrections, the time patients spend in full brackets is substantially reduced and a more balanced profile is achieved.

References

1. Pancherz H. Treatment of class II malocclusions by jumping the bite with the Herbst appliance. A cephalometric investigation. Am J Orthod 1979;76:423–442.

2. Wieslander L, Lagerstrom L. The effect of activator treatment on class II malocclusions. Am J Orthod 1979;75:20–26.

3. Mayes JH. Improving appliance efficiency with the cantilever Herbst. Clin Impressions 1994; 3:2–5,17–19.

4. Faulkner J. An interview with Dr Joe Mayes on the Cantilever Bite Jumper. Orthodontic CYBERjournal, 1997. Available online at: www.oc-j.com/issue5/mayes.htm

5. McNamara JA Jr. Components of class II malocclusion in children 8–10 years of age. Angle Orthod 1981;51:177–202.

6. Valant JR, Sinclair PM. Treatment effects of the Herbst appliance. Am J Orthod Dentofacial Orthop 1989;95:138–147.

7. Mayes JH. The single-appointment preattached Cantilever Bite-Jumper. Clin Impressions 1996; 5:14–17,23. Available online at: www.ormco.com/learning/publications/ci/index.cfm

8. Sachdeva R. Orthodontics for the next millennium. Orange, CA: Ormco; 1987: 301–309.

9. Mayes JH. Bite jumper enhancements. Clin Impressions 1998;7:12–15. Available online at: www.ormco.com/learning/publications/ci/index.cfm

CHAPTER 6

The Ritto Appliance® — an easy way to treat Class II malocclusions

António Korrodi Ritto

CONTENTS

Introduction

In orthodontics there are multiple options available for treating Class II malocclusions. The degree of difficulty for Class II treatment depends on the accompanying disorder. Class II division 1 malocclusions are considered to be the most frequent problem encountered in orthodontics.[1] McNamara[2] and Bass[3] consider that skeletal mandibular retrusion is the most common characteristic in this type of malocclusion.

Functional appliances have been used for many years and the selection of which to use varies with the type of skeletal and dental anomaly, the growth pattern, and the operator's preference.[4] The appearance of fixed functional appliances dates from the beginning of the 1900s, when Emil Herbst presented his system to the International Dental Congress in Berlin. Very little was published on this appliance until the 1970s, when Hans Pancherz rekindled interest with the publication of several articles on Herbst's appliance (Dentaurum, Ispringen, Germany).[5] It was only towards the end of the 1980s that different systems, derived from Herbst's appliance, began to appear, which have drawn special attention.

This chapter will describe the author's approach to this type of malocclusion. From the experience gained after many years of using different techniques, a simplified treatment approach will be presented. In addition to giving the patient the best treatment possible, the procedure adopted needs to be as easy as possible for all parties involved, including the patient. The approach detailed below not only gives the patient the best results but also keeps them happy, which is satisfying for everyone.

When to Treat

Early Class II treatment has provoked a controversial debate. There has been considerable discussion in the orthodontic literature regarding the biologic and clinical advantages and disadvantages of early orthodontic treatment. Early treatment for Class II malocclusion is frequently undertaken with the objective of correcting skeletal disproportion by altering the growth pattern.[6]

The timing of early treatment involves intervention in primary dentition, early mixed dentition (permanent first molars and incisors present), and late mid-mixed dentition (intertransitional period, before the emergence of first premolars and permanent mandibular canines). On one hand, the public is increasingly asking for interceptive care and general dentists are alerted to orthodontic problems, referring patients in deciduous or mixed dentition, while at the same time orthodontists know that some problems cannot be fully corrected until all teeth have erupted.

Early treatment can take advantage of normal growth to correct malocclusions before they become severe. It seems desirable to stimulate mandibular growth as much as possible in young patients with severely retrognathic mandibles in the hope of avoiding more complex treatment after maturity. For this reason, many orthodontists prefer to intervene early with orthopedic treatment in order to decrease skeletal dysplasia before patients with Class II malocclusions reach their teens.[6,7] There is a greater ability to modify the growth process with the added possibility of having a second stage to repeat the procedure (better use of growth potential). Treatment in late mixed dentition gives the clinician only one chance at correction and, if cooperation is poor, the result may be unsatisfactory. Other benefits of early treatment include improvement in the patient's self-esteem and parent satisfaction.

Facial esthetics has been found to be a significant determinant of self and social perceptions and attributions, which may influence psychologic development from early childhood to adulthood. The individual's interactions with and responses from others may influence the development of the self-concept.

Early treatment of deleterious habits is easier than treatment after years of habit reinforcement. Compliance is also believed to be greater because younger patients are considered to be more cooperative and attentive than adolescents.

The opposite view is that we cannot be certain that the results of early treatment will be sustained. Early treatment may not only cause damage or prolong therapy; it may also exhaust the child's spirit of cooperation and compliance. The total treatment time is longer when the observation period between the two stages is also considered. Sometimes it is very difficult to explain to parents that 6–8 years is not a long treatment period. Two or three phases of treatment lead to patient burnout and parent dissatisfaction.

When esthetic aspects are involved, motivation for treatment may also be higher than during earlier periods of development because the adolescent is often more concerned about facial appearance.

Conversely, a number of factors discourage early treatment, including decalcification under bands left for too long, impaction of maxillary canines by prematurely uprighting the roots of the lateral incisors, impaction of maxillary second molars from distalizing first molars, and the need for a second phase of treatment after eruption of the permanent teeth.

There is no clinically important difference in the outcomes of two-stage and one-stage Class II treatment except for a longer treatment time in two-stage samples.[8] As these authors note, "For children with moderate to severe Class II problems, early treatment followed by later comprehensive treatment on average does not produce major differences in jaw relationship or dental occlusion, compared with later one-stage treatment." We cannot as yet find any evidence data to refute these conclusions.

In recent years general opinion on this issue has been to treat Class II discrepancies during growth. However, some authors have shown that it is possible to treat such patients in late adolescence or as young adults, stating that:

> It is now time to revise the above concept in skeletal Class II therapy using age as a decisive factor when choosing between a growth adaptive or surgical approach. This is because of the fact that research has disclosed that growth in the temporomandibular joint (TMJ) region can continue for many years after the age of 20 or it can be reactivated at this later age.[9]

Paulsen & Karle investigated morphologic changes in the TMJs of two patients with Class II division 1 malocclusion in adulthood after cessation of endochondral growth (union of the radius epiphysis) with an asymmetric sagittal molar occlusion, treated with the Herbst appliance and followed for 2 years.[10] They concluded that TMJs exhibit asymmetric, adaptive bone growth, normalizing the sagittal molar occlusion.

The main objective of therapy with functional appliances is to induce supplementary lengthening of the mandible by stimulating increased growth at the condylar cartilage. The effectiveness of functional treatment of mandibular growth deficiencies strongly depends on the biologic responsiveness of the condylar cartilage, which in turn depends on the growth rate of the mandible.[11] It is well known that the growth rate of the human mandible is not constant throughout development. A peak in mandibular growth velocity (pubertal growth spurt) has been described in many previous cephalometric studies.[12,13] Clinical research has demonstrated that the greatest effects of functional appliances take place when the mandibular growth peak is included in the treatment period. Hagg & Pancherz found that sagittal growth at the condyle in patients treated with the Herbst appliance at the pubertal growth peak was twice that observed in patients treated 3 years before or 3 years after the peak.[14]

Petrovic et al revealed that some removable functional appliances (activator, Frankel, and bionator) are more effective when they are used during the ascending portion of the individual pubertal growth spurt.[15] Malmgren et al demonstrated significantly greater skeletal effects induced by the Bass appliance in boys treated during the peak period than in those treated in the pre-peak period.[16] McNamara et al described less dramatic changes in mandibular length in subjects who started treatment with the Frankel FR-2 appliance during early to mid-mixed dentition (average age 8.8 years) than in those starting treatment during late mixed to early permanent dentitions (average age 11.6 years).[17] Baccetti et al revealed that the optimum treatment timing for twin-block therapy for Class II disharmony appears to be during or slightly after the onset of the pubertal peak in growth velocity.[18]

It has been claimed that the functional correctors promote forward growth of the mandible[19–21] and restriction of the maxilla,[22–24] while others claim that the effects are purely dentoalveolar with few or no skeletal effects.[25,26] The majority of researchers agree that there is retroclination of the upper incisor teeth during treatment[27–29] and that proclination of the lower incisors is a common finding, although it is maintained that this is an effect of a poorly constructed and handled appliance.[30,31] We find this controversial debate in the literature, but very few authors report advantages of the functional treatment.[32]

Why Use a Functional Approach?

The benefits of using a fixed functional appliance include the 24-hour growth stimulus, but there are other, more important factors.

- Immediate alteration of the profile, smile and facial expressions that helps to improve psychologic problems.
- Improvement of skeletal disharmony.
- Periodontal problems caused by deep overbite can be prevented.
- Traumatic injuries on upper incisors have less opportunity to occur.
- Sucking habits immediately disappear.
- Labial competence is established and mastication is improved.
- Oropharyngeal space is increased, as well as space for the tongue.
- Functional problems like mouth breathing and speech difficulties are improved.

There are some psychologic, traumatic, and functional factors that could influence the decision for early treatment.[33] It is important to note that with removable functional appliances or elastics, many of the improvements described will not happen immediately after fitting the appliance. With the fixed devices, this is different due to a constant change in mandibular position and free palatal space for the tongue.

Psychological Factors

The early orthodontic correction of the morphologic and functional problems that adversely affect a patient's psychology could help eliminate a potential inferiority complex and also have a beneficial effect on general personality development. The appearance of the mouth and smile plays an important role in physical attraction. Nobody doubts that the visible aspects of Class II malocclusions can lead to low self-esteem.

Facial esthetics are a determining factor in social perception and influence psychologic development from childhood to adolescence. Individual interaction with peer groups has a great influence on the development of self-esteem. For example, during school life, being singled out and taunted with nicknames could contribute to the development of psychologic problems.

Sometimes the child has a "strange" appearance and parents force them to close their mouth, and make derogatory observations such as "You look weird." Constant pressure of this nature can promote negative feelings to the patient.

Due to the anatomic skeletal position of the mandible, maxilla, and teeth, together with lip incompetence, mastication is sometimes very difficult and food can fall from the mouth. Saliva can also appear at the corners of the lips during nonmasticatory movements. It is common to hear from parents that their child has difficulties masticating and takes a long time to eat. Frequently, parents state that "My child eats as though he was backward" and that they are embarrassed to take them to restaurants. Furthermore, this can contribute to psychologic problems. It is worse when parents force the child to close their lips during mastication, saying "It is not good manners to chew with your mouth open." When faced with a patient going through such difficulties or psychologic problems, early treatment is called for.

Traumatic Factors

Due to its anatomo-geographic situation, the anterior area is the most affected zone in facial trauma. When dentition protrudes, as in Class II division 1 malocclusion, the possibility of trauma in this area increases.

It is important to evaluate the personality of the patient. The probability of injury is greater if the child is energetic or highly active, absent-minded, inattentive or with a debilitated motor system or if they take part in active sports. It is advisable to be careful with front teeth and orthodontic treatment can be justified in such situations.

In the same way, in deep overbite cases lower incisors can injure the palatal mucosa and the degree of severity can vary from just an impression to gingival recession. Thus, in these cases it is also important to make an evaluation and decide if treatment should be started.

Functional Factors

All problems related to respiratory functions, phonation, deglutition, and mastication should be evaluated so as to establish an adequate treatment plan. This type of malocclusion is often accompanied by problems of buccal respiration, atypical deglutition with lingual interposition, deficient mastication (with little lateral movement), and incorrect pronunciation of certain words.

Oral habits as primary etiologic factors of malocclusion may lead to abnormal growth and development of craniofacial structures and may interfere with the successful progress of orthodontic treatment. The most common oral habits are finger sucking, lip biting, nail biting, tongue sucking, infantile swallowing, and oral respiration. It is important to know that the advance of the mandible in Class II cases can help to improve functions and eliminate habits.

In open bite and large overjet cases, a tongue-thrust swallow pattern is present as well as altered tongue posture. Resting tongue posture can be easily assessed by visual inspection when the teeth are slightly apart immediately following deglutition, or by more sophisticated methods. It is also essential to have a conversation with the patient and check tongue posture during speech. The lingual pearl is the appliance of choice to treat tongue posture problems during Class II therapy.[34-38]

True macroglossia is rare and an apparently large tongue is presumably the result of a forward tongue posture. Proffit[39] and Graber[40] demonstrated that forces from the tongue and lips in the rest position are primary factors in dental equilibrium. Tongue posture usually depends on anatomic relationships in the pharynx. Also mouth respiration is common in patients with adenoidal tissue blockage of the nasal airway.

Correction of such dysfunctions may involve long treatment periods. The degree of difficulty in correcting these dysfunctions varies from patient to patient. All oral dysfunctions should be eliminated so as to avoid residual etiologic factors after concluding treatment.

It is important to evaluate the severity of the existing problems and estimate the improvement that could result from orthopedic correction at an earlier stage of growth or with a two-phase treatment.

How to Treat

Fixed and removable appliances have various advantages and disadvantages.

Removable appliances are quite large, have unstable fixation and cause discomfort. There is no tactile sensibility and space for the tongue is reduced, which can cause swallowing and speech difficulties. Due to their large size, they can easily affect esthetics. They are for use at night and for partial daytime sessions so the clinician does not have good control over patient cooperation.

In contrast, fixed functional appliances can often produce undesirable dental movements, such as teeth rotations and lower incisor proclination. It is essential to have good anchorage, so it is necessary to include a large number of teeth in the fixed appliance and sometimes additional anchorage devices are required.

The main advantage of treatment with functional appliances and elastics is the possibility of advancing the mandible in a correct position, thus contributing to the enhancement of oral functions, rapid improvement of profile, and the elimination of psychologic problems.

The Ritto Appliance® (KS 2400-194 Leiria, Portugal) is recommended for correction of Class II malocclusion with mandibular deficiency in mixed or permanent dentition using only conventional bands on the upper molars and two tubes on the lower molars with brackets on the lower incisors.[32,33,35,41–44] The Ritto Appliance can be described as a miniaturized telescopic device with simplified intraoral application and activation. It has been developed over a 12-year period with the goal of creating an efficient appliance with a telescopic action that is both miniature and versatile[33] (Fig. 6.1). It is supplied in a single format, which allows it to be used on both sides, and it is available in only two sizes.

The appliance does not come apart (no disengagement after achieving maximum extension) which provides enormous advantages: it eliminates the time lost in measuring length before fitting, as is the case with competitor appliances. This facility makes it possible to fit the appliance in around 5 minutes and only about half that time is required to remove it. This also contributes to the avoidance of posterior impingement of the cheek. The smaller size facilitates adaptation, it is simple to use, comfortable, cost-effective, fracture resistant, it does not affect esthetic appearance or speech and requires no patient cooperation.

Fixing accessories consist of a steel ball-pin and a lock (Fig. 6.2). Upper fixing is carried out by placing a steel ball-pin into the tube

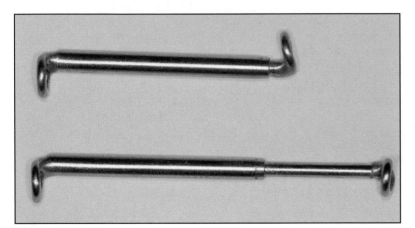

Figure 6.1 The Ritto Appliance is a miniaturized telescopic device.

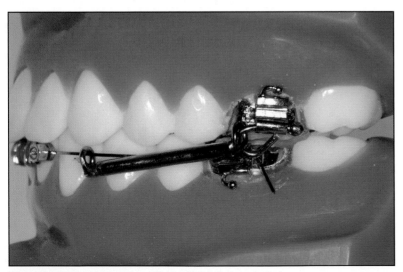

Figure 6.2 Fixing accessories consist of a steel ball-pin and a lock.

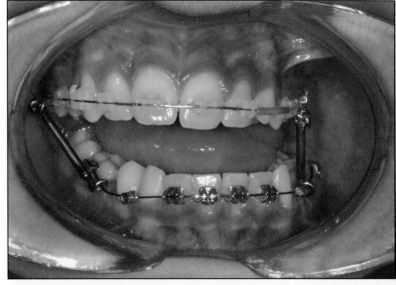

Figure 6.3 This fixation gives freedom to the appliance.

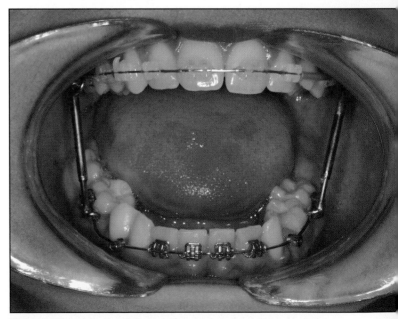

Figure 6.4 The patient can fully open the mouth and make lateral movements.

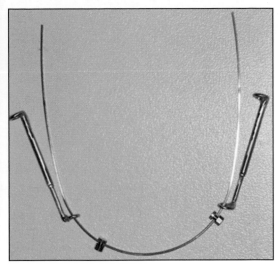

Figure 6.5 Preparation of the lower arch before fitting into the lower molar tubes.

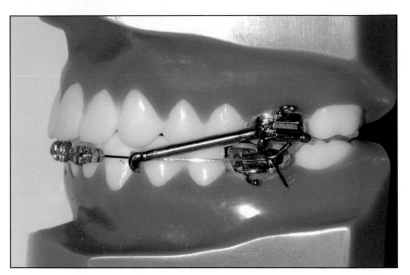

Figures 6.6, 6.7 Activation is achieved by sliding the lock along the lower arch in the distal direction and then fixing it against the Ritto Appliance.

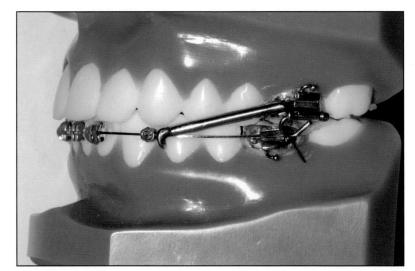

Figure 6.7

0.045″ from the upper molar band crossing the appliance, which is then totally bent over. With this fixation the patient can perform lateral movements without limitation (Figs 6.3 and 6.4). The appliance is fixed onto the lower arch, which has to be prepared before insertion. The thickness and type of archwire are chosen, its length is adjusted, locks are fitted and the Ritto Appliance is then inserted (Fig. 6.5). The size of the lower archwire should be a 0.017 × 0.025″ stainless steel, which should be replaced every 3–4 weeks, with a 0.022″ lower tube slot and a 0.018″ lower incisor bracket slot. Activation is achieved by sliding the lock along the lower arch in the distal direction and then fixing it against the Ritto Appliance (Figs 6.6 and 6.7).

The following factors are important for the success of treatment and the biomechanical considerations.[33]

Choice of Patient

Choosing a patient for orthopedic correction with a fixed functional appliance is not complicated as long as a few important guidelines are taken into consideration. It is possible to make an unsuitable choice and in this case other solutions have to be sought.

Type of Malocclusion

The Ritto Appliance was initially developed with the aim of treating Class II division 1 malocclusions with mandibular deficiency that present an overjet over 6 mm. The candidate should still be growing, have a brachy- or mesofacial skeletal pattern and be preferably in transition from mixed to permanent dentition (see Patient 2, below).

Facial Profile

Analysis of facial esthetics is highly valuable in patient evaluation. If there is an improvement in profile when the mandible is advanced to

Class I, then it will be advantageous to carry out this type of correction (see Patient 1, below).

Dental Contacts

The condyle and incisor guide may be responsible for the appearance of a posterior open bite when the mandible is advanced. If there are no significant sagittal and transversal problems, then when advancing the mandible, contact of the posterior teeth will appear. The greater the Spee curve, the greater the space will be that is created between the premolars and molars. However, if it is important to start the treatment early without the alignment phase, artificial contacts can be created on upper molars and the transversal and sagittal dimension corrected at the same time (Figs 6.8–6.10). It is possible to advance

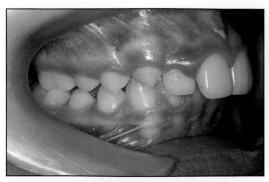

Figure 6.8 If the curve of Spee is severe before treatment, when the mandible is advanced there is a posterior open bite.

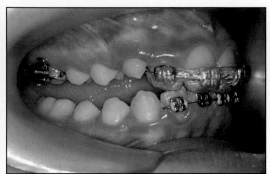

Figure 6.9 The mandible is advanced.

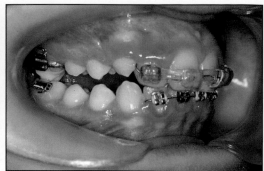

Figure 6.10 Composite artificial contacts can be bonded on molars to give more comfort and stability when chewing.

a mandible with a pronounced Spee curve and use the advantages gained from the correction carried out at the expense of the extrusion of the posterior sectors in a meso- or brachyfacial patient. If anterior contact is made on a bite plan (as with a lingual technique), an intrusion of the incisors can also be achieved. This investigation should be carried out during the first appointment and the more contact there is, the greater the initial stability will be.

Muscular Elasticity

Good muscular elasticity can be appreciated when the patient is asked to advance the mandible with lips touching. In these patients, there is no great muscular contraction. Another manner of checking is through the lip separators when intraoral photographs are taken. If elasticity is good then the first molars and sometimes even second molars will be seen. These patients demonstrate greater adaptation ability. Electromyography can be used to evaluate the patient's capacity to maintain the mandible advanced.

Cooperative Ability

Although this is a fixed appliance, cooperation is important throughout the whole treatment process. The explanation given to parents about correction usually prompts immediate responses about their child's behavior (whether they are careful, obedient, etc.).

The Secret of Success

Negative opinions are sometimes expressed by colleagues who have tried fixed functional appliances unsuccessfully. Many orthodontists have experienced the frustration of continual breakage that discourages the use of fixed functional appliances (FFA). Fracture is cited as the most common cause for dissatisfaction. After one bad experience, some orthodontists are unwilling to try again and conceive a great dislike of this form of treatment.

The keys to success have never been properly described but they are essential in order to keep the patient motivated and focused. When they are properly followed, the risk of fracture in support

systems is considerably reduced as well as the risk of lower incisor proclination.

1 The choice of patient is fundamental. However, it is always possible to make a bad judgment (see Choice of patient, above).

2 After the orthodontic stage (with the arches coordinated), the patient should use a mini stimulator for mandibular advancement for 2 months. In functional treatment with FFAs, it is necessary to prepare the patient for 1–2 months before fitting the appliance so as to stimulate musculature and avoid the patient exerting too much force on the support systems, fracturing them or originating unwanted dental movement. For this reason, the use of a mini stimulator for mandibular advancement is advised.[33] This is a thermoformed splint of 0.7 mm in thickness, only for the upper incisors, and incorporates an acrylic bite block for the lower incisors constructed with the mandible in a forward position (Figs 6.11–6.13). For the first 15 days or 1 month, the patient should wear the splint for as long as possible and maintain the lower incisors fitted into the bite block. In the following weeks, the patient should start to carry out swallowing exercises, with lips in contact and incisors against the bite block.

Only after this stage should therapy be started with the Ritto Appliance, given that the musculature has already been stimulated and the patient has memorized the forward position of the mandible. Deblocking of the occlusion is also achieved.

It is possible to fit the Ritto Appliance in conjunction with the mini stimulator for the first few weeks (Fig. 6.14).

3 Arch coordination must be done so that when the mandible is advanced, the maximum possible number of posterior contacts is obtained. These contacts provide stability and comfort when chewing and help to achieve faster adaptation. It is through the initial orthodontic stage that the necessary leveling out is done. Posterior contacts contribute to comfort and rapid patient adaptation after the advance of the mandible. This also creates a posterior proprioceptive sensibility. It is not always

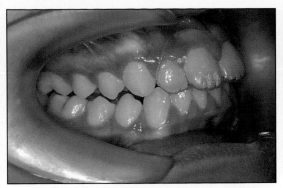

Figure 6.11 The mini stimulator is a thermoformed splint with an acrylic bite block for the lower incisors, made with the mandible advanced in Class I.

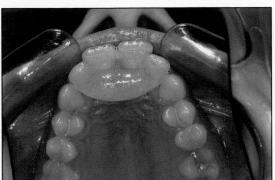

Figure 6.12 Acrylic bite block on the lower incisors.

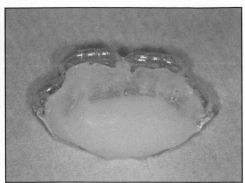

Figure 6.13 Acrylic bite block.

necessary to have perfect coordination of the arches before starting functional treatment. Sometimes, even with a pronounced Spee curve, therapy can be started as long as some artificial contacts are constructed with composite on the molars (see Fig. 6.10). The extrusion of the premolars can be beneficial in the correction of a vertical problem.

Activation

There are no scientific data available on how many millimeters the mandible should be advanced. There are authors who prefer to carry out an immediate advance from edge to edge.[5] There are others who carry out progressive advances every month and even those who follow the two-thirds rule of the condyle test.[45]

An initial exaggerated advance of the mandible would provoke intolerance to the appliance and there would be a tendency to fracture. With the Ritto Appliance, the activation will be dependent on the severity of the malocclusion, treatment stage and, above all, on good clinical sense (acquired experience and knowledge of the patient). Usually, the mandible is advanced to Class I canine relationship, in one step. This activation is similar to the position memorized by the patient during the first stage with the mini stimulator.

However, the plan that should be followed is as follows.[33]
- For the first week the patient merely has the appliance fitted, i.e. without forced mandibular advance. This is the *adaptation stage*.
- In the second week the appliance is activated 2–3 mm. This is known as the *adjustment stage*, where the lower support system (lower arch) adapts to the pressure exercised by the activation and opening and lateral movements carried out.
- In the third week the *activation stage* is started. The degree of mandibular advancement is dependent on the number of contacts in forced protrusion (the more there are, the better the adaptation) and on the severity of the malocclusion (when the initial overjet is too great, total advancement should not be attempted in only one step, because there will be considerable effort involved in adaptation and exaggerated stresses on the support systems).

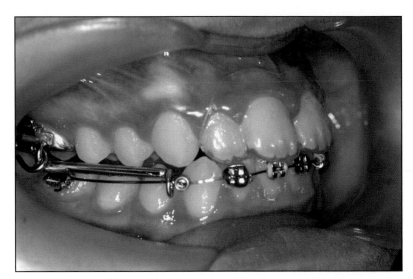

Figure 6.14 It is possible to use the mini stimulator in conjunction with the Ritto Appliance for the first 2 weeks.

On average, an activation of 6–7 mm is carried out and repeated 3 weeks later. In summary, a slight activation is carried out at the beginning, which is then progressively increased during treatment and adaptation. When a Class I relation with acceptable intercuspation is achieved (usually 4–6 months later), the functional appliance may be removed and the remaining treatment can be carried out by applying Class II elastics at night or simply by using small fixed mechanical details.

Retention

The retention is dependent on many factors, such as age, amount of crowding at the beginning, mixed or permanent dentition, etc. The best way to finish a case is to remove the wires or place thin round wires (0.12″ NiTi) 2 months before the end of treatment. With this procedure we can better evaluate the stability of the case.

Overtreatment is not indicated. If the teeth are well placed in Class I, with a nice intercuspation, and all the functions are well balanced, without novice habits, infantile deglutition and mouth breathing, it is not crucial to perform overcorrections or place activators or retainers.

Treatment Considerations

Permanent Dentition

Upper Jaw
- No upper incisor crowding—thermoformed splint with 0.7 mm thickness, from canine to canine, during the night and only three times per week for 6 months.
- Upper incisor crowding—thermoformed splint with 0.7 mm thickness, from canine to canine, at night for 6 months, followed by discontinuous use (three times per week for the next 6 months).
- Open bite at the beginning—the rest position of the tongue should be checked, as well as the swallow. If there is a tendency to push the tongue forward, a bonded lingual pearl is recommended for at least 4 months before the end of treatment, and 4 months after treatment. The lingual pearl should be used in conjunction with the other retainers.
- Severe deep bite at the beginning—the same protocol as described above but sometimes an artificial contact in composite on the palatal surfaces of the upper incisors is placed or lingual brackets to prevent deep bite relapse.
- In patients without good intercuspation, due to lack of growth, poor cooperation, etc., the use of an activator is recommended until the settling of occlusion in Class I.

Lower Jaw
Lingual arch bonded on #33 and #43, until third molars in occlusion, or extracted.

Mixed Dentition

The same protocol is followed but if the treatment is finished at the end of the mixed or transitional period, an activator can be fitted to maintain the same relation. If the treatment is finished in an early stage of the mixed dentition, some relapse should be expected during the next phase. Instability in the intercuspation due to teeth abrasion and less growth in this period compared to puberty are among the related factors.

Problems

1 The main problem with this appliance is *fracture of the lower arch*. This kind of fracture is very important because it occurs when the patient puts too much force on the appliance. To avoid this problem, the patient should be prestimulated beforehand. The fracture can also occur if the wire is not changed in 3 or 4 weeks. Usually a 0.017 × 0.025″ stainless steel wire is placed at the beginning with a 0.018″ slot on the anterior brackets and 0.022″ on lower molars.
Solution. Change the lower arch. Only the half part of the wire broken should be replaced until the next appointment. With this procedure the time lost is around 5 minutes (Figs 6.15–6.17).

2 Another problem that can occur is *fracture of the ball-pin*. This is not common because it is made of 0.045″ stainless steel. However, if the bend is too tight or if the bend was opened and closed a few times, a fracture can happen (Fig. 6.18).
Solution. Change the ball-pin and make the correct bend in two or three steps. Never forget that the upper part of the Ritto Appliance should be inserted mesial to the upper molar tube.

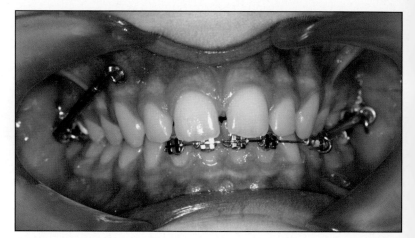

Figures 6.15–6.17 In a case of lower archwire fracture, it is possible to replace only half of the arch until the next appointment.

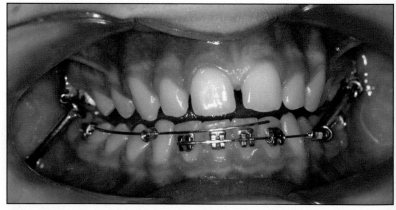

Figure 6.16

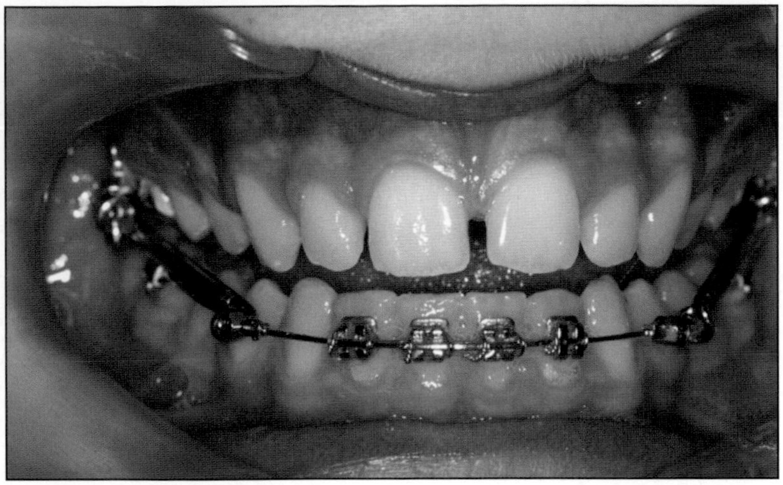

Figure 6.17

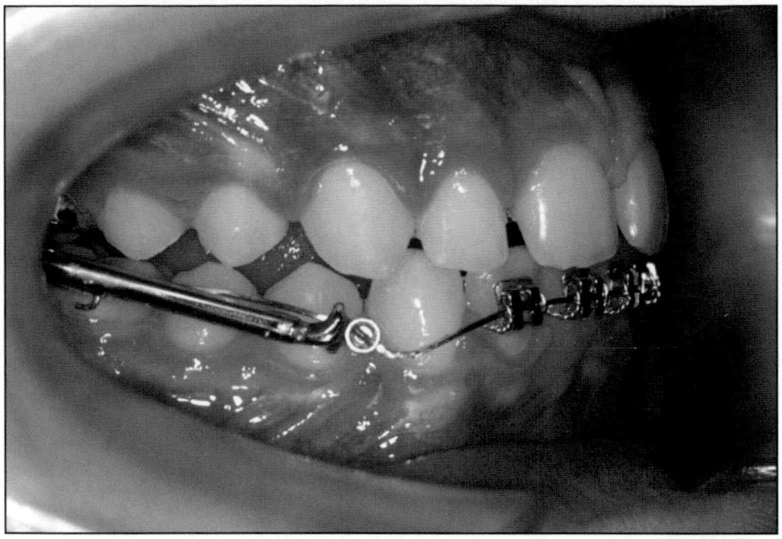

Figure 6.19 An incorrect distal bend will increase the possibility of lower incisor proclination as well as archwire distortion.

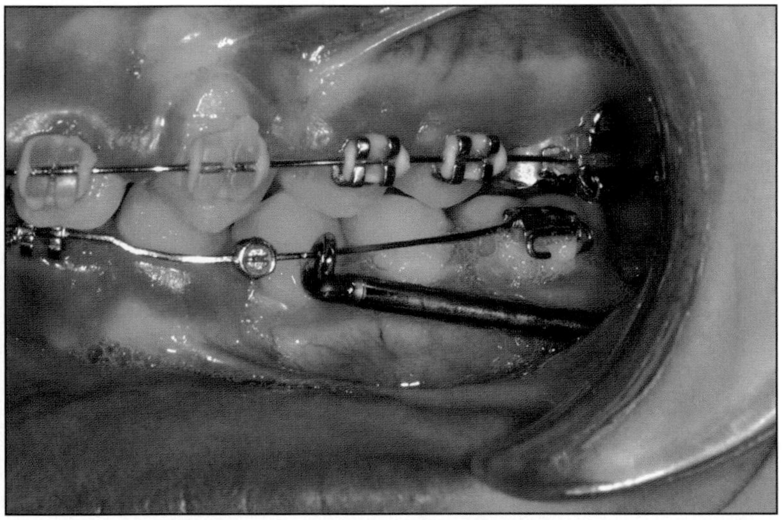

Figure 6.18 A ball-pin fracture is not common but it can happen if it is opened and closed a few times.

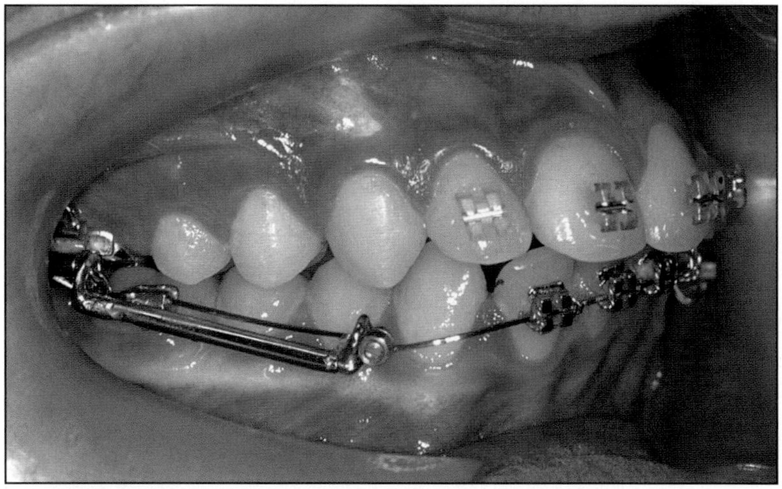

Figure 6.20 Proclination of lower incisors can happen in uncooperative patients or those not prestimulated with the mini stimulator.

3 *Lower arch distortion* can happen due to an incorrect distal bend or thin arch (0.016 × 0.016″ stainless steel). In this situation the clinician should evaluate whether it is necessary to change the arch or not. An incorrect distal bend will increase the possibility of lower incisor proclination (Fig. 6.19).

4 *Protrusion of lower incisors* due to noncooperation. If the patient is not prestimulated or does not cooperate, the lower incisors will procline (Fig. 6.20).
Solution. Use the mini stimulator for 2 months and motivate the patient. Electromyography is a good tool to evaluate the degree of adaptation to a new position of the mandible. Sometimes it is necessary to remove the appliance for 1 month and motivate the patient. After that the appliance is fitted again. If this does not work, the treatment plan should be reevaluated.

5 *The appliance comes out* of the upper fixation due to an incorrect ball-pin bend.
Solution. Avoid any gap between the ball-pin and the upper band (see Fig. 6.2).

6 *The lock slides* along the lower arch due to a thin archwire or unscrew.

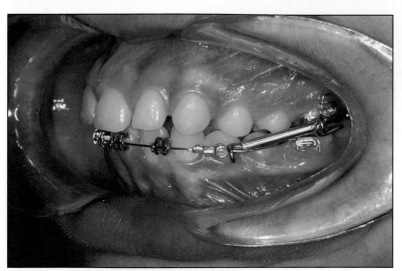

Figure 6.21 A crimpable hook can be placed mesial to the lock if it has a tendency to slide mesially.

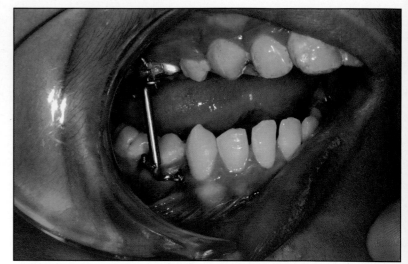

Figure 6.22 Fixed functional appliances could be attached to mini-implants for bone support.

Solution. Change the arch or place a crimpable hook mesial to the lock (Fig. 6.21).

7 *Bracket debonding* is not a common problem. Use lower bands instead of brackets.

Relapse Patients

There are many reasons for Class II treatment relapse. Among them we can include unfavorable growth, lack of patient cooperation, lack of muscular adaptation, instable posttreatment occlusion, persistence of labiolingual dysfunction or harmful habits, and lack of posttherapy contention.

Very often it is difficult to decide on the best approach for particular patients. Among removable and fixed appliances there are activators, positioners, retainers or full fixed therapy. Cooperation is a drawback in such patients and sometimes retreatment with a removable activator or positioner is hard work.

The Ritto Appliance can help in this situation. With only two upper bands and brackets on lower canines and first premolars, retreatment can be easily achieved. Lower incisors are free because the lingual retainer is bonded (see relapse patient, below).

The Future of Orthopedic Treatment

The main problem of orthopedic treatment with fixed appliances is the difficulty in controlling the proclination of lower incisors and the advancement of all mandibular teeth, which can compromise the mandibular advancement and the final esthetic result. In recent years the problem has been reduced with the introduction of the mini stimulator as an obligatory part of the treatment, as discussed above. In the future, new techniques using mini-implants and mini-plates will allow lower bone support to advance the mandible (Fig. 6.22).

Case Studies

Relapse Patient

This patient had a deep bite Class II malocclusion which was treated with fixed appliances and Class II elastics for 23 months (Figs 6.23–6.28). Retention was achieved with a Hawley Appliance and a bonded lower 3/3 wire. Some artificial composite contacts were bonded on the palatal surfaces of the upper incisors to prevent the deep bite relapse. After 1 year of treatment, the overjet was 6 mm (4 mm of relapse) and an infantile swallow appeared (Figs 6.29–6.32). The patient had a dual bite. After advancement of the mandible to Class I, an intercuspation in the premolar area was not present. The relapse was probably due to inadequate use of the Hawley Appliance, i.e. discontinued use and night-time only for 2 months. Another factor that could be involved is the early treatment period. This male patient started the treatment at 9 years old and finished the treatment at 11 years old, before the growth peak. However, all the permanent teeth were present.

It was decided to use the Ritto Appliance to retreat the patient at 13 years of age, during the growing peak. The main advantage of this system is that the treatment can be carried out with only brackets on lower canines and molars, because the lower fixed 3/3 lingual retainer is still in place. On the upper arch, upper molar bands were fitted.

Class I intercuspation was achieved in 4 months (Figs 6.33–6.35). The appliance was removed and a Hawley Appliance was fitted for use at night for 1 year. One year after the retreatment, the occlusion remained stable (Figs 6.36–6.38). The retainer was removed. Two years after the retreatment everything was stable, with a good Class I intercuspation (Figs 6.39–6.41).

This approach to Class II relapse patients is very easy, comfortable, and esthetic. It has the advantage of being a fixed, 24-hour appliance,

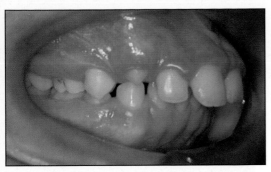 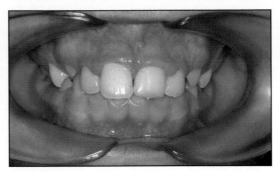 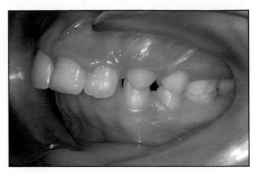

Figures 6.23–6.25 This patient had a Class II malocclusion with deep bite.

Figure 6.24

Figure 6.25

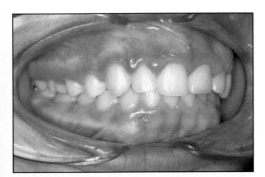 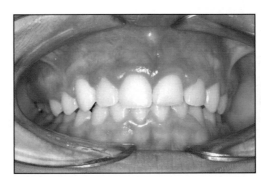 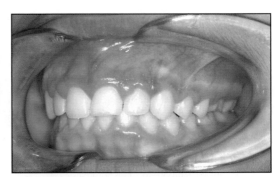

Figures 6.26–6.28 After treatment with fixed appliances and Class II elastics for 23 months.

Figure 6.27

Figure 6.28

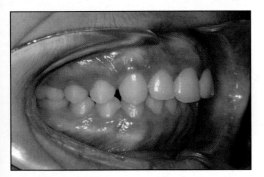 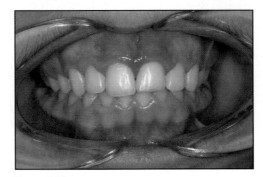 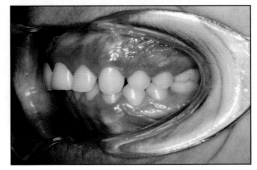

Figures 6.29–6.32 Relapse 1 year after the treatment.

Figure 6.30

Figure 6.31

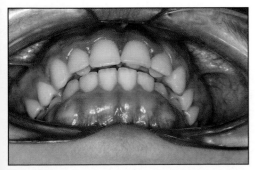

Figure 6.32

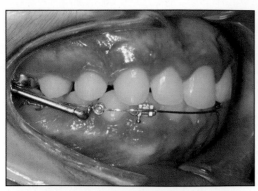
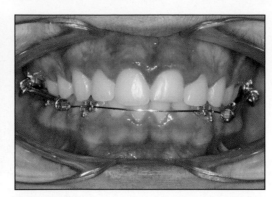
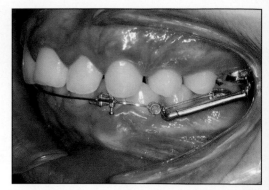

Figures 6.33–6.35 After 4 months Class I intercuspation was achieved.

Figure 6.34

Figure 6.35

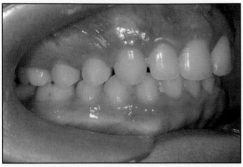
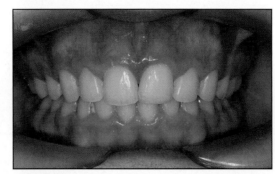
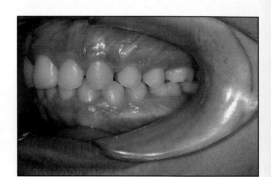

Figures 6.36–6.38 One year after the retreatment, the occlusion remains stable. The retainer was removed.

Figure 6.37

Figure 6.38

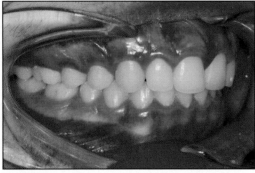
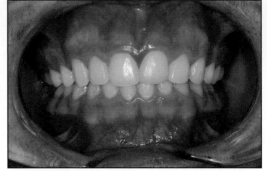
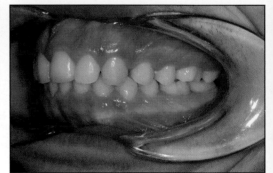

Figures 6.39–6.41 Two years after the retreatment, the occlusion is stable.

Figure 6.40

Figure 6.41

allowing growth and the settling of occlusion in Class I. The retreatment can be carried out in a few months and a retainer can be placed only at night.

Patient 1

This 8.5-year-old female patient presented with a severe Class II division 1 malocclusion in early mixed dentition, as a consequence of sucking habits and lingual dysfunction (Figs 6.42–6.46). She could not close her lips without an effort of muscular chin contraction, due to a big overjet (13 mm). Her profile was retrognathic and convex.

Cephalometric Radiograph

The cephalometric analysis showed a severe skeletal mandibular deficiency and a convex profile (ANPg 8°, SNPg 72°) (Fig. 6.47). In relation to the anterior cranial base, the upper jaw was in correct position, while the mandible was retrognathic, determining a distal sagittal relation, as shown by the ANPg variable (Table 6.1). The overjet was augmented (13 mm) and the overbite was 4 mm.

Treatment Plan

Due to the large overjet and convex profile, which was improved when the mandible was advanced, treatment with a fixed

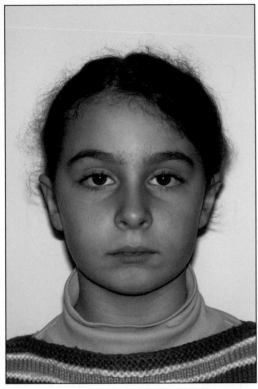

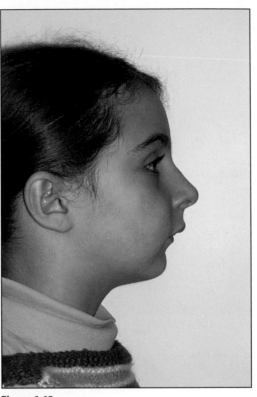

Figures 6.42–6.46 Severe Class II division 1 malocclusion in a female patient 8 years and 5 months old. Early mixed dentition.

Figure 6.43

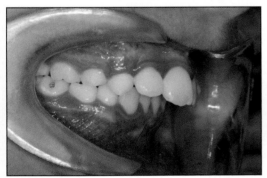

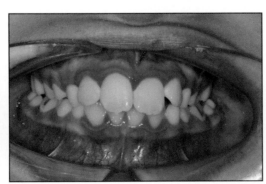

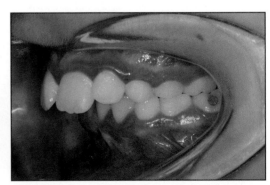

Figure 6.44

Figure 6.45

Figure 6.46

functional appliance was planned. A further retreatment at the age of 12 in permanent dentition will probably be necessary. Treatment was planned first with a mini stimulator for 2 months followed by the Ritto Appliance. The appliance would be fixed to the lower archwire (only with incisors and lower molars bonded), and on the upper bands. A transpalatal arch would also be inserted. After reaching a Class I intercuspation, a multibracket appliance would be placed to level and align the upper incisors. At the end of the treatment an activator would be placed as a retainer for use at night, for 1 year.

Treatment

A mini stimulator was placed for 2 months to stimulate muscles before the fixed therapy. After this first step, the Ritto Appliance was fitted as well as a transpalatal arch, and the mandible was positioned in Class I relationship (Figs 6.48–6.50). Three months later a multibracket appliance was bonded on the upper arch. The Ritto Appliance was maintained for 7 months, followed for a period of 3 months with Class II elastics (at night) to stabilize the Class I relationship. The appliance was removed (12 months of treatment) and an activator was placed for use at night.

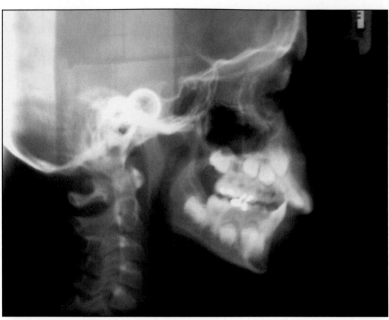

Figure 6.47 Cephalometric radiograph before treatment.

Posttreatment Results

At the end of the treatment the profile was improved as well as the occlusion (Figs 6.51–6.55). The cephalometric radiograph (Fig. 6.56) shows an improvement in the skeletal relationship (see Table 6.1).

Patient 2

This female patient, aged 8 years and 11 months, was referred by her dentist because she had an open bite. She had a skeletal Class II division 1 malocclusion in late mixed dentition (Figs 6.57–6.59). A thumb-sucking habit was maintained since early childhood. Normally she kept the lips apart. Increased mentalis muscle activity could not be seen when lips were closed. Good labial elasticity. Swallowing with interposition of the tongue between the anterior segments of the dental arches. She could breathe through nose and mouth without any noticeable impairment.

Table 6.1. Patient 1. Cephalometric measurements before and after treatment.

	Before treatment	After treatment	Mean ± SD
Sagittal skeletal relations			
Maxillary position			
SNA	80°	80°	82° ± 3.5°
Mandibular position			
SNPg	72°	76°	80° ± 3.5°
Sagittal jaw position			
ANPg	8°	4°	2° ± 2.5°
Vertical skeletal relations			
Maxillary inclination			
SN/ANS-PNS	11°	12°	8° ± 3.0°
Mandibular inclination			
SN/GoGn	34°	31°	33° ± 2.5°
Vertical jaw relation			
ANS-PNS/GoGn	23°	20°	25° ± 6.0°
Dentobasal relations			
Maxillary incisor inclination			
1 – ANS-PNS	120°	121°	110° ± 6.0°
Mandibular incisor inclination			
1 – GoGn	100°	104°	94° ± 7.0°
Mandibular incisor compensation			
1 – APg	−2 mm	3 mm	2 ± 2.0 mm
Dental relations			
Overjet	13 mm	2 mm	3.5 ± 2.5 mm
Overbite	4 mm	2 mm	2 ± 2.5 mm
Interincisal angle	118°	111°	132° ± 6°
Mandibular length (Co/Gn)	101 mm	107 mm	

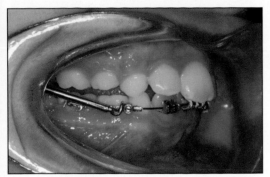

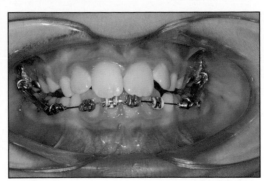

Figure 6.49

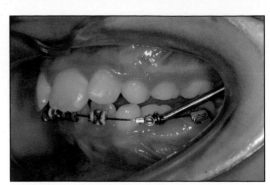

Figure 6.50

Figures 6.48–6.50 The Ritto Appliance was fitted to the upper bands and to the lower archwire. Four brackets on the lower incisors and two lower tubes on the molars are enough. The mandible is positioned in Class I relationship.

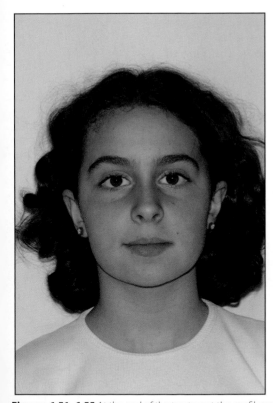

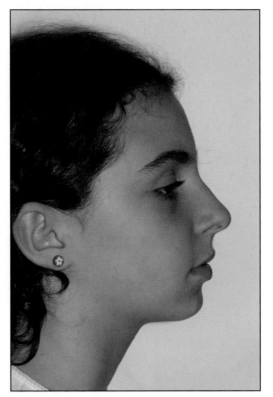

Figures 6.51–6.55 At the end of the treatment the profile was improved as well as the occlusion.

Figure 6.52

Cephalometric Radiograph

The cephalometric evaluation showed a skeletal mandibular deficiency and a convex profile (Fig. 6.60). In relation to the anterior cranial base, the upper jaw was in an anterior position, while the mandible was retrognathic, determining a distal sagittal relation, as shown by the ANPg variable (Table 6.2). The lower incisors were 1 mm in front of the A/Pg line. The overjet was augmented (9 mm) and the overbite negative: −2 mm (open bite).

Treatment

Due to the convex profile which was improved when the mandible was advanced, an advancement of the mandible was planned.

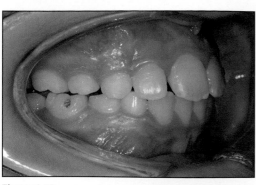

Figure 6.53

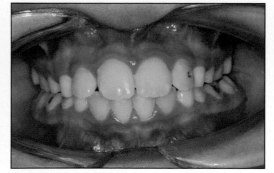

Figure 6.54

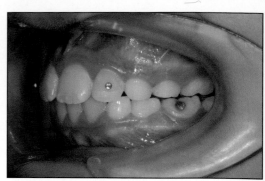

Figure 6.55

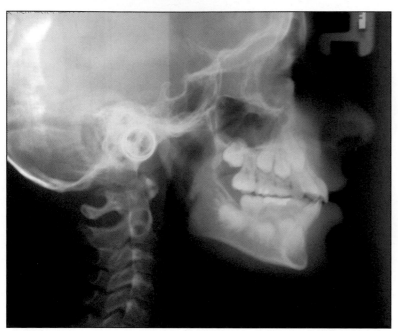

Figure 6.56 Cephalometric radiograph after treatment.

Treatment was done with a mini stimulator for 1 month followed by a Ritto Appliance, leaving the lateral area free for eruption in Class I intercuspation. The appliance was fixed to the lower archwire and to the upper bands (Figs 6.61–6.63). A transpalatal arch was inserted. Six months later, the Class I intercuspation was achieved and a multibracket appliance was placed to level and align the teeth. During the first months of treatment the patient was encouraged to eliminate the thumb-sucking habit.

Posttreatment Results

The malocclusion was corrected through dentoalveolar and skeletal movements (Figs 6.64– 6.67). A reduction in the SNA angle and an increase in the SNPg angle could be noticed. The ANPg decreased 4°. These modifications contributed to the overjet reduction. The maxilla rotated posteriorly 3° (SN/ANS-PNS), and the mandible anteriorly 2° (SN/CoGn) (see Table 6.2). This modification helped to close the bite. The upper incisors inclined to palatine and the lower incisors inclined 1° to vestibular. Regarding the soft tissues, the profile was improved and the patient could close her lips without muscular contraction at rest position.

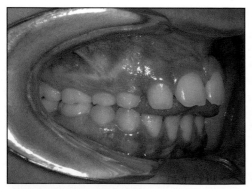

Figures 6.57–6.59 Skeletal Class II division 1 open bite malocclusion in late mixed dentition.

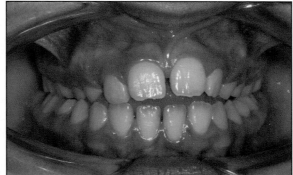

Figure 6.58

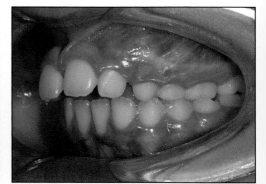

Figure 6.59

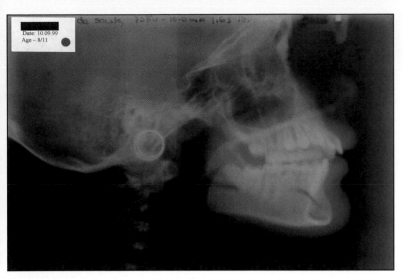

Figure 6.60 Cephalometric radiograph before treatment.

Retention

The combination of a good intercuspation achieved by the treatment, the elimination of novice habits, and the patient's strong cooperation and intention to maintain the result (good retainer wear) gave some confidence in this treatment's stability. Retention in the lower arch was done with a lower 3-3 bonded retainer and in the upper with a thermoformed splint retainer (#13 to #23).

Postretention Evaluation

The retention period demonstrated stability of the treatment effects (Fig. 6.68). The overjet did not relapse, the overbite increased, and the intercuspation remained excellent, with all teeth well aligned and in good contact (Figs 6.69–6.71). From the frontal view, facial symmetry and harmony were good, with an attractive smile. Retention has been done with the lower bonded 3-3 retainer. No retention on the upper jaw.

Table 6.2. Patient 2. Cephalometric measurements before treatment, after treatment and 2 years later.

	Before treatment	After treatment	After retention	Mean ± SD
Sagittal skeletal relations				
Maxillary position				
SNA	83°	82°	83°	82° ± 3.5°
Mandibular position				
SNPg	77°	80°	81°	80° ± 3.5°
Sagittal jaw position				
ANPg	6°	2°	2°	2° ± 2.5°
Vertical skeletal relations				
Maxillary inclination				
SN/ANS-PNS	5°	8°	8°	8° ± 3.0°
Mandibular inclination				
SN/GoGn	34°	32°	30°	33° ± 2.5°
Vertical jaw relation				
ANS-PNS/GoGn	30°	25°	22°	25° ± 6.0°
Dentobasal relations				
Maxillary incisor inclination				
1 – ANS-PNS	106°	104°	101°	110° ± 6.0°
Mandibular incisor inclination				
1 – GoGn	103°	104°	102°	94° ± 7.0°
Mandibular incisor compensation				
1 – APg	1 mm	3 mm	2.5 mm	2 ± 2.0 mm
Dental relations				
Overjet	9 mm	2 mm	2 mm	3.5 ± 2.5 mm
Overbite	−3 mm	2 mm	3.5 mm	2 ± 2.5 mm
Interincisal angle	123°	127°	135°	132° ± 6°

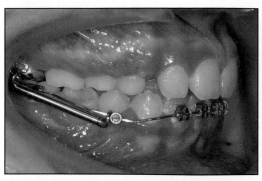

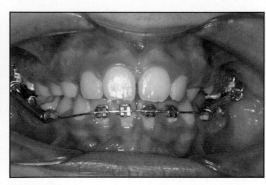

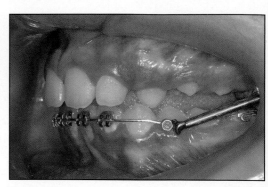

Figures 6.61–6.63 Sequence of treatment with the Ritto Appliance for 3 months.

Figure 6.62

Figure 6.63

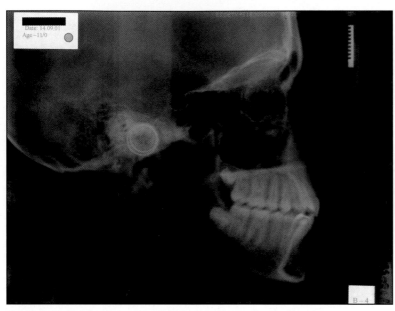

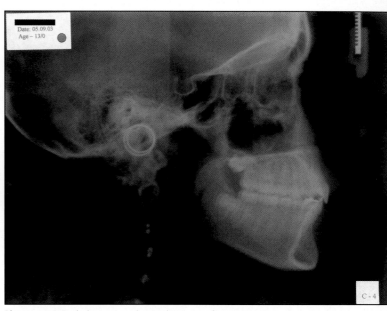

Figure 6.64 Cephalometric radiograph after treatment.

Figure 6.68 Cephalometric radiograph 2 years after treatment.

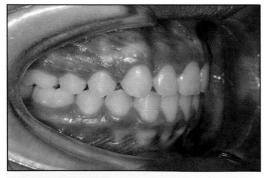

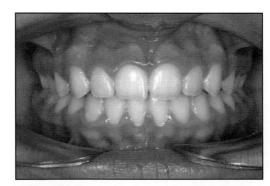

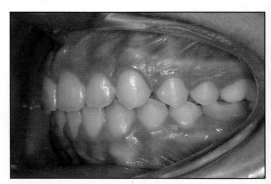

Figures 6.65–6.67 Patient after treatment.

Figure 6.66

Figure 6.67

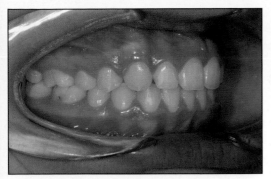
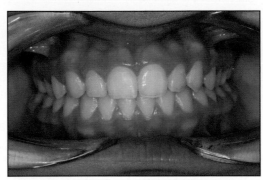
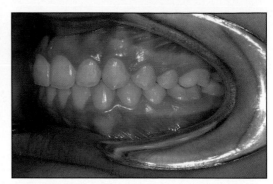

Figures 6.69–6.71 Patient 2 years after treatment.

Figure 6.70

Figure 6.71

Patient 3

This male patient, aged 14 years and 3 months, presented a skeletal Class II division 1 malocclusion in permanent dentition with 12 mm overjet (Figs 6.72–6.75). The patient had passed the peak of growth, as can be seen by the vertebral maturation (Fig. 6.76).

Due to the mandibular deficiency (Table 6.3), it was decided to treat the patient with the Ritto Appliance in the same way as in the other patients presented above. After 1 month with the mini stimulator, the fixed functional appliance was fitted on the upper bands and on the lower molar tubes and incisors brackets (Figs 6.77–6.79). After 6 months a multibracket appliance was placed. The duration of treatment was 24 months.

The profile improved (Figs 6.80–6.83), but the treatment was carried out mainly by dental movements, as was expected due to having missed the main skeletal growth period (Fig. 6.84). Retention was done with a bonded lingual wire #33 to #43, and a thermoformed splint retainer (#13 to #23). Two years after the treatment, the occlusion remains stable (Figs 6.85–6.88).

Concluding Remarks

In functional treatment with fixed functional appliances, it is necessary to prepare the patient for 1–2 months before fitting the appliance so as to stimulate the musculature and avoid the patient

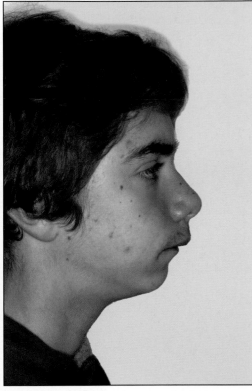

Figures 6.72–6.75 Class II division 1 malocclusion in permanent dentition. Male patient 14 years and 3 months old.

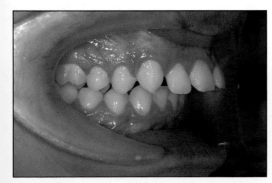
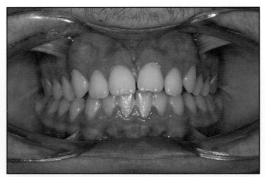
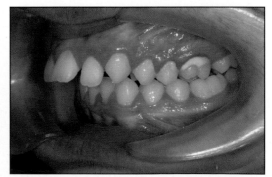

Figure 6.73

Figure 6.74

Figure 6.75

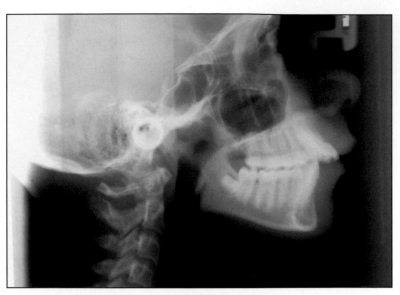

Figure 6.76 Cephalometric radiograph before treatment.

exerting too much force on the support systems, thus fracturing them or originating unwanted dental movement.

For this reason, the use of a mini stimulator for mandibular advancement is advised. This is a thermoformed splint of 0.7 mm in thickness, used only for the upper incisors, and incorporates an acrylic bite block for the lower incisors constructed with the mandible in a forward position. For the first 15 days or 1 month, the patient should wear the splint for as long as possible and maintain the lower incisors fitted into the bite block. In the following weeks, the patient should start to carry out swallowing exercises with lips in contact and with incisors against the bite block. Only after this stage should therapy be started with the Ritto Appliance.

The Ritto Appliance can be described as a miniaturized telescopic device. It enables the correction of skeletal Class II division 1 and 2 malocclusions (mixed or permanent dentition) and mandibular asymmetries, and is an excellent anchorage system in Class I and II treatment (extraction or nonextraction).

Table 6.3. Patient 3. Cephalometric measurements before and after treatment.

	Before treatment	After treatment	Mean ± SD
Sagittal skeletal relations			
Maxillary position			
SNA	82°	81°	82° ± 3.5°
Mandibular position			
SNPg	74°	75°	80° ± 3.5°
Sagittal jaw position			
ANPg	8°	6°	2° ± 2.5°
Vertical skeletal relations			
Maxillary inclination			
SN/ANS-PNS	9°	10°	8° ± 3.0°
Mandibular inclination			
SN/GoGn	38°	38°	33° ± 2.5°
Vertical jaw relation			
ANS-PNS/GoGn	30°	30°	25° ± 6.0°
Dentobasal relations			
Maxillary incisor inclination			
1 – ANS-PNS	118°	103°	110° ± 6.0°
Mandibular incisor inclination			
1 – GoGn	100°	103°	94° ± 7.0°
Mandibular incisor compensation			
1 – APg	0 mm	3 mm	2 ± 2.0 mm
Dental relations			
Overjet	12 mm	2 mm	3.5 ± 2.5 mm
Overbite	−2 mm	2 mm	2 ± 2.5 mm
Interincisal angle	112°	124°	32° ± 6°
Mandibular length (Co/Gn)	111 mm	114 mm	

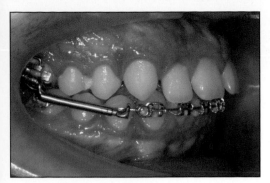

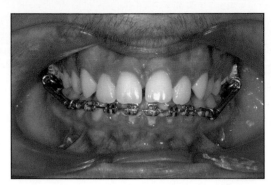

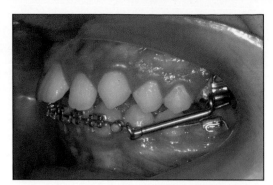

Figures 6.77–6.79 Sequence of treatment with the Ritto Appliance for 3 months.

Figure 6.78

Figure 6.79

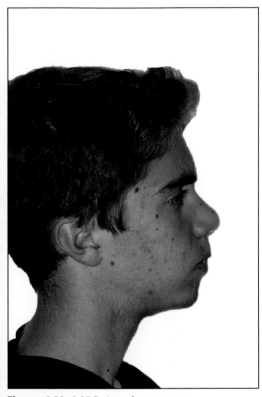

Figures 6.80–6.83 Patient after treatment.

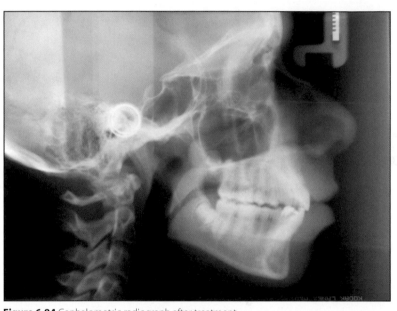

Figure 6.84 Cephalometric radiograph after treatment.

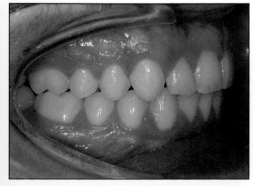

Figure 6.81

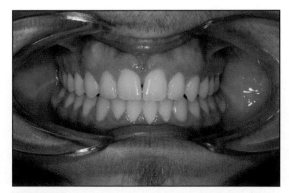

Figure 6.82

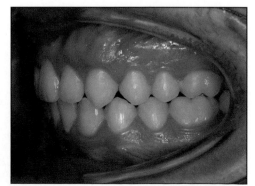

Figure 6.83

The main differences when compared to competitor appliances are:

- the appliance does not come apart (no disengagement after achieving maximum extension)
- the smaller size facilitates adaptation and it does not affect esthetic appearance or speech.

The Ritto Appliance comes in a single format, which allows it to be used on both sides, and is available in only two sizes. It is simple to use, comfortable, cost-effective, breakage resistant, and requires no patient cooperation. The fact that the appliance does not disengage has enormous advantages. It eliminates the time lost in measuring length before fitting, as is the case with competitor appliances. This facility makes it possible to fit the appliance in around 5 minutes and about half that time is sufficient to remove it.

The Ritto Appliance does not require any laboratory stage, which means a reduction in both time and costs. Nor does it require any prior measurement due to the manner in which it is activated. Preparation of the lower arch is the only prefitting procedure suggested by the author.

Upper fixing is carried out by placing a steel ball-pin into the 0.045″ tube from the upper molar band crossing the appliance, which is then totally bent over. The appliance is fixed onto the lower arch, which has to be prepared before insertion. The thickness and type of arch are chosen, its length is adjusted, locks are fitted and the Ritto Appliance is then inserted. The lower arch must always remain bent behind the tube for the molars so that protrusion of the lower incisors is avoided. It is necessary first to bend from one side then connect the brackets to the arch, swivel the arch to the other side so as to eliminate any gaps that are present around the first bend, then finally bend from the other side as close as possible to the tube. The appliance should slide free of contact in the premolar area. Activation is achieved by sliding the lock along the lower arch in the distal direction and then fixing it against the Ritto Appliance.

Another important factor that contributes to comfort and rapid patient adaptation is the achievement of posterior contact after the advancement of the mandible. This also creates a posterior proprioceptive sensibility.

It is not always necessary to have perfect coordination of the arches before starting functional treatment. Sometimes, even with a pronounced Spee curve, therapy can be started as long as some artificial contacts are constructed with composite on the molars. The extrusion of the premolars can be beneficial in the correction of a vertical problem.

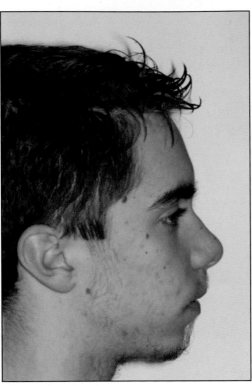

Figures 6.85–6.88 Two years after the treatment, the occlusion remains stable.

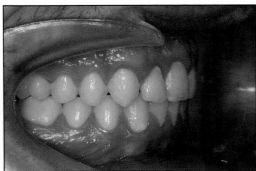

Figure 6.86

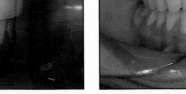
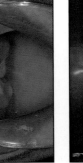

Figure 6.87

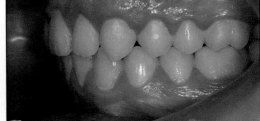

Figure 6.88

References

1. Fisk RO. When malocclusions concern the public. J Can Dent Assoc 1960;26:397–412.

2. McNamara JA. Components of Class II malocclusion in children 8–10 years of age. Angle Orthod 1981;51:177–202.

3. Bass NM. Dentofacial othopaedics in the correction of Class II malocclusion Br J Orthod 1982;9:3–31.

4. Schmuth GPF. Milestones in the development and practical application of functional appliances. Am J Orthod Dentofacial Orthop 1983;84:48–53.

5. Pancherz H. Treatment of Class II malocclusions by jumping the bite with the Herbst appliance. A cephalometric investigation. Am J Orthod 1979; 76:423–442.

6. Ritto AK. Class II malocclusion: why, when and how to treat this anomaly in mixed dentition with fixed functional appliances. J Gen Orthod 2001; 12:9–21.

7. Ritto AK. The use of model templates for Class II treatment. Orthodontic CYBERjournal, 2001. Available online at: www.oc-j.com

8. Tulloch JF, Philips C, Proffit WR. Benefit of early Class II treatment: progress report of a two-phase randomized clinical trial. Am J Orthod Dentofacial Orthop 1998;113:67–72.

9. Pancherz H. Dentofacial orthopedics or orthognathic surgery: is it a matter of age? Am J Orthod Dentofacial Orthop 2000;117:571–574.

10. Paulsen HU, Karle A. Computer tomographic and radiographic changes in the temporomandibular joints of two young adults with occlusal asymmetry, treated with the Herbst appliance. Eur J Orthod 2000;22:649–656.

11. Franchi L, Baccetti T, McNamara J. Mandibular growth as related to cervical vertebral maturation and body height. Am J Orthod Dentofacial Orthop 2000;118:335–340.

12. Hunter WS. The correlation of facial growth with body height and skeletal maturation at adolescence. Angle Orthod 1966;36:44–54.

13. Nanda RS. The rates of the growth of several facial components measured from serial cephalometric roentgenograms. Am J Orthod 1955;41:658–673.

14. Hagg U, Pancherz H. Dentofacial orthopaedics in relation to chronological age, growth period and skeletal development: an analysis of 72 male patients with Class II Division 1 malocclusions treated with the Herbst appliance. Eur J Orthod 1988;10:169–176.

15. Petrovic A, Stutzman J, Lavergne J. Mechanism of craniofacial growth and modus operandi of functional appliances: a cell-level and cybernetic approach to orthodontic decision making. In: Carlson DS, ed. Craniofacial growth theory and orthodontic treatment. Craniofacial Growth Series, vol. 23. Ann Arbor: Center for Human Growth and Development, University of Michigan; 1990.

16. Malmgren O, Omblus J, Hagg U, Pancherz H. Treatment with an appliance system in relation to treatment intensity and growth periods. Am J Orthod Dentofacial Orthop 1987;91:143–151.

17. McNamara J, Bookstein FL, Shaughnessy TG. Skeletal and dental changes following functional regulator therapy on Class II patients. Am J Orthod 1985;88:91–110.

18. Baccetti T, Franchi L, Toth LR, McNamara J. Treatment timing for Twin-block therapy. Am J Orthod Dentofacial Orthop 2000;118:159–170.

19. Frankel R. The theoretical concept underlying the treatment with functional correctors. Trans Eur Orthod Soc 1966:223–250.

20. McNamara JA. On the Frankel appliance. Part 1. Biological basis and appliance design. J Clin Orthod 1982;16:320–337.

21. McNamara JA. On the Frankel appliance. Part 2. Clinical management. J Clin Orthod 1982; 16:390–406.

22. Owen AH. Clinical application of the Frankel appliance: case reports. Angle Orthod 1983;53:29–88.

23. Owen AH. Clinical management of the Frankel FR-II appliance. J Clin Orthod 1983;18:605–618.

24. Owen AH. Morphologic changes in the transverse dimension using the Frankel appliance. Am J Orthod 1983;83:200–217.

25. Gianelly AA, Brosnan P, Martignoni M, Bernstein L. Mandibular growth, condyle position and Frankel appliance therapy. Angle Orthod 1983;53:131–142.

26. Righellis EG. Treatment effects of Frankel, activator and extra-oral traction appliances. Angle Orthod 1983;53:107–121.

27. Schulhof RJ, Engel GA. Results of Class II functional appliance treatment. J Clin Orthod 1982; 16:587–599.

28. Creekmore TD, Radney LJ. Frankel appliance therapy: orthopaedic or orthodontic? Am J Orthod Dentofacial Orthop 1983;83:89–108.

29. Robertson NRE. An examination of treatment changes in children treated with the functional regulator of Frankel. Am J Orthod Dentofacial Orthop 1983;83:299–310.

30. Eirow HL. The bionator. Br J Orthod 1981; 8:33–36.

31. Frankel R. Concerning recent articles on Frankel appliance therapy. Am J Orthod 1984;85: 441–445.

32. Ritto AK. Fixed functional appliances – trends for the next century. Func Orthod 1999;16: 122–135.

33. Ritto AK. Aparelhos funcionais fixos – novidades para o próximo século. Ortodontia 1998;2:124–150.

34. Ritto AK. Pérola lingual – construção e colagem. Revista Virtual de Ortodontia 1997;1(1).

35. Ritto AK. El Aparato de Ritto: colocacion y activation. Ortodoncia Clin 1999;2:145–150.

36. Ritto AK. The Ritto Appliance – a new fixed functional device. Orthodontic CyberJournal, 1999. Available online at: www.oc-j.com

37. Ritto AK. The lingual pearl. Ortodoncia 2000; 5:68–71.

38. Ritto AK, Leitão P. The lingual pearl. J Clin Orthod 1998;32:318–327.

39. Proffit WR. Equilibrium theory revisited: factors influencing position of the teeth. Angle Orthod 1978;48:175–186.

40. Graber TM. The three "M's": muscles, malformation, and malocclusion. Am J Orthod 1963; 49:418–450.

41. Ritto AK. Aplicação da perola lingual na terapia da fala. Ortodontia 2000;5:35–40.

42. Ritto AK. Fixed functional appliances – a classification. Func Orthod 2000;17:2–32.

43. Ritto AK. Fixed functional appliances – a classification (updated). Orthodontic CYBERjournal, 2001. Available online at: www.oc-j.com

44. Ritto AK, Ferreira AP. Hybrid fixed appliances. Ortodontia 2001;6:74–82.

45. Chateau M. Orthopédie dento-faciale, vol. 2. Paris: Editions CDP; 1993.

CHAPTER 7

The Mandibular Protraction Appliance in the treatment of noncompliant Class II patients

Carlos Martins Coelho Filho, Fabio Oliveira Coelho

CONTENTS

Introduction

Noncompliance in wearing prescribed auxiliary accessories such as headgear and intermaxillary elastics is among the main factors responsible for compromising treatment of patients presenting with Class II malocclusion. The reintroduction of the Herbst appliance (Dentaurum, Ispringen, Germany) to the orthodontic community by Pancherz[1] brought new hope to the profession regarding noncompliance, since this appliance was fixed and did not depend on the patient's collaboration to wear it. The reports of Class II treatment with the use of the Herbst appliance looked impressive and this seems to have inspired the development of several appliances belonging to the same category, i.e. fixed dentofacial orthopedic appliances.

Coelho Filho published an article in 1995 in which he presented the mandibular protraction appliance (MPA), a fixed dentofacial orthopedic noncompliant device that could be fabricated by the clinician and permitted easy application to the patient.[2] Although he considered his treatment results with the MPA satisfactory, he reported frequent breakage of the appliances. This led him to introduce several modifications[3–5] until the appliance reached its fourth version,[6,7] which was more resistant to breakage and much more stable during functioning than the previous ones.

The Appliance

The first MPA design was extremely simple, consisting of only a 0.036″ sectional stainless steel wire with one circular loop at each end. Each circular loop ran mesially and distally along the maxillary and mandibular archwire during opening and closing of the mouth. The length of the appliance was equal to the distance measured from mesial of the upper molar tube to a stop made in the lower archwire distal to the lower cuspid and was capable of maintaining the patient in an incisor edge-to-edge position when the mouth was closed.

During opening of the mouth, the upper loop moved mesially along the maxillary archwire while the lower moved distally along the mandibular archwire. During mouth closing, each loop moved in the opposite direction (Fig. 7.1A). However, this model interfered with mouth opening, causing too many breakages of archwires as well as loosening of bands.

The author then developed a second design aimed at solving the limitation in mouth opening. It consisted of two pieces of 0.036″ stainless steel wire, each with a circular loop at one of its tips. After slipping one piece of coil into one of the components, the tip of each component was reciprocally inserted into the circular loop belonging to the other. The piece of tubing or coil placed between them was meant to prevent too much approximation of the two circular loops belonging to each part, since this might cause undesirable movement between the parts. With this configuration, each part could slide along the other without too much instability between them. This new design was named the MPA II (Fig. 7.1B).

Although it represented an improvement over the original MPA, the MPA II still suffered from instability during functioning. The author believed this was due to the way the appliance was adapted to the archwire in each jaw. He realized that stability could be attained only if the appliance could move around an axis in each jaw and not run along the archwires as it did until then. This was partly achieved in the MPA III, which had a mandibular rod rotating within a circular loop placed in the lower archwire distally to the lower cuspid. The longer section of the mandibular rod ran within a telescopic tube that was introduced in this design (Fig. 7.1C).

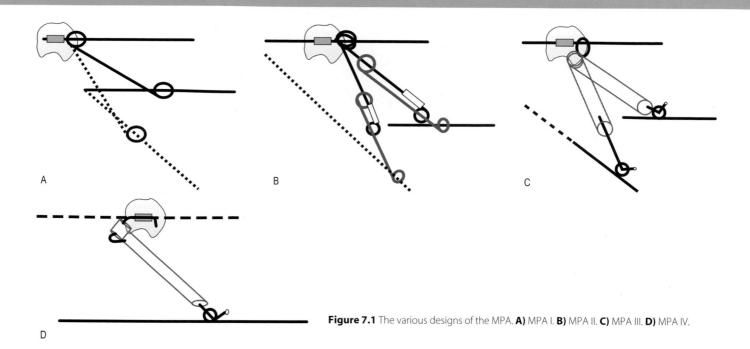

Figure 7.1 The various designs of the MPA. **A)** MPA I. **B)** MPA II. **C)** MPA III. **D)** MPA IV.

Stability was greatly increased in the MPA III but the author considered that it could be improved even more if the adaptation of the appliance to the upper jaw also resembled a rotation around an axis. This was achieved only in the MPA IV, in which the maxillary extremity of the appliance ran around a 1 mm sectional stainless steel wire that was bent 90° before entering the distal side of the 0.045″ round molar tube and was locked in its mesial side (Fig. 7.1D). The MPA IV thus achieved the maximum stability possible and a near-total absence of breakages.

Mode of Action

The main expected action resulting from the use of the MPA is the attainment of Class II correction, including overbite, overjet and other related features, such as subdivision asymmetries and the frequently associated dental midline shifts. The mode of action appears to be basically through dentoalveolar alterations. The results obtained with its use thus far have been stable for 5 or more years.

Although young patients treated with the appliance have shown considerable amounts of mandibular growth, the author does not attribute such growth solely to the appliance's influence. He prefers to link it to the hypothesis that MPA installation generates a "normality environment" that facilitates function to accomplish the necessary modifications to correct the case. The reason for such caution in attributing the growth occurring during treatment only to the influence of the MPA lies in the fact that overjets as large as 10–12 mm have been reduced to normal in a period as short as 6–8 months and that does not comply with the average growth increments related to that period of time seen in any growth age. Besides, such overjet reduction is equally seen in adults who have no

growth. When the MPA is activated, the mandible is brought forward initially and later reverses by the action of the retracting musculature, concomitantly retracting the maxillary dentoalveolar complex. During this process, intrusion of the upper occlusal plane often occurs, permitting mandibular counterclockwise rotation and mandibular anterior translation.

Since the incisors are placed in an edge-to-edge position as recommended by Pancherz[8] when activating the Herbst, overbite is reduced to zero at the moment of the MPA installation and activation. This leads to the temporary surging of a posterior open bite, which gradually closes by itself due to progressive dentoalveolar leveling.

When the mandible has finished returning to its most distal position, upper and lower incisors are still edge to edge, suggesting that the maxillary dentition is also in its most distal position. Being at its most distal position, the mandible cannot go backwards farther so as to permit reappearance of the overjet. The stability of the overbite is attributed to the reciprocal support between the incisors, which was generated after upper dentition distalization.

Management of the Appliance

Before installation, the MPA IV must have its length adequately defined so as to keep upper and lower incisors in an edge-to-edge relationship when the patient closes the mouth. This measurement corresponds to the distance from distal of the upper first molar tube to the circular loop placed in the archwire distal to the lower cuspid and is taken in the incisor edge-to-edge position with midlines coincident. The MPA can also be installed from mesial of the upper first molar tube, provided the patient's maximum mouth aperture does not cause disengagement of the MPA parts. This can be evaluated during measurement. Upon installation of the MPA, a posterior open bite appears and causes discomfort to the patient due to the difficulties in chewing with the posterior teeth. The patient must be informed that this open bite gradually closes by itself with time and within about 1.5 weeks, mastication with the posterior teeth will be possible even though the open bite will not be completely closed yet.

After installation, the MPA must be supervised for breakage and any other undesirable occurrences. If activation is necessary, it is done by slipping a section of coil-spring between the mandibular rod and the telescopic tube. It is not necessary to remove the appliance for activation. Activation can also be done by pressing the prongs of a three-prong plier against the mandibular rod at an adequate distance from the circular loop existing in the archwire distal to the lower cuspid, so as to make a light bend that will serve as a stop and reduce its running distance within the telescopic tube.

In our experience, the MPA has fulfilled its function in periods of 6–8 months for growing patients and up to 1 year for adults, although this time difference is not always deemed necessary. When the MPA is discontinued, labial inclination of the lower incisors may be too accentuated. This is self-corrective, returning to normal in about 1–2 months. Ruf et al reported the same phenomenon following use of the Herbst appliance.[9]

The MPA can be activated with different amounts of force per side, with the objective of correcting midline shifts. It can also be used on only one side with the same objective. In both situations, upper and lower archwires must be cinched back on all quadrants behind the molar tubes.

If archwires are not cinched back distal to upper molar tubes, the MPA works as an efficient individual molar distalizer. When the archwires are cinched back, upper teeth will move distally en masse. It must be remembered that the lower archwire must be locked behind the molar tubes in any situation.

Both growing patients and adults respond well to MPA treatment. Recently, the authors have been dealing with several first molar extraction cases both in adults and in growing patients. When the lower first molars are absent, the lower anterior anchorage provided by the MPA is often used to support forward movement of the second and lower third molars without the risk of undesirable lingual inclination of lower incisors.

Patients' reactions to the MPA vary on an individual basis. Some complain strongly about the initial discomfort, while others accept it without difficulty. Just after installation some patients say they cannot close their mouth. They are instructed to lightly project their mandible forward and start closing from that point on. From then on, they start to get accustomed to the appliance and each passing day they feel more at ease with it. Something that can be annoying is the posterior open bite that appears just after installation. This is due to placing the incisors in an edge-to-edge position for maximum activation in the presence of a Spee curve.[8] Patients are advised not to try to chew strongly with their posterior teeth in the presence of an open bite, which would risk loosening of the upper molar tubes from their bands.

The most critical discomfort occurs between the first and third days, although it can last up to 1 week. During that adaptation period, we are fully available to the patient, hearing their complaints and encouraging them. If they have doubts regarding cessation of the discomfort, we like to show them video-clips from other patients of the same age who describe their own experience with the appliance. Usually, the patient interviewed in the clip says that they also felt a lot of discomfort in the beginning but 3 days later they could already tolerate it without a problem, and that after 30 days they felt as if they had nothing within their mouth. This certainly gives new patients a lot of reassurance.

We like to install MPAs on Friday afternoons, because after leaving the office the patient goes home and normally does not have to go to school until the following Monday, which gives them a weekend period to adapt to the appliance. This is very useful for those patients whose faces became stressed after MPA installation. By Monday their faces should be relaxed again. Curiously some patients, regardless of the discomfort felt, insist on keeping their MPAs. In their opinion their faces become so much better after installation that they want to keep the improvement obtained, in spite of knowing that such improvement is artificial, at least temporarily.

Indications for Use

The MPA has proved its efficacy in the treatment of:
- late mixed dentition malocclusions
- growing patients in the pubertal period
- upper molar distalization
- asymmetric cases (Class II division 1 or 2)
- adult patients
- first molar extraction cases.

Late Mixed Dentition Treatment

The utilization of the MPA in the mixed dentition is possible provided labial inclination of lower incisors is closely monitored. Since in most cases lower canines are not yet present and lower second molars are far from erupting, available lower anchorage at that moment is less than desirable. This may cause too much labial inclination of the lower incisors. One alternative to diminish such risk could be the gradual activation of the appliance. Mixed dentition cases treated by the authors are selected according to the severity of the malocclusion and its effect on the child's facial disharmony, which may cause psychologic problems. The risk of damaging procumbent incisors if the child is not treated is also taken into consideration. If such aspects are not too severe, it is preferable to postpone treatment. It must be borne in mind that very young patients still have much growth ahead, a fact that may cause the malocclusion to relapse if the correction of the maxillomandibular relationship is not maintained by an appropriate functional removable appliance.

Growing Patients

Growing patients' responses to MPA treatment are usually positive, often demonstrating great increments of mandibular growth, with an apparent restriction in growth of the maxilla.[3] This is often associated with widening of the maxillary dental arch resulting from the expansive distal vector that occurs when the mandible is returning to the distal position it occupied before the appliance activation. In spite of this expansive vector, we do not combine the MPA with palatal bars, considering the frequent observation of the aperture of the heavy stainless steel 0.019 × 0.025″ archwire to be enough. We also take into consideration that such effect is sometimes desirable.

Just as with patients in the mixed dentition, future growth may indicate the need to maintain the maxillomandibular correction by means of a functional intermaxillary removable appliance.

Upper Molar Distalization

If upper molars are free to slide along the archwire when pushed by the MPA, their individual distal movement obtained by this means is normally very large. This has been used advantageously in several situations of maxillary dentoalveolar discrepancies, such as blocked out cuspids or palatal blocking of bicuspids.

Asymmetric Cases (Class II Division 1 or 2)

Class II division 1 or 2 cases associated with midline shifts respond well to MPA treatment through its unilateral or bilateral use with greater activation on the discrepancy side.[10] The correct management depends on the malocclusion situation. The correction may occur by

distal movement of the upper first and second molars on the Class II side and then lateral movement of the other teeth to the space created by the MPA. For this individual molar distal movement to occur, it is necessary not to lock the upper archwire behind the molar tubes. On the other hand, if the decision is to correct the Class II side and midline discrepancy simultaneously through "en masse" movement of the entire dentoalveolar bone, both the upper and lower archwires must be cinched back behind their molar tubes on all quadrants. The choice of the most appropriate procedure depends mainly on the professional treatment plan for the case.

Adult Patients

Since the alterations induced by the MPA are apparently dentoalveolar in nature, there is no conventional limit to treatment based on age if the teeth and their support are healthy.[11,12] For adults, the length of time for which the MPA must stay in the mouth does not differ much from the time applied to growing juvenile patients: around 6–8 months. Adult patients have demonstrated much better stability than younger patients. Their retention aims solely at the maintenance of teeth alignment. The author's appliance of choice for this procedure is the Essix Retainer (Raintree Essix, Metairie, LA).

First Molar Extraction Cases

Due to the absence of adequate decay prevention programs, many communities throughout the world present great prevalence of lost or indicated-for-extraction first molars. Frequently, such teeth are still present but are carrying large restorations, endodontic root treatment or prosthetic crowns.

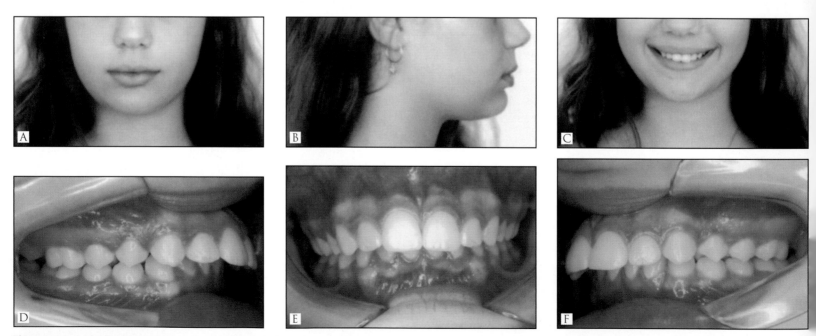

Figure 7.2 Patient 1. Pretreatment intraoral and extraoral photographs.

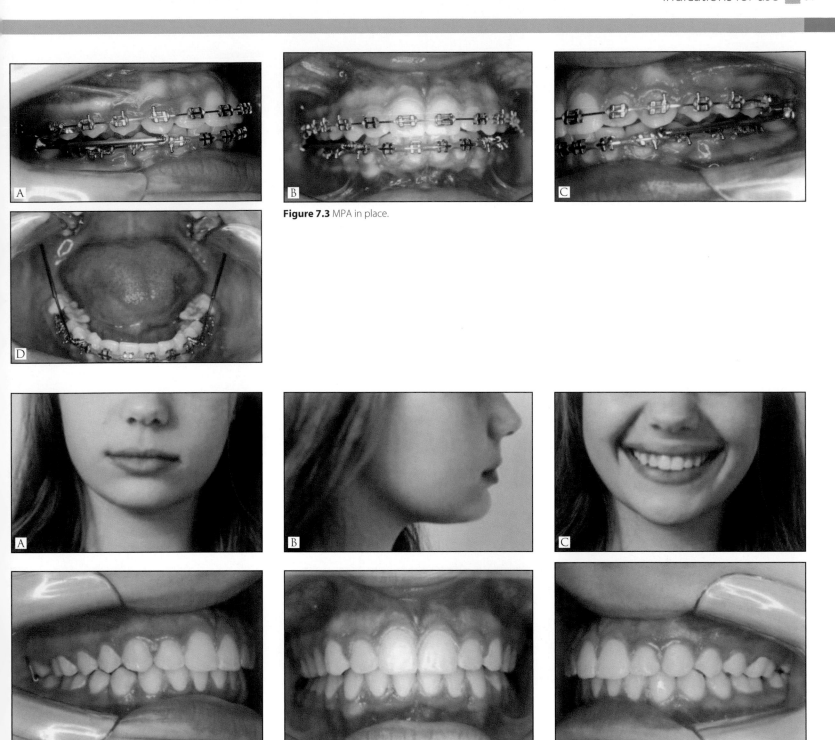

Figure 7.3 MPA in place.

Figure 7.4 Posttreatment intraoral and extraoral photographs.

If it is decided that the longevity of those teeth is not promising and third molars are demonstrated radiographically to be normal in size and anatomy, the compromised first molars are selected for extraction. If the case is a Class I with bimaxillary protrusion, the treatment protocol is simple and includes retracting sliding mechanics in the lower jaw until the desired axial inclination of lower incisors is attained. Then an MPA is used to anchor the upper second molars while maxillary anterior teeth are retracted also by sliding mechanics. If there is still some space left mesial to the lower second molars when the lower incisors have reached their desirable axial inclination, such space is closed by bringing those second molars forward by means of activated bull-loops. There

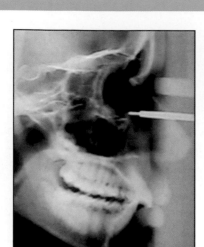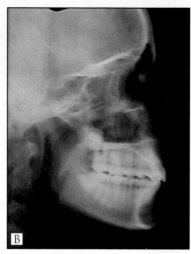

Figure 7.5 Lateral cephalometric radiographs. **A)** Initial. **B)** Final.

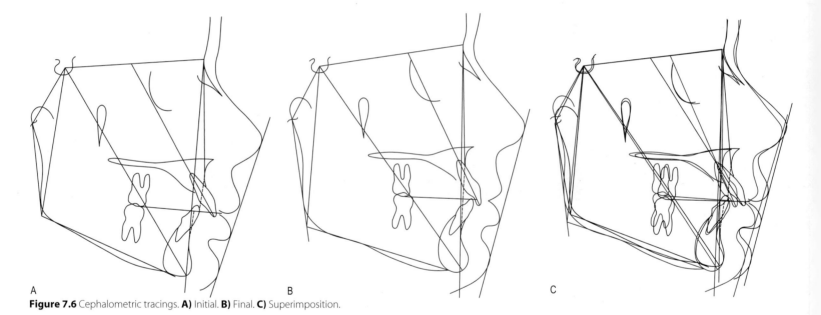

A   B   C

Figure 7.6 Cephalometric tracings. **A)** Initial. **B)** Final. **C)** Superimposition.

is no danger of undesirable lingual inclination of the lower incisors during this process, since they are heavily anchored by the MPA.

During all such procedures, the activation of the MPA is light, barely sufficient for the appliance to work as an anchor device. On the other hand, if after all spaces are closed the teeth are in Class II relation, activation must be adequately increased so that Class I is attained by "en masse" dentoalveolar movement.

Contraindications

The MPA is not indicated for use in the deciduous and early mixed dentition. This is due to the lack of adequate dental support to resist the heavy muscular force derived from the activation of the appliance. Even in late mixed dentition cases, the MPA must be used with

caution for the same reason. Cases with excessive labial inclination of lower incisors are also contraindicated if such inclination cannot be corrected before MPA installation. This is because the increase in the labial inclination of the lower incisors is the main adverse effect generated by the MPA. Finally, each individual case must be carefully analyzed to decide if it belongs in the surgical category, which would contraindicate the use of the MPA.

Clinical Cases

Patient 1

This patient was a 13-year-old girl presenting with a Class II division 1 malocclusion. A nonextraction treatment plan was decided upon and a MPA was applied. The treatment time was 28 months (Figs 7.2–7.6; Table 7.1).

Patient 2

The patient was a 13-year-old boy transferred from another orthodontist. He presented with a Class II division 1 malocclusion associated with severe space deficiency for the upper cuspids, which were impacted. The upper left cuspid appeared to be severely rotated in the X-ray, which cautioned us against extracting the first bicuspids in case we could not bring the upper left canine to normal occlusion due to its compromised position.

Regardless of the patient's biprotrusion, we decided upon a nonextraction treatment plan. An MPA was utilized for upper molar distalization. When sufficient space was created, the cuspid was exposed surgically and brought orthodontically to the occlusal plane. In such configuration upper archwires were not locked behind their molar tubes. Biprotrusion was diminished through anterior and posterior dental stripping. The treatment time was 34 months (Figs 7.7–7.12; Table 7.2).

Patient 3

This case of a 12-year-old girl is presented to illustrate the correction of a Class II division 1, subdivision condition in which all right teeth were in Class II relationship, while all left teeth were in Class I. There was also dental crowding and a light upper dental midline deviation to the left side. Her treatment was carried out without extractions by utilizing an MPA with heavier activation on the Class II side. The treatment time was 28 months (Figs 7.13–7.17; Table 7.3).

Table 7.1. Patient 1. Cephalometric measurements before and after treatment.

Variable	Before treatment	After treatment
SN	75 mm	75 mm
SAr	33 mm	33 mm
ArGo	49 mm	56 mm
GoGn	77 mm	79 mm
Y axis	127 mm	128 mm
Witts	+4 mm	−0.5 mm
^SNA	87°	82°
^SNB	82°	80°
^ANB	5°	2°
>S	125°	127°
>AR	144°	144°
>GO	119°	115°
U1 to SN	116°	115°
L1 to NB	4 mm	4 mm
Pg to NB	2 mm	2 mm

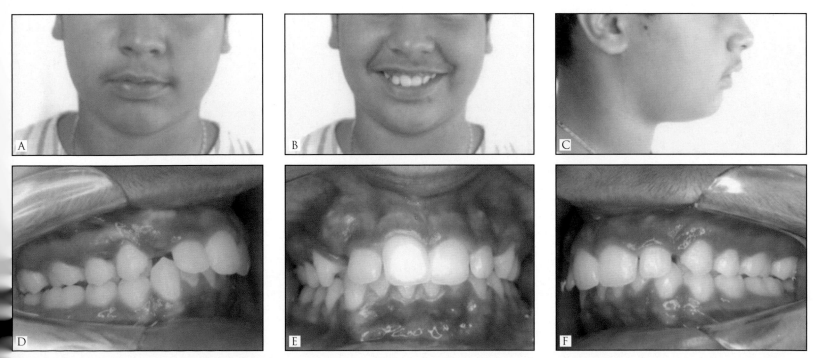

Figure 7.7 Patient 2. Initial intraoral and extraoral photographs.

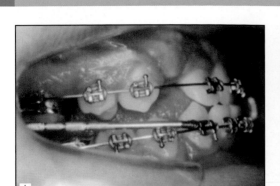

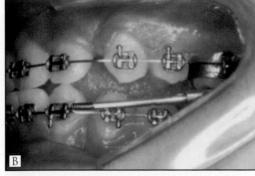

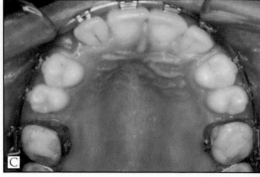

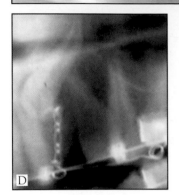

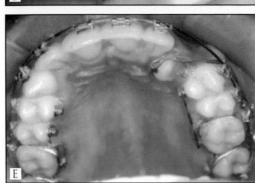

Figure 7.8 A–C) Space being generated by upper molar distalization through the use of MPA. **D)** Orthodontic traction of the upper left cuspid after creation of the necessary space. **E)** Derotation of the upper left cuspid after orthodontic traction.

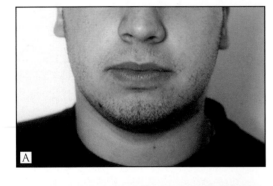

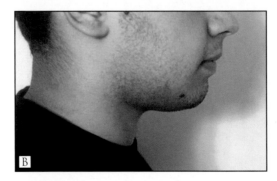

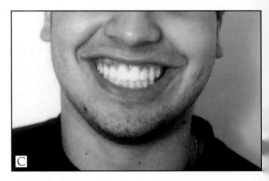

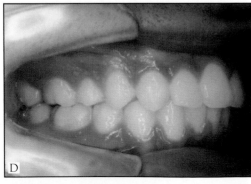

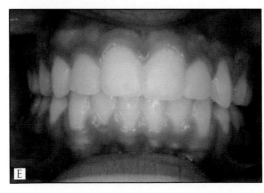

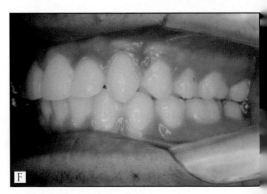

Figure 7.9 Posttreatment intraoral and extraoral photographs.

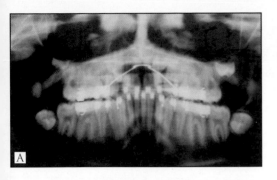
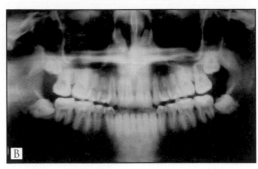

Figure 7.10 Panoramic radiographs. **A)** At the time of transfer. **B)** Final.

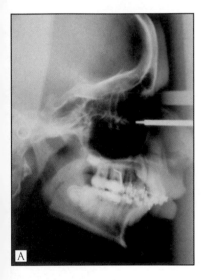
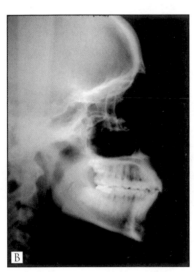

Figure 7.11 Lateral cephalometric radiographs. **A)** At the time of transfer. **B)** Final.

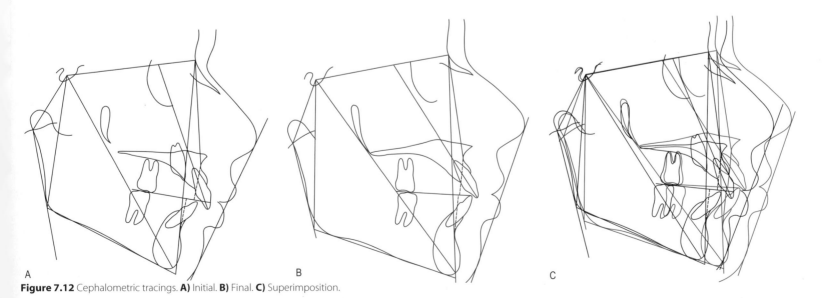

A   B   C

Figure 7.12 Cephalometric tracings. **A)** Initial. **B)** Final. **C)** Superimposition.

Table 7.2. Patient 2. Cephalometric measurements before and after treatment.

Variable	Before treatment	After treatment
SN	74 mm	78 mm
SAr	37 mm	38 mm
ArGo	46 mm	50 mm
GoGn	78 mm	84 mm
Y axis	125 mm	135 mm
Witts	4 mm	2 mm
^SNA	86°	87°
^SNB	78°	82°
^ANB	8°	5°
>S	128°	121°
>AR	138°	147°
>GO	108°	108°
U1 to SN	107°	112°
L1 to NB	7 mm	9 mm
Pg to NB	1.5 mm	3 mm

Table 7.3. Patient 3. Cephalometric measurements before and after treatment.

Variable	Before treatment	After treatment
SN	70 mm	71 mm
SAr	41 mm	41 mm
ArGo	48 mm	54 mm
GoGn	75 mm	75 mm
Y axis	123 mm	123 mm
Witts	+3 mm	+2 mm
^SNA	87°	86°
^SNB	83°	82°
^ANB	4°	4°
>S	126°	123°
>AR	135°	140°
>GO	121°	115°
U1 to SN	110°	90°
L1 to NB	8 mm	6 mm
Pg to NB	4 mm	2 mm

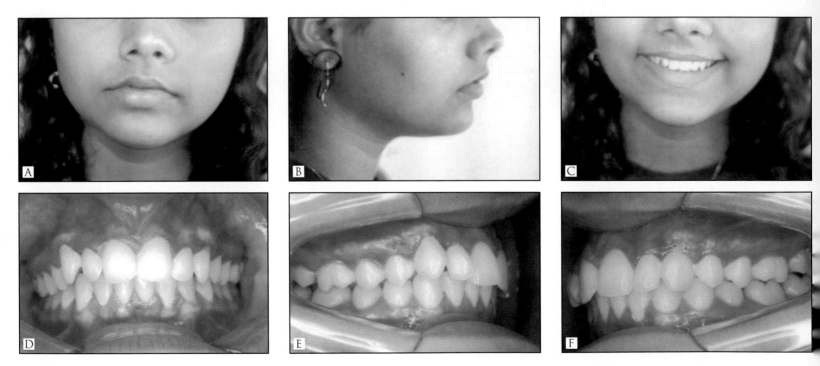

Figure 7.13 Patient 3. Pretreatment intraoral and extraoral photographs.

Additional Considerations

After utilizing the mandibular protraction appliance for 15 years we cannot overstate our satisfaction with it. This satisfaction includes several features such as reduced cost, ease of construction and installation, acceptance by the patient, lightness, reduced failure occurrence and, most of all, the predictability of its results. It is as if, during the MPA activation, you construct a template around which

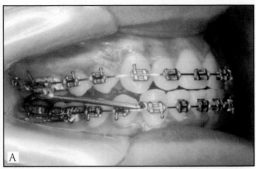

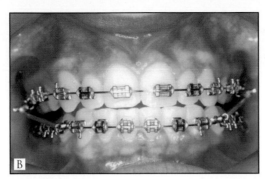

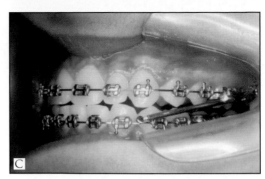

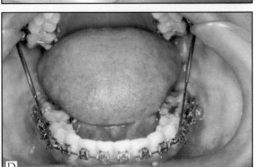

Figure 7.14 MPA in place activated to exert a heavier force on the Class II side with the objective of rotating the entire upper dentoalveolar bone to the right, thus correcting the Class II. Activation also placed upper and lower midlines coincident.

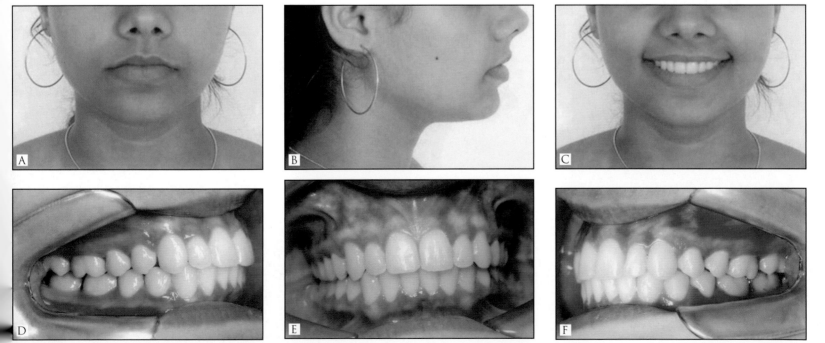

Figure 7.15 Posttreatment intraoral and extraoral photographs.

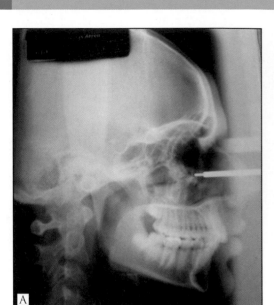

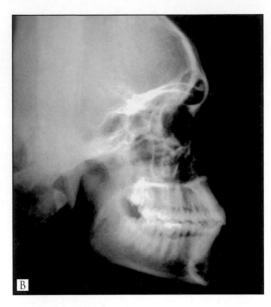

Figure 7.16 Lateral cephalometric radiographs. **A)** Pretreatment. **B)** Posttreatment.

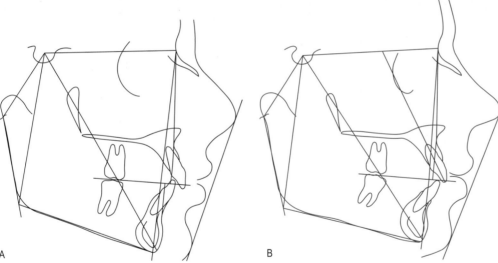

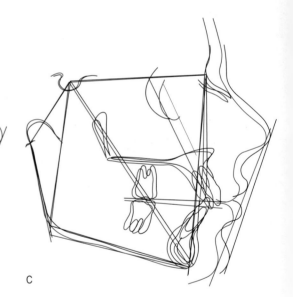

Figure 7.17 Cephalometric tracings. **A)** Initial. **B)** Final. **C)** Superimposition.

function may correct the existing deviations, building the occlusion around a "normality" template.

However, we consider it necessary to mention that the principles governing MPA performance are the same as those for other similar fixed functional appliances. The differences are merely a question of mechanics. What really seems to count is the concept of utilizing forces generated by the anterior or lateral positioning of the mandible to reciprocally adjust upper and lower dental arches. The appliance per se is only a secondary detail and success with it can be achieved only via the expertise of the conscious clinician. Many aspects of the MPA's mode of action are not clear but once the clinical results have proved more than satisfactory, basic research can be undertaken to further investigate its clinical efficacy.

References

1. Pancherz H. Treatment of Class II malocclusions by jumping the bite with the Herbst appliance. Am J Orthod 1979;76:423–442.

2. Coelho Filho CM. Mandibular protraction appliances for Class II treatment. J Clin Orthod 1995; 29:319–336.

3. Coelho Filho CM. Clinical application of the Mandibular Protraction Appliance. J Clin Orthod 1997;31:92–102.

4. Coelho Filho CM. The Mandibular Protraction Appliance N° 3. J Clin Orthod 1998;32:379–384.

5. Coelho Filho CM. Emprego Clínico do Aparelho para Projeção da Mandíbula. R Dental Press Ortodon Ortop Facial1998;3:69–130.

6. Coelho Filho CM. Mandibular Protraction Appliance IV. J Clin Orthod 2001;35:18–24.

7. Coelho Filho CM. Aparelho de Protração Mandibular IV. R Dental Press Ortodon Ortop Facial 2002;7:49–60.

8. Pancherz H. The mechanism of Class II correction in Herbst appliance treatment. A cephalometric investigation. Am J Orthod 1982;82:104–113.

9. Ruf S, Hansen K, Pancherz H. Does orthodontic proclination of lower incisors in children and adolescents cause gingival recession? Am J Orthod Dentofacial Orthop 1998;114: 100–106.

10. Coelho Filho CM. Clinical application of the mandibular protraction appliance in upper lateral agenesy and in asymmetric cases. Tex Dent J 2002;119:618–626.

11. Coelho Filho CM. O Aparelho de Protração Mandibular (APM) no tratamento de pacientes adultos. In: Sakai E, ed. Nova visão em ortodontia – ortopedia facial. São Paulo: Editiones Santos; 2002: 457–463.

12. Coelho Filho CM, White L. Treating adults with the Mandibular Protraction Appliance. Orthodontic CYBERjournal, 2003. Available online at: www.oc-j.com/jan03/MPA2.htm

CHAPTER 8

The Mandibular Anterior Repositioning Appliance (MARA™)

James E. Eckhart

CONTENTS

Brief Description of the MARA™

The MARA™ (Allesee Orthodontic Appliances, Sturtevant, WI) is a Class II corrective device which does not require compliance to be effective. It can be considered to be a fixed twin block. It is "fixed" in that it is cemented, not removable. It is similar to a twin block in that it has two opposing vertical surfaces positioned to keep the lower jaw forward. By holding the lower jaw forward long enough, growth and/or remodeling of the jaws and migration of the teeth result in a permanent change in the bite, from Class II to Class I (Fig. 8.1).

Historical Perspective

The earliest reference which may illustrate the use of opposing vertical surfaces to correct a Class II is in Angle's textbook of 1900.[1] Herbst mentioned that he tried but discarded the concept of inclined planes.[2] McCoy showed what may have been two opposing surfaces in his text.[3] Clark introduced the twin block in 1988.[4] Hanks wrote and illustrated a review of significant inclined plane functional Class II treatment predecessors.[5]

Toll developed the modern concept and the name of the MARA and taught it to others via study clubs (1985–1989). Dischinger relayed the concept to another study club (1990), where the current author learned of it and developed it to become commercially feasible (1990–1996). Other persons influential in its development were Damon (the vertical leg of the elbow, 1994), Kent Smith (the use of large square wire and tubes for torque control of elbows, 1994), Simon (the ball hook tieback and the buccal shield, 1998), Engelbart (the square wire lower arm, 2000), and Fuller (the e-MARA™, 2001).

Biologic Basis and Overview of Treatment Effects

Since there are some lecturers who advocate posturing the mandible downward and forward on the articular eminence and leaving it there as a method of treating Class II malocclusions, it should be clarified that this is not what the MARA is intended to do. The goal of MARA treatment is that the mandibular condyles, although displaced anteriorly and downward initially, eventually will be relocated in the approximate centers of the fossae. For years this has been confirmed by the author by TMJ-oriented tomograms before removing the MARAs.

One published study of the MARA shows that the treatment effects are quite similar to the effects of the Herbst.[6] A group of 30 children treated for 10.7 months, when compared to similar untreated controls, was found to have experienced 2.4 mm distal upper molar movement, 0.7 mm mesial lower molar movement, 0.0 mm posterior upper jaw movement, and 2.7 mm anterior lower jaw movement. However, in this study tomograms were not taken to ascertain the condyle position, so the last measure of lower jaw movement might be suspect.

Detailed comparison of the lateral cephalograms and tomograms taken before and after MARA treatment of Eckhart's patients shows considerable differences between boys, girls, and adults. Without comparing to untreated controls but only comparing the before-treatment records to the mid-treatment records, boys and girls both show considerable growth of the mandible but girls show much less than boys, presumably because they are closer to skeletal maturation. Adults show essentially no growth, only dentoalveolar remodeling changes in both jaws. Small changes are seen in the porion (suggesting movement of the temporal bone) and in the glenoid fossa, and larger changes are seen in the maxilla and mandible and in the dentition, depending on the timeframe of the study.

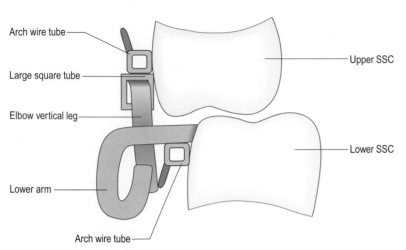

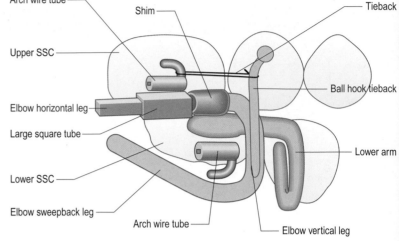

Figure 8.1 The names of the parts of the MARA.

Parts of the MARA

Maxillary Parts

Stainless Steel Crowns and Bands

The MARA attaches to the first permanent molars via either stainless steel crowns or very thick or reinforced bands. Crowns are preferred by many because they are so strong and resist tearing from the leverage forces of the elbows and arms. Further, the high heat involved in soldering the attachments to the buccal surface can be better dissipated by conduction with crowns than with bands, thus avoiding annealing and weakening. Also, crowns provide superior retention by covering more of the molar crown.

Bands are preferred by some because they do not cover the occlusal surface and therefore do not cause intrusion of the molars from occlusion. Some fear that the TMJ would be adversely affected by occlusal coverage, although this has not been found to be true by this author. Some dislike fitting stainless steel crowns due to unfamiliarity, although it is easy (five crown sizes cover the range of 20 band sizes). More than one manufacturer makes very thick molar bands which are suitable. There is not quite as much room on a band vertically for soldering. Some prefer bands because crowns can be so difficult to remove but conversely, bands can come off too easily, whereas techniques exist to remove crowns easily. At this time, most users prefer crowns. Some crown users remove much of the occlusal of the crown prior to cementing, leaving only a lip-rim on the occlusal surface.

Large Square Tube

The large square tube has an internal dimension of 0.063″ on each side, accepting a large square wire elbow of 0.060″. The tube is 4 mm long and its wall thickness is 0.015″. It is soldered onto the buccal surface of the crown, occlusal to the archwire tube. Prior to

soldering, the tube is laser-welded to the crown to reinforce the solder.

Archwire Tube

A single edgewise archwire tube (0.022 × 0.028″) with a hook is welded in the center of the buccal surface to the crown or band (0.018 × 0.028″ is available upon request).

Occlusal Rests

Occlusal rests may be soldered to the distal occlusal of the upper crown, extending onto the mesial occlusal of the second molar. This extension may or may not be bonded onto the surface of the second molar. The purpose is to keep the marginal ridges of the molars at the same height, discouraging distal tip-back of the first molar, which is more likely to happen while treating adults, who have greater dentoalveolar movement due to less growth.

Rapid Palatal Expander, Transpalatal Arches

RPEs can be placed on upper MARA crowns or bands if the upper jaw needs preliminary expansion. However, most users find that 80% of the time a separate traditional RPE is best, followed by a separate MARA. If the entire MARA is delivered at once with a RPE, it is possible that the elbows will be difficult to adapt to the lower crowns due to the upper width insufficiency. Some users deliver only the upper crowns and RPE, leaving out the lower crowns and the elbows until after the expansion is completed. Other users have placed all the components at once, adapting the elbows with a dog-leg bend (Fig. 8.2) and seeing the patient more often to torque the elbows inward as the upper widens.

TPAs are optional. If present, they assure that the crowns are cemented in the same rotational position in which the lab fabricated them; they maintain the width and torque of the first molars and

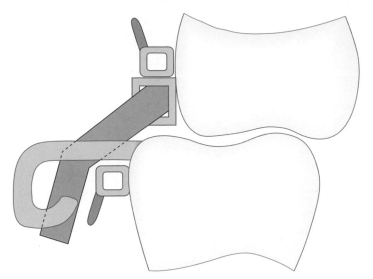

Figure 8.2 If the upper molar is too narrow, the elbow can have a dog-leg bend to engage the lower arm.

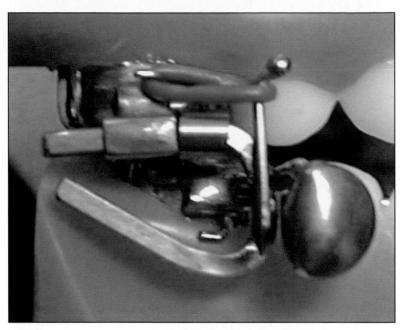

Figure 8.3 The elbow is triangular, with the horizontal leg, the vertical leg, and the sweepback leg.

they help assure that if one crown loosens, it will not fall out and be swallowed. They are not necessary to prevent distal buccal rotation of the first molar, because that does not happen very much and if it does happen, that usually helps to correct the Class II.

Elbows

Standard Elbows

Elbows are made of square stainless steel wire 0.060″ on a side. They are bent roughly into a triangle shape. The top portion of the triangle is the horizontal leg which slides into the large square tube on the upper molar. The horizontal leg is 20 mm long initially, but usually gets trimmed shorter to fit the mouth. From its anterior end, the vertical leg drops straight down and it is 10 mm long. The inferior end of the vertical leg curls backward and upward and becomes the sweepback leg which extends distally diagonally toward the posterior end of the horizontal leg (Fig. 8.3).

Onto the lateral surface of the vertical leg is welded a ball hook. The ball end faces upward and the ball hook is ligated to the archwire tube hook, to prevent the elbow falling out of the large square tube.

The elbows are the movable part of the MARA. They slide into the large square tubes from the mesial and are tied in. The vertical leg forms one of the vertical interfaces which hold the lower jaw forward. The anterior–posterior position of the vertical leg varies because spacers (also called shims, washers or bushings) are placed onto the horizontal leg to limit how far it can slide into the large square tube.

Shims

The shims are made of stainless steel round tubing with an inner diameter of approximately 0.085″ and a wall thickness of around

0.015″. They come in lengths of 1, 2, 3, 4, and 5 mm. They are standard Herbst shims (Fig. 8.4). Shims are used both to produce the advancement and to control the midline. By varying the length of the shims asymmetrically, one can align the midlines in cases where they are not aligned.

Very Long, Very Tall Elbows

Very long elbows (long in the anterior–posterior dimension), in which the horizontal leg is 25 mm long, have been used in some cases where the lower molar is unusually far forward, such as when the lower second premolar is missing and the first molar is forward into its space. There is some disadvantage to the long lever arms of long elbows easily getting out of control, or jacking the stainless steel crowns loose from the molars, so that a better approach in such a case would be to place the lower arms further back toward the distal of the lower molars and to use standard elbows.

Very tall elbows (tall in the vertical leg dimension) have been tried, especially in cases with big posterior open bites, with vertical legs of 15 mm, but they are usually unsatisfactory because the lower portion of the vertical leg and the sweepback leg hit the lower alveolar mucosa and cause pain. They cannot be successfully torqued laterally to avoid the mucosa because then the lower arms bite inside them.

Jackscrew Elbows

Elbows have been made out of jackscrews and they have some advantages. They offer a broad, flat surface to the cheek which helps

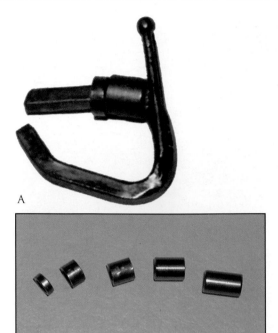

Figure 8.4 The shims come in varying lengths and slide onto the horizontal leg of the elbow.

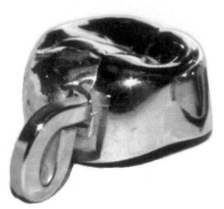

Figure 8.6 The lower arm provides the second vertical surface.

shield the cheek from the lower arm projection. They can be advanced by both shimming and turning the jackscrew, so they have a longer range of action. Further, they are easily adjusted because just like regular elbows, they are removable and can have their spindle turned extraorally. They sometimes need the distal occlusal corner ground down to avoid impingement on the lower alveolar mucosa (Fig. 8.5). They cost a bit more than standard elbows.

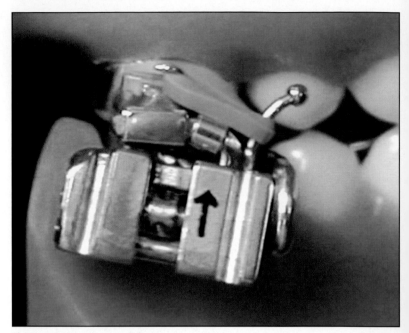

Figure 8.5 The jackscrew elbow.

Mandibular Parts

Stainless Steel Crowns and Bands

Either crowns or bands can be used on the lower molars. If bands are used, they should be the very hefty thick bands (or reinforced bands).[7] On at least one brand of stiff band, there is sufficient room vertically for both the arm and an archwire tube. However, crowns are more commonly used than bands.

Arms

The lower arms are soldered onto the buccal surface of the crown or band in a horizontal mesial-distal solder joint near the occlusal, above the archwire tube. Prior to soldering, the arms are laser-welded to the crown to reinforce the solder. The anterior of the solder joint gives rise to the buccally perpendicular projecting arm, which is normally located flush with the mesial of the crown or band. The arm projects buccally 8 mm and then curves downward into a flattish loop around 8 mm tall, which tucks inward. The arm is made out of 0.060″ square stainless steel wire (Fig. 8.6).

Buccal Shields

Some users request a sagittal loop to be soldered onto the vertical loop and then to be filled with solder, creating a pad or shield to protect the cheek from the projection of the lower arm (Fig. 8.7).

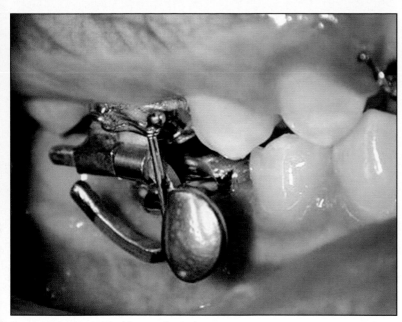

Figure 8.7 The buccal shield option for the lower arm.

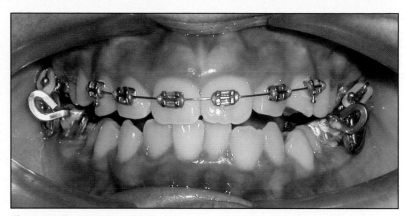

Figure 8.8 The MARA™ U, with the lower arms pointing upward, very good for incisor deep bite cases.

Upside-Down Arms

The lower arms can be inverted so that the loop points upward instead of downward. This has the advantage of increasing the vertical overlap between the elbow and the arm, making it more difficult for the patient to disengage from the guiding surfaces when they open their mouth part-way. This is called the MARA™ U (for upside down). It is particularly useful in posterior open bites caused by advancing incisor deepbite cases into Class I (Fig. 8.8).

Archwire Tubes

A single edgewise archwire tube (0.022 × 0.028″ or 0.018 × 0.028″ upon request) with a hook is welded in the center of the buccal surface, to the crown or band, and then the arm is soldered above it after being laser-welded.

Lower Lingual Arch

The lower molars always need to be stabilized with a lower lingual arch (LLA), usually 0.036″ stainless steel. The lingual arch may be fastened via a lingual sheath or by solder. If the lower molars are not stabilized, the pressure of the vertical leg of the upper elbows pushing anteriorly on the back side of the lower arms causes the lower molars to rotate mesiolingually, and as they do so, the buccal projection of the lower arm diminishes and the elbow is unable to stay engaged behind it, so the mandible drops back into Class II. It has also been found that braces alone on the lower teeth are insufficient to prevent this unwanted molar rotation, and that a lingual arch is required even if lower braces are present.

Occlusal Rests

Provided that a lower lingual arch is used, there is no need for occlusal rests on the lower crowns. The molars do not tip or rotate unfavorably if stabilized by a lower lingual arch. There is also no need for occlusal rests from the lower lingual arch to the lower first premolars, such as are used with Herbst treatment, because there is no vertical vector of force with the MARA.

Clinical Management

Decompensation, Expansion

In this author's experience, it is unusual to extract in Class II cases, so crowding is usually treated with arch expansion, widening the arches, and advancing the incisors.

Crowded incisors need to be unraveled either before or early during MARA treatment so they may be used as references for where to move the lower jaw. Similarly, in deepbite cases the incisors may need intrusion before MARA placement, so as not to increase the posterior vertical dimension more than necessary.

If the posterior upper jaw would be narrow relative to the lower when the lower jaw is advanced, then upper posterior widening should precede lower jaw advancement.

Separators

To place a MARA, the first molars must first be separated and the separators must be in place for 1–3 weeks. There are different possibilities for where the MARA will come from at the delivery appointment. It may come from a commercial lab or it may come from a kit within your own office but whichever source is used, preparatory instructions are written at the separator appointment. Either a lab slip or e-mail or fax must be sent to the commercial lab, or an in-house lab slip must be made for the lower lingual arch, which can be made on a new model or on the original hard copy study model.

Lab-fabricated MARA

Impressions, Separators, Preparing Models

If models are going to be sent to a commercial lab for MARA fabrication, alginate impressions are made and separators are then placed and left for the 2–3 weeks that the lab requires. The impressions are poured in plaster or hard stone with minimal bases. The heels are carved so the models can be hand-articulated without interferences, and the models are held together in the occlusion where you want the lab to make the case. Vertical pencil lines record that position on the models. The lab will slice-cut the mesial and distal contacts of the first molars on the models and will select and fit MARA crowns or bands directly onto the models. They will use bands or crowns from their inventory, so it is not necessary to prefit bands or crowns in the mouth to send to them. The distals of the molars should not be partly covered by gums (such as in partial eruption of immature molars), as that makes size selection by the lab unreliable. In such a case, you should fit a crown or band in the mouth (after separation) and tell the lab which size fits.

Lab Slip

For most commercial labs, the standard MARA comes with stainless steel crowns, standard elbows and shims, no buccal shields on the lower arms, a lower lingual arch, and no holes in the occlusal surfaces.

The lab slip should specify if you requested bands, jackscrew elbows, RPE, TPA, lower arms pointing upward, buccal shields, occlusal rests, and holes in the occlusal surfaces. You may be able to arrange a standing prescription that would be understood for each of your cases.

e-MARA fabricated MARA

One commercial lab (the primary lab) has developed a reliable method of providing MARAs electronically (e-MARA™), without receiving models through the mail. This enables that lab to send correctly fitting parts to orthodontists anywhere in the world or to a lab that the orthodontist chooses if they want MARAs fitted to models by a lab other than the primary lab.

The primary lab has determined that the mesial–distal width of a first molar can reliably predict the size of stainless steel crown that is required to fit that molar. The customer (orthodontist or sub-lab) can send the mesial–distal width information to the primary lab, either by sending an image of the occlusal surfaces of the study models with a millimeter ruler embedded in the image or by simply measuring the molar dimensions on the study model and sending that measurement. A data transmission form (hard copy or electronic) has been designed to facilitate the information transfer either by fax (hard copy) or e-mail (electronic) (Fig. 8.9). Upon receipt, the primary lab sends presoldered laser-welded crowns from existing inventory, and the customer solders the lingual arch (which they make to fit their original study model) to the crowns, after trying the crowns in the mouth. Many customers order one size larger and one size smaller, for insurance that one of the crowns will fit, and keep the remaining inventory in a kit for future delivery to another patient. In this manner, before long the customer is fitting patients from existing inventory and only ordering replacements.

Study Models, Separators

When using an e-MARA, the orthodontist would either take the beginning study models or new models made the day the separators are placed, and measure the mesial–distal width of the first molars to within a half millimeter, which will be transmitted to the primary lab. The same models would then be sent to a nearby or in-house lab for lower lingual arch bending. The patient would be sent home with separators in place, a handout explaining the separators and an appointment for 2–3 weeks later.

Transmission Form, E-Mail

The e-MARA transmission form can be either hard copy or electronic. A hard-copy version can have the blanks filled out, including the crown size selections wanted (the form itself has a table showing which millimeter measurements correspond to which crown sizes), with instructions on whether to place holes in the occlusals, whether extra sizes of crowns are wanted, or extra elbows or shims (all of which is listed on the form). Once completed, that form can be faxed or scanned and e-mailed.

If an electronic submission is preferred to hard copy, the electronic form can have the necessary information typed into it, can be saved under the patient's name, and can then be attached to an e-mail to the primary lab.

Kit-Fabricated MARA

Orthodontists can buy a kit of MARA parts, with enough inventory in it to treat several patients, thus enabling them to fit MARA crowns onto the patient directly from the kit as soon as the teeth are adequately separated. The kit contains multiple presoldered laser-welded crowns of each of the common sizes (sufficient inventory to treat a maximum of 13 patients, as of 2004). It also has right and left standard elbows, shims of several lengths, and a torquing tool. The kit is preferred by doctors outside the US who want to minimize customs duties and also by doctors anywhere who want the MARA made in their own office by their own lab technician. As parts are used from the kit, replacements can be ordered by e-mail using the

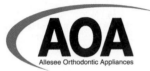

e-MARA

Communication Center
13931 Spring Street, PO Box 725, Sturtevent, WI 53177
1.800.262.5221
e-mail john.fuller@sybrondental.com

Dr. _____

Address _____

City, State, Zip _____

Tel. _____ Fax _____

Dr.'s e-mail _____

Patient _____

Date Transmitted _____ Placement Date_____

☐ Use crown sizes Upper R _____ L _____
　　　　　　　　　Lower R _____ L _____

☐ Remove occlusal of the crowns

☐ Vent holes in the occlusal of the crowns (3mm. diameter)

How to Use This Form:

From your accurate study models, measure the mesial-distal dimensions of each first molar to within a half millimeter. Using the table below, select the Ormco crown sizes corresponding to those dimensions, and enter those sizes into the box above. If you want openings in the occlusals of the crowns, enter that information above also.

From your lower study model, select a lower lingual arch size using the overlay acetate shapes template, and enter that size in the space below.

Standard MARA _____　　with buccal shields _____　　MARA U (with lower _____ Jack-screw upper elbows _____
　　　　　　　　　　　　　　　　　　　　　　　　　　　　　　arms pointing upward)

Tall Upper Elbows _____　　Short Upper Elbows _____　　Custom Elbows _____
(10mm vertical leg)　　　　　　(7mm vertical leg)　　　　　　(20mm long horizontal leg, 10mm vertical leg)
(most commonly ordered)　　　(not often used)　　　　　　　 (if 2 lower teeth missing, or if cantilevered lower arms)

Lower Lingual Arch size _____ LLA length left side _____　　LLA length right side _____

Vertical loops in LA _____　　Do solder the LLA _____　　Removable LLA _____

Additional Instructions: (Type here)

Occlusal Mesial-Distal Width of Molars:							
Upper 1st Molar	9.5mm = Ormco size	3R	3L	Lower 1st Molar	10.0 mm = Ormco size	3R	3L
	10.0 mm =	4R	4L		10.5 mm =	4R	4L
	10.5 mm =	5R	5L		11.0 mm =	5R	5L
	11.0 mm =	6R	6L		11.5 mm =	6R	6L
	11.5 mm =	7R	7L		12.0 mm =	7R	7L
	12.0 mm =	8R	8L		12.5 mm =	8R	8L

Please forward Extra MARA parts - (select parts and sizes, indicate quantity in parentheses)

Torquing Tool ( )
Upper Crown/MARA Assembly　Right side size 3 ( ) 4 ( ) 5 ( ) 6 ( ) 7 ( ) 8 ( )
　　　　　　　　　　　　　　　Left side size 3 ( ) 4 ( ) 5 ( ) 6 ( ) 7 ( ) 8 ( )
Lower Crown/MARA Assembly　Right side size 3 ( ) 4 ( ) 5 ( ) 6 ( ) 7 ( ) 8 ( )
　　　　　　　　　　　　　　　Left side size 3 ( ) 4 ( ) 5 ( ) 6 ( ) 7 ( ) 8 ( )
Upper Elbows:　Standard R ( ) L ( ) Short R ( ) L ( )　　　　Jack-screw Elbows R ( ) L ( )
Advancement Shims　　1mm ( ) 2mm ( ) 3mm ( ) 4mm ( )

September, 2005

Figure 8.9 The e-MARA™ transmission form.

e-MARA concept (see above). Lingual arches, TPAs, RPEs, and occlusal rests can be prefitted to the patient's study model and soldered once the crowns are selected from the kit, using an in-house lab.

Appointment Scheduling

Once separators have been placed and working models or study models have been obtained, the next appointment will be to deliver the MARA, from whichever source it is being supplied. If the crowns have been fitted by a lab to models, and any necessary soldering has already been done on models, the delivery appointment consists only of trying the completed appliance into the mouth, removing it and cementing it, and then educating the patient, which might require 45–60 minutes. If the crowns are being fitted from the e-MARA or the kit system, once fitted they will need some soldering prior to re-trying them in, and then the same following steps as above. The extra soldering might add around 20 minutes to that appointment. The interval between separator placement and MARA delivery should be at least 1 week to allow enough separation, but not longer than 3 weeks or the separators will start falling out.

Appliance Delivery

Removal of Separators and Trial

Once the separators have been in place at least a week, and the MARA parts are on hand, the separators are removed and the crowns are tried on.

Laboratory Fabricated

If the MARA was made in a lab to fit a model, the assembled parts (lower crowns with LLA, upper crowns with TPA, perhaps) are tried on the teeth. If the crowns fit too loosely, they can have their gingival margins crimped in with a Tweed plier. Before cementing, the upper crowns (with elbows) and lower crowns are observed in the mouth to verify that right and left elbows both touch the lower arms and that the dental midlines are aligned. When the patient bites in their retruded Class II bite, the lower arms should hit the sweepback legs of the elbows, interfering with bite closure. If the lower arms bite inside (medial to) the sweepback legs while the patient is attempting to bite in Class II, the elbows need to be torqued inward to correct that. The patient cannot be allowed any possibility of biting in Class II, or they will.

e-MARA or Kit Fabricated

If the MARA is being fitted onto the patient's teeth *without* having been prefit to a working model, using instead specific e-MARA crowns sent from the primary lab or crowns selected from your kit, once the separators are removed, a crown is chosen, pushed onto the molar with finger pressure, and evaluated for fit. If it is obviously too large, impinging on the gums and not snug on the tooth, a smaller size is selected. If it seems too snug, a larger crown can be tried. The proper sized crown is further seated by having the patient squeeze it into place using a bite stick. If a hole has been ground in the occlusal (to aid removal later) it enables one to see if the crown is seated fully. The properly seated crown will usually have its gingival margins slightly sub-gingival, but the margins rarely need to be trimmed shorter. Sometimes the gingival margins need to be crimped in tighter to eliminate minor rocking or gum impingement. Once the correct size is known, it is recorded in the patient's chart, in case a crown has to be replaced later. The rotation of the crowns can usually be adjusted somewhat so that the right and left sides have approximately the same distance between the mesial of the upper large square tubes and the back side of the lower arms when the patient is biting in Class I with the midlines centered over each other. This helps provide for the elbows to be extended the same on both sides.

Soldering Lower Lingual Arch

The preformed lingual arch should have bilateral vertical loops to allow adjustment of the anterior portion of the lingual archwire after soldering, in case a small error occurs in soldering. Those vertical loops should be placed opposite the lingual of the first premolars, so that the heat of soldering will not weaken the wire in the bending-stressed loop area, leading to a fracture later. After soldering the lower lingual arch, and grinding and polishing the solder joint, the arch is tried back into the mouth to adjust the torque of the crowns and to see what adjustment of the loops is needed.

Preparation for Cementing

Recording Sizes, Creating Removal Holes, Sandblasting, Waxing

After recording the crown sizes, the crowns are prepared for cementing. For easiest crown removal at the end of treatment, it is helpful to have already placed (prior to cementing) occlusal holes to accommodate a crown removal plier. In lower crowns, the occlusal hole is in the mesial *buccal* of the occlusal surface, about 3 mm diameter. In upper crowns, the occlusal hole is in the mesial *lingual*, also about 3 mm diameter. Also, on upper crowns it helps before cementing to have created a 0.5×2.0 mm horizontal slit in the mesial lingual axial corner halfway between the gingival and occlusal, to enable the crown removal plier beak to bite into the crown at removal time (Fig. 8.10). When glass ionomer cements are used, cement washout from these holes has never been a problem and decay under the crowns is not seen. The benefit of the holes is that crown removal is much less stressful to the patient, and is quite quick.

The crowns have been internally microetched (sandblasted) by the manufacturer but if a blaster is available in the office, it helps to reblast, to rid the interior of the crowns of any oxides that

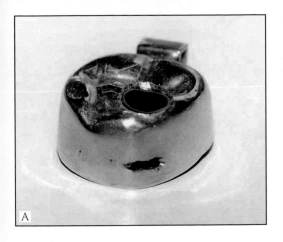
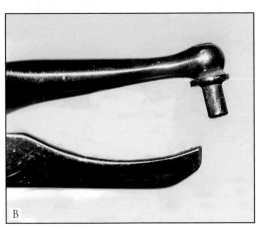

Figure 8.10 A horizontal slit in the mesial lingual corner facilitates later removal of the crown with the crown-removing plier.

might have accumulated over time and during try-in. The archwire tubes and large square tube are waxed to keep cement out of them.

Cementing

Teeth Preparation, Cement to Use, How to Mix, Cleanup

The teeth do not need to be etched to aid retention. They are only isolated and dried.

A good cement to use is gold-colored glass ionomer (Protech Gold, Ormco, Orange, CA) because it is easy to distinguish it from tooth enamel during cleanup and after crown removal. The cement should be mixed on a refrigerated glass or aluminum slab, using six drops of liquid per crown and spreading the cement out over the slab for maximum cooling. Six drops allows generous loading of the crown, preventing voids. If occlusal holes have been placed in the crowns, the cement will partly escape out the holes during seating and is easily wiped up. The crowns should be quickly bitten into place with a bite stick and then the excess cement wiped away. The patient should bite on cotton rolls for 5–10 minutes while waiting for the cement to harden. After the cement is hard and strong, the final scaling of cement from the crown margins can proceed.

Elbow Fitting

Once the cement is strong, elbows can be tried in. If they have not already been prepared by the lab, they can be prepared as follows. Before placing an elbow, the patient is guided to bite in Class I and an estimate is made of how many millimeters of shim are needed. The shims are selected from the kit or parts box and slid onto the horizontal leg of the elbow. The elbow is inserted into the large square tube and the patient is guided into the desired bite.

The vertical leg of the elbow is inspected to see how well it falls distal to the lower arm. If necessary, the elbow is removed and adjustment bends are placed in the horizontal leg to move the vertical leg medially or laterally, and up or down (Fig. 8.11). These bends are made with a small-beak three-prong plier (one which has space between the beaks, so the heavy wire has room to flow when being bent). The torque of the vertical leg (relative to the horizontal leg) is adjusted by sliding the torquing tool onto the horizontal leg, to hold it, while torquing the vertical leg with a utility plier (Fig. 8.12).

Next the sweepback leg is adjusted. It cannot be so medial that it hits the lower archwire tube when closing in Class I, nor the lower alveolar mucosa. Its distal extension cannot flare out into the cheek, but should be bent with the small-beak three-prong plier so that it curls up to nearly touch the horizontal leg, thus nearly completing a circle with the elbow so that no ends are poking out (see Fig. 8.4). The distal end of the horizontal leg can be cut shorter and then green-stoned to smooth the burred end.

After the elbows seem to be engaged correctly behind the lower arms and are not protruding into the cheeks, the final test is to have the patient briefly bite back in Class II and make sure the sweepback legs hit the top of the lower arms and that the lower arms do not bite inside (medial to) the sweepback legs, nor behind (distal to) them. Once these criteria are met, tie in the elbows, tying the ball hooks to the upper archwire tube hooks, using twisted-double steel ligatures, and tuck in the pigtail ends of the ligatures.

It should be emphasized that there is no requirement that the patient be advanced to Class I at the initial delivery appointment, particularly if the patient is a big Class II. It is wise to give the patient a minor advancement they can tolerate without too much difficulty, so they will not get a negative idea about the MARA. In big Class II cases, if they are advanced too far, they will be able to bite behind the sweepback leg when they relax back into Class II and the device will be ineffective. Do not advance a patient more than 4 mm at a time. They can come back in 2 months and they will easily tolerate additional advancement.

Home Care Instructions

Show the patient where to bite; it usually helps to say "Bite on your front teeth." Tell them that this is their new permanent jaw position

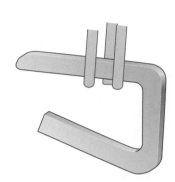

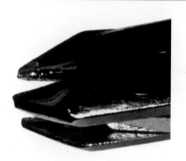

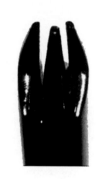

Figure 8.11 The legs of the elbow can be bent up, down, in or out to fit correctly behind the lower arm, using a small-beak three-prong plier with sufficient room between its beaks for the thick wire to flow.

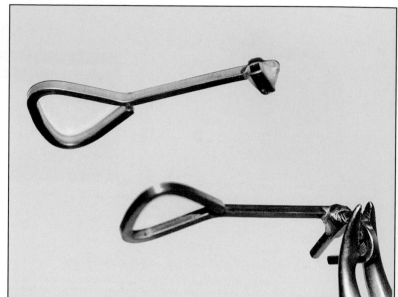

Figure 8.12 The torquing tool slides onto the horizontal leg to hold it, while the vertical leg is bent with a utility plier.

and they are not to bite in the overbite position any more. Tell them they will not be able to chew as well as they are used to and they had better try soft foods for a while until their skill returns. Warn them that accidental cheek biting is common for the first couple of days and that they will learn how to avoid it. For children, tell them not to "bang" on the arms because it leads to breakage, but for adults, tell them to keep the vertical surfaces in contact, because that pressure is what will cause the dentoalveolar remodeling necessary. Tell the patient to bring any loose parts with them if something breaks.

Well-adjusted arms and elbows do not cause cheek sores but if the patient experiences soreness inside the cheeks, they can place cotton wool over the area until they can come in for an adjustment.

The improvement in chin projection is worth pointing out to children, because a lot of it will become reality over the next year, but with adults, all the initial chin change relapses as the teeth migrate through the jaws and the muscles of mastication pull the mandible back distally.

Subsequent Advancements

The patient is usually scheduled for a 12 week appointment. At that point, the Class II has often partly returned, presumably due to migration of the molars. Usually the bite has also deepened somewhat. The canine relationship should be inspected; if the canines are Class II, advance the elbows with more shims. Also pay attention to the

relationship between the elbow vertical leg and the lower arm; if they are not well engaged, adjust the elbow. If the lower crowns are supported by a lower lingual arch, the positions of the lower arms should not change but it is common to have to adjust the elbows for better engagement.

In this manner, the patient is seen at 3–4 month intervals for a year. The MARA should have been in place without any advancement or repair for 4 months immediately prior to removal, in order to have confidence that the condyles are centered in the fossae and stable. TMJ tomograms help confirm this. In the absence of tomogram evidence, the ability to protrude the mandible 11–13 mm beyond where the MARA is holding the patient may indicate that the condyles are centered in the fossae.

User's Kit of Elbows, Shims, and Torquing Tool

Even if the orthodontist does not have a MARA kit, they should have a kit of extra parts, including elbows, shims, and a torquing tool. Patients sometimes come in having lost elbows, even though they were warned to bring any loose parts with them, so it is necessary to have replacement inventory. Also, longer elbows are sometimes needed during the progress checkups, and frequently more shims are needed.

The torquing tool is a piece of 0.063 square tubing laser-welded and soldered onto a handle of 0.060 square wire (see Fig. 8.12). The tool is slid onto the horizontal leg of an elbow in order to hold that leg without damaging its square corners while torquing the vertical leg. If the horizontal leg were held with a plier instead, it would tend to roll in the plier beaks and damage the corners of the wire.

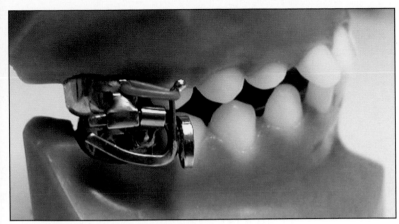

Figure 8.13 The lower arms cantilevered forward to the middle of the mesial tooth, so the elbow legs do not have to extend so far distally.

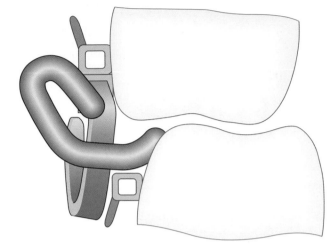

Figure 8.14 When the lower arm extends upward, it increases the vertical interface so that the patient is less likely to escape engagement by partially opening.

The kit of extra parts is normally provided by the primary lab with the initial MARA order. Replacement parts for it can be ordered by the e-MARA system.

Avoiding Trouble

Avoid using the MARA in young children unless the lower arms are cantilevered forward (Fig. 8.13), because with too little room in the posterior cheek area, there will be more emergencies. Do not attach the MARA to deciduous molars, because the long lever arms tend to loosen the teeth sooner and the crowns are very hard to remove from loose teeth. The first permanent molars must be erupted, with no gum coverings over the distal, in order to size the necessary crowns properly.

In high angle cases, do not extend an upper archwire from the anterior teeth to the first molar crown, because any distal tipping of the upper molar would tend to extrude the anterior teeth, making the face longer. In high angle cases, a cervical collar can be worn several hours per day to keep an intrusive force on the posterior teeth, preventing the face from lengthening.

Be sure the patient cannot bite behind the sweepback leg; it must extend distally enough that the patient cannot get behind it and do not advance them too far at first or they will bite behind it. Also, the vertical interface between the vertical leg of the elbow and the lower arm must be sufficient that the patient cannot easily open their mouth enough to disengage. Often it helps to have the lower arm loop point upward to increase the vertical interface (Fig. 8.14).

Do not let the distal extensions of the horizontal leg of the elbows extend more than 3 mm out of the large square tube, and be sure the sweepback leg approaches that distal extension, so that they shield each other. Do not let the lower arm extend too far buccally without good shielding from the elbow, or a cheek sore may develop.

Allow enough time before removing the MARA. Plan on severe Class IIs and adults taking longer than 12 months. Even if the condyles are recentered in the fossae, if the muscles attached to the mandible are still stretched because they have not had enough time for their periosteal attachments to migrate, they may pull the mandible distally after MARA removal, causing resorption on the posterior wall of the fossae and a relapse of the Class II correction.

The absence of posterior occlusion (posterior open bite) when the MARA is removed may allow too much loading of the immature new condylar bone, resulting in resorption and Class II relapse. Hence rapid closure of the posterior open bite with vertical elastics is recommended.

Removal

Provided that the removal holes were placed before cementing, removing the MARA is simple using the crown removal plier (Ormco, Orange, CA). For upper crowns, the beak of the plier inserts into the horizontal slit in the mesial lingual axial corner of the crown, and the post of the plier pushes through the 3 mm diameter hole in the mesial lingual portion of the occlusal surface of the crown. A firm squeeze will usually pop the crown loose without significant pain for the patient. The elbow does not need to be removed separately; it comes out with the crown. Since the teeth were not etched, but the interior of the crown was sandblasted, most of the cement comes off inside the crown, but usually there is some cement to clean off the occlusal of the tooth. If gold-colored cement was used, it is easy to detect and can be removed with a scaler or handpiece.

The lower crown is removed by placing the plier beak under the buccal archwire tube and arm, and placing the plier post into the 3 mm diameter hole in the mesial buccal portion of the occlusal surface of the crown, and then squeezing with a firm grip. The lingual arch comes out with the lower crowns.

After removing the MARA crowns, the posterior teeth are bonded with brackets, the archwire is extended back to the new brackets, and posterior vertical elastics are started, to close the posterior open bite.

Treatment Effects

Treatment Changes

The following information is derived from an unpublished study performed by the author of this chapter. A sample of 14 boys, 20 girls, and eight adults was used. For boys, the average start age was 13.1 years (range 11–15); for girls, the average start age was 11.7 years (range 9–15); for adults, the average start age was 30.8 years (range 16–49). The average headfilm interval was 21 months for boys (range 13–44); for girls it was 17 months (range 12–30); for adults it was 23 months (range 14–32). The T1 headfilm was taken before any treatment was started. The T2 headfilm was taken before the completion of orthodontic treatment, but when it was judged that the mandible seemed stable in the fossae, and it included TMJ tomograms to confirm that the condyles were centered in the fossae. The headfilm tracings were superimposed on sella–nasion at sella, and the antero-posterior measurements were made relative to a line drawn through sella, 20° posterior to perpendicular to sella–nasion.

Maxilla

The effect on the maxilla depends on the time period studied. There is a headgear-like backward movement of A-point due to the pressure on the vertical leg of the upper elbow from the lower arm. This movement is detectable when comparing treated patients to untreated controls, but not when looking only at treated children because forward growth overpowers the backward movement in both boys and girls in the short and longer term. Adults do show a small backward movement of A-point.

Mandible

The largest component of MARA Class II correction in children is mandibular growth, more so in boys than in girls (three times more), probably because girls are nearing skeletal maturation sooner than boys. In adults, mandibular growth does not happen with MARA treatment; in fact, the horizontal projection of pogonion seems to decrease as the mandible hinges vertically open a little.

Upper Molar

The upper molar moves backward within the maxilla around 2 mm equally in boys, girls, and adults. In children, this backward movement is concealed in longer-term studies because the molar later moves forward, so that without controls to compare with, the effect is not as clear.

Lower Molar

In children there is very little movement of the lower molar within the mandible. In girls the lower molar moves slightly forward; in boys it moves slightly backward. The group average is very negligible movement. In adults the lower molar moves around 2 mm forward within the mandible.

Fossa

The normal growth of the fossa is down and backward from sella in untreated children. With treatment, the fossa moves slightly but inconsequentially forward in the short run, but then resumes its backward descent. These changes can be seen by observing porion on lateral headfilms and also by tracing the outlines of the fossa from tomograms. The effects on the fossae for adults and children are less than 1 mm change.

Vertical Changes

In adults, vertical changes with the MARA tend to be counter-intuitive. Those adults with a high occlusal plane angle relative to SN (average 24°) before treatment tended to have their occlusal plane angle close during treatment, whereas those with a low occlusal plane angle relative to SN (average 16°) before treatment tended to have their occlusal plane angle open during treatment.

The MARA has no vertical vector of force on the molars because there is no connection between the jaws, only the interface between the vertical abutment surfaces. There is nevertheless an intrusive force on both upper and lower molars due to occluding on the stainless steel crowns, and this fact can cause the mandible to hinge downward initially, increasing the vertical dimension and opening the bite. Furthermore, advancing a deepbite incisor case forward to nearly end-to-end incisors increases the vertical height of the face. If braces are present concurrently, they will tend to intrude the incisors, shortening the face. If braces are not present concurrently, the posterior teeth will tend to erupt, until the posterior open bite closes and the face has been lengthened.

Posttreatment Changes

Class II Relapse

Similar to the Herbst, for reasons not well documented but hypothetically explained below, some Class IIs corrected with the MARA relapse to a greater or lesser degree. An easy explanation would be that the condyles were left down and forward on the eminence, and if this were true it would be understandable enough. However, nearly every case treated by this author had tomograms of the TMJs before removal of the MARA in order to verify that the condyles were centered in the fossae, and all patients were held in the MARA at least 1 year, usually longer. Yet occasionally a patient will relapse into a severe Class II, either unilaterally or bilaterally (more

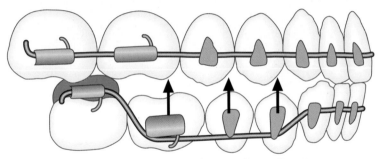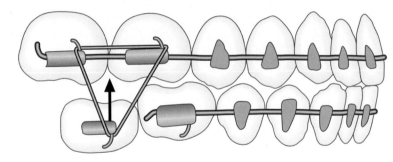

Figure 8.15 Bite closing wire and elastics configuration for rapid bite closing.

frequently but still only occasionally they relapse into a *slight* Class II and need Class II elastics as part of finishing, especially adults).

Allow enough time before removing the MARA. Plan on severe Class IIs and adults taking longer. Even if the condyles are recentered in the fossae, if the muscles attached to the mandible are still stretched because they have not had enough time for their periosteal attachments to migrate, they may pull the mandible distally after MARA removal, causing resorption on the posterior wall of the fossae or on the condylar head and a relapse of the Class II correction. Similarly, the absence of posterior occlusion (posterior open bite) when the MARA is removed may allow too much loading of the immature new condylar bone, resulting in resorption and Class II relapse.

To prevent a Class II relapse, one can use bite-advancing bite ramps bonded onto the lingual of the upper incisors (Ortho Organizers, San Marcos, CA). It is also possible to create a "distal shoe horn" hanging down vertically from the distal of the upper second molar, engaging the distal of the lower second molar and holding the mandible forward. Class II elastics can be used to a greater or lesser degree. One can also support the posterior occlusion with composite build-ups on the second molars while vertical elastics are worn to the first molars, and then remove the build-ups and apply elastics to the second molars, or by using an extruding wire configuration as shown in Figure 8.15.

References

1. Angle EH. Treatment of malocclusion of the teeth and fractures of the maxillae – Angle's system, 6th edn. Philadelphia: The S.S. White Dental Manufacturing Company; 1900: 162.

2. Herbst E. Atlas und Grundriss der Zahnarztlichen Orthopadie, vol 26. In: Lehmann JF, ed. Lehmann's Medizinische Handatlanten. Munich: J.F. Lehmann Verlag; 1910.

3. McCoy JD. Applied orthodontia. Philadelphia: Lea and Febiger; 1922: 292.

4. Clark WJ. The twin block technique. A functional orthopedic appliance system. Am J Orthod Dentofacial Orthop 1988;93:1–18.

5. Hanks SD. Trying to get out of the 20th century: a partial translation of Emil Herbst's 1910 text. World J Orthod 2000;1:9–16.

6. Pangrazio-Kulbersh V, Berger JL, Chermak DS, Kaczynski R, Simon ES, Haerian A. Treatment effects of the mandibular anterior repositioning appliance on patients with Class II malocclusion. Am J Orthod Dentofacial Orthop 2003;123: 286–295.

7. Rogers MB. The banded Herbst appliance. J Clin Orthod 2001;35:494–499.

CHAPTER 9

Energy management: the philosophy behind fixed intermaxillary mechanics

James J. Jasper

Introduction

Virtually everything an orthodontist does to treat their patients involves the application of physical pressures of a measured amount and direction to the teeth and jaws. These mechanical force vectors are usually produced by intraoral or extraoral machines that are called appliances. The energy required to power up the appliances that generate these oral force vectors can come from a variety of sources and is vitally important if the treatment plan is to proceed on time or indeed at all. It is, therefore, wise to develop a management awareness to control and protect these energy sources.

Difficulty of the Task

The facial deformity known as malocclusion is extremely stable. If left untreated, a large overjet at age 10 will persist and be present as a large overjet at age 20. Even if the malocclusion is treated orthodontically, there is a well-documented tendency of the face and teeth to return to their original stable state. The body calls this healing; orthodontists call it relapse.

The reason for this stability and the ongoing threat of relapse is that the original malocclusion is being created by two extremely powerful forces of nature: heredity and environment.

Force Vectors

Centuries ago, people realized that living things respond to physical pressure. Practitioners have used force vectors to create culturally determined versions of beauty. Force vectors were used by the Mayans to change head shapes, by the Chinese to change foot shapes, and by Bonsai gardeners to change plant shapes.

In the 1930s, a machine was invented by Dr Angle to deliver precise force vectors to individual teeth. Fixed edgewise mechanics gave orthodontists absolute control over tooth position and arch shape as long as the archwire, the energy source, was in place. In that era, most orthodontics was being done with removable appliances and there was considerable debate and controversy about whether using a fixed system was advantageous or safe. There were concerns about appliance breakage and iatrogenic damage from the constant force vectors that fixed edgewise was able to deliver. As Dr Angle admonished his contemporaries who were slow to change to fixed edgewise mechanics, "All you can do is push or pull or rotate teeth. I've given you a machine to do just that. Now, by God, use it." This fixed system recognized the need to manage energy input in order to control the output of results. A skilled practitioner of edgewise orthodontics would never think of using removable archwires and thus allowing the patient to control the energy sources that power these excellent tooth-straightening machines.

The dilemma, of course, is that malocclusion is an intermaxillary problem and to correct intermaxillary problems, one requires intermaxillary force vectors. The edgewise system that Dr Angle developed is, in reality, two separate intramaxillary machines: one for the maxilla and one for the mandible. Facial deformities, however, produce poor profiles, overjet, and soft tissue abnormalities that having straight teeth does very little to correct. Can the principles of edgewise mechanics (fixed energy source) be extended to the intermaxillary level by thinking in terms of an intermaxillary archwire?

Vector Generation Machines

The machines most commonly used for producing intermaxillary force vectors are still headgears and elastics. These appliances were popularized in the 1950s and are now routinely used by thousands of orthodontists on hundreds of thousands of patients every year. These machines utilized the technology that was available at that time and used rubber products to pull between the teeth or around the neck to pull the maxilla toward the neck. These pulling forces, however, produce vectors that have some very unfortunate side effects. Pulling forces, as a category, all tend to produce extrusion as a side effect simply due to the geometry of their vector diagrams. As excessive vertical development has been implicated as a primary etiologic factor in the majority of Class II malocclusions, it is bizarre to think of adding yet more extrusion during treatment with this category called pulling mechanics.

Cervical headgears pull down and back on the upper molars, which autorotates the chin distally and worsens the profile. Class II elastics also place extrusive vectors upon the upper incisors, which is normally contraindicated due to gummy smiles. When rubber products are used to pull between the dental arches, the resulting extrusive vectors also produce a lingual tipping moment which tries to narrow the often crowded dental arches. In fact, this early rubber-based pulling technology gave orthodontists vectors that seemed to be contrary to 90% of their treatment plans!

But by far the most serious complaint with the pulling force category is that these appliances are usually removable. Simply because an elastic is pulling between two points, it is forced to pull in too close to the teeth, which necessitates its removal during eating and brushing. How ironic it is to have a precise fixed machine to straighten individual teeth (which is of secondary importance) and then use an imprecise removable rubber band with poor vectors to treat the malocclusion (which is extremely important).

Practitioners have learned to compensate for the irregular usage of these removable appliances by increasing the force levels. Headgears are typically used at over one pound of force at night and then removed all day to have zero force. Modern research and centuries of experience have proven that this heavy, intermittent force is precisely the wrong kind of force to be using to reshape living things. It is damaging, painful, slow, and may cause root resorption. Ideally, what orthodontists need is a continuous source of energy to continuously power their intermaxillary machines.

Energy Sources

The practice of orthodontics involves the skillful application of force vectors to transform the teeth and jaws. Teeth are moved for precise distances and in precise directions. This activity is described in physics by the formula Force × Distance = Work. As Energy is defined as the capacity to do Work, one can see that no Energy = no Work = no treatment results.

The search for a source of this energy initially led to the patients themselves. It was assumed that the patient would have an interest in their own successful treatment and be willing to work toward that goal. Early attempts at intermaxillary appliances relied entirely upon the patient to manually power their own intermaxillary mechanics by

stretching elastic bands around the neck and head or between the arches. This chore ultimately fell upon the parents of the patient who were forced to diligently police and monitor the use of these removable energy sources.

The Face as Energy

Ironically, the very area of the face that orthodontists are attempting to reshape is energy rich! The lower face is constantly in a state of activity. Speaking, swallowing, emoting, and eating all involve bringing the teeth into occlusion. And to do so produces significant levels of force that are generated via the facial muscles. It has been estimated that the face can generate thousands of ft.lbs of work per day.

Until the 1980s, no one had discovered a way of harnessing this natural source of energy. Other forces of nature have been captured using the principle of resistance. A dam resists the flow of a river and thus builds up potential energy to power generators. A sail resists the flow of wind to power the boat. Certain types of metals resist the flow of electrons to produce heat energy.

To apply this principle of resistance to the face muscles, one must think in terms of pushing the jaws apart while the muscles are attempting to bring the jaws together. And thus, the concept of flexible pushing mechanics was born. My first attempt at making a pushing force module was actually a length of very resilient edgewise wire soldered between the two normal archwires.

Research has shown us that, on average, the teeth close together with about 10 pounds of force when powering into centric. If, for example, the pushing force modules are set at 4 ounces of resistance per side, then the face muscles must bite down with an extra 8 ounces of force to bring the teeth into occlusion. This extra one-half pound of force then represents a 5% increased workload on the face musculature ($10/100 : 0.5/\times$). As the jaws come together towards centric, a pushing force module can then capture this extra energy from the face muscles by deflecting into a curved shape which also stores this energy temporarily. It can then be delivered as needed to the teeth and jaws as light continuous force vectors.

Resistance Training for the Facial Muscles

The entire human body, from the neck down at least, responds very favorably to the exercise provided by resistance training. The science of physical therapy, the trend for personal trainers, and the narcissistic "body sculptors" of Muscle Beach all use the same general principle to achieve their goals—through rigorous movement and exercise of the muscles (pumping iron), the body can be made more healthy and beautiful. Therefore, resisting the closure of the jaws with a fixed flexible force module may have an enormously beneficial effect on the face muscles themselves.

The muscles of mastication (temporalis, buccinator, masseter, obicularis oris, etc.) are what you see when you look at the face. Their primary design function is to squeeze the jaws together. By resisting this closure, these muscles are forced to work a little harder, thus increasing blood flow, oxygen, nutrients, neuromuscular coordination, etc.

All other fields of medicine have recognized the need for exercise to assist in normal growth and development and to maintain optimal health. However, the orthodontic profession has historically shown very little interest in facial exercise simply because a resistance unit, the pushing force module, had not been invented. The few studies we have all suggest that biting down harder increases the strength and mass of the muscles which in turn affects the size and density of the facial bones. This is just what orthodontists usually like to see in an underdeveloped lower face. Every other part of the body is made more beautiful through exercise—the face is no exception.

Vector Quality of Pushing Mechanics

Now that we have captured energy from the face muscles and given them a workout in the process, let's examine the quality of the vectors produced and compare them to the extrusive vectors produced with the pulling mechanics of removable neck straps and rubber bands as discussed above.

In general, the force vectors of flexible pushing mechanics are intrusive in nature and thus avoid all the treatment-damaging effects of extrusive pulling mechanics. Intrusive vectors assist in the correction of overerupted lower incisors and protect against any unwanted extrusion typically induced by closing loops or other orthodontic activity.

Although the jaws can close with up to 10 pounds of force, the Jasper Jumper, which is a commercially available pushing force module, can be adjusted to capture a range of light forces between 0 and 8 ounces per side, depending on what is called for in the treatment plan. These forces can be used to distalize individual teeth or groups of teeth.

Pushing forces also lead to a tendency to expand the dental arches. Since the point of attachment is on the buccal, intrusive vectors tend to tip the teeth toward the buccal. This side effect is generally thought to be positive as the amount of expansion typically experienced is in the 2–3 mm range and indeed, for upper molars to move distally, they must expand.

With ideal growth and development, the face and jaws follow a well-documented path downward and forward along the growth axis. Regardless of what the specific etiology is for each different malocclusion, it typically manifests itself orthodontically as an abnormality along this growth axis.

By using flexible pushing mechanics, the force module is placed in parallel to the problematic growth axis in an attempt to harmoniously use force vectors that mimic nature in direction and magnitude and thus are potentially more biologically acceptable to the developing face.

Converting from removable pulling mechanics to fixed pushing mechanics and the use of a force module that harvests energy from the face is quite simple but it does require a learning curve. Getting used to anything new or different is always a challenge. It is hoped that the amount and quality of the vectors that this system can produce will make it worth the effort.

The Jasper Jumper™

Frank J. Weiland

Introduction

Class II, division 1 malocclusion has been called "the most frequent treatment problem in the orthodontic practice".[1] Droschl found the frequency to be 37% among school children.[2] McNamara investigated 277 children showing Class II malocclusions.[3] He concluded that mandibular skeletal retrusion was the most common single characteristic of the Class II sample, whereas maxillary skeletal protrusion was not a common finding. In most cases the incisors were well positioned. The same conclusions were drawn by other authors.[2,4]

A treatment approach aiming at modification of direction and amount of mandibular growth rather than restriction of maxillary development would therefore be indicated in many Class II patients. This concept plays a primary role in functional jaw orthopedics. Various types of appliances have been developed over the last eight decades. Most of these have in common that they are removable and, as a consequence, demand very good cooperation of the patient. Noncompliance of patients in general, however, has been increasing over the years,[5] a trend that does not exclude orthodontics.[6] Investigations showed that patients often fulfill just half of the orthodontist's requirements regarding wearing time of the appliance.[7]

Consequently, a primary advantage of fixed functional appliances is their independence of cooperation. One of the oldest examples is the Herbst appliance,[8] which proved to be very effective in treating Class II, division 1 malocclusions.[9–17] Another example is the Jasper Jumper™ (American Orthodontics, Sheboygan, WI), a flexible intraoral force module, which may be seen as a modification of the Herbst appliance. It was introduced to the market in 1987, having received a United States Patent in the same year. In this chapter the application and the treatment effects of the Jasper Jumper will be described.

The Jasper Jumper

The Jasper Jumper consists of two parts: the force module and the anchor parts. The force module is flexible and consists of a stainless steel coil spring that is attached to stainless steel caps at both ends. The inner construction is shown in Figure 10.1 (original source: United States Patent no. 4,708,646, 1987). The caps have holes to which the anchoring parts can be attached. The spring core is surrounded by an opaque gray polyurethane material that covers part of the anchoring ends. The original design did not have this overlap, which led to frequent breakage of the modules. The modules are designed for use on the right or the left side of the arch. They are available in seven lengths, ranging from 26 to 38 mm in 2 mm increments. The sizes are marked on the maxillary end of the module (UR means upper right, UL upper left; sizes 1 through 7) (Fig. 10.2).

To determine the correct length of the module, the distance between the mesial of the upper molar tube and the point of insertion to the mandibular arch is measured. Adding 12 mm to this measurement will give the appropriate length of the jumper (Fig. 10.3).

Usually, the jumpers are attached to previously placed fixed orthodontic appliances. The parts needed are shown in Figure 10.4. The force module is attached posteriorly to the maxillary arch by a ball-pin that is placed through the distal attachment of the force module and then extends anteriorly through the face-bow tube on the upper first molar band (Fig. 10.5). The ball-pin is anchored in

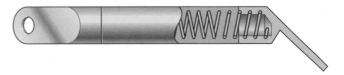

Figure 10.1 Schematic drawing of the construction of the force module.

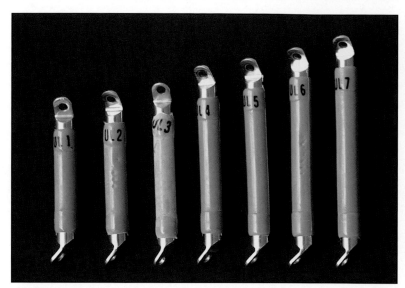

Figure 10.2 Collection of the seven available left force modules (UL 1 through 7).

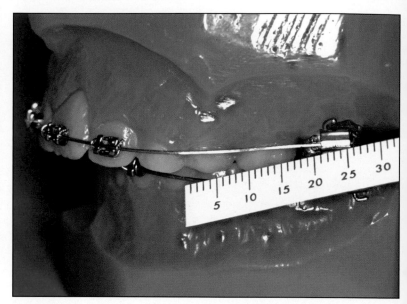

Figure 10.3 Determining the correct length of the force module: distance 21 mm + 12 mm = 33 mm. In order to have some spare length for reactivation, it is advised to take size 5 (34 mm).

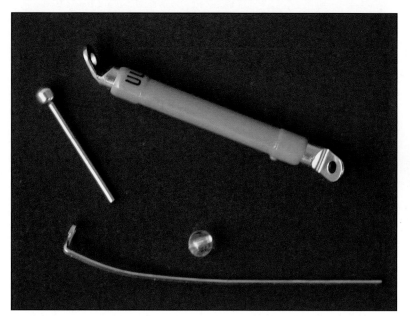

Figure 10.4 Force module, ball-pin for maxillary attachment, auxiliary arch and plastic bead for mandibular attachment.

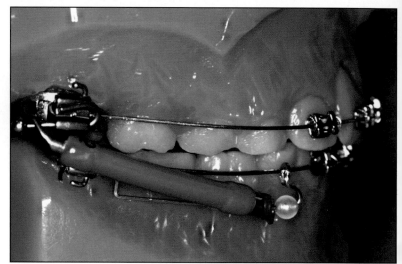

Figure 10.5 Attachment of distal end of force module to maxillary molar through the use of ball-pin. Appliance can be activated by moving the ball-pin anteriorly. In this case, in the mandibular arch the module is attached to an auxiliary wire.

position by placing a return bend in the ball-pin at its mesial end. The upper end of the module is marked UR (upper right) or UL (upper left) and a number (1–7) representing the size; the corresponding lengths are marked on the box containing the modules.

The jumpers can be attached to the mandibular arch in several different ways. Originally, it was suggested that the practitioner slide the anterior cap of the force module onto the main archwire. Bayonet bends are placed distal to the mandibular canines and small plastic beads are slipped over the archwire to provide an anterior stop. In order to allow the patient freedom of movement, it is important to remove the first and second premolar brackets. Figure 10.6 shows an example in the mixed dentition.

Alternatively, the jumpers can be attached to auxiliary sectional archwires, that are attached posteriorly through an auxiliary tube located on the lower first molar band and hooked anteriorly to the main archwire between the first premolar and canine (Fig. 10.7).[18] It is recommended to use 0.018 × 0.025″ stainless steel wire in both the 0.018″ and 0.022″ slot. Alternatively, the auxiliary wire can be ordered (0.017 × 0.025″ sectional wire, American Orthodontics, Sheboygan, WI). This method with the sectional wire allows the

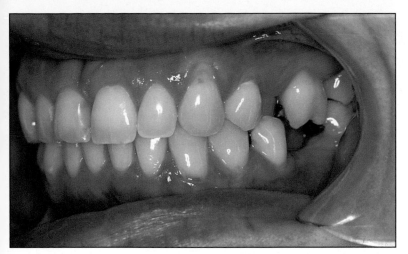

Figure 10.17 Class I malocclusion with missing lower left first molar, elongated upper first molar and cross-bite of second premolar.

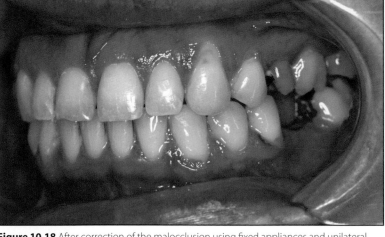

Figure 10.18 After correction of the malocclusion using fixed appliances and unilateral Jasper Jumper. Active treatment time was 9 months.

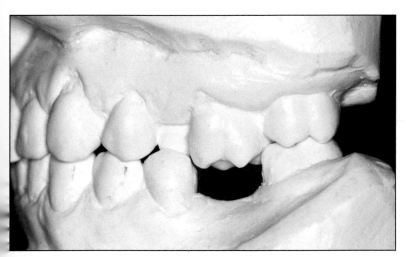

Figure 10.19 Study models before correction.

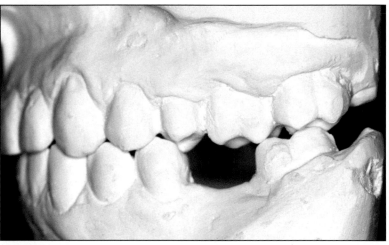

Figure 10.20 Study models after correction. Note the vertical and sagittal dentoalveolar correction compared to Fig. 10.19.

arch[25] or to removable functional appliances.[26] The latter technique in particular is beyond the scope of this book.

If proclination of the mandibular incisors combined with mesial movement of the cuspids is indicated, in the first phase the auxiliary arch should contact the lower cuspid bracket and not be cinched back directly behind the molar slot. The auxiliary arch may now slide forward, driven by the mesially directed force from the module, at the same time tipping the anterior lower segment forward. After this segment is in the planned position, the auxiliary arch is activated by sliding it through the molar slot in a distal direction and cinching it back. In this second phase, the lower buccal segments are moved mesially. It is advised to use a slot-filling archwire. In order to reduce friction in the posterior segment, the wire should be reduced in dimension distal to the cuspid. Alternatively, as is preferred by the author, a bidimensional bracket system (cuspid to cuspid: 0.018″ slot, buccal segments: 0.022″ slot) can be used.

Accordingly, space closure in the lower arch in a mesial direction (e.g. after extractions in the lower arch or agenesis of premolars) can be performed with a Jasper Jumper without having to fear loss of anterior anchorage.

En masse retraction of the six upper anterior teeth can be done routinely using the jumpers as anchorage. As the horizontal force component reaches from 200 to over 300 g, depending on the length of the force modules, an absolute sagittal anchorage can be expected if the retraction forces do not exceed this amount of force. In contrast to the original recommendation to attach a spring or a tie from a hook on the archwire to the anterior part of the upper ball-pin, it is advised to attach this to the hook on the molar attachment. On opening the mouth, the forces exerted by the Jasper Jumper decrease. As a consequence, the ball-pin tends to be pulled anteriorly, if this is used as an anchoring point for en masse retraction. This has been reported by patients as being very unpleasant.

Case Studies

Two cases will be presented in detail to demonstrate the typical effects of treatment of Class II malocclusions with fixed appliances and the Jasper Jumper.

Patient 1 (Figs 10.21–10.39)

This boy was 9 years and 6 months old when he came for clinical evaluation. The face made a symmetric impression; he lacked lip closure at rest and his lower lip was interposed between the upper and lower teeth most of the time (Figs 10.21 and 10.22). Clinically, the mandible made a retrognathic impression. The dentition exhibited a full Class II molar relationship; the overjet was 9 mm, the overbite 6 mm with palatal impingement (Figs 10.23 and 10.24). In the upper buccal segments, three premolars erupted prematurely due to early loss of deciduous teeth. The left upper second deciduous molar showed a carious lesion (Fig. 10.25). The lower arch exhibited some crowding in the anterior part and a deepened Spee curve (Fig. 10.26). The panoramic radiograph showed the mixed dentition and the early development of the third molars (Fig. 10.27). Cephalometric analysis revealed an ANB angle of 5° in a bimaxillary retrognathic and hyperdivergent skeletal pattern. The position of the upper incisors was judged to be normal, whereas the lower incisors were retroclined (Fig. 10.28).

A two-phase treatment plan was developed. Treatment was started at the age of 9 years and 9 months. The upper and lower first molars were banded and brackets were bonded to the incisors. The lower incisor brackets had 5° labial root torque. A transpalatal arch and a lower lingual arch were inserted. After leveling and aligning, which took 6 months, full-sized archwires were inserted. Jasper Jumpers were selected and fitted according to the manufacturer's instructions. After 6 months, overcorrected Class I occlusal relationships were achieved. Appliances were removed. Phase 1 lasted 1 year. One year later all permanent teeth had erupted and a second phase of treatment was started using preangulated and pretorqued fixed appliances. The occlusal relationships were stable; therefore the detailing of the occlusion took only 6 months. Total active treatment time therefore was 1.5 years with a break between the two phases of 1 year. Retention was performed with bonded retainers in both arches.

Post treatment, lip closure at rest was possible without strain. The gummy smile increased. The profile was harmonious (Figs 10.29–10.31). Stable Class I relationship was achieved (Figs 10.32–10.36). Clinically, no difference between RCP and ICP could be detected. The panoramic radiograph showed a satisfactory alignment of the roots (Fig. 10.37). Cephalometric analysis revealed that the ANB angle reduced to 0° in a bimaxillary retrognathic, hyperdivergent pattern. The incisors were well positioned (Fig. 10.38). The superimposition shows the overall changes: distal relocation of the maxillary anterior border, anterior development of the

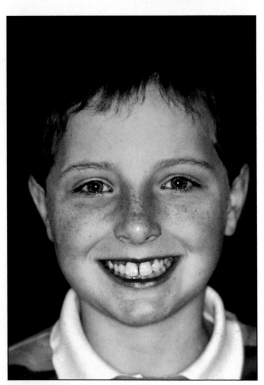

Figures 10.21–10.28 Typical Class II treatment using fixed appliances and Jasper Jumper in the mixed dentition: initial records at 9 years 6 months.

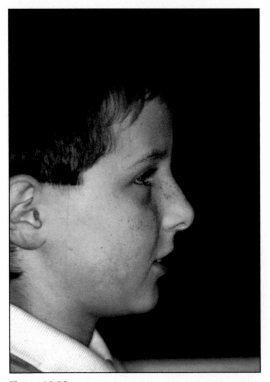

Figure 10.22

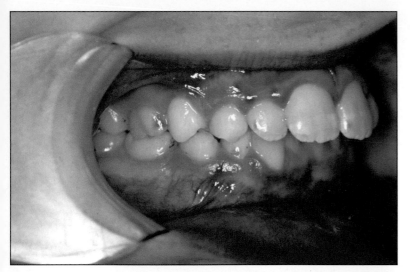

Figure 10.23

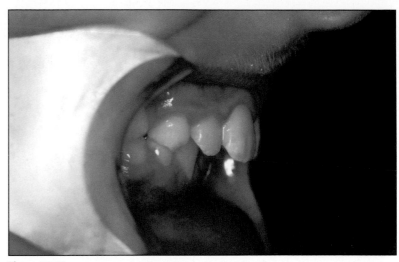

Figure 10.24

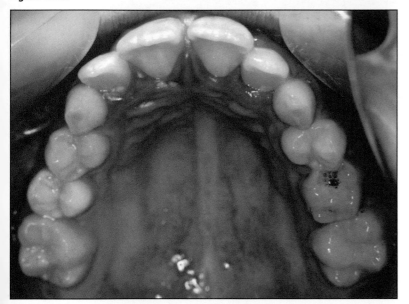

Figure 10.25

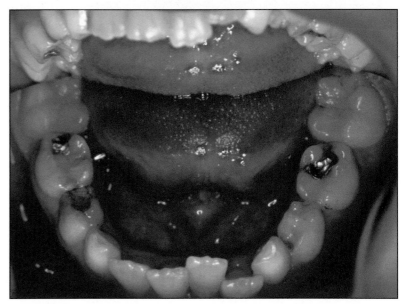

Figure 10.26

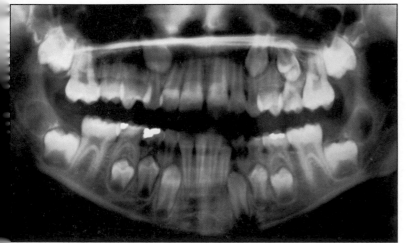

Figure 10.27

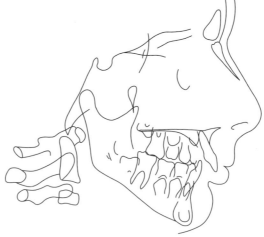

Figure 10.28

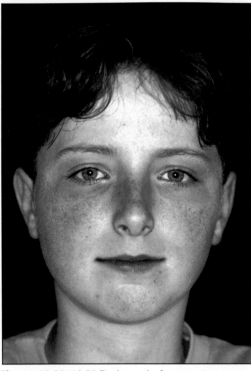

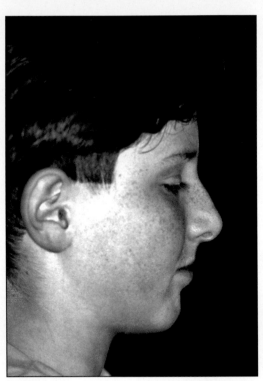

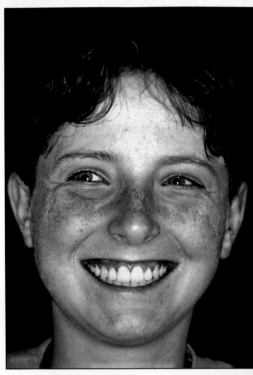

Figures 10.29–10.38 Final records after treatment.   **Figure 10.30**   **Figure 10.31**

mandible, combined with retraction of the upper incisors and a slight protrusion of the lower incisors. A marked tipping of the occlusal plane occurred, due to intrusion of the lower incisors, extrusion of the upper incisors and minimal intrusion of the upper molars (Fig. 10.39). As a consequence, the gummy smile deteriorated (see Fig. 10.30). The changes seen in this patient are typical for the treatment of this type of malocclusion using the Jasper Jumper.[20,27,28]

Patient 2 (Figs 10.40–10.57)

The second case report shows a modification in the use of the Jasper Jumper to reduce some typical side effects. This 11-year-old boy presented with a moderate Class II, division 1 malocclusion. The lower anterior face height was increased, as was the nasolabial angle (Figs 10.40 and 10.41). The occlusion was Class II on both sides. Overjet was 6 mm, overbite 1 mm (Figs 10.42 and 10.43). No crowding was present in upper and lower arch (Figs 10.44 and 10.45). The panoramic radiograph showed a late mixed dentition with early development of the third molars (Fig. 10.46). Cephalometric analysis displayed a slightly retrognathic maxilla and a clearly retrognathic mandible; the ANB angle was 6°. The skeletal pattern was hyperdivergent. The upper incisors were proclined, the lower incisors were well positioned in relation to the lower and anterior border of the mandible (Fig. 10.47).

It was decided to treat this malocclusion with fixed appliances and the Jasper Jumper. Upper and lower incisor brackets were bonded, molar bands were inserted. An upper transpalatal arch and a lower lingual arch were fitted. After leveling and aligning the arches, a full-sized archwire was inserted in the lower arch. This initial phase lasted 4 months. After eruption of the upper premolars, the buccal segments were stabilized. Jasper Jumpers and an intrusive base arch[29] were inserted. The Jasper Jumpers were fitted mesial to the upper molar tube and to an auxiliary wire in the lower arch. This was done to keep the distal tipping moment to the molar as a result of the base arch mechanics and the Jasper Jumpers within certain limits. The resulting force system (Fig. 10.48) made us expect an improved vertical control in the upper incisor area. As a result, the development of a gummy smile in this vertically growing patient might be avoided. A second advantage we expected was that through the improved vertical anterior control, a better sagittal skeletal reaction would take place.[20,30]

The Jasper Jumpers were in place for 6 months. Sixteen months after starting treatment, appliances were removed. Good facial esthetics were seen. The nasolabial angle increased slightly (Figs 10.49 and 10.50). A solid Class I occlusion with overjet and overbite within normal limits was achieved (Figs 10.51–10.54). The panoramic radiograph revealed suboptimal root alignment of the upper lateral incisors and a retarded eruption of the upper second molars (Fig. 10.55). Cephalometric analysis showed a reduction of the ANB angle to 1°. The anterior development of the

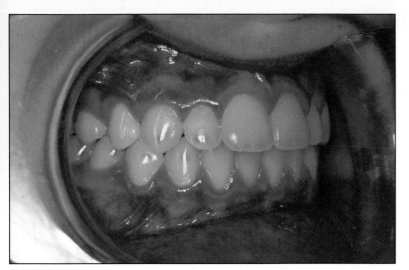

Figure 10.32

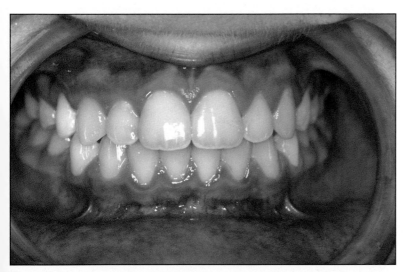

Figure 10.33

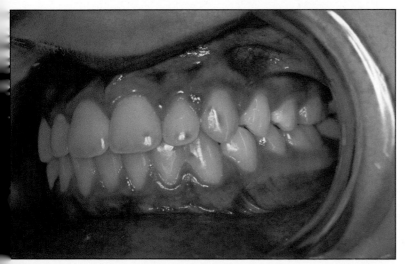

Figure 10.34

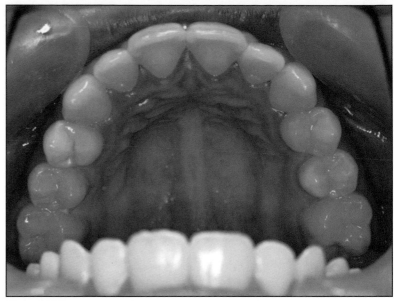

Figure 10.35

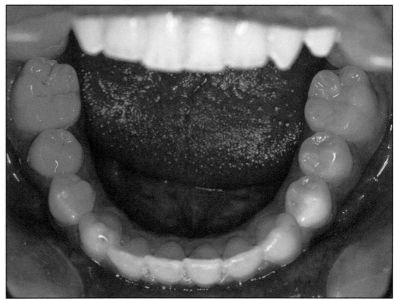

Figure 10.36

maxilla was clearly reduced, whereas the bony chin and mandibular length increased more than could be expected during normal growth. The lower incisors protruded by 4°. Due to the very good vertical control of the upper incisors, the tipping of the occlusal plane was minimal (Figs 10.56 and 10.57).

This case demonstrates that by slight modifications compared to the normal use of the Jasper Jumper, the effect of the appliance can be enhanced in hyperdivergent patients by improving vertical and sagittal control.

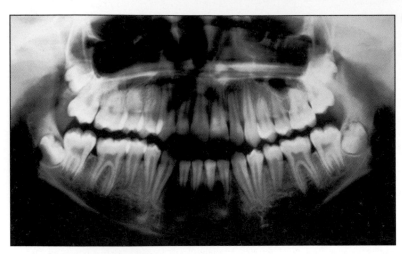

Figure 10.37

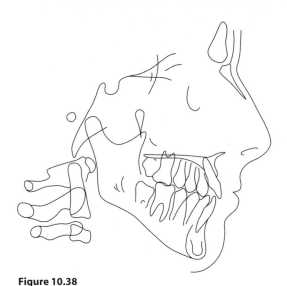

Figure 10.38

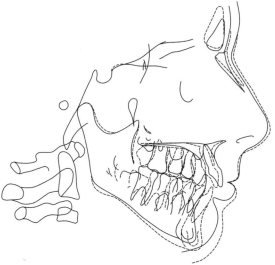

Figure 10.39 The cephalometric superimposition reveals the changes that occurred during therapy. Active treatment time was 1.5 years.

Treatment Effects

Several studies were performed to quantitate the average skeletal and dentoalveolar reactions to Class II treatment using fixed appliances and the Jasper Jumper force modules. In a pilot study, the effects during treatment in growing patients were evaluated.[27] The sample consisted of 17 consecutive Class II, division 1 malocclusion cases in the mixed dentition (10 boys and seven girls) treated with the Jasper Jumper. The mean pretreatment age was 11 years 4 months (SD = 1 month). Before treatment, all patients showed a bilateral Class II molar relationship and a deep overbite. The average time that elapsed between insertion of the Jasper Jumpers and achievement of a Class I molar relationship was 6 months (SD = 1 month). To evaluate the effects of Jasper Jumper treatment on the dentofacial complex in relation to normal growth changes, the Bolton standards of dentofacial developmental growth were used.[31]

In all patients the first molars were banded, using bands with triple attachments and slots for a transpalatal arch in the upper, and a lingual arch in the lower jaw, respectively. Pretorqued brackets (0.018″ slot) were bonded to the incisors (upper central: + 14°; upper lateral: +7°; lower incisors: −5°). After an initial leveling phase 0.017 × 0.025″ stainless steel archwires were inserted and cinched back. In addition, transpalatal and lingual arches (0.9 mm stainless steel) were put in passively to enhance stability. The Jasper Jumpers were selected according to the manufacturer's instructions and inserted. After approximately 3 months the jumpers were renewed in all but one patient, because they lost elasticity.

Sagittal skeletal and dental changes that occurred during treatment were analyzed on lateral cephalograms. One was made before insertion of the Jasper Jumpers, a second one immediately after removal of the appliance. In addition to a number of angular

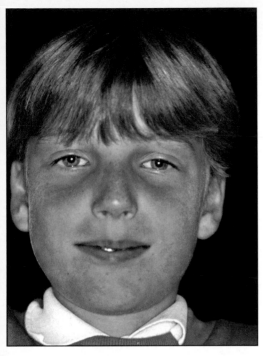

Figures 10.40–10.47
Eleven-year-old boy with a moderate Class I division 1 malocclusion. Initial records.

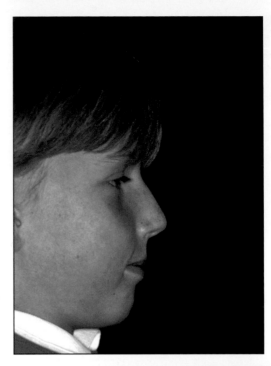

Figure 10.41

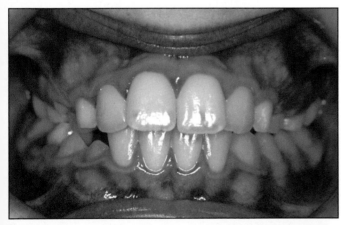

Figure 10.42

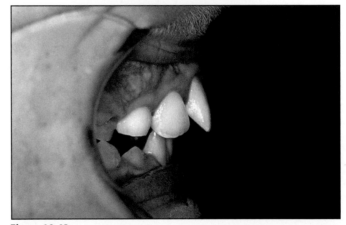

Figure 10.43

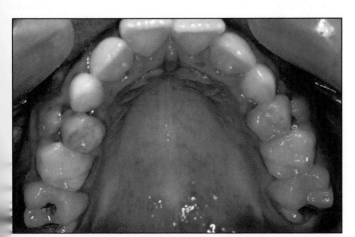

Figure 10.44

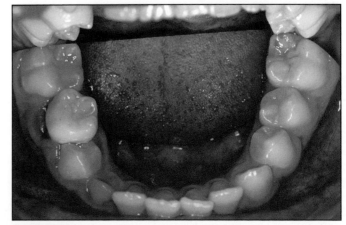

Figure 10.45

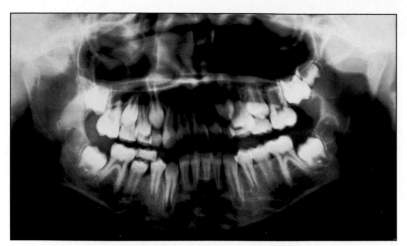

Figure 10.46

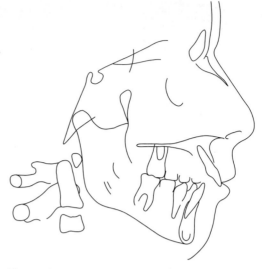

Figure 10.47

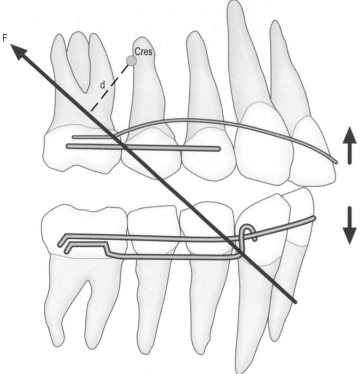

Figure 10.48 The force system designed to treat the malocclusion.

measurements, the analysis of linear changes was made according to the method of Pancherz (Fig. 10.58).[32] A reference grid, consisting of the occlusal line (OL) and the occlusal line perpendicular (OLp), was drawn on the tracing of the first headfilm. This grid was transferred to the second headfilm by superimposing on the nasion–sella line (NSL) at sella (S). All measurements were made parallel with OL to OLp. From the Bolton standards, the composite headfilm tracings at 11 years and at 12 years were traced in the same manner. The changes during this 1-year period of normal growth

were registered and subsequently halved. In this way it was possible to compare the effects of our treatment regimen with normal growth changes that occur in a period of 6 months in a sample of the same age. The data were statistically analyzed. (For more details of the investigation, see Weiland & Bantleon.[27])

Clinically, in all 17 patients, Class I dental relationships with correction of overjet were established after 6 months. The difference between RCP and ICP was within 1 mm in all patients. The angular and linear cephalometric measurements revealed that the Jasper Jumper had only limited, nonsignificant skeletal effects on the maxilla (SNA: −0.8°, A-OLp: +0.1 mm). Dentoalveolar changes, however, were more marked, as can be seen by the retroclination of the upper incisors by almost 6° and distal movement of the incisal edge by 2.4 mm. The maxillary molars moved distally by approximately 1.5 mm. In contrast, there was a significant effect on the mandible: the SNB angle increased (+1.2°) and pogonion moved forward more than 2 mm. In combination with a slight forward movement of the condyle as represented by point articulare (Ar), a significant increase in mandibular length of 1.7 mm resulted. The lower incisors (0.8 mm) and molars (1.6 mm) moved forward in relation to the mandibular base, the lower incisors proclining by 4°. No significant tipping of maxilla and mandible took place, whereas the occlusal plane tipped in a backward-upward/forward-downward direction significantly by 3°, due to the intrusive movement of the upper molars and lower incisors, which is a consequence of the force vector of the modules. Additionally, the intrusion of the lower incisors led to a reduction in overbite, which may have a bearing in patients showing an anterior open bite before treatment.[28] The sagittal linear changes are shown in Figure 10.59.

An analysis of the relative maxillary and mandibular skeletal and dental contribution to the correction of overjet and molar relationship revealed that 40% of the change in incisor and molar relationship was

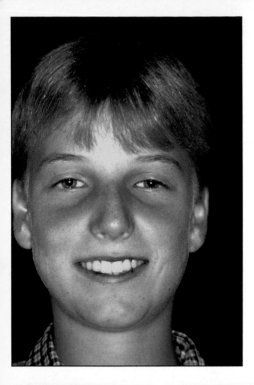

Figures 10.49–10.56 Final records show an adequate correction of the original malocclusion.

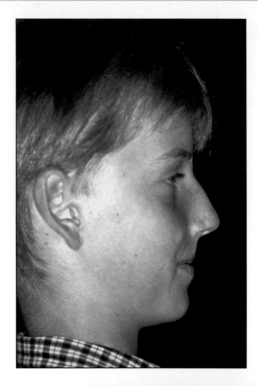

Figure 10.50

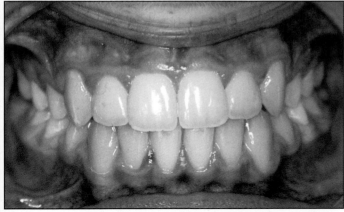

Figure 10.51

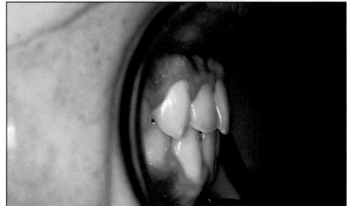

Figure 10.52

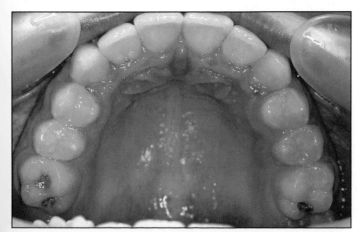

Figure 10.53

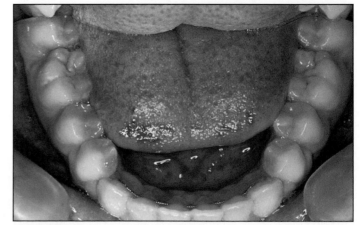

Figure 10.54

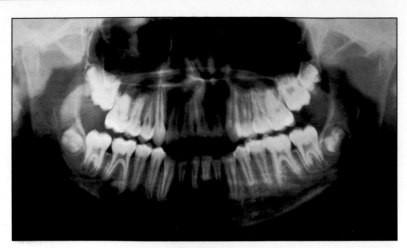

Figure 10.55

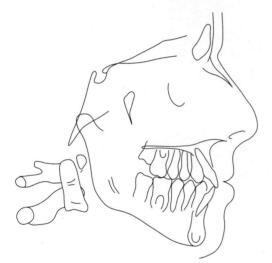

Figure 10.56

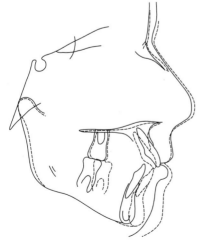

Figure 10.57 The cephalometric superimposition shows the good upper incisor vertical control and a very good anterior displacement of the bony chin, combined with posterior movement of the upper incisors.

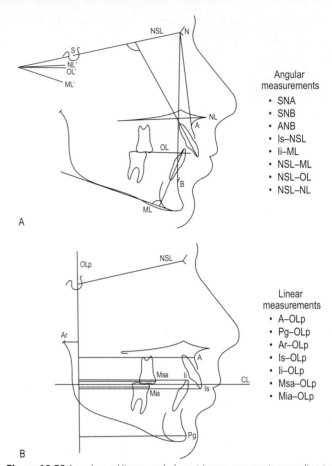

Angular measurements
- SNA
- SNB
- ANB
- Is–NSL
- Ii–ML
- NSL–ML
- NSL–OL
- NSL–NL

A

Linear measurements
- A–OLp
- Pg–OLp
- Ar–OLp
- Is–OLp
- Ii–OLp
- Msa–OLp
- Mia–OLp

B

Figure 10.58 Angular and linear cephalometric measurements according to the method of Pancherz. *(From Weiland & Bantleon 1995,[27] with kind permission of the American Association of Orthodontists)*

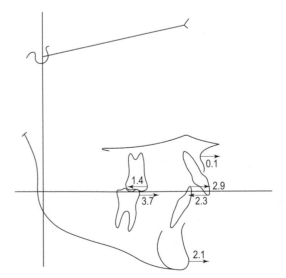

Overjet correction   5.2 mm
Molar correction   5.0 mm

Figure 10.59 Schematic diagram illustrating mean changes in dentofacial structure of experimental sample occurring with Jasper Jumper therapy. *(From Weiland & Bantleon 1995,[27] with kind permission of the American Association of Orthodontists)*

due to skeletal changes, whereas 60% was a result of dentoalveolar adaptations. Overjet correction was mainly due to mandibular growth that was greater than maxillary growth and a retrusion of the maxillary incisors. Molar correction was a result of the greater mandibular growth, distal movement of the upper and mesial movement of the lower molars.

Compared with the normal developmental changes (Bolton standards) that can be expected, the maxillary anterior development is slightly reduced and mandibular growth appears to be increased. In addition, in contrast to normal development the mandible as a whole is moved anteriorly slightly. The latter change might partly be the result of remodeling processes in the articular fossa area.[33–37] The upper dentition is distalized in relation to the maxillary base and the lower teeth are moved mesially to the mandibular base, combined with a marked tipping of the occlusal plane.

Comparing the ratio of correction (60% dentoalveolar, 40% skeletal) to data from the literature and from our own investigations[20,27] concerning the treatment effects using removable or fixed functional appliances, it appears that the changes occurring with the Jasper Jumper compare very well with the average of the reported ratios. An overview of data from the literature is shown in Table 10.1.

Stucki & Ingervall investigated the effects of the Jasper Jumper in the treatment of Class II, division 1 malocclusions in the young permanent dentition.[38] The mean treatment time with the force modules was 5 months, followed by a median period of observation of 7 months. The authors found similar results as described above. After the period of observation, the dentoalveolar effects (especially the intrusion of the upper molars and lower incisors and the retroclination of the upper incisors) had partially or totally relapsed. The remaining effect contributing most to the correction was the skeletal effect on the mandible, i.e. the increase in mandibular prognathism. In contrast, Covell et al found hardly any skeletal effect in the mandible.[39] The authors concluded that the Jasper Jumper corrected Class II discrepancies largely through maxillary and mandibular dentoalveolar effects and, to a limited extent, by restraint of forward maxillary growth.

In the young permanent dentition, the amount of mandibular skeletal change seems to be age independent.[38] The age range of their sample was 13–25 years. As a consequence, the indication to use the Jasper Jumper to induce skeletal changes does not seem to end in late adolescence. Similar effects were seen in young adult patients treated with the Herbst appliance, although the authors found fewer skeletal effects and more mandibular dental adaptations contributing to overjet correction compared to younger patients.[40]

The mechanism of correction of Class II malocclusions in adult patients treated with the Jasper Jumper is a combination of distal movement of the upper dentition, anterior movement of the lower dentition, and a distinct tipping of the occlusal plane.[41] In

Table 10.1. Comparison of dentoalveolar and skeletal contribution to Class II correction as recorded in various studies (from Weiland 1994).

Author	Appliance	Dentoalveolar (%)	Skeletal (%)
Jakobsson (1967)[48]	Activator	65–70	30–35
Dietrich (1973)[48]	Activator	80	20
Righellis (1983)[50]	Activator	70	30
Pancherz (1984)[32]	Activator	52	48
Remmer et al (1985)[51]	Activator	73	27
Looi & Mills (1986)[52]	Activator	90	10
Weichbrodt (1990)[53]	Activator	31	69
Weiland (1994)[20]	Activator	55	45
Teuscher (1988)[54]	Headgear-activator	50	50
Weiland (1994)[20]	Headgear-activator	46	54
Creekmore & Radney (1983)[55]	FR II	63	37
Righellis (1983)[50]	FR II	60	40
Gianelly et al (1984)[56]	FR II	70	30
Remmer et al (1985)[51]	FR II	77	23
Pancherz et al (1989)[15]	Bass appliance	23	77
Pancherz (1982)[12]	Herbst	44	56
Pancherz et al (1989)[15]	Herbst	77	23
Wieslander (1984)[17]	Herbst + headgear	28	72
Weiland (1994)[20]	Jasper Jumper	38	62
Weiland & Bantleon (1995)[27]	Jasper Jumper	40	60

Posttreatment Development

Seven months after removing the force modules, approximately 60% of the overjet reduction and 75% of the molar correction remained.[38] This confirms clinical experience and seems comparable to posttreatment development using the Herbst appliance.[42] In Herbst appliance therapy, it is advised to overcorrect occlusal relationships to an end-to-end incisor position. In the following 6 months, the occlusion settles.[43] In the long term, relapse seems to be clearly related to unstable occlusion, as is usually seen in mixed dentition cases. Therefore, it is recommended to retain the achieved occlusal relationships for at least 2 years with an activator.[43] As it is very difficult to overcorrect occlusal relationships with a flexible module, it is advisable to retain the achieved sagittal occlusal relationships with light Class II elastics during ongoing fixed appliance therapy after removing the Jasper Jumpers.

An interesting question is whether it is possible to normalize basal jaw relationship long-term in Class II patients compared to subjects exhibiting normal growth. It has been demonstrated that mandibular length increased more than in subjects with ideal occlusions (Bolton standards)[31] with fixed functional appliances like the Jasper Jumper[20,27,28] or the Herbst appliance.[10–12,43] Moreover, the increase of sagittal condylar growth in Herbst patients was significantly greater than in untreated Class II control subjects.[44–46] At the end of the growth period, however, the treatment effect compared to the Bolton standards is no longer evident. It can be concluded that the long-term total amount of mandibular growth is almost identical in subjects treated with the Herbst appliance and in subjects with ideal occlusion.[43]

In conclusion, it can be stated that Herbst treatment improves the basal jaw relationship, but does not normalize it compared with ideal occlusion subjects exhibiting normal growth. Reanalysis of Class II patients treated with Jasper Jumpers at least 7 years earlier revealed a similar result (Weiland, unpublished data). Stable Class I occlusal relationships, however, were seen in 17 of 20 (85%) consecutive Jasper Jumper patients. This compares very well to long-term results with the Herbst appliance.[47]

Conclusion

The Jasper Jumper is a very versatile auxiliary for the correction of Class II malocclusion with fixed appliances. Its major advantage is its independence from patient cooperation. In order to justify the use of "noncompliance appliances," however, these should not just simplify treatment for the clinician but also maintain or enhance the quality of the treatment results as achieved with "conventional" treatment. Therefore, a thorough understanding of the force system, the treatment effects in growing and nongrowing patients and the side effects is a prerequisite and enables the clinician to treat suitable malocclusions very efficiently. The number of fixed flexible appliances now on the market that are based on similar design considerations show that Jasper's considerations in the 1980s have been widely accepted.

References

1. Fisk RO. When malocclusions concern the public. J Can Dent Assoc 1960;26:397–412.

2. Droschl H. Die Fernröntgenwerte unbehandelter Kinder zwischen dem 6. und 15. Lebensjahr. Berlin: Quintessenz; 1984.

3. McNamara JA. Components of Class II malocclusion in children 8–10 years of age. Angle Orthod 1981;51:177–202.

4. Bass NM. The aesthetic analysis of the face. Eur J Orthod 1991;13:343–350.

5. Koltun A, Stone GC. Past and current trends in patient noncompliance research: focus on diseases, regimes programs, and provider-disciplines. J Compl Health Care 1986;1:21–32.

6. Sahm G, Bartsch A, Witt E. Reliability of patient reports on compliance. Eur J Orthod 1990;12:438–446.

7. Sahm G, Bartsch A, Witt E. Micro-electronic monitoring of functional appliance wear. Eur J Orthod 1990;12:297–301.

8. Herbst E. Dreissigjährige Erfahrungen mit dem Retentionsscharnier. Zahnärztl Rundschau 1934;43:1515–1524, 1563–1568, 1611–1616.

9. McNamara JA, Howe RP, Dischinger TG. A comparison of the Herbst and Fränkel appliances in the treatment of Class II malocclusion. Am J Orthod Dentofacial Orthop 1990;98:134–144.

10. Pancherz H. Treatment of Class II malocclusions by jumping the bite with the Herbst appliance. Am J Orthod 1979;76:423–442.

11. Pancherz H. The effect of continuous bite jumping on the dentofacial complex: a follow-up study after Herbst appliance treatment of Class II malocclusions. Eur J Orthod 1981;3:49–60.

12. Pancherz H. The mechanism of Class II correction in Herbst appliance treatment. Am J Orthod 1982;82:104–113.

13. Pancherz H. The Herbst appliance – its biologic effects and clinical use. Am J Orthod 1985;87:1–20.

14. Pancherz H. Dentofacial orthopedics in relation to somatic maturation. Am J Orthod 1985;88:273–287.

15. Pancherz H, Malmgren O, Hagg U, Omblus J, Hansen K. Class II correction in Herbst and Bass therapy. Eur J Orthod 1989;11:17–30.

16. Valant JR, Sinclair PM. Treatment effects of the Herbst appliance. Am J Orthod Dentofacial Orthop 1989;95:138–147.

17. Wieslander L. Intensive treatment of severe Class II malocclusions with a headgear-Herbst appliance in the early mixed dentition. Am J Orthod 1984;86:1–13.

18. Blackwood HO. Clinical management of the Jasper Jumper. J Clin Orthod 1991;25:755–760.

19. Pancherz H, Hansen K. Mandibular anchorage in Herbst treatment. Eur J Orthod 1988;10:149–164.

20. Weiland FJ. Distalbiss-Therapie mit Jasper Jumper und Aktivator – eine vergleichende kephalometrische Studie. Doctorate degree thesis. Bern: Bern University; 1994.

21. Jasper JJ, McNamara JA Jr. The correction of interarch malocclusions using a fixed force module. Am J Orthod Dentofacial Orthop 1995;108:641–650.

22. Jasper JJ. The Jasper Jumper – a fixed functional appliance. Sheboygan, WI: American Orthodontics; 1987.

23. Cassady CW. Case report. PCSO Bulletin 2004:40–42.

24. Carano A, Machata WC. A rapid molar intruder for "non-compliance" treatment. J Clin Orthod 2002;36:137–142.

25. Mills CM, McCulloch KJ. Case report: modified use of the Jasper Jumper appliance in a skeletal Class II mixed dentition case requiring habit correction and palatal expansion. Angle Orthod 1997;67:277–282.

26. Sari Z, Goyenc Y, Doruk C, Usumez S. Comparative evaluation of a new removable Jasper Jumper

27. Weiland FJ, Bantleon HP. Treatment of Class II malocclusions with the Jasper Jumper appliance – a preliminary report. Am J Orthod Dentofacial Orthop 1995;108:341–350.

28. Weiland FJ, Ingervall B, Bantleon HP, Droschl H. Initial effects of treatment of Class II malocclusion with the Herren activator, activator-headgear combination, and Jasper Jumper. Am J Orthod Dentofacial Orthop 1997;112:19–27.

29. Burstone CJ. Deep overbite correction by intrusion. Am J Orthod 1977;72:1–22.

30. Williams S, Melsen B. The interplay between sagittal and vertical growth factors. An implant study of activator treatment. Am J Orthod 1982;81:327–332.

31. Broadbent BH, Broadbent BH Jr, Golden W. Bolton standards of dentofacial development growth. St Louis, MO: Mosby; 1975.

32. Pancherz H. A cephalometric analysis of skeletal and dental changes contributing to Class II correction in activator treatment. Am J Orthod 1984;85:125–134.

33. Birkebaek L, Melsen B, Terp S. A laminographic study of the alterations in the temporo-mandibular joint following activator treatment. Eur J Orthod 1984;6:257–266.

34. Ruf S, Pancherz H. Temporomandibular joint growth adaptation in Herbst treatment: a prospective magnetic resonance imaging and cephalometric roentgenographic study. Eur J Orthod 1998;20:375–388.

35. Ruf S, Pancherz H. Temporomandibular joint remodeling in adolescents and young adults during Herbst treatment: a prospective longitudinal magnetic resonance imaging and cephalometric radiographic investigation. Am J Orthod Dentofacial Orthop 1999;115:607–618.

36. Stöckli PW, Willert HW. Tissue reactions in the temporomandibular joint resulting from anterior displacement of the mandible in the monkey. Am J Orthod 1971;60:142–155.

37. Woodside DG, Metaxas A, Altuna G. The influence of functional appliance therapy on glenoid fossa remodeling. Am J Orthod Dentofacial Orthop 1987;92:181–198.

38. Stucki N, Ingervall B. The use of the Jasper Jumper for the correction of Class II malocclusion in the young permanent dentition. Eur J Orthod 1998;20:271–281.

39. Covell DA, Trammell DW, Boero RP, West R. A cephalometric study of Class II Division 1 malocclusions treated with the Jasper Jumper appliance. Angle Orthod 1999;69:311–320.

40. Ruf S, Pancherz H. Dentoskeletal effects and facial profile changes in young adults treated with the Herbst appliance. Angle Orthod 1999;69:239–246.

41. Cash RG. Adult nonextraction treatment with a Jasper Jumper. J Clin Orthod 1991;25:43–47.

42. Pancherz H. The nature of Class II relapse after Herbst appliance treatment: a cephalometric long-term investigation. Am J Orthod Dentofacial Orthop 1991;100:220–233.

43. Hansen K, Pancherz H. Long-term effects of Herbst treatment in relation to normal growth and development: a cephalometric study. Eur J Orthod 1992;14:285–295.

44. Hagg U, Pancherz H, Taranger J. Pubertal growth and orthodontic treatment. In: Carlson DS, Ribbens KA, eds. Craniofacial growth during adolescence. Monograph 20, Craniofacial Growth Series. Ann Arbor, MI: Center for Human Growth and Development. The University of Michigan; 1987;87–115.

45. Pancherz H, Hagg U. Dentofacial orthopedics in relation to somatic maturation. An analysis of 70 consecutive cases treated with the Herbst appliance. Am J Orthod 1985;88:273–287.

46. Pancherz H, Litmann C. Somatische Reife und morphologische Veränderungen des Unterkiefers bei der Herbst-Behandlung. Inf Orthod Kieferorthop 1988;20:455–470.

47. Hansen K, Iemamnueisuk P, Pancherz H. Long-term effects of the Herbst appliance on the dental arches and arch relationships: a biometric study. Br J Orthod 1995;22:123–134.

48. Jakobsson SO. Cephalometric evaluation of treatment effect on Class II, division 1 malocclusions. Am J Orthod 1967;53:446–455.

49. Dietrich UC. Aktivator – mandibuläre Reaktion. Schweiz Monatschr Zahnheilk 1973;83:1093–1104.

50. Righellis EG. Treatment effects of Fränkel, activator and extraoral traction appliances. Angle Orthod 1983;53:107–121.

51. Remmer KR, Mamandras AH, Hunter WS, Way DC. Cephalometric changes associated with treatment using the activator, the Fränkel appliance, and the fixed appliance. Am J Orthod 1985;88:363–372.

52. Looi LK, Mills JRE. The effect of two contrasting forms of orthodontic treatment on the facial profile. Am J Orthod 1986;89:91–109.

53. Weichbrodt L. Distalbisstherapie mit Begg-Technik und Aktivator. Doctorate degree thesis. Bern: Bern University; 1990.

54. Teuscher U. Quantitative Behandlungsresultate mit der Aktivator-Headgear-Kombination. Heidelberg: Hüthig; 1988.

55. Creekmore TD, Radney LJ. Fränkel appliance therapy: orthopaedic or orthodontic? Am J Orthod 1983;83:89–108.

56. Gianelly AA, Arena SA, Bernstein L. A comparison of Class II treatment changes noted with the light wire, edgewise, and Fränkel appliances. Am J Orthod 1984;86:269–276.

CHAPTER 11

The Flex Developer

Heinz Winsauer, Alfred Peter Muchitsch

CONTENTS

Design and Construction Features

The Flex Developer (FD) is a most powerful and indestructible noncompliance intermaxillary Class II mechanism (Fig. 11.1). The force of the FD arises from a 3.0 mm diameter (D) elastic polyamide minirod that is clipped on to a standard fixed appliance. The unique anterior hooklet module makes the FD adaptable to any length. The hooklet is relockable and allows the orthodontist to take the device out easily for adjustments.

Because of its ability to produce high intermaxillary forces, the FD can be compared in some respects with the Herbst appliance. Only a few millimeters of mandibular protrusion will instantly reduce the force to zero. As the therapeutic force vector runs mainly parallel to the occlusal plane, there are only minimal vertical side effects in clinical use.

The FD is customarily combined with a prebent bypass arch, which allows delivery of forces up to 1000 cN and gives additional stability. This bypass arch also has an antirotational and antitipping effect on the attached molar. But using the FD does not necessarily mean only using high forces. The possibility to reduce the FD's minirod diameter and therefore achieve lower forces (as low as 50 cN) for single tooth movements or for periodontal reasons is another outstanding feature.

Observed clinically, the FD produces up to 1.0 mm tooth movement per month with no particular patient cooperation.

Pulling or Pushing Class II Mechanics?

At first it may not seem that the difference between these two types of mechanics is particularly relevant, since it is clear that both aim at the correction of Class II situations. However, the effects are different and important.

Pulling intermaxillary Class II mechanics, such as elastics or closed superelastic coil springs, may lead to open bite situations due to the extrusion of teeth and an increasing force when opening the mouth. As extrusion happens much faster than intrusion, this is a common threat.

In contrast, *pushing* intermaxillary Class II mechanics have an intruding side effect on upper molars and lower anterior teeth. As mentioned above, this vertical effect (intrusion) is much smaller than the extrusion created by *pulling* appliances. At the same time, it must be realized that the greatest force levels in the pushing devices are achieved in the final stages of mouth closing and include therefore a significant horizontal component. Taking this one stage further, it is interesting to contrast the effect of the Jasper Jumper™ and the FD. Experiments and clinical evidence show clearly that the effect of the FD is similar to that of the Herbst appliance, whereas the Jasper Jumper develops its maximum force while the force vector is in a less optimal (more vertical) direction.

Using rigid constructions such as the Herbst appliance or the FD, an immediate decrease of force is observed when the patient moves the mandible forward or opens the mouth only slightly. Therefore the FD can be applied even in high angle Class II or in open bite cases (see Figs 11.20–11.36).

More than 2000 orthodontists are now using the FD because of its simple insertion and outstanding durability.

Indications and Contraindications for Use of the Flex Developer

Indications

- Class II correction of dental arches (removable or fixed appliances)
- Mesial movement of lower molars and premolars after extraction or in cases of aplasia

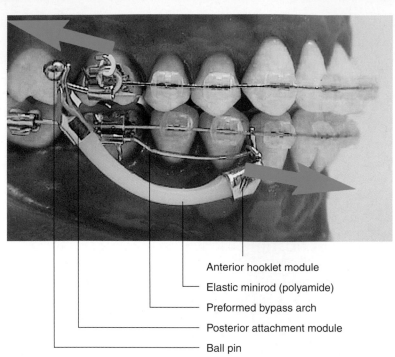

Anterior hooklet module
Elastic minirod (polyamide)
Preformed bypass arch
Posterior attachment module
Ball pin

Figure 11.1 The general design and components of the FD system. The FD itself is attached to the bypass arch in the lower anterior region and the posterior part is attached from the distal side of the headgear tube on the maxillary first molar.

- Distalization of upper molars (headgear effect)
- Retraction of anterior teeth (upper molar anchorage)
- Protrusion of lower teeth (presurgical decompensation of Class III cases)
- Mandibular development (orthopedic effect)
- Midline correction (asymmetric use of FD)
- Unilateral dental Class II correction (unilateral FD)

Contraindications

- Proclination of lower incisors
- Steep occlusal plane
- Gummy smile
- Extreme anterior open bite

Excessive protrusion of the lower incisors will probably lead to loss of alveolar bone and gingival recessions. Especially in patients in whom these teeth are protruded prior to treatment, a further proclination represents a risk of instability and iatrogenic damage. In this context the thickness of the symphyseal area can give information as to how much the lower incisors may be protruded during treatment.[1–3]

Like any other intermaxillary treatment mechanism, the FD produces a slight tipping of the occlusal plane which could worsen a gummy smile. Nevertheless, worsening of these situations should be avoided.

History

The concept of jumping the bite is not new in Class II correction; in fact, it is nearly as old as orthodontics itself. The Herbst appliance was first presented by Emil Herbst at the International Dental Congress in Berlin in 1905 and reviewed in a later article.[4] After a long period of relative anonymity, the Herbst appliance experienced a revival in the 1970s[5] and, because of exhaustive research studies concerning its skeletal and dentoalveolar effects, is probably one of the most investigated and documented mechanisms in orthodontics. The original design of the Herbst appliance involved the creation of a strong, stable framework on which the telescopes, the active part of the appliance, were mounted. One of the disadvantages of the Herbst appliance is a relatively limited lateral movement, which results from the stiff telescopic system.

The Jasper Jumper was introduced as a flexible alternative, allowing better lateral movement and at the same time being used in conjunction with a standard fixed appliance. There is some discussion about the relationship of skeletal and dentoalveolar effects. An investigation by Weiland & Bantleon described a 40% skeletal and 60% dentoalveolar effect for the Jasper Jumper.[6] One of the drawbacks most frequently observed with this appliance was the risk of fracture. The soldered connection between the eyelets and the open coil represents a weak point where fracture is most likely to occur.[7] The need to stock various lengths, both for the left and right side, increases the risk of not having the right size available when needed. The applicable force is limited to approximately 250 cN (38 mm JJ) and cannot be reduced much.

In 1995, Dr Williams from the Royal Dental College, University of Aarhus, Denmark, presented for the first time an alternative device for jumping the bite (the Sagittal Developer), in which the rubber-coated spring of the Jasper Jumper was replaced by a polyamide minirod, eliminating the risk of fracture (S Williams, personal communication, 1995). The polyamide minirod was unbreakable, stable, and found to deliver a constant force. Williams also developed an adjustable anterior hooklet module to shorten the polyamide minirod to the patient's individual need. For easier insertion, this hooklet could be opened and relocked by the orthodontist. It was suggested that the appliance slid on a bypass arch as published earlier by Blackwood.[8] The anterior hooklet module of the Sagittal Developer at that time was not able to withstand the power development, often causing unexpected repair appointments. In spite of numerous successful clinical results, the reliability of the metal components was difficult to predict. The Williams sagittal developer was the first appliance on the market that could be shortened to any individual length and was able to deliver a high and continuous force.

Design and Use

In 1997, Winsauer optimized this concept by adding more than 18 improvements (Fig. 11.2). He redesigned the metal components

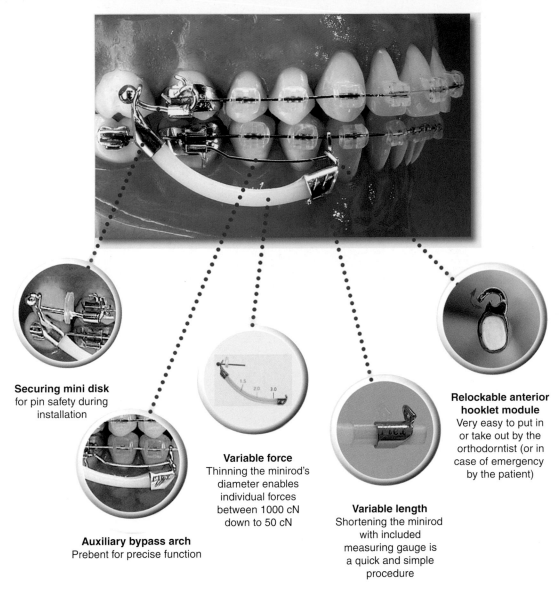

Figure 11.2 Features of the FD also have an antirotational effect on the attached molar.

Securing mini disk
for pin safety during installation

Auxiliary bypass arch
Prebent for precise function

Variable force
Thinning the minirod's diameter enables individual forces between 1000 cN down to 50 cN

Variable length
Shortening the minirod with included measuring gauge is a quick and simple procedure

Relockable anterior hooklet module
Very easy to put in or take out by the orthodorntist (or in case of emergency by the patient)

and made them more reliable and functional. Plasma welding (no solder) guarantees long-lasting robustness along with inert quality. A *starterkit* for standardized and simplified insertion was added (Fig. 11.3). The adjustability of the appliance length was maintained, in that the anterior hooklet module could slide along the polyamide minirod and be fixed at an appropriate length. Moreover, Winsauer introduced the possibility of *reducing the minirod's diameter* in order to obtain an individually adjusted power range.

At this time a more powerful and color-stable polyamide material came into use. In order to avoid time-consuming and individual bending procedures, a *standardized prebent bypass arch* was added to each FD. The prebent auxiliary bypass arch has a precise form enabling optimal use. Besides letting the FD slide forward and backward, it also serves as an antirotational and antitipping device. Another well-liked feature of the FD is the *security disk* mounted on the posterior pin

which eliminates the danger of a dropped pin during its insertion into the rear end of the headgear tube. Another security feature is the patient's ability to open the hooklet in case of emergency (claustrophobia, technical defect) and this way for convenience the FD can be hooked onto the upper archwire.

Due to the average insertion time being less than 4 minutes and the minirod being guaranteed to last a lifetime, the FD has become a widespread and highly accepted Class II intermaxillary treatment device. In addition to its high efficiency, the FD requires no compliance from the patient.

The appliance is offered for sale together with a starter kit of instruments, etc., which facilitates the fitting of the FD. Force adjustment is achieved by reducing the diameter of the polyamide rod (see Fig. 11.3). For this purpose a special Gyroform™ *grinding wheel* is included in the kit. This wheel is also able to produce a

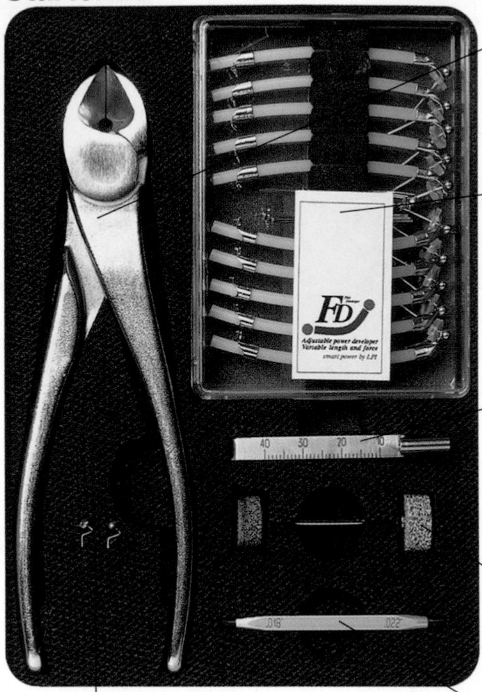

Starterkit

Sharpened side cutter
Trimming of elastic
minirods, crimp stop for
anterior hooklet module

Flex Developer – box
5 left FD
5 right FD (red)
Complete with 5+5
preformed bypass arches

Measuring ruler
Intraoral measurement
to determine the
length and to
shorten the elastic
minirod

Gyroform® buffer
Brown for reducing
FD-minirod (metal, FD)
green for polishing
FD-minirod (FD)

Headgear pins
For the attachment of the FD to auxiliary
tube. This way the HG-tube remains free for
simultaneous HG or lip bumper use

Torquing key
Fine adjustment of
preformed bypass arch

Figure 11.3 Toolbox with a set of FDs, cutter, ruler, gyroform grinding wheel, torquing wrench and headgear pins.

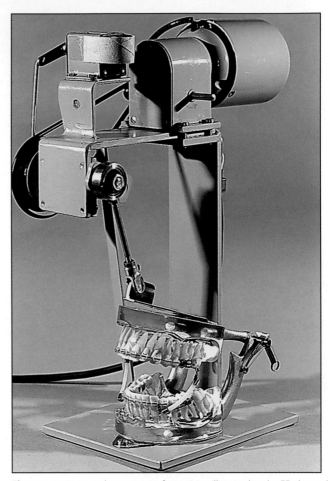

Figure 11.4 In an endurance test of over 2.5 million cycles, the FD showed virtually no loss of power (less than 5%). The test was performed in artificial saliva at 38°C.

smooth rounded finish to the end of the polyamide rod. The desired force can easily be measured with a Correx force gauge.

A *torquing wrench* is also included for fine adjustments of the prebent bypass arch. If the anterior end of the bypass arch and the hooklet module are too close to the gingiva, this wrench allows third-order bends in the posterior region without distorting other parts of this segmented arch.

A *ruler* enables intraoral measurements to determine the length of the elastic minirod and at the same time serves as a gauge to determine the appropriate length of the FD. It also ensures an automatic activation of the FD corresponding to 8 mm. An extra sharp *cutter* helps to shorten the minirod and to crimp the anterior module to the rod.

Durability of the Flex Developer during Occlusal Function

Two FDs underwent an endurance test of 2 million cycles (Fig. 11.4). One had a length of 36 mm and no reduction in diameter (3 mm). The initial force was set at 640 cN. The second FD was 38 mm long and its diameter reduced by 1 mm (diameter 2 mm). The initial force was set at 210 cN. Assuming a patient is opening and closing

the mouth 8000 times per day, this would equal 250 days of continuous treatment time.

The bench testing was interrupted after 2 million cycles without failure or breakage (Fig. 11.5). After this test the force reduction of the FD (original diameter 3 mm) was less than 5%. The reduced FD (2 mm) showed no change of elasticity.

Comparison of Different Noncompliance Class II Treatment Appliances

Due to the possibility of adjusting the FD's resilience to any amount between 50 and 1000 cN, a wide range of treatment applications is possible. These findings encourage the use of the FD in numerous types of appliances in removable and permanent orthodontic treatment techniques.

All measured samples were 38 mm in length (Fig. 11.6). In Figure 11.6, the yellow curve displays the rapid increase of power typical for rigid Herbst telescopes. The red lines represent the spectrum of force of three FDs with different diameters (3 mm, 2 mm, 1.5 mm). Note that a 38 mm FD (D 3 mm) develops 300 cN (approximately 300

Endurance test: 2 million cycles

In order to prove its reliability two sets of FDs were tested under standardized conditions (artificial saliva, 37°C)

	3.0 FD 36 mm ø = 3 mm = 100%	2.0 FD 38 mm ø = 2 mm = 66%
Force before testing	640 cN	210 cN
Force after 2 million cycles	620 cN	210 cN

Calculating 8000 chewing cycles per day is equal to 250 treatment days of continuous FD action (7 months)

Figure 11.5 The results of bench testing of the FD.

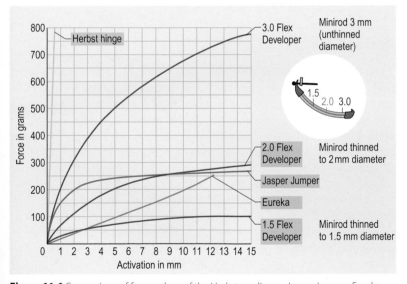

Figure 11.6 Comparison of force values of the Herbst appliance, Jasper Jumper, Eureka Spring and FD (all 38 mm length).

pond) after only 2 mm of activation. The blue line is the Jasper Jumper, quite similar to a FD with a diameter of 2 mm. The smooth and gradual ascent of the green curve is typical of the Eureka Spring.

It is important to know that the use of shorter FDs will cause higher treatment forces and therefore steeper ascents of all red curves (see FD instruction manual, available at: www.flexdeveloper.com).

Because of the greater stiffness of the FD, there is good reason to assume that the skeletal effect is higher than that of the Jasper Jumper or other Class II pushing devices.[6]

Clinical Use

The following is a short review of the FD fitting process. Prior to insertion of the FD, the dental arches should be well aligned and full-sized rectangular stainless steel wires should be fitted. An exception to this rule could be the case of anterior maxillary crowding, where the crowding is to be relieved by distal movement of the maxillary molars using the FD.

Before installation, the little hook of the lower molar attachments should be bent forward, caudal and gingivally. This way, the sticking of the elastic minirod under the molar attachment is avoided.

Bypass Arch

Insert the prebent bypass arch so that its hooklet is situated on the treatment arch between the lower canine bracket and the lower first premolar bracket. The position of the hooklet of the bypass arch is critical. Where the appliance is to induce forward tipping of the mandibular incisors and canines, e.g. in the decompensation of the mandibular arch in Class III cases, the hooklet of the bypass arch may rest against the canine bracket and the distal end of the bypass arch must remain straight (see Fig. 11.62). However, if forward tipping of the lower anterior teeth is to be avoided, the hooklet must not touch the canine bracket and the distal end of the bypass arch should be bent coronally to avoid the arch slipping forward. Using the fine three-prong pliers, a step bend is made and the hooklet is closed with a Weingart plier.

This way the anterior part of the bypass arch is able to move forward, making space closure or anterior movement of posterior teeth possible. The bypass arch also serves as an antitipping and antirotational device for the lower first molars. If spaces are to be closed during treatment (aplasia), the bypass arch will be shortened continuously by pulling it through the auxiliary tube, while moving the step bend more anteriorly.

Determining the Length of the FD

The distance between the anterior surface of the headgear tube and the anterior end of the bypass arch is measured with the FD ruler. The FD is thereafter inserted into the tube of the ruler, so that the posterior module lines up with the number that was just measured. The excess minirod is cut off and the anterior module slid forward into position and crimped with the side cutter. The use of this ruler assures an automatic activation of the FD corresponding to 8.0 mm. Now the FD is at its ideal length and can be inserted into the mouth.

Activation During Treatment

There are four different ways to activate the FD:
- shortening of the bypass arch
- shortening of the pin in the headgear tube

- placing a stop (composite resin) at the anterior part of the bypass arch
- use of a longer FD.

Further details are given in the instruction booklet (available at: www.flexdeveloper.com).

Case Studies

Patient 1 (Figs 11.7–11.12)

A 15-year-old girl showing dental Class II with increased overjet of 8.0 mm, poor vertical overlap (0.0 mm) and spaces in the upper incisor region. Cephalometrically, a slight protrusion of the maxillary incisors was observed (112°) and a slight increase in mandibular plane angle (Figs 11.7–11.10). The patient was treated using the FD for 6 months, retracting the upper incisors and normalizing canine relationships. Note the overcorrection before removing the FD, which is generally recommended for this type of treatment. The results in Figure 11.11 show good sagittal relationship and space closure. The patient obtained a FD-splint positioner with integrated headgear tubes and bypass arches as an active removable retainer (Fig. 11.12).

Patient 2 (Figs 11.13–11.19)

This patient, a very athletic 38-year-old man, asked for treatment because of increasing discomfort in the TMJ and continuous enamel abrasion on his anterior teeth. The Class II malocclusion was slightly more severe on the right side than on the left (Figs 11.13 and 11.15). The lateral cephalometric radiograph revealed no skeletal discrepancy but obvious retroclination of the maxillary incisors (81°) (Fig. 11.14). Treatment was started using fixed appliances initially with maxillary incisor torque using the torquing rod technique.[9] The functional freeway space thus created permitted dentoalveolar correction of the Class II situation using the FD. The force applied was 350 cN per side (Fig. 11.16).

Immediately after the removal of the FD, a good relationship was observed (Fig. 11.17), which later settled to a perfect Class I. After treatment the patient's dentist started to reconstruct the original cusps of the buccal teeth. The lateral cephalometric radiograph and analysis showed a good inclination of the maxillary incisors (108°) together with a moderate protrusion of the lower incisors (Fig. 11.18).

Note that directly after the FD was placed in the mouth, the patient was encouraged to eat a piece of apple to experience the reliability of the appliance (Fig. 11.19).

Patient 3 (Figs 11.20–11.36)

The patient was a 22-year-old woman with an open bite and contact only in the posterior region. The upper central incisors were root-filled and restored with crowns after previous trauma (Figs 11.20, 11.21, 11.24 and 11.25). The lateral cephalometric analysis (Figs 11.22 and 11.23) demonstrated a slight increase in the vertical jaw relationship and a moderate ANB discrepancy (4°). Due to a relatively large mandible and tongue, it was planned to expand the maxilla to permit correction of the buccal occlusion. During the 6 month period of rapid maxillary expansion, posterior bite plates were used in addition to a vertical chin cap (Figs 11.26 and 11.27). Tongue function was modified by a combination of increased bite opening (bite blocks of the RME device) and logopedic training support.

After removal of the rapid maxillary expansion device and dental arch leveling, the left side was in Class I occlusion, although the right side was still in ½ premolar-width Class II relationship. A unilateral FD was used for the correction (Figs 11.28 and 11.29). Figure 11.30 shows the situation before removal of the FD. As already mentioned above, the vertical side effect of the FD is negligible. The minor bite opening in the right buccal region closed 3 weeks after removal of the FD. Figures 11.31–11.34 show the patient at the end of treatment. The lateral cephalometric analysis demonstrated the tremendous changes (Figs 11.35 and 11.36). The comparison of the two analyses shows a slight distalization of the maxillary molars with mild protrusion of the lower incisors.

Patient 4 (Figs 11.37–11.56)

This patient was a 15-year-old girl with a Class II, division 1 malocclusion with protrusion and crowding in the maxillary arch. The lower right second premolar was aplastic and the lower right first molar was mesially tipped. There were large restorations in the first molars (Figs 11.37–11.42). The panoramic X-ray (Fig. 11.43) confirmed the presence of upper third molars, although both lower ones appear to be impacted. The lateral cephalometric analysis revealed a high angle situation and an apparently small maxillary apical base.

The treatment plan included extraction of the upper first premolar on the right side, showing a one premolar-width Class II relationship, and extraction of the upper left first molar, because of the deep filling and ½ premolar-width Class II on the left side. The lower right first molar was to be moved upright and the space anterior to it closed (Figs 11.43 and 11.44). Using segmental arches, spaces were closed with the upper right first molar serving as anchorage. This tooth moved a little too far mesially. On the other side, the upper left first molar moved forward, losing anchorage as well. Somewhat later, as a result of the very deep restoration, a pulpitis developed by the upper right first molar and the treatment plan was modified so that this tooth had to be extracted (Fig. 11.45). At this point it was decided to extract the lower first molars as well, because of the large restorations and the presence of well-shaped third molars (Fig. 11.46).

Later, after eruption of the second molars, intense FD treatment was performed for space closure in the lower arch and to achieve a Class I canine relationship. The force was adjusted to 350 cN, reactivating the FD 1.0 mm every 4 weeks. Note the elongated bypass arch extending underneath the canine bracket (Figs 11.47 and 11.48),

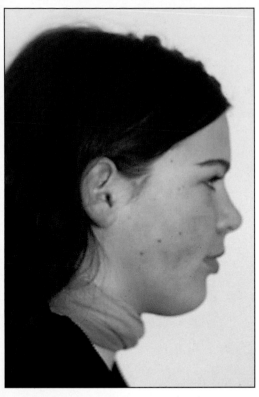

Figures 11.7–11.12 Case 1, Patient LO. Profile view before treatment.

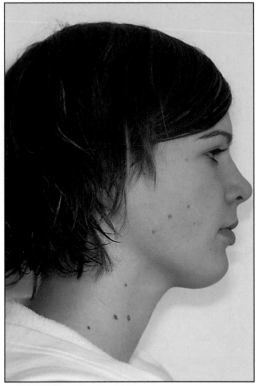

Figure 11.8 Profile view after treatment.

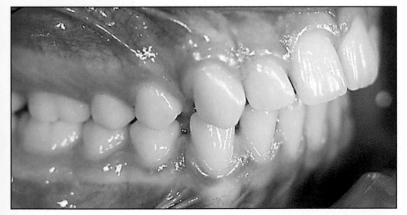

Figure 11.9

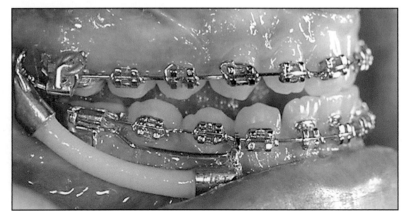

Figure 11.10

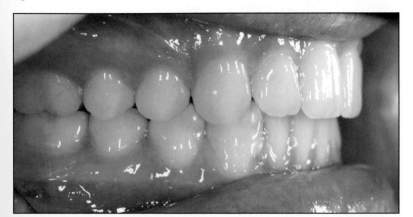

Figure 11.11

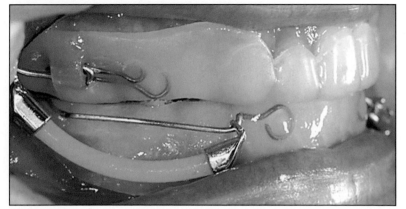

Figure 11.12

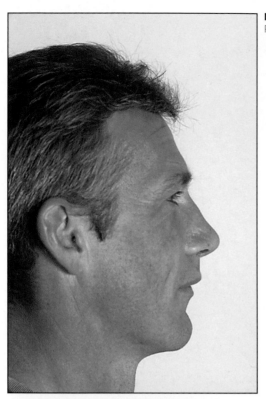

Figures 11.13–11.19 Case 2, Patient HR.

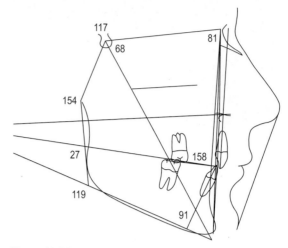

Figure 11.14

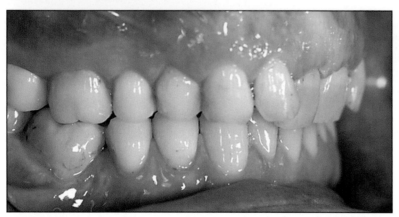

Figure 11.15

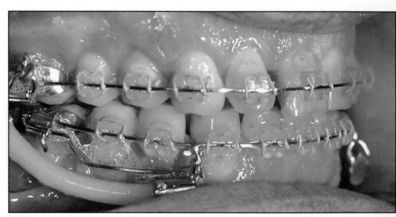

Figure 11.16

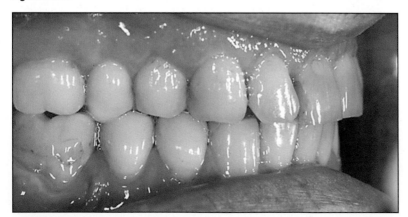

Figure 11.17

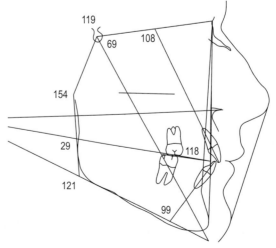

Figure 11.18

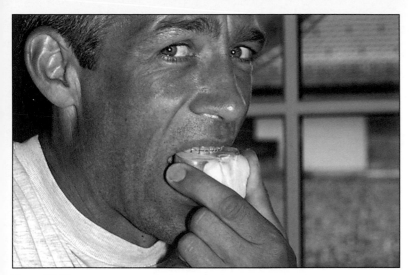

Figure 11.19

giving the FD a longer range of action. A splint positioner with bypass arches and FDs created a reliable active retention device (Fig. 11.49). The results are shown in Figures 11.50–11.56 with harmonious dental arches in Class I relationship.

Patient 5 (Figs 11.57–11.69)

A 44-year-old man presented with severe mandibular prognathism and reversed overjet before presurgical orthodontic treatment (Figs 11.57–11.61). The lateral cephalometric radiograph (Figs 11.58 and 11.59) demonstrated severe retrusion of the mandibular incisors. Therefore a presurgical decompensation was necessary at the same time as the buccal teeth were moved mesially. Two FDs, each delivering a force of 340 cN, were applied over a period of 5 months (Figs 11.62 and 11.63). In Figure 11.62 it can be seen that spaces anterior to the first molar have been developed, since the entire force was pushing on the canine bracket. Space closure was performed by continuously shortening and retracting the bypass arches. Figure 11.64 demonstrates the robustness of the elastic minirods as in such treatments continuous abrasion through adjacent brackets is common. The treatment was completed with only one set of FDs. These pictures demonstrate the presurgical decompensation.

The posttreatment results are presented in Figures 11.65–11.67. The lateral cephalometric radiographs and the comparison of the analyses reveal the change in lower incisor angulation from 66° to 85° (Figs 11.68 and 11.69).

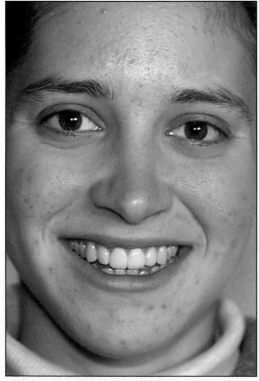

Figures 11.20–11.36 Case 3, Patient CZ.

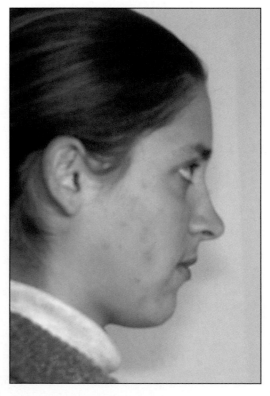

Figure 11.21

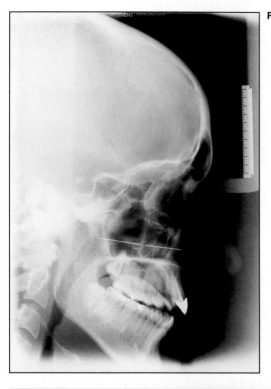

Figure 11.22

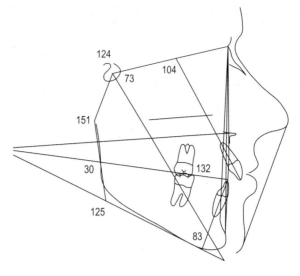

Figure 11.23

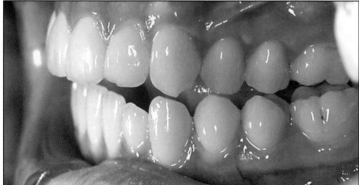

Figure 11.24

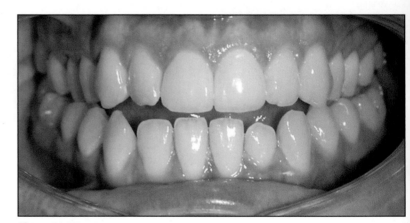

Figure 11.25

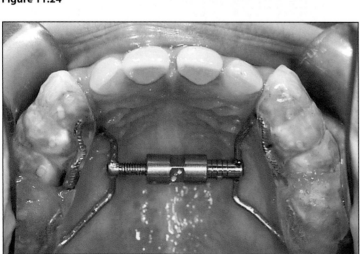

Figure 11.26

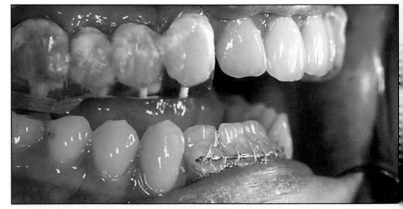

Figure 11.27

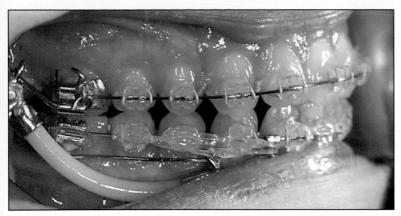

Figure 11.28

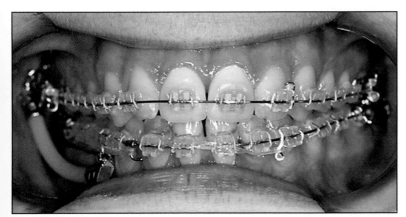

Figure 11.29

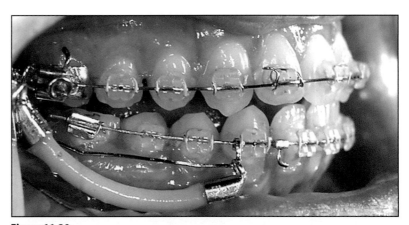

Figure 11.30

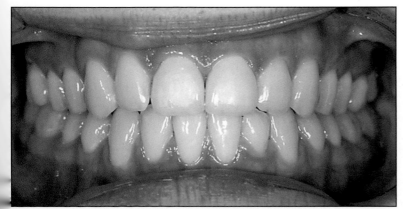

Figure 11.31

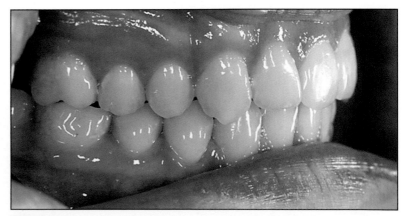

Figure 11.32

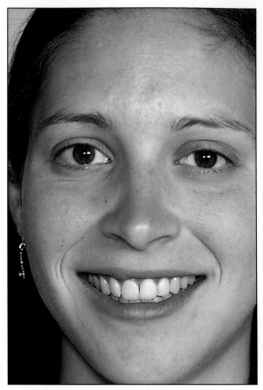

Figure 11.33

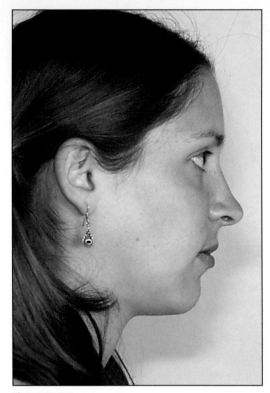

Figure 11.34

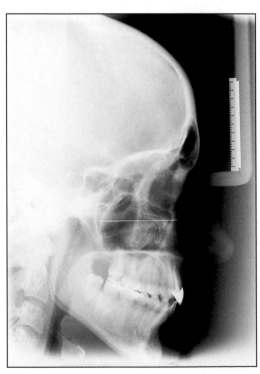

Figure 11.35

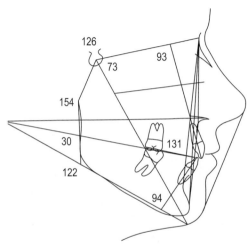

Figure 11.36

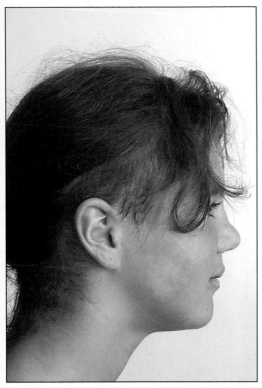

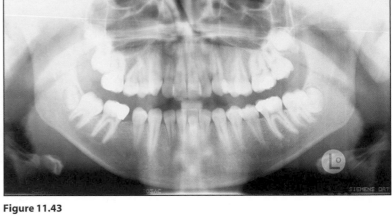

Figure 11.43

Figures 11.37–11.56 Case 4, Patient MG.

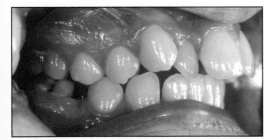

Figure 11.38

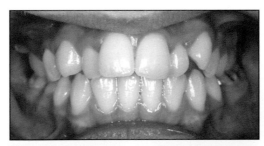

Figure 11.39

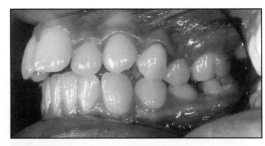

Figure 11.40

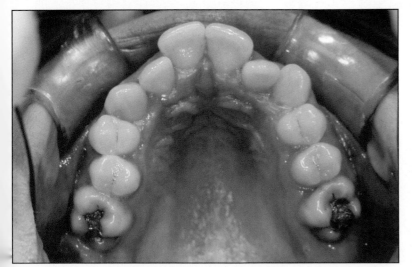

Figure 11.41

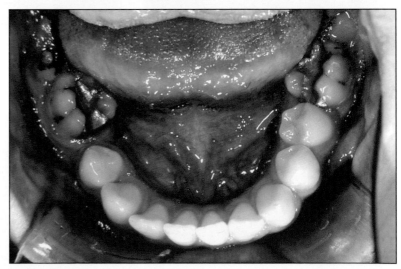

Figure 11.42

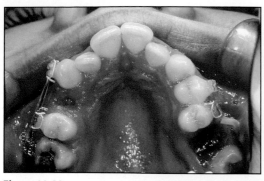

Figure 11.44

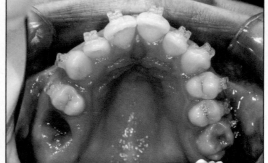

Figure 11.45

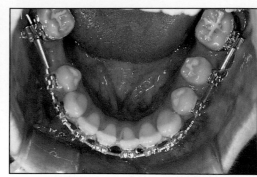

Figure 11.46

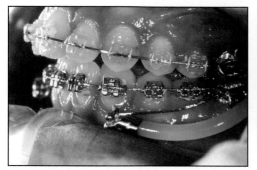

Figure 11.47

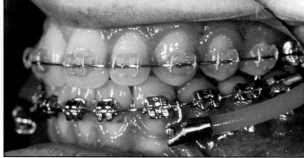

Figure 11.48

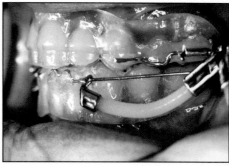

Figure 11.49

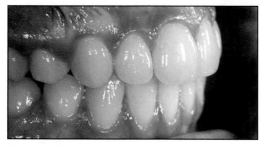

Figure 11.50

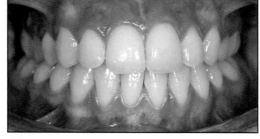

Figure 11.51

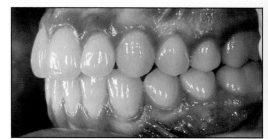

Figure 11.52

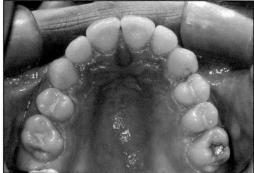
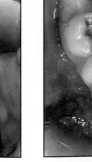

Figure 11.53

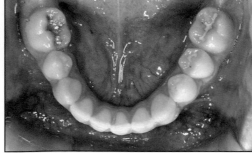

Figure 11.54

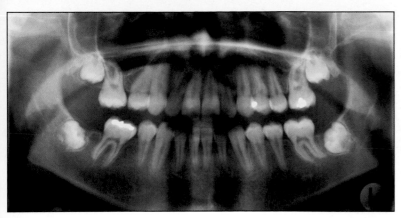

Figure 11.55

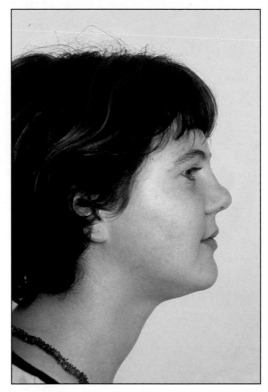

Figure 11.56

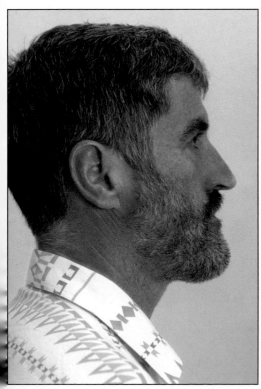

Figures 11.57–11.69 Case 5, Patient HZ.

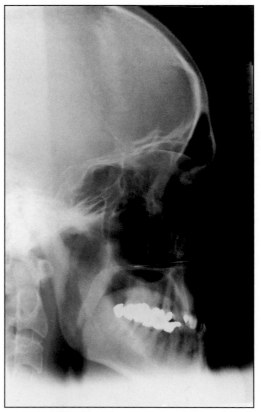

Figure 11.58

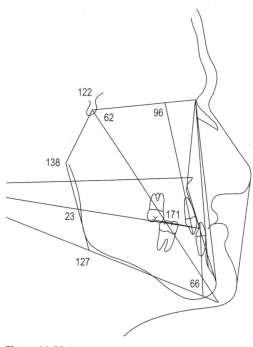

Figure 11.59

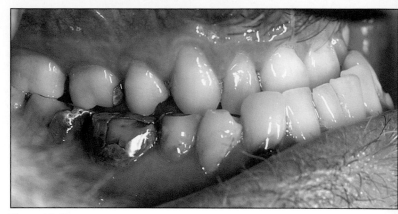

Figure 11.60

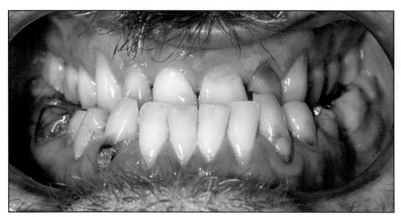

Figure 11.61

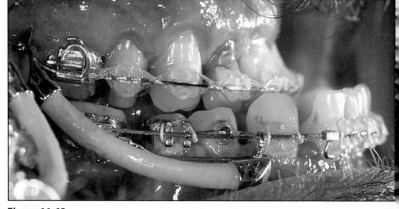

Figure 11.62

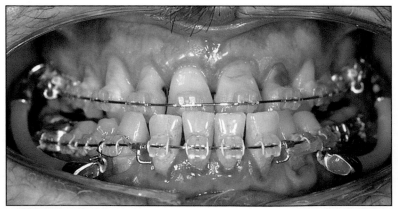

Figure 11.63

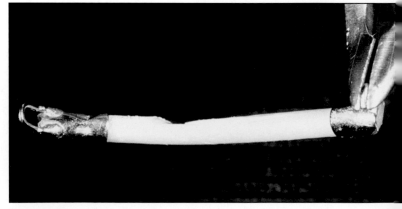

Figure 11.64

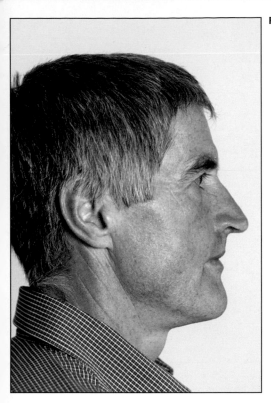

Figure 11.65

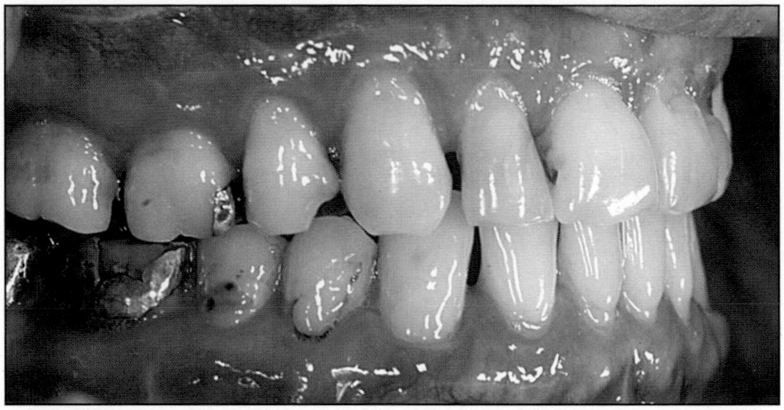

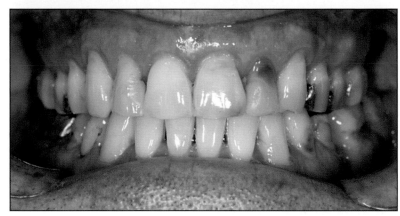

Figure 11.66

Figure 11.67

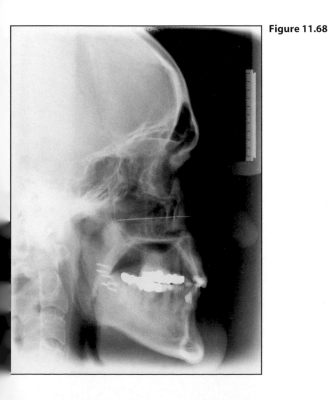

Figure 11.68

Figure 11.69

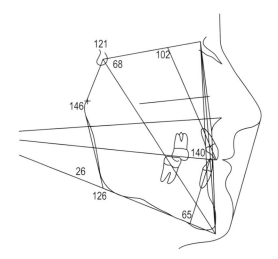

Acknowledgments

The authors would like to express their gratitude to Dr Steven Williams (Vienna) and Dr Claudia Ruopp (Munich) for their substantial support in structuring and proof-reading this chapter.

References

1. Fuhrmann R. Three-dimensional interpretation of alveolar bone dehiscences. An anatomical-radiological study. Part I. J Orofac Orthop 1996;57:62–74.

2. Fuhrmann R. Three-dimensional interpretation of labiolingual bone width of the lower incisors. Part II. J Orofac Orthop 1996;57:168–185.

3. Fuhrmann R. Three-dimensional interpretation of periodontal lesions and remodeling during orthodontic treatment. Part III. J Orofac Orthop 1996;57:224–237.

4. Herbst E. Dreissigjährige Erfahrungen mit dem Retentions-Scharnier. Zahnärztl Rundschau 1934;43:1515–1524, 1563–1568, 1611–1616.

5. Pancherz H. The Herbst appliance – its biologic effects and clinical use. Am J Orthod 1985;87:1–20.

6. Weiland F, Bantleon HP. Treatment of Class II malocclusion with the Jasper Jumper appliance – a preliminary report. Am J Orthod Dentofacial Orthop 1995;108:341–350.

7. Schwindling P. Jasper Jumper™. Merzig: Edition Schwindling, 1997.

8. Blackwood HO. Clinical management of the Jasper Jumper. J Clin Orthod 1991;12:755–760.

9. Winsauer H, Richter M. Das Innsbrucker Toquekonzept. Prakt Kieferorthop 1989;3:17–24.

CHAPTER 12

The Eureka Spring™: a compact, versatile, and cost-effective Class II corrector

John P. DeVincenzo

Introduction

Diminished compliance among adolescents is a major concern of all healthcare providers. Even in such life-threatening conditions as sickle cell anemia,[1] renal transplant,[2,3] cancer,[4,5] and diabetes,[6,7] adolescent noncompliance is significant and approaches 50%,[2,3,8] with only 10% of patients showing excellent cooperation.[8] Additionally, it is difficult to predict the level of compliance at the onset of treatment[5,9,10] and clinicians experience waxing and waning levels of compliance over an extended treatment period.[2]

The initial motivation for trying a Eureka Spring™ will most likely come from working with the noncompliant patient who has consistently demonstrated insufficient wear of Class II elastics or extraoral headgear. With the resultant extended treatment time and inability to obtain the desired correction force, the clinician has to make one of two choices. First, treatment can be terminated with resignation that Class II correction will be incomplete. Second, a Class II correction appliance can be fitted which does not rely on patient cooperation.

Most of the appliances described in this book assume that noncompliance will be experienced and hence the treatment is planned accordingly from the onset. This applies to all the appliances described in Sections III and IV and most of those included in Section II. Some might argue that a number of those in Section II,

such as the Herbst, Cantilever Bite Jumper, Mandibular Protraction Appliance, MARA, Sabbagh and Twin Force Bite Corrector, if used as a mandibular repositioning device, were chosen because of an orthopedic effect on the mandible resulting in a portion of the Class II correction derived from increased mandibular length.

However, long-term longitudinal evaluations of previously obtained increases in mandibular length by repositioning question the durability of the initial mandibular orthopedic gains.[11–14] If this is true, then only the dentoalveolar changes, at least in the mandible, are lasting and therefore these appliances were selected, for all practical purposes, in anticipation of noncompliance. Thus, only the Eureka Spring, Jasper Jumper, and the Twin Force, when not used to reposition the mandible anteriorly, can be used by the clinician who is experiencing unanticipated noncompliance during treatment.

The Eureka Spring should be thought of, at least initially, as an alternative to Class II elastics. Thus, Class II elastics and/or headgear are prescribed first. If cooperation is lacking and treatment time extended, a Eureka Spring can be offered to the patient. If compliance does not improve on the subsequent appointment, a Eureka Spring is placed.

The Eureka Spring differs from Class II elastics in many ways, including mechanism of action, insertion, management and relapse, and these differences will be discussed below. Because the Eureka Spring exerts a push rather than the pull force of Class II elastics, a Class II Eureka Spring attaches in the direction of a Class III elastic (Fig. 12.1). Given the same point of attachment, the horizontal component of the Class II vector will be similar in the two systems while the vertical component will be opposite, with Class II elastics extruding maxillary anterior and mandibular posterior teeth and potentially causing downward and backward mandibular rotation. With the Eureka Spring, the vertical component intrudes the maxillary molars and mandibular incisors, resulting in stable and upward and forward mandibular rotation.[15]

A further difference exists in mouth breathers and those patients with a tendency to keep their teeth apart. In these the extrusive component of the Class II vector increases when elastics are used while the intrusive component of the Eureka Spring diminishes.

The force vectors and duration of wear of Class II elastics can be varied by the clinician. These can also be varied with the Eureka

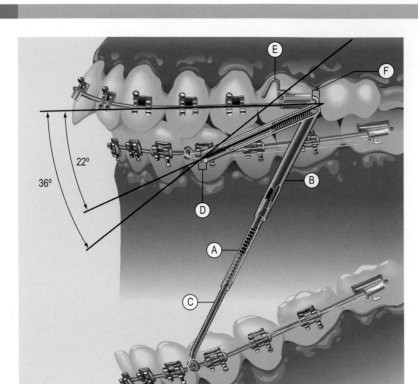

Figure 12.1 Components of the Class II Eureka Spring illustrated in a complete Class II occlusion with a 50 mm open-mouth position as produced by a hinge axis recorded articulator. The essential aspects include spring module A, molar attachment tube B, push rod C, free distance D, molar attachment wire E, free distance F.

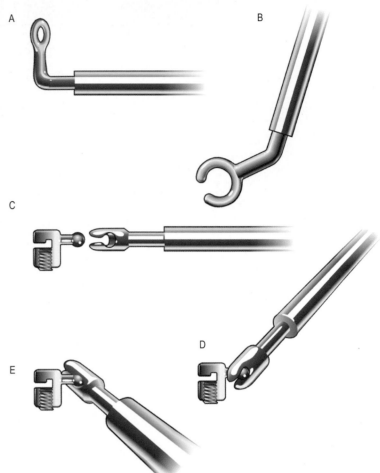

Figure 12.2 Choice of archwire attachments. Classic closed ring A, Classic open ring B, and Quick-Connect C, D, and E. In C, the spring module is inserted at its large opening E, then rotated 180° as shown in D, so the neck engages the narrow portion.

Spring. If the Eureka Spring was viewed as an adjunct or alternative to Class II elastics, it would be prescribed frequently and the cumulative cost in an orthodontic practice would become significant and possibly limit its use to the most severe conditions. Fortunately, simplicity of design and manufacture permits the Eureka Spring to be relatively inexpensive, very cost-effective in comparison to extended treatment with Class II elastics, and hence could enjoy frequent use. I use the Eureka Spring on about 25% of patients during some portion of their active orthodontic treatment.

The Eureka Spring was first described in 1997 and treatment results on a variety of noncompliant Class II patients were presented.[16] The impetus behind its development was frustration with the increasing number of noncompliant patients and the frequent breakage of the Jasper Jumper, the best noncompliant treatment appliance available at that time.

Description

The essential components of the Eureka Spring are shown in Figure 12.1, in which the mouth is closed into a completed Class II condition and also opened to 50 mm. The spring module (A) slides within a molar attachment tube (B). A compression spring

is encased within the spring module and drives the push rod (C) against the mandibular anterior teeth. It is important at insertion that the free distance (D), the distance from the elbow of the push rod to the open end of the molar attachment tube, be at least 2 mm when the mouth is closed. This free distance will extend the life of the spring and permit lateral excursions during mouth movements.

Several attachments to the mandibular archwire are available and illustrated in Figure 12.2. The *Classic closed ring* (A), the most popular model, requires archwire removal for insertion and removal, whereas the *Classic open ring* (B) permits attachment without archwire removal (the ring is gently crimped after insertion and one arm bent open for removal). The *Quick-Connect model* (C, D, and E) utilizes a block attached to the archwire from which a neck and sphere protrude. The spring module (A, Fig. 12.1) has been fitted with a receiving end on one side of which is an entrance slightly larger than the sphere on the block, while on the other side and joining the larger entrance is a slit slightly larger than the neck of the sphere. By inserting the sphere into the larger opening of the receiving end and then rotating the spring module 180° so that the narrow slit now engages the neck of the sphere (D), the spring module becomes fixed to the block. The Quick-Connect model permits rapid insertion without archwire removal and easy replacement of the spring module to one of greater or lesser force and/or distance as treatment progresses. When the desired Class II correction has been obtained, the spring module can be removed and the block used for intraoral elastics. Dental auxiliaries can easily place a Quick-Connect module in 1–2 minutes and remove it in half the time. This is comparable to the time taken to place Class II elastics if patient instruction time is included.

Figure 12.3 illustrates both the Classic and Quick-Connect models in a Class I molar relationship, in contrast to the Class II relationship depicted in Figure 12.1. Note the change in the angle of the force vector when going from Class II to Class I and also the slightly more horizontal vector of the Quick-Connect compared to the Classic model. It is also important to observe the very unfavorable vector generated when the maxillary attachment is placed mesial of the first molar (see Fig. 12.1). This becomes particularly important in severe Class II conditions.

Light (150 g) and heavy (225 g) spring force modules, depending on the configuration of the internal spring, are available. In adult patients requiring significant Class II corrections, the heavy spring module should be considered. In very young patients the light force module is preferred. In mid- to late-adolescent patients, both modules are used. If there is a bilateral Class II, more severe on one side, the heavy force spring module may be placed on that side while the light force module can be used contralaterally. The heavy force module will correct sagittal discrepancies more rapidly and will also produce more maxillary posterior dental intrusion.[17]

Extending from the distal aspect of the molar attachment tube (B, Fig. 12.1) is an 0.85 mm attachment wire (E, Fig. 12.1) with a ball end enclosed within the molar attachment tube. This attachment wire inserts from the distal into an auxiliary molar tube which must be at least 0.90 mm ID. At its anterior end it is secured to the hook on the molar tube. Adjustments in the attachment wire permit alterations in the vertical component of the force vector, as shown in Figure 12.4. Bending the attachment wire as in (A) will produce the largest intrusive component, whereas bending as in (C) will produce the least intrusive component. (Avoid bending the attachment wire completely vertical, because the hinge motion of the ball on opening may be limited.)

The ability to manipulate the force vector can be invaluable in obtaining rapid orthodontic treatment and is often overlooked. For example, in an anterior deep bite a vector producing more vertical intrusion as in (A) (Fig. 12.4) should be generated, whereas where no anterior overbite is present the clinician would be wise to create a vector nearly parallel to the occlusal plane, as depicted in (C). In the transverse dimension, if no transpalatal arch is used, greater buccal crown torque will occur in attachment method (A) than in (C). This would be desirable for correction of some malocclusions but very undesirable for others.

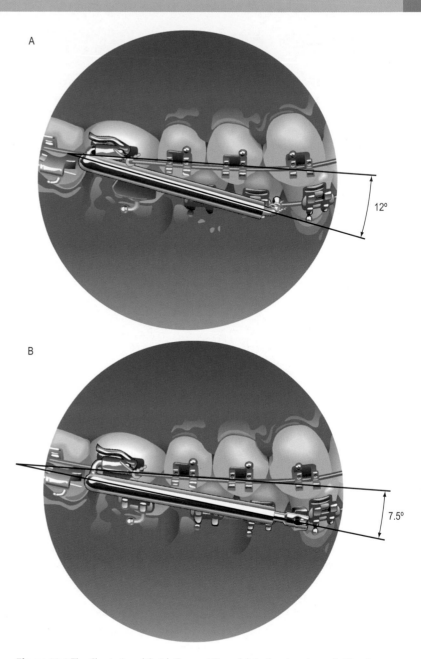

Figure 12.3 The Classic A and Quick-Connect B models in the closed-mouth Class I position. Note the change in the vectors (black lines), particularly comparing Fig. 12.1 Class II with Fig. 12.3 Class I.

Moments, Forces, and Vectors

The three dimensions of forces acting on the dentition can be seen in Figure 12.5, and close examination will indicate the expected clinical results of Eureka Spring therapy. In the buccal vector, the larger horizontal component will produce the desired sagittal Class II correction while the vertical component should produce maxillary molar and mandibular anterior intrusion.[15] This secondary intrusion effect which would facilitate correction of a severe Spee curve or

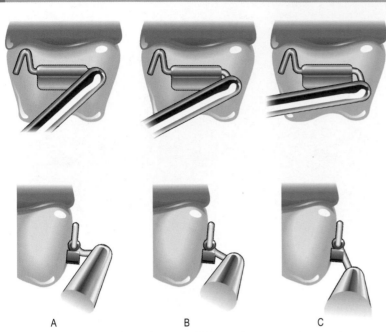

Figure 12.4 By changing the configuration of the attachment wire, the vertical component of the vector can be manipulated.

anterior overbite, often associated with Class II malocclusions, can be increased by manipulating the buccal vector as shown in Figure 12.4. However, if little curve of Spee exists along with a tendency for anterior open bite, Eureka Spring treatment should be combined with anterior vertical elastics, an increase in the curve of Spee in the mandibular archwire or a decrease in the vertical component of the buccal vector (see Fig. 12.4). The molar intrusive component would be welcomed in dolichofacial types, who are just the patients in whom Class II elastics are frequently contraindicated. However, in severe brachyfacial Class II patients, maxillary molar intrusion may not be desirable and the Eureka Spring contraindicated.

Manipulation of the vertical component of the buccal vector can be important. This is accomplished easily either at insertion or on subsequent appointments by modifying the direction the attachment wire (E, Fig. 12.1) takes as it emerges from the distal of the molar tube (see Fig. 12.4). It is noteworthy that the teeth drawn in Figure 12.5 are in a Class I relationship. The more Class II the original malocclusion, the greater will be the vertical (intrusive) component of the buccal vector. Likewise, the more anteriorly the maxillary attachment is placed, the greater the vertical component and the slower that sagittal correction will occur. This combination of sagittal and vertical effects explains why the Eureka Spring is not attached at the mesial of the maxillary molar.

The clinician should consider extension of the maxillary archwire through the second molars if prolonged Eureka Spring therapy is anticipated. Additionally, the heavy Eureka Spring will produce a larger vertical component than that resulting from a light Eureka Spring.[17] However, shorter treatment time with the heavy Eureka

Spring may reduce the total vertical force exerted on the dentition over the timespan of Eureka Spring treatment.

The sagittal correction produced by the horizontal component of the buccal vector will mesialize the mandibular dentition while causing posterior migration in the maxilla. To some extent differential movement can be obtained. For example, a large rectangular archwire (0.43 × 0.64 in a 0.46 × 0.61 slot) with palatal root torque to the maxillary incisors and second molars engaged along with a small mandibular rectangular archwire (0.41 × 0.56 in a 0.46 × 0.61 slot) with anterior lingual root torque and without second molars will result in as much as 80% of the correction occurring in the mandibular dentition. Likewise, with the reverse anchorage the clinician can expect as much as 80% of correction to occur in the maxillary dentition.

Stromeyer et al found all of the above-mentioned expectations at clinically significant levels.[15] When 10–15° of labial root torque was placed in the anterior region of the mandibular 0.41 × 0.56 archwire in 0° 0.46 × 0.64 slots and a similar sized wire and amount of palatal root torque was placed in the maxillary anterior archwire in Roth prescription anterior 0.46 × 0.64 slot brackets, the maxillary dentition migrated distally an amount equal to the anterior migration of the mandibular dentition. Likewise, for every 3 mm of sagittal correction, 1 mm of maxillary molar and mandibular incisor intrusion was measured. Also, as expected, in the subset of the dolichofacial patients neither the mandibular plane angle nor anterior face height increased during sagittal correction.

An examination of the occlusal vector (see Fig. 12.5) would increase the clinician's awareness of the potential for the afore-mentioned sagittal correction along with maxillary molar expansion and mesiobuccal rotation and mandibular anterior constriction. This is readily observed in practice. Therefore, if some maxillary constriction along with mesiobuccal rotation is present initially, the Eureka Spring will aid in this correction. However, if the buccal maxillary molar relationship is acceptable, either the maxillary arch must be constricted or a transpalatal arch placed. Clinical experience has shown that a 0.41 × 0.56 constricted maxillary archwire with 15° of buccal root torque has insufficient resistance to counter the expansive force of the light Eureka Spring.

When bilateral Eureka Springs are used, the expected constriction in the mandibular arch is not observed. However, if a unilateral Class II Eureka Spring is placed, visible skewing of the arch, lingual on the treatment side and buccal on the contralateral side, is observed frequently with small rectangular archwires (0.41 × 0.56).

From the frontal view (see Fig. 12.5) one can recognize the impacts of the Eureka Spring in the three dimensions. Maxillary molar expansion caused by buccal crown torque, mandibular anterior constriction resulting from lingual crown torque, and varying degrees of intrusion depending on the vector direction are apparent.

Focusing on the three moments acting on the maxillary molars (see Fig. 12.5) reveals the increased adverse effects of Eureka Spring therapy on these teeth. These undesirable effects can be clinically negated by using a transpalatal bar and archwire engagement into the second molars. This should always be considered if more than

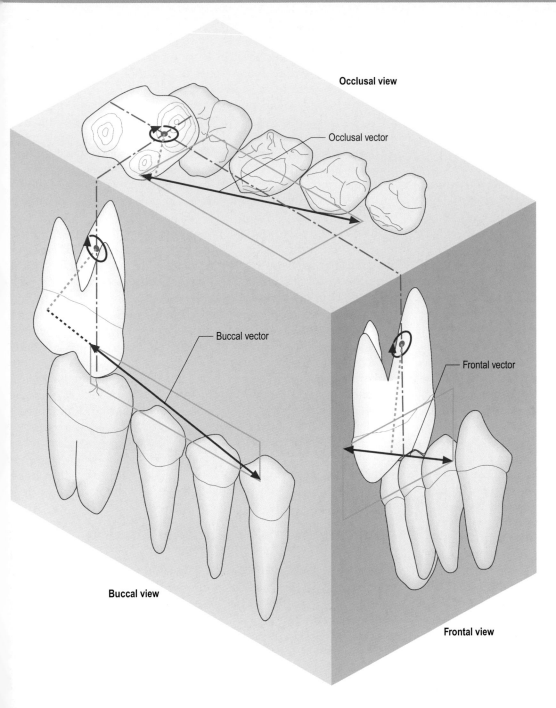

Occlusal view

Occlusal vector

Buccal vector

Buccal view

Frontal vector

Frontal view

Figure 12.5 Three-dimensional model of the forces acting on the dentition, with primary emphasis on the molar. The centerline (alternating long and short dashes) connects the approximate center of resistance (blue spot) of the molar in each view. The short dashed blue line going through the center of resistance is used to demonstrate the produced moment, which is represented as the red circular arrow around each center of resistance. The components of the vectors in each view are shown by the green rectangles.

2.5–3 mm of sagittal correction is needed. In other words, if active Eureka Spring treatment is expected to extend past 3–4 months (rate of sagittal correction is about 0.7 mm per month at 150 g of force and 0.85 mm at 225 g),[15] the treatment plan should include a transpalatal arch and incorporation of second molars.

Some clinicians use a 0.35 ligature wire engaging the first or second molar and functioning as both a tieback and tiedown of the push rod, as shown in Figures 12.1 and 12.3. Others prefer a short piece of power chain attached mesially on the cuspid and distally at a bicuspid or molar, whereas some attach the power chain directly to

the archwire mesial of the push rod, going occlusally over the push rod and then attaching to a bicuspid or molar.

Insertion, Routine Management, and Patient Motivation

The Eureka Spring should not be placed on a round wire in the mandibular arch. The smallest mandibular rectangular wire should be 0.41 × 0.56. In the maxillary arch, rectangular wires are generally preferred but if a transpalatal bar is used and maxillary second molars engaged, no anterior archwire or bonding is required, although interarch anchorage manipulation then becomes limited.

The most important step in insertion of a Eureka Spring is to obtain 2 mm of free distance between the push rod (D, Fig. 12.1) and the anterior edge of the molar attachment tube (B, Fig. 12.1). Other important insertion aspects include stabilizing the push rod (C, Fig. 12.1) in the Classic models, to prevent its rotating occlusally. The attachment wire can be adjusted either at insertion or during treatment to influence the magnitude of the vertical component of the Class II vector (see Fig. 12.4). Generally a more horizontal vector, i.e. as parallel to the occlusal plane as possible, is preferred (C, Fig. 12.4) but in severe overbite caused by extrusion of mandibular anterior teeth, a more vertical vector (A, Fig. 12.4) may be utilized.

Depending on the angulation of the molar attachment or the arch form (more tapered than ovoid), more offset of the molar tube than provided by the manufacturer's initial bend of the attachment wire may be required. Occasionally this offset must be increased to prevent occlusal interference with the attachment on the mandibular first molars. This is discussed in the instruction manual or can be viewed on the web page: www.eurekaortho.com

Other important steps include securing the mesial aspect of the attachment wire to the hook on the molar band and maintaining at least 2 mm of free distance in the attachment wire (F, Fig. 12.1). Complete instructions accompany the product and can be viewed on the web page.

After insertion, the most important management practice is the evaluation of the push rod on each subsequent appointment to assure that the remaining force of the internal spring is adequate. The greatest weakness of the Eureka Spring is premature breakage of the internal spring, and hence reduced force. This will not be apparent to the patient or on casual clinical evaluation. The tension should be checked and if the remaining force is deemed inadequate, the spring module should be replaced. Frequently there is sufficient force remaining to complete the Class II correction even if the spring within the spring module (A, Fig. 12.1) has broken.

If using Class I forces in combination with Eureka Spring, as occurs often in extraction cases, alterations in these two force systems during treatment should be considered so that pretreatment goals can be obtained. One or two progress cephalograms may be valuable to aid in these adjustments.

Tissue irritations are infrequent at the corners of the mouth but are more common in the buccal corridor distal to the maxillary molar. Often this is on one side only and corresponds to the patient sleeping on the irritated side. To help alleviate this problem, the molar attachment tube can be positioned more horizontally or the patient can be instructed to press against this tube occlusopalatally and in so doing bend the attachment wire.

In some patients with mouth opening wider than 55 mm, the spring module can occasionally become disengaged from the molar attachment tube. Instructions at insertion include how to reinsert these parts.

It is not uncommon to schedule appointment intervals of 2 months when Eureka Spring therapy is in progress. More frequent appointments permit the clinician to make archwire adjustment bends with the goal that within 3–5 months of cessation of Eureka Spring therapy, active treatment should be completed.

As the Class II correction occurs and the free distance increases, the force from the Eureka Spring will diminish. To decrease the free distance to its initial 2 mm, the clinician may pull the attachment wire mesially and rebend, distalize the anterior contact on the mandibular archwire, or crimp the molar attachment tube with a ligature cutter just mesial of the inserted ball. (The mouth must be opened wide during this crimping to avoid also crimping the sliding spring module.)

A final comment on patient motivation may be helpful. In my practice the Eureka Spring is frequently viewed as an alternative to interarch elastics, with the added benefit of no extrusive vertical component. For the average patient Class II elastics and/or neck gear are prescribed for one appointment. If wear is inadequate, the patient is given the choice of Eureka Spring or another try at elastics and/or neck gear. On the subsequent appointment, if wear is still inadequate, Eureka Springs are inserted or two or more bicuspids are removed. Later, should the patient wish to try elastics again, the opportunity is given. Because of its small size, appealing esthetics, speed of treatment, and elimination of the need for constant replacement of Class II elastics, the Eureka Spring alternative is initially selected by about half of patients.

In the dolichocephalic patient with initial gingival display on smiling, the Eureka Spring is always prescribed at the onset. Likewise, in the brachycephalic patients, Class II elastics are the treatment of choice and Eureka Springs offered only as a later alternative.

Applications and Treatment Planning

Once the clinician has become comfortable with the insertion and management of the Eureka Spring appliance and office protocol utilizing this versatile tool has become routine, thoughts regarding actual treatment planning will naturally follow and information on this can be found in previous[18] or upcoming publications.[19]

In the nonextraction Class II patient, leveling and aligning are first accomplished. This should include engagement of the maxillary second molars if possible and the placement of a transpalatal arch. The Eureka Spring should not be inserted until rectangular wires of at least 0.41 × 0.56 are in place. Appropriate sizes and torques, to accomplish desired anchorage and obtain necessary anterior root angulations, are made at this time.

If much maxillary arch retraction is desired, a headgear or cervical gear can be worn 10 hours per day. This combination of intermittent heavy extraoral force coupled with continuous light intraoral Eureka Spring force routinely corrects full Class II malocclusions into Class I dental relationships in less than 6 months. To accomplish this, either two sufficiently large tubes or modified bending of the attachment wire, as shown in Figure 12.6, is required if a single large

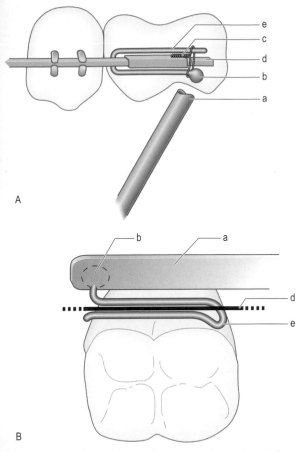

Figure 12.6 Configuring the attachment wire when only a single rectangular tube is present on the molar. **A)** Buccal view: a) molar attachment tube partially cut away, b) ball at end of attachment wire which fits into molar attachment tube, c) ligature wire encircling d) archwire and e) attachment wire. **B)** Occlusal view with molar tube cut away.

molar tube exists. If only a small molar tube is present, a Eureka Spring can still be used by making the attachment wire into a similar configuration, but then no extraoral force can be applied.

Figures 12.7–12.12 shows the initial severe Class II malocclusion (Figs 12.7 and 12.8) and rapid correction in 4 months (Fig. 12.9) using the combination of light Eureka Spring continuous force coupled with 10 hours per day intermittent cervical extraoral force. An additional 2.5 months of treatment resulted in obvious overcorrection (Fig. 12.10), while significant relapse occurred in the ensuing 4 months (Figs 12.11 and 12.12) during which no Class II elastics or extra anchorage were used.

The use of the Eureka Spring appliance in Class II nonextraction treatment will result in anterior movement of the mandibular incisors and posterior movement of the maxillary incisors, the extent of which can be somewhat modified by archwire selection and torque but never completely avoided unless coupled with titanium bony anchors. These anchors can prevent dental movement in whichever arch they are placed.

An example is shown in Figure 12.13 where the second molar, soldered onto the transpalatal bar from the first molar, is attached to an anchor to prevent the maxillary dentition from migrating distally while a Class II Eureka Spring and class I interarch force protract the mandibular dentition and mesialize the first molar into a Class III relationship because of a congenitally missing second bicuspid.

The Eureka Spring is particularly suited to correction of a unilateral Class II. This treatment can be initiated when rectangular archwires are placed but more rapid correction and overall reduced treatment time can occur if the unilateral condition is first corrected.

The patient shown in Figures 12.14–12.17 had only selected teeth bonded initially, and the maxillary anterior teeth were bonded

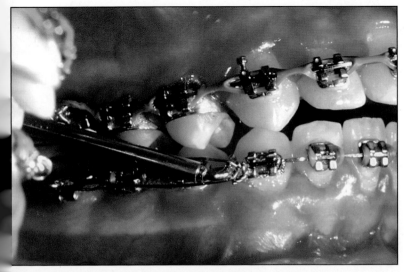

Figure 12.7 Eureka Spring and neck gear. After leveling and aligning.

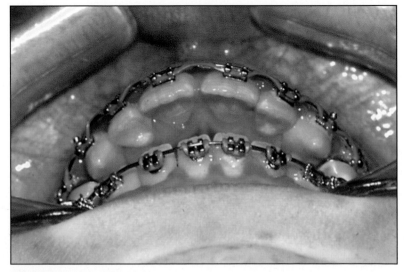

Figure 12.8 Insertion of Eureka Springs.

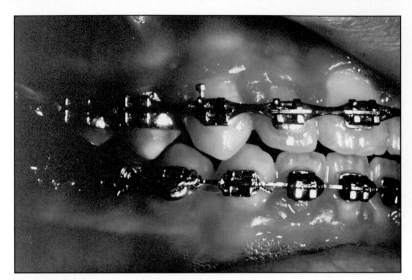

Figure 12.9 Four months later at correction of Class II.

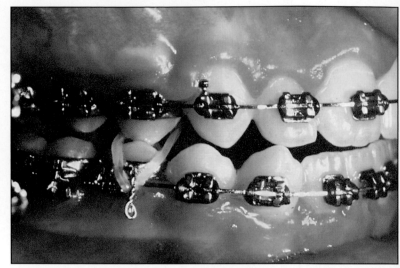

Figure 12.10 Two and a half months' additional treatment to overcorrect.

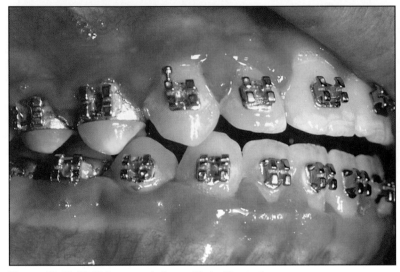

Figures 12.11, 12.12 Four months later, with significant relapse.

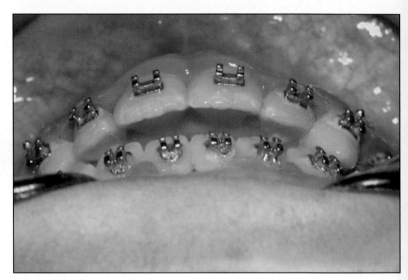

Figure 12.12

Figure 12.13 Partial Class II cuspid relation and congenitally missing second bicuspid. Class II interarch Eureka Spring and Class I intraarch force to move molar mesially. Bony anchor connected to maxillary second molar to prevent maxillary molar distalization.

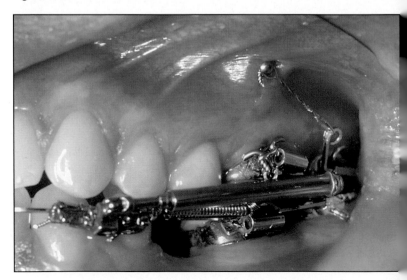

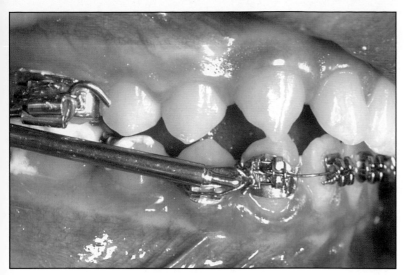

Figure 12.14 Rapid unilateral correction of Class II with minimal initial bonding. Delivery of Eureka Spring.

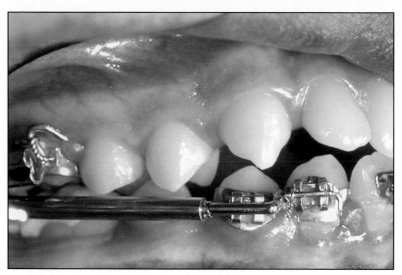

Figure 12.15 Three and a half months later, with increased free distance.

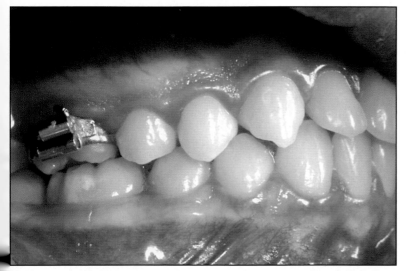

Figures 12.16, 12.17 At completion 8 months later. Total treatment time 12 months.

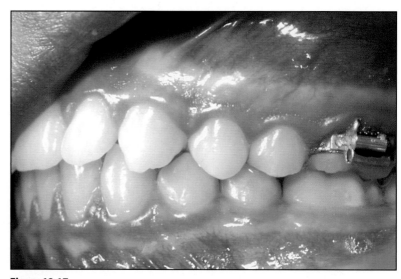

Figure 12.17

for only the last 8 months of treatment. Soldering the maxillary first and second molars together without a transpalatal arch distalizes the center of resistance while providing sufficient anchorage to counteract most of the predicted intrusion and moments that would be expected. Without the resistance to posterior movement afforded by the transpalatal arch, the molar relationship is corrected rapidly. Utilizing a cuspid-to-cuspid fixed lingual bar in the mandible helps maintain intercanine width while encouraging mesial migration on the affected side.

The patient illustrated in Figures 12.18–12.21 presents a more conventional, full-bonded treatment in conjunction with a unilateral Class II Eureka Spring. Although the end results in both patients represented by Figures 12.14–12.17 and 12.18–12.21 are similar,

the total treatment times and side effects of extended Eureka Spring wear are obvious differences.

Often patients begin treatment with an acceptable degree of cooperation but then it diminishes and treatment time extends. The patient presented in Figures 12.22 and 12.23 started with a cervical extraoral force with an additional Class II elastic on the left, and treatment progressed well for 10 months. Then cooperation vanished. Six weeks later, after a firm conversation and no improvement, the patient elected to have a unilateral Eureka Spring in lieu of elastics.

At the time of Eureka Spring placement, 1 year of treatment had elapsed, the crossbite had been corrected by an auxiliary expansion wire, and the cervical gear and Class II elastics had partially corrected

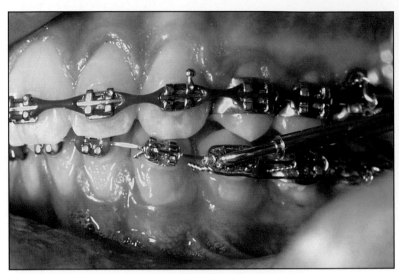

Figure 12.18 Conventional unilateral correction of Class II with initial complete bonding. Delivery of Eureka Springs preceded by 4 months of leveling.

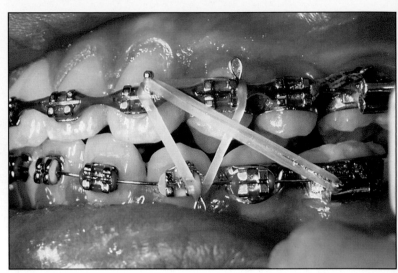

Figure 12.19 At removal of Eureka Springs 10 months later. Note generalized open bite in posterior region.

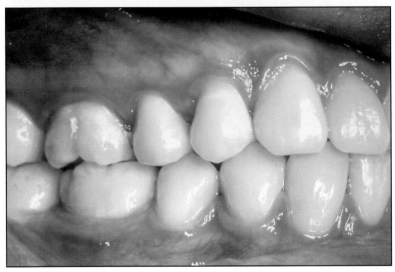

Figures 12.20, 12.21 At completion 6 months later. Total treatment time 20 months.

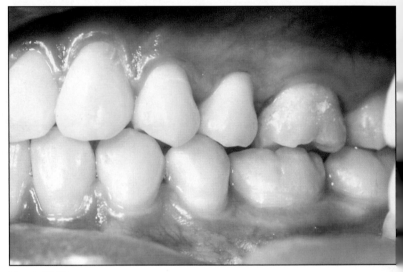

Figure 12.21

the initial Class II condition (Fig. 12.24). After 4 months the Eureka Spring was removed (Fig. 12.25), and active treatment completed 3 months later (Figs 12.26 and 12.27).

Eureka Springs are used frequently in bicuspid extraction cases and, depending on the anchorage preparation and teeth extracted, pretreatment anterior tooth positions generally can be obtained. The patient shown in Figures 12.28–12.33 had four first bicuspids extracted. After 10 months of treatment, during which leveling, aligning and space closure were accomplished, Eureka Springs were placed (Figs 12.28 and 12.29) for 3 months (Figs 12.30 and 12.31), followed by 4 months of detailing and light Class II elastic wear at night and then the appliance was removed (Figs 12.32 and 12.33).

At the time Eureka Springs were placed, the patient was given the choice of Class II elastics or Eureka Springs. During treatment the mandibular plane angle remained unchanged, the lower incisor to mandibular plane decreased from 105.5° to 93°, and the lower incisor to the A-Po line decreased 2 mm to +3. The maxillary incisor to SN decreased from 117° to 105°.

The patient in Figures 12.34–12.39 had extraction of maxillary first and mandibular second bicuspids. A severe dolichofacial pattern existed with the SN-MP angle at 46°. After 11 months of treatment during which only intraarch forces were used to close extraction sites, the occlusion was as shown in Figures 12.34 and 12.35. At this time Eureka Springs were placed for 3 months (Figs 12.36 and 12.37)

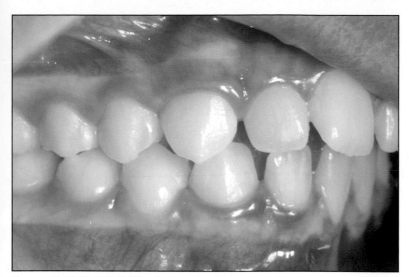

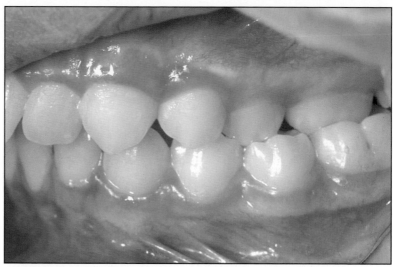

Figures 12.22, 12.23 Initial Class II.

Figure 12.23

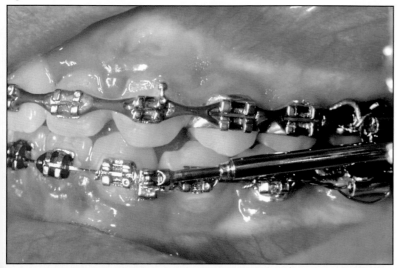

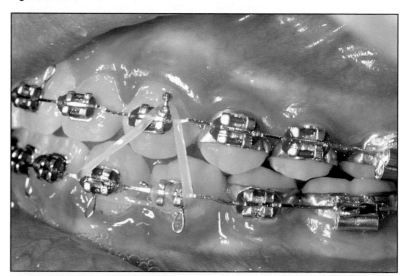

Figure 12.24 After 1 year of treatment with no improvement at last appointment. Class II Eureka Springs placed.

Figure 12.25 After 4 months of Eureka Spring treatment.

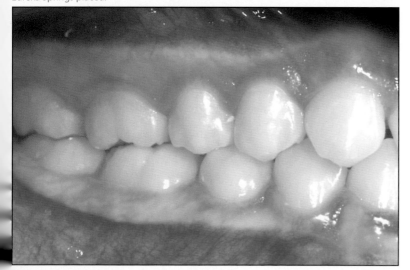

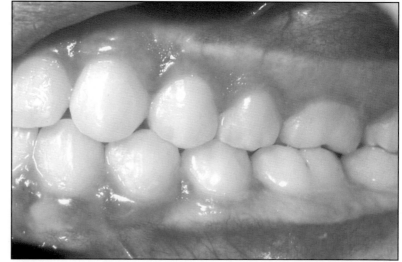

Figures 12.26, 12.27 Treatment completed 3 months later. Total treatment time 19 months.

Figure 12.27

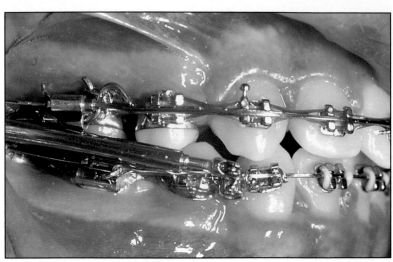
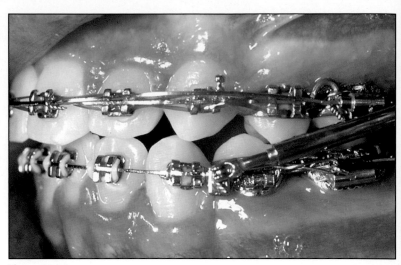

Figures 12.28, 12.29 Four first bicuspid extraction case. At insertion of Class II Eureka Springs.

Figure 12.29

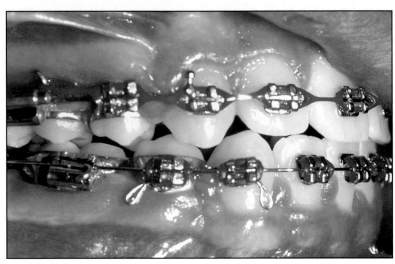
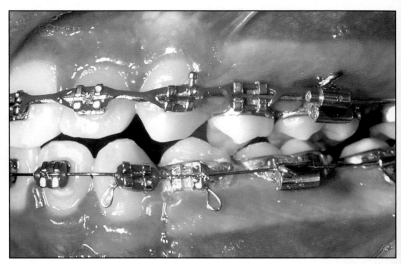

Figures 12.30, 12.31 After 3 months of Eureka Spring treatment.

Figure 12.31

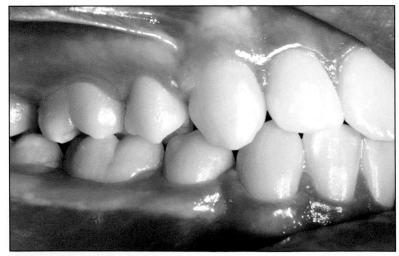
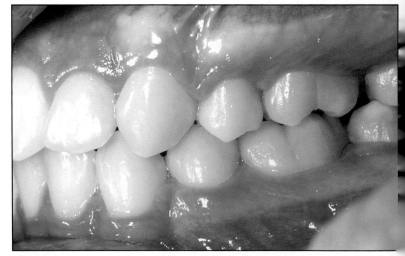

Figures 12.32, 12.33 At appliance removal 4 months later.

Figure 12.33

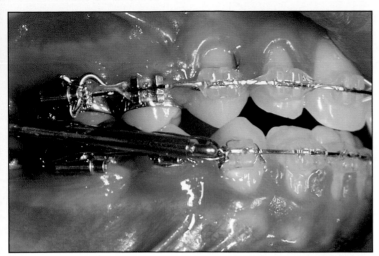

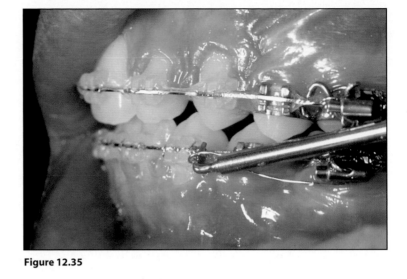

Figures 12.34, 12.35 Extraction of maxillary first and mandibular second bicuspids in a severe dolichofacial pattern. After 11 months of intraarch force and at placement of Eureka Springs.

Figure 12.35

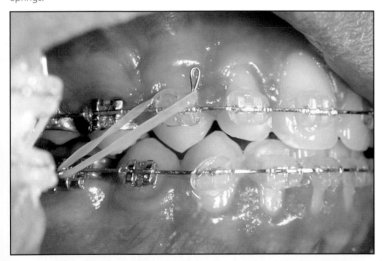

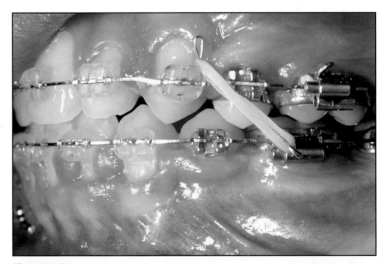

Figures 12.36, 12.37 At removal of Eureka Springs 3 months later, followed by 3 months of Class II elastics.

Figure 12.37

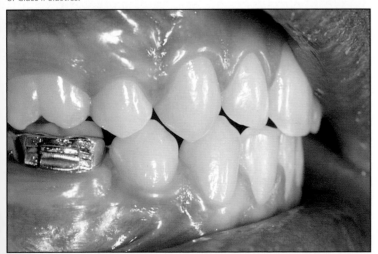

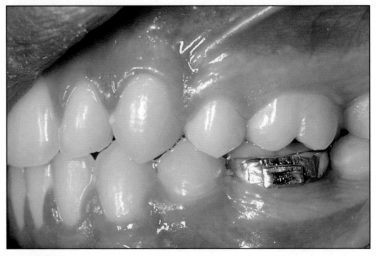

Figures 12.38, 12.39 At appliance removal 3 months after completion of Eureka Spring treatment. Note fixed mandibular 6 × 6 retainer.

Figure 12.39

followed by light Class II elastics till appliance removal 3 months later (Figs 12.38 and 12.39). During treatment the lower incisor to mandibular plane decreased from 92.5° to 87.5° and the lower incisor to the A-Po line went from +3 mm to +2 mm. The maxillary incisor to SN decreased from 98.5° to 94° and the mandibular plane angle remained unchanged. Eureka Springs work very well in high angle cases and do not increase anterior face height in this facial type.[15]

Figures 12.40–12.45 are selected photographs of a patient in whom all second bicuspids were extracted and inadequate Class II elastic wear occurred for two consecutive appointments (Figs 12.40 and 12.41). The patient was then given the choice of continuing treatment for 2 more years, based on the past rate of correction, or 1 more year using the Eureka Spring, and chose the latter. Five months later (Figs 12.42 and 12.43) the springs were removed and detailing and finishing continued with cooperative wear of Class II elastics, in part because of the understanding that Eureka Springs would be placed again if needed. Active treatment was completed (Figs 12.44 and 12.45). Cephalometric measurements revealed an unchanged mandibular plane angle while the lower incisor to mandibular plane increased from 88.5° to 94.5°, the lower incisor to A-Po line from 0.5 to 1 mm, and the upper incisor to SN line from 102° to 104.5°.

Frequently during the course of orthodontic treatment the need for Class II elastics becomes obvious. At that moment what options exist for the clinician? We usually think of only cooperation with Class II elastics and/or extraoral force. It is hoped that the three patients discussed above illustrate that a third option exists: utilizing the Eureka Spring.

Giving the patient ample time, one or two appointments, in which to demonstrate a level of cooperation prior to Eureka Spring placement has been a good practice management policy. Patient realization that Eureka Springs could always be replaced if subsequent cooperation wanes has also been a valuable motivational tool.

The value of differential force magnitudes depending on the extent of necessary correction is illustrated in Figures 12.46–12.49. Considerably more Class II correction was needed on the right side (Fig. 12.46) and therefore a heavy Eureka Spring was placed, while on the left side a light Eureka Spring was inserted (Fig. 12.47). After 4.5 months the right Eureka Spring was removed (Fig. 12.48) and an up-and-down elastic placed while the lighter left-side Eureka Spring remained for one more appointment. With the Quick-Connect model the spring module (A, Fig. 12.1) can be easily changed to heavy or light force.

The increased intrusive component of the heavy Eureka Spring (see Fig. 12.48) is clearly expressed. Note the increased open bite as compared to the light and slow action of the left Eureka Spring. This increased intrusion is apparent in both the maxillary posterior and mandibular anterior regions. Imagine the extent of this intrusion had the vector angle, as measured from the occlusal plane, been increased because of insertion at the mesial of the maxillary first molar.

Additional discussion of Eureka Springs in noncompliant patients can be found in Chapter 17 of *Orthodontics: current*

principles and techniques, 3rd edition, edited by Graber and Vanarsdall,[18] and in their upcoming 4th edition as well. A chapter in Graber and Rakosi's soon-to-be-published work, *Color atlas on orthodontic treatment*, contains much detailed information and many clinical examples of treatment planning with the Eureka Spring.[19]

Completion of Orthodontic Treatment Following Eureka Spring Therapy

As the desired sagittal correction approaches, the clinician may want to lessen the force. Often this occurs naturally as the distance between the mandibular anterior and maxillary posterior teeth increases. At times the internal breakage of the spring lessens the force sufficiently.

The clinician can lessen the force to about 100 g by increasing the free distance distal of the molar tube (F, Fig. 12.1) or by permitting the anterior attachment to touch the distal of the mandibular cuspid.

The clinician may also elect to maintain full force until all sagittal correction has been obtained and then either lessen the Eureka Spring force to 100 g and hold for 2–3 months or remove the Eureka Spring.

Upon Eureka Spring removal, Class II and/or up-and-down elastics should be prescribed and maintained through completion of orthodontic treatment. Even in initially noncompliant patients, compliance is surprisingly good during this time because the patient is informed that noncompliance will result in resumption of Eureka Spring therapy and that completion of active treatment is expected within 4 months of removal of Eureka Springs.

The more rapid the Class II treatment, the more important becomes the management of the potential subsequent relapse. Bone changes occur faster than soft tissue adaptation[20] and clinicians would do well to read the excellent review of relapse by Thilander.[21] It is my clinical experience that the more rapid and extensive the correction, the more pronounced will be the ensuing relapse. This is clearly illustrated by the dramatic relapse depicted in Figures 12.11 and 12.12 which should be a reminder to all in clinical orthodontics that, in varying degrees, Class II relapse will come back to haunt us.

In an evaluation of more than 100 patients utilizing Eureka Spring therapy, about 25% experienced subsequent relapse of at least 2 mm.[22] The direction of the relapse closely mimicked the direction of previous correction. That is, if in a particular patient most of the correction occurred by maxillary tooth distalization, most of the subsequent relapse also occurred there. If correction was equally distributed in both arches, so was the subsequent relapse.

The heavy Eureka Spring produces more rapid correction than the light Eureka Spring (see Figs 12.46–12.49).[23] However, the extended treatment required after heavy Eureka Spring removal to maintain the Class I position and correct the often accompanying adverse movement of buccal root torque and/or intrusion frequently results in similar completion times.

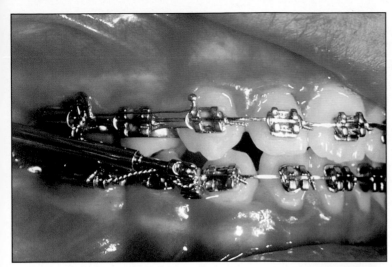

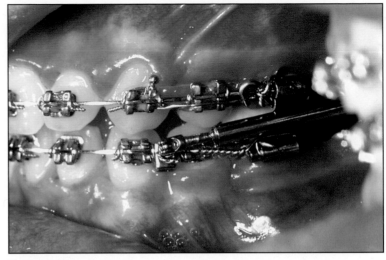

Figures 12.40, 12.41 An uncooperative patient, with extraction of all second bicuspids. After 12 months of treatment and two appointments of inadequate Class II elastic wear.

Figure 12.41

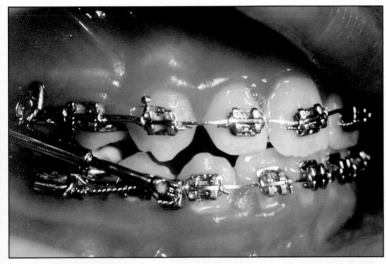

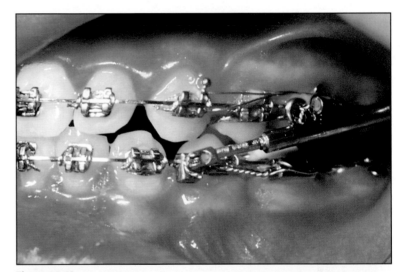

Figures 12.42, 12.43 After 5 months of Eureka Spring wear.

Figure 12.43

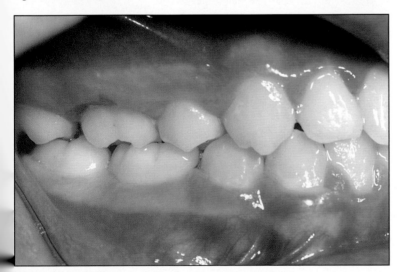

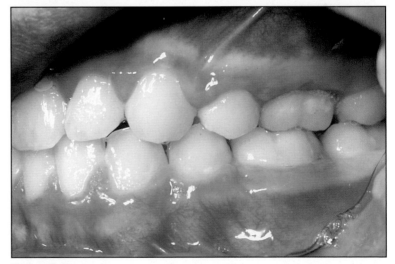

Figures 12.44, 12.45 After appliance removal 4^1/$_2$ months later.

Figure 12.45

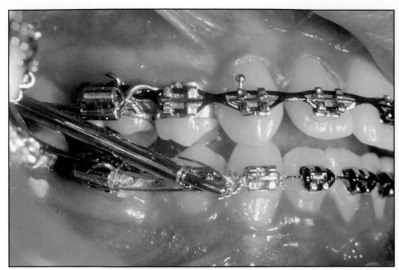

Figure 12.46 Heavy forces utilized to correct varying degrees of Class II condition.

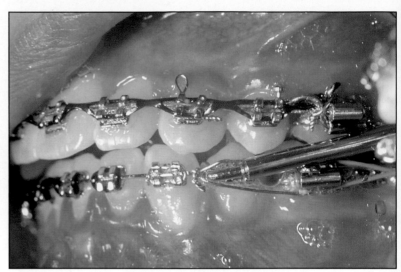

Figure 12.47 Light forces utilized to correct varying degrees of Class II condition.

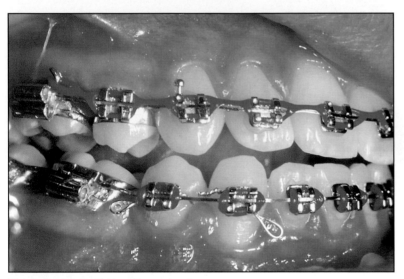

Figures 12.48, 12.49 After 4^1/$_2$ months of treatment.

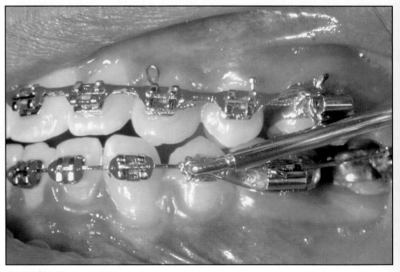

Figure 12.49

Overcorrection of the initial Class II condition, as illustrated in Figures 12.7–12.12, has not proven to be an attractive option and is no longer recommended. A more detailed discussion of relapse and remedial treatment can be found in DeVincenzo.[19] Rather, a slowing of the rate of treatment as the end approaches, a diminishing of the force as suggested previously or light continuous or intermittent Class II elastics wear during the final detailing and finishing stage of active treatment is preferred.

Conclusion

The Eureka Spring can be a valuable auxiliary in the correction of Class II sagittal conditions. Its compact size permits it to be used in most patients. Its versatility for use in both the Class II and Class III modes when coupled with Class I force extends the treatment planning options available for Class II corrections. When coupled with titanium bony anchors, very selective movement can be obtained and by altering the direction of the vector, more or less intrusion can accompany the sagittal correction. Light and heavy spring modules are available along with three archwire attachment mechanisms, providing the clinician with a great variety of interchangeable options either in treatment planning or as may arise during the active phase.

I have found the Eureka Spring to be a compact, versatile, and cost-effective Class II dentoalveolar corrector for noncompliant patients and it is a mainstay of my practice.

References

1. Teach SJ, Lillis KA, Grossi M. Compliance with penicillin prophylaxis in patients with sickle cell disease. Arch Pediatr Adolesc Med 1998;152: 274–278.

2. Blowey DL, Hebert D, Arbus GS, Pool R, Korus M, Koren G. Compliance with cyclosporine in adolescent renal transplant recipients. Pediatr Nephrol 1997;11:547–551.

3. Ettenger RB, Rosenthal JT, Marik JL, et al. Improved cadaveric renal transplant outcome in children. Pediatr Nephrol 1991;5:137–142.

4. Festa RS, Tamaroff MH, Chasalow F, Lanzkowsky P. Therapeutic adherence to oral medication regimens by adolescents with cancer. I. Laboratory assessment. J Pediatr 1992;120:807–811.

5. Tebbi CK. Treatment compliance in childhood and adolescence. Cancer 1993;71(10 Suppl): 3441–3449.

6. Jacobson AM, Hauser ST, Lavori P, et al. Adherence among children and adolescents with insulin-dependent diabetes mellitus over a four-year longitudinal follow-up: I. The influence of patient coping and adjustment. J Pediatr Psychol 1990; 15:511–526.

7. Thomas AM, Peterson L, Goldstein D. Problem solving and diabetes regimen adherence by children and adolescents with IDDM in social pressure situations: a reflection of normal development. J Pediatr Psychol 1997;22:541–561.

8. Michaud PA, Frappier JY, Pless IB. Compliance in adolescents with chronic disease. Arch Fr Pediatr 1991;48:329–336.

9. Nanda RS, Kierl MJ. Prediction of cooperation in orthodontic treatment. Am J Orthod Dentofacial Orthop 1992;102:15–21.

10. Scarfone RJ, Joffe MD, Wiley JF 2nd, Loiselle JM, Cook RT. Noncompliance with scheduled revisits to a pediatric emergency department. Arch Pediatr Adolesc Med 1996;150:948–953.

11. Pancherz H, Fackel U. The skeletofacial growth pattern pre- and post-dentofacial orthopedics: a long-term study of class II malocclusions treated with the Herbst appliance. Eur J Orthod 1990; 12:209–218.

12. DeVincenzo JP. Changes in mandibular length before, during, and after successful orthopedic correction of Class II malocclusions, using a functional appliance. Am J Orthod Dentofacial Orthop 1991;99:241–257.

13. Wieslander L. Long-term effect of treatment with the head gear-Herbst appliance in the early mixed dentition: stability or relapse? Am J Orthod Dentofacial Orthop 1993;104:319–329.

14. Pancherz H. The effects, limitations, and long-term dentofacial adaptations to treatment with the Herbst appliance. Semin Orthod 1997;3:232–243.

15. Stromeyer EL, Caruso JM, DeVincenzo JP. A cephalometric study of the class II correction effects of the Eureka spring. Angle Orthod 2002; 72:203–210.

16. DeVincenzo JP. The Eureka spring: a new inter-arch force delivery system. J Clin Orthod 1997; 31:454–467.

17. Gunduz E. Skeletal and dentoalveolar responses to light and heavy inter-arch forces delivered by Eureka springs. Masters thesis. Vienna: Medical University of Vienna; 2004.

18. DeVincenzo JP. Treatment options for sagittal corrections in noncompliant patients. In: Graber TM, Vanarsdall RL Jr, eds. Orthodontics: current principles and techniques, 3rd edn. St Louis: Mosby; 2000: 779–800.

19. DeVincenzo JP. Inter-arch compression springs in orthodontics. In: Graber TM, Rakosi T, eds. Color atlas on orthodontic treatment. Stuttgart: Thieme Medical Publishers; 2005 (in press).

20. Reitan K. Principles of retention and avoidance of post-treatment relapse. Am J Orthod 1969;55: 776–790.

21. Thilander B. Biological basis for orthodontic relapse. Semin Orthod 2000;6:195–205.

22. DeVincenzo JP, Smith KD. Analysis of relapse following rapid class II correction with Eureka springs. Eur J Orthod 2001;23:449.

23. Braga GC, Machado GB. Eureka spring for finishing correction of class II and improving anchorage. R Dental Press Orthodon Orthop Facial 2001;6:51–60.

CHAPTER 13

The Twin Force Bite Corrector in the correction of Class II malocclusion in adolescent patients

Flavio Uribe, Jeff Rothenberg, Ravindra Nanda

Introduction

The extraction/nonextraction debate has been a subject of controversy since the early days of modern orthodontics. The balance between these two treatments has moved from one side to the other throughout the years. Currently it seems that the balance has shifted to the nonextraction side.[1,2]

This debate is simplistic since neither of these two therapies clearly defines an outcome. Hence, the goal in orthodontics is objective-based therapy.[3] Therapies such as distalization of maxillary molars, extraction, growth modification, surgery, etc. will only make sense if substantiated by clearly defined objectives. None of the aforementioned therapies defines specifically the final skeletofacial, soft tissue, incisor or molar position in the three planes of space.[4] If these specific objectives are determined, the decision between treatment modalities will be easier. Moreover, the appliance that more closely meets the desired objectives can then be selected based on the evidence available in the literature.[5]

Therefore understanding the biomechanics allows the clinician to decide whether the appliance selected for the correction of the orthodontic problem complies with the predetermined objectives of treatment. Thus, the effects of the appliance will not only be measured in the anteroposterior direction, i.e. occlusal Class II correction, but also in relation to the skeletofacial, vertical, transverse, etc. objectives.

Correction of a Class II malocclusion can be accomplished by modifying the skeletal or dental components or both. The great majority of young patients with this malocclusion are corrected by the normal differential maxillomandibular growth and a combination of treatment effects in the dentition and facial complex. However, it is only through surgery that a pure skeletal effect can be obtained. And even when this mode of treatment is selected, dental presurgical movements are still required.[6] Orthopedic movement in a growing patient also attempts to achieve a pure skeletal change. However, most of these appliances at best obtain a 50% skeletal effect in the short term.[7]

The appliances for Class II correction can be divided into two broad categories: intraarch and interarch. In the intraarch category, only the headgear is tailored to obtain an orthopedic effect. This appliance has fallen into disfavor due to the compliance needed from the patient to achieve a positive result. The other intraarch appliances are aimed at correcting the malocclusion dentally, by distalizing the upper molars through a reciprocal force. The great advantage is that compliance is not an issue as these appliances are usually fixed to the upper arch. However, no orthopedic change is expected.

Interarch mechanics for Class II correction can be divided in fixed and removable appliances. Most of the purely functional appliances by definition are within the removable category. The patient is not actively pushed in a protrusive position but guided to it through function. Some of the most common are the Twin Block, Bionator, Activator, Frankel, etc.[8] On the other hand, some of the most commonly used fixed appliances are the Jasper Jumper™ (American Orthodontics, Sheboygan, WI), the Herbst (Dentaurum Inc., Newtown, PA), the Twin Force Bite Corrector (Ortho Organizers Inc., San Marcos, CA), Eureka Spring™ (Eureka Orthodontics, San Luis Obispo, CA), MARA™ (Allesee Orthodontic Appliances, Sturtevant, WI), etc. These fixed appliances are also known as bite-jumping appliances.

The classic interarch Class II corrector that has been used since the early days of orthodontics is the intermaxillary elastic.[9] The effects of Class II elastic wear are very well documented and can be summarized as predominantly dental. Most of the Class II correction is obtained by a clockwise rotation of the occlusal plane with uprighting of the upper incisors and flaring of the lower incisors.[10] Negligible orthopedic change has been reported with Class II elastics.[11] Additionally, one major disadvantage is the need for patient compliance.

The Jasper Jumper was developed to deal with this very issue of patient compliance and elastic wear. This appliance delivers a constant light force to the upper molar and lower arch via a compressed coil within a plastic housing. Although the rationale is adequate, the major problem encountered with this appliance is the tremendous amount of breakage. In a thesis project, Rankin found a significant amount of breakage.[12] The effects produced by this appliance resembled those of a Class II elastic, i.e. occlusal plane rotation with flaring of lower incisors and retrusion of the upper incisors.[13]

The classic interarch fixed appliance for Class II correction is the Herbst appliance popularized by Pancherz.[14] Its reported effects are a combination of orthopedic and dental.[7] Arguably, it can be considered as the gold standard in terms of most favorable orthopedic and dental effects. Therefore, most published research involving functional appliances in Class II malocclusions compare the findings to the effects produced by this appliance.[15,16]

The Twin Force Bite Corrector (TFBC)[17] was developed from a combination of concepts from the Herbst and Jasper Jumper. The appliance incorporates the Herbst concept by having a constant anterior protrusion of the mandible by means of a plunger system with a fixed distance. Additionally, an active push coil delivers a constant force of approximately 210 g.

Description

The TFBC is a bilateral interarch push-type appliance that is individually tied to the archwires on each side. Each element is made up of two 16 mm telescopic cylinders parallel to each other (Figs 13.1–13.3). Within each cylinder and in opposite ends, a plunger is incorporated. An active nickel titanium coil within the cylinder pushes each plunger outside the cylinder a distance of 15 mm (see Figs 13.1–13.3). At the free end of each plunger, a double-sided housing attachment is secured with a titanium hex bolt to the archwire. The attachment is a free movable ball joint that allows easy intraoral attachment from a coronal or gingival direction.

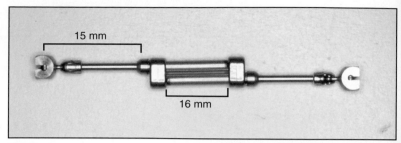

Figure 13.2

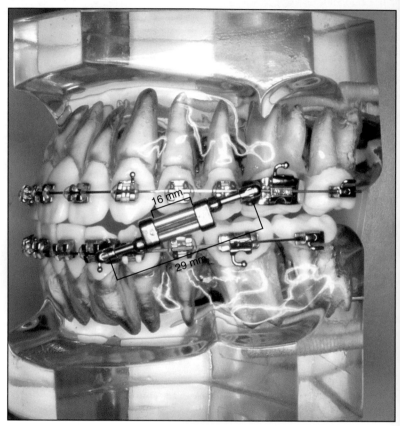

Figure 13.3

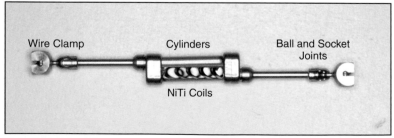

Figures 13.1–13.3 Components and dimensions of the standard Twin Force Bite Corrector. The appliance at full compression should protrude the mandible into an edge-to-edge anterior relationship.

When the plungers are fully compressed within the cylinders, the appliance measures 29 mm from one attachment to the other (see Figs 13.1–13.3). A short version of the appliance that measures 27 mm is also available. This version is indicated in patients with congenitally missing premolars or in patients who underwent extraction of these teeth and a Class II malocclusion still persists.

Mode of Attachment

The TFBC is attached mesial to the first maxillary molar and distal to the lower canine (Figs 13.4 and 13.5). When it is fully compressed, the patient should have the mandible protruded to an edge-to-edge

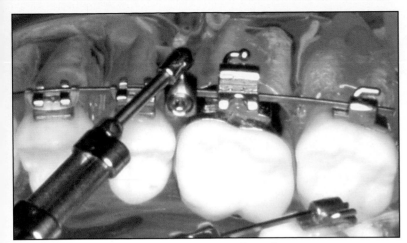

Figure 13.4 Mesial point of attachment to the upper first molars.

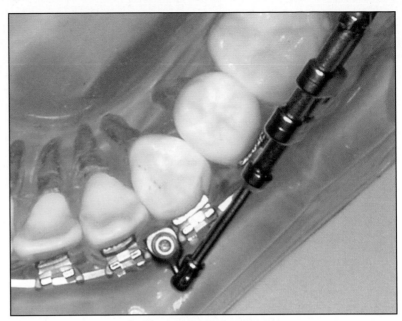

Figure 13.5 Distal point of attachment to the lower canines.

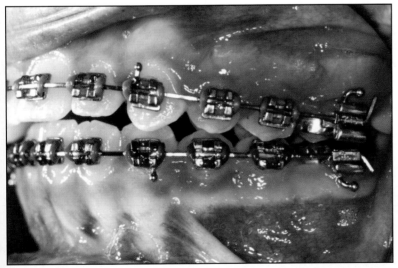

Figure 13.6 Tightly cinched stiff archwires are needed in upper and lower arches before TFBC insertion.

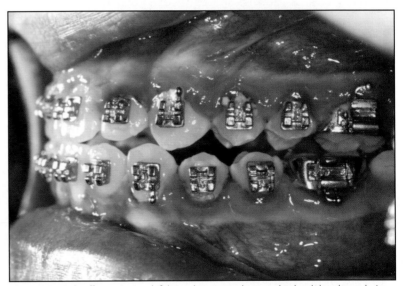

Figure 13.7 Side effect on upper left buccal segment due to palatal arch breakage during active TFBC treatment.

incisor relationship. The push coil within the plunger adds an oscillating force with normal masticatory function. The force of this coil when fully compressed is 210 g.

Setting for the TFBC

The appliance should be delivered with stiff upper and lower archwires. Additionally, due to the expected flaring effect of the lower incisors, a 6° torque lower bracket prescription is recommended. Ideally, the lower archwire should have dimensions of 0.021 × 0.025″ and the upper archwire a minimum of 0.019 ×0.025″. Both archwires

should be in stainless steel and cinched back to prevent space opening (Fig. 13.6). A palatal arch is also inserted to prevent the molars from tipping labially (Fig. 13.7).

Biomechanics

From a lateral view the appliance exerts an equal and opposite force on the maxilla and the mandible. Since the maxilla has a stiff archwire, the entire maxilla is considered as a unit. The center of resistance of the maxillary dentition is close to the apex of the root of the first and second premolars. The mandibular dentition also holds a stiff lower archwire and reacts as a single unit. The center of resistance of the lower denture base is also considered to be located between the first and second bicuspids. It is important to understand the forces and moments that are generated with this appliance.

Force

Point of Force Application

Point of force application is mesial to the upper first molars on the maxilla and distal to the canines in the mandible.

Direction of Force

The direction of the force on the maxillary denture base is posterior and apical. The distal component of the force is larger than the apical component when the patient is in occlusion. The direction of the force in the mandible is anterior and apical. The anterior component is also greater than the apical component when the patient occludes (Fig. 13.8). It should be noted that the patient does not occlude in maximum intercuspation but in a protruded mandibular relationship due to the inherent fixed distance of the superposed cylinders in the appliance.

Magnitude of Force

The appliance generates an oscillating force so it is difficult to quantify its magnitude. When the patient is in occlusion (with an edge-to-edge anterior relationship) the force is muscle driven, dependent on the reciprocal force of the muscles that want to bring the mandible into centric relation. Additionally, the NiTi coils inside the cylinders generate a force of approximately 210 g in this occlusal relationship when fully compressed. During function, the direction and the magnitudes of forces intervening are difficult to determine.

Moments

The forces in relation to the center of resistance of both dentitions produce a clockwise moment on the maxilla and the mandible (Fig. 13.9). Due to the indeterminate nature of the force magnitudes, the magnitudes of the moments are also indeterminate. However, since the point of application of force is known, the direction of the moments can be determined.

The moments generate a clockwise rotation of the occlusal plane responsible for some of the Class II correction. This rotation has some important implications at the level of the incisors in their vertical and anteroposterior component. This clockwise rotation of the occlusal plane has been shown to relapse and will be discussed later in further detail.

Prospective Study to Evaluate Skeletal and Dental Effects of the TFBC

A prospective study to evaluate the short- and long-term effects of the TFBC has been part of two thesis projects at the Department of Orthodontics at the University of Connecticut.

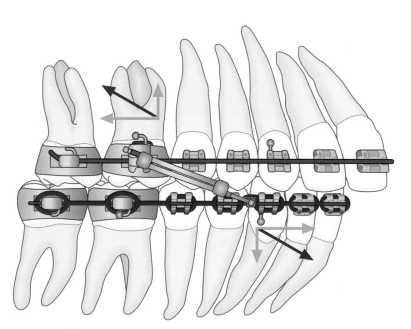

Figure 13.8 Forces generated by the TFBC. Although there is a vertical component to the force, the anteroposterior components are greater.

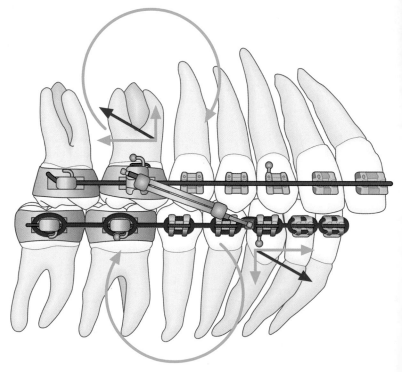

Figure 13.9 Moments on the denture bases generated from the forces with the TFBC.

Twenty patients with a Class II malocclusion, who underwent TFBC therapy for 3 months followed by an additional 4-month period involving seating of the occlusion with intermaxillary elastics, were evaluated at TFBC removal and end of treatment for skeletal and dental changes. The treatment sample was compared with matched controls for skeletal age and gender from the Bolton Growth Study with Class II and Class I malocclusions.

Inclusion Criteria

- Young female or male patients between 11 and 16 years of age
- Full permanent dentition
- Convex skeletal profile due to a retrognathic mandible
- Class II division 1 malocclusion
- Minimum end-on molar relationship
- Four millimeters of overjet after aligning and leveling procedures

Exclusion Criteria

- Missing teeth other than the third molars
- Syndromic condition
- Significant dental or skeletal asymmetry
- Skeletal open bite characteristics
- Clinically or radiographically detectable temporomandibular joint dysfunction
- Previous growth modification therapy
- Excessive proclination of the lower incisors

Based on the selection criteria, 12 males (age range 12.5–16.4) and eight females (age range 12.8–14.1) comprised the sample (Table 13.1).

Alignment and leveling procedures started in every patient with a 0.022 slot Nanda Prescription (Ortho Organizers Inc., San Marcos, CA), including a lower incisor bracket prescription of 6° in torque in order to minimize flaring. Wire progressed up to a 0.019×0.025 stainless steel archwire on the upper arch and a 0.021×0.025 archwire on the lower arch. Both archwires were cinched back to prevent space opening. Additionally, a 0.032 CNA (beta titanium) (Ortho Organizers Inc., San Marcos, CA) transpalatal arch was placed to control upper molar width.

Skeletal age of the patients was assessed after leveling and alignment procedures, through a cervical vertebrae maturation stage (CVMS)

Table 13.1. Age distribution in treated group.

	n	Age (years)	Range
Male	12	13.8	12.5–16.4
Female	8	13.3	12.8–14.1
Total	20	13.5	12.5–16.4

analysis in the lateral cephalogram.[18] This film was the baseline X-ray for the treatment group and was considered as the initial time point (T1). At this time point, models and photographs of the patients were also taken.

Patients at this visit had the TFBC delivered to position the mandible into an incisor edge-to-edge relationship. Patients maintained the fixed appliance for an average 3-month period with monthly evaluation visits. During each of these visits, the appliance was unattached to allow the patient's muscles to relax for a 30-minute period. At this time, the occlusion was evaluated. The majority of the patients exhibited an edge-to-edge incisor relation at the time of appliance removal. The palatal arch was also removed to facilitate settling of the occlusion.

A new set of records were taken that included a lateral cephalometric X-ray, a set of models, and photographs (T2). The upper archwire was maintained and the lower archwire was changed to a 0.017×0.025 SS. The patients were instructed to wear intermaxillary Class II elastics for a 3-month period from upper canine and first premolars to lower first and second premolars. The objective of this elastic was to maintain the Class II correction and allow a proper interdigitation of the posterior occlusion.

Patients were finished with standard finishing procedures with coordinated upper and lower 0.018×0.025 CNA archwires. An upper wrap-around retainer and a lower 0.0175 braided fixed lingual archwire canine to canine were delivered after fixed appliances removal. At the deband visit, a new set of records (T3) was taken. Figures 13.10–13.39 show the treatment progress of one patient from start to finish.

Cephalometric Analysis

Lateral cephalometric X-rays from pre appliance (T1), post appliance (T2), and after deband (T3) time points were hand traced on acetate paper and verified by a second investigator. Any discrepancy between the tracings of both evaluators was reanalyzed and retraced.

Twenty-four landmarks (nine skeletal, eight dental and seven points in the soft tissue) were used to evaluate 20 angular and linear relationships (Figs 13.40 and 13.41). It is important to note that the occlusal plane definition in the treatment group varied slightly from the conventional. The occlusal plane in the treatment group in this study was based on the upper archwire clearly depicted on the lateral cephalogram. The occlusal plane on the control group was determined by a perpendicular line to the longitudinal axes of the buccal segments.

Measurements were made by hand using a protractor and a Boley gauge. Cranial base, maxillary, and mandibular superimpositions were done by hand by both investigators using the best fit method.[19]

Two methods were used to evaluate treatment changes over the different treatment periods (T1–T2, T2–T3, and T1–T3). The first method was a direct angular or linear measurement change between time periods. The second method involved evaluating the vertical and anteroposterior skeletal changes on cranial base superimpositions using a SN-7 horizontal axis. This horizontal axis for the pair of lateral

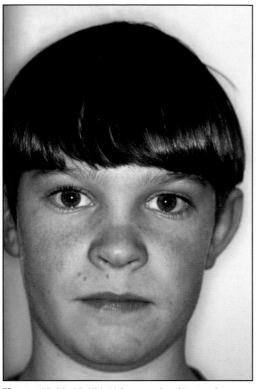

Figures 13.10–13.17 Initial extraoral and intraoral photographs of patient LK.

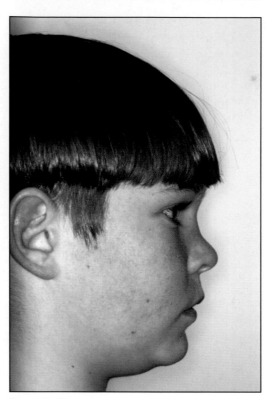

Figure 13.11

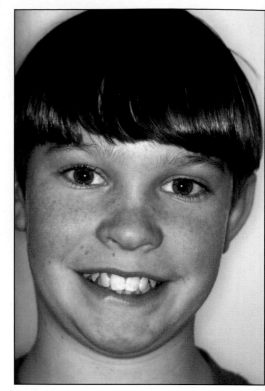

Figure 13.12

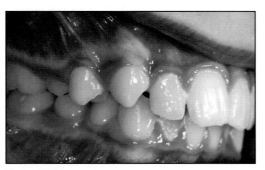

Figure 13.13

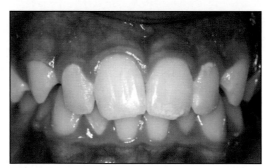

Figure 13.14

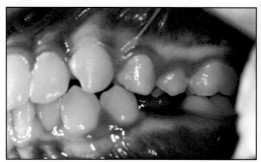

Figure 13.15

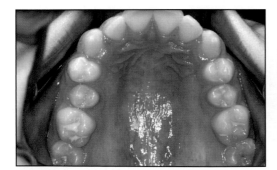

Figure 13.16

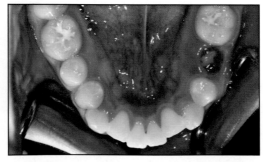

Figure 13.17

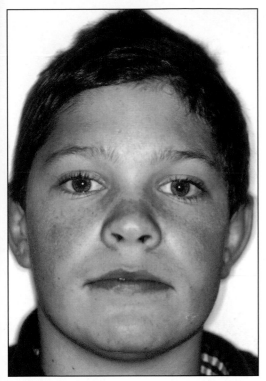

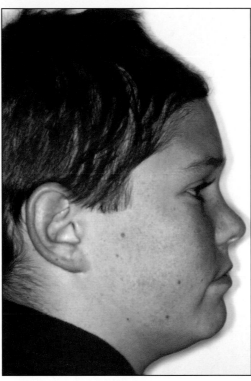

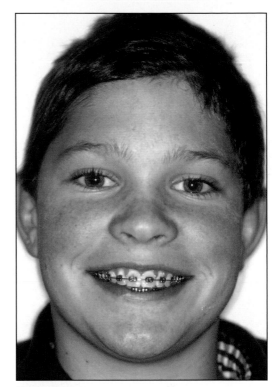

Figures 13.18–13.25 T1 photographs taken before TFBC insertion with leveled and aligned arches.

Figure 13.19

Figure 13.20

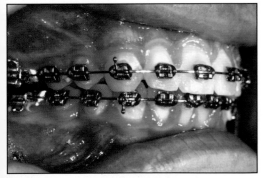

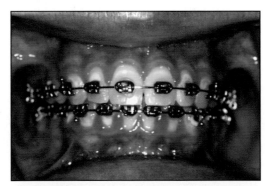

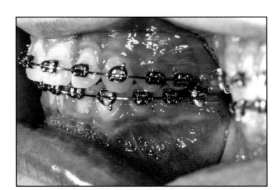

Figure 13.21

Figure 13.22

Figure 13.23

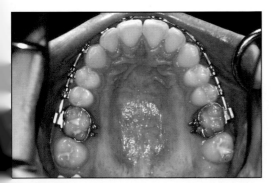

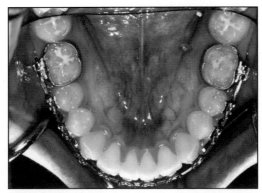

Figure 13.24

Figure 13.25

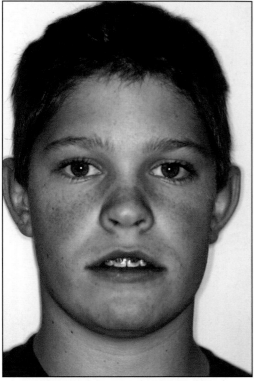
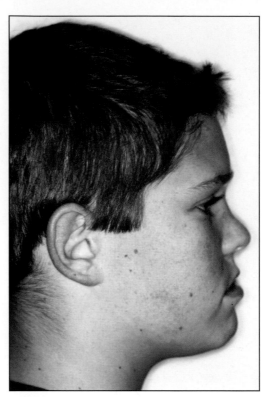
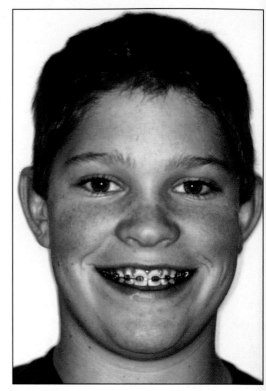

Figures 13.26–13.31 T2 photographs at completion of 3 months' TFBC therapy, prior to removal of the appliance.

Figure 13.27

Figure 13.28

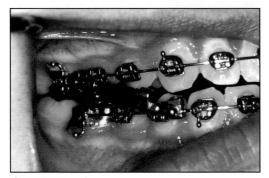
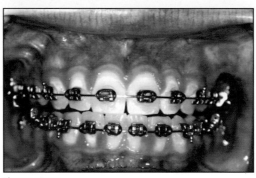
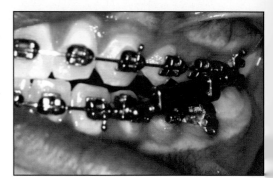

Figure 13.29

Figure 13.30

Figure 13.31

cephalograms was transferred to graph paper and changes measured on the grid. Dental changes were evaluated using a similar method where the occlusal plane was the horizontal line or *x*-axis.[20] Changes in the anterior and inferior direction were deemed as positive values. As aforementioned, changes were compared to the controls in the Bolton Growth Study. The data from this study were normalized for time (3 months) and size (magnification).

Descriptive statistics was used for comparisons between treatment and control group at T1–T2, T2–T3, and T1–T3 changes. An independent samples *t*-test was used to determine significance of the differences at a level of $p<0.05$, $p<0.01$, and $p<0.001$.

Results

T1 (Initial Time Point)

The treatment and control groups had some significant differences at the skeletal (N-A-Pg, A-B/OP, LFH/TFH, UFH), dental (OJ, molar discrepancy, upper incisor inclination, interincisal angle), and soft tissue (LL-SnPg and NL) levels at the initial time point (Table 13.2). These differences are accounted for by Class II division 1 malocclusion in the experimental group compared to a combination of Class I and Class II skeletal patterns in the control group from the Bolton Growth Study.

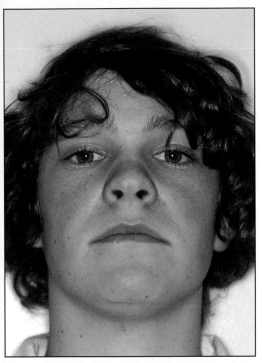

Figures 13.32–13.39 T3 photographs at the removal of fixed appliances.

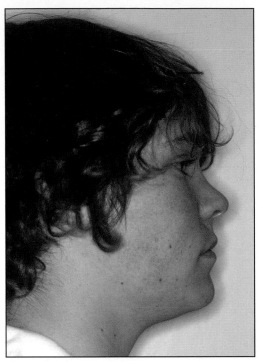

Figure 13.33

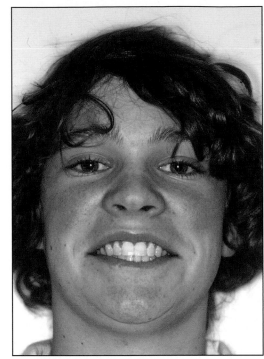

Figure 13.34

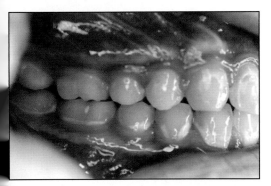

Figure 13.35

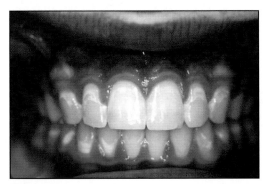

Figure 13.36

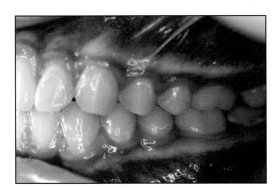

Figure 13.37

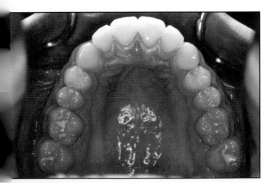

Figure 13.38

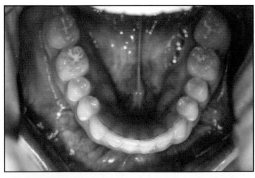

Figure 13.39

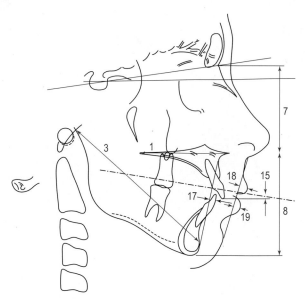
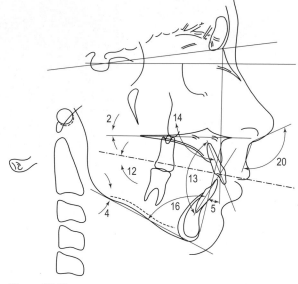

Figures 13.40, 13.41 Independent (T1, T2, T3) cephalometric measures. (See Box 13.1)

Figure 13.41

T1–T2

All 20 subjects in the experimental group had an improvement in the Class II relationship reflected in the overjet, skeletal convexity, and molar discrepancy reduction. Results for this treatment period are summarized in Table 13.3.

Dental Findings

Molars The upper first molar moved distally 0.8 mm at the coronal level and 0.3 mm at the apical level from T1. Mean intrusive movement of the upper molar was 1.1 mm at the coronal and apical level. The control group had a slight opposite anterior and extrusive movement of the molar of 0.2 mm.

The lower molars demonstrated a mesial crown movement of 1.9 mm and a mesial root movement of 0.7 mm. Extrusive movement of the molar was 1.2 mm. The control group had a 0.2 mm anterior movement and a 0.1 mm extrusive movement.

Incisors Upper incisor inclination decreased 7.4° compared to a 0.1° increase for the control group. The nature of the movement was uncontrolled tipping, with 1.8 mm of posterior crown movement and 0.6 mm of anterior root movement.

Lower incisor proclination was evidenced by a mean change of 2.7° and 7.7° for the Mn1-APg and IMPA measurements respectively. No significant difference was noted at the anteroposterior movement at the apical level. The lower incisor intruded 2.5 mm at the coronal level and 1.2 mm at the apical level.

The uprighting of the upper incisor and the proclination of the lower incisors accounted for no difference in the interincisal angle between groups.

Overjet and Molar Discrepancy The mean overjet was reduced 5.6 mm in the treatment group compared to 0.1 mm in the control group. Molar discrepancy was reduced 3.9 mm in the study group compared to no change in the controls.

Dentoalveolar Findings

The occlusal plane showed a clockwise 4.8° rotation compared to a negligible change in the controls. This was a major contributor to the 5 mm A-B/OP in the treated group compared to the controls in whom no change was observed.

Skeletal Findings

Skeletal Convexity The skeletal convexity of the treatment group was reduced 1.7° compared to a 0.3° reduction in the controls.

Size and Position of the Maxilla and Mandible A point moved 0.5 mm posteriorly in the experimental group compared to a 0.1 mm anterior movement for the controls. Vertically, A point moved 1.7 mm inferiorly in the experimental group compared to 0.4 mm in the controls. A 0.5° clockwise rotation of the palatal plane was noticed in the experimental group compared to 0.1° for the control group. B point had a significant vertical change compared to controls (2.6 mm compared to 0.5 mm). The horizontal change in B point was not significant between groups.

Mandibular length (Ar-Pg) increased 2.1 mm in the study group compared to 0.7 mm for the control group. No significant difference was observed in the anteroposterior position of pogonion between groups.

Vertical Dimension No significant difference in mandibular plane angle was noticed between groups, although the mean LFH increased 1.2 mm in the experimental compared to 0.4 mm in the controls.

Box 13.1

Craniofacial Relationship	Measures
Maxillary Skeletal	
1. ANS-PNS (mm)	Anterior-posterior dimension of mandible
2. PP-SN7 (deg)	Angle of palatal plane/nasal floor to constructed Frankfort
Mandibular Skeletal	
3. Ar-Pg (mm)	Effective length of mandible
4. MP-SN7 (deg)	Angle of mandible to constructed Frankfort
5. N-A-Pg (deg)	Facial convexity angle; actually 180° (N-A-Pg)
Maxillo-mandibular	
6. A-B(OP) (mm)	Position of maxillary denture base relative to mandibular denture base along respective (T1, T2, T3) functional occlusal plane reference axes
Vertical	
7. N-ANS y (mm)	Upper facial height, measured along perpendicular to SN7
8. ANS-Me y (mm)	Lower facial height, measured along perpendicular to SN7
9. LFH(100)/TFH (%)	Lower facial height percentage of total facial height
Interdental	
10. OJ (mm)	Overjet – measure of Mx1 incisal edge relative to Mn1 incisal edge along respective (T1, T2, T3) functional occlusal plane reference axes
11. Molar (mm)	Molar relationship – measure of Mx6 mesiobuccal cusp tip relative to Mn6 buccal groove point along respective (T1, T2, T3) functional occlusal plane reference axes
12. FOP-SN7 (deg)	Angle of functional occlusal plane to constructed Frankfort
13. Inter-Inc (deg)	Angle between upper and lower central incisors
Maxillary Dental	
14. Mx1-SN7 (deg)	Angle between upper central incisor and constructed Frankfort
15. Inc-Stm y (mm)	Incisal show – measure from stomion superius to incision along perpendicular to constructed Frankfort
Mandibular Dental	
16. Mn1-MP (deg)	Angle between lower central incisor and mandibular plane
17. Mn1-APg (mm)	Protrusion of lower central incisor (along perpendicular to A-Pg line)
Soft Tissue	
18. UL-SnPg (mm)	Measure along a perpendicular to subnasale-soft tissue pogonion to labrale superius
19. LL-SnPg (mm)	Measure along a perpendicular to subnasale-soft tissue pogonion to labrale inferius
20. NL (deg)	Angle between nose and philtrum of upper lip

Soft Tissue

There was a significant reduction in the upper lip protrusion measured at the UL-SnPg (−0.7 mm in the treatment group compared to 0.1 mm in the controls) and in the nasolabial angle (2.1° increase in the treatment group compared to 0.1° in the controls).

T2–T3

Results for this treatment period showing the changes from the removal of the TFBC to the removal of all appliances are summarized in Table 13.4.

Dental Findings

Molars Horizontal and vertical changes for the upper molars were significant between the experimental and control groups. No horizontal change at the crown level was observed in the experimental group compared to a 0.6 mm anterior change in the control group. At the apical level, the study group had 0.1 mm of posterior movement compared to 0.4 mm of anterior movement in the controls. Vertical crown and apical movement was 0.1 mm downward for the experimental group compared to 0.5 mm movement in the same direction for the controls.

The mandibular molars had no significant difference with the controls in anteroposterior movement. Vertically, the molars

Table 13.2. Initial form (T1) comparison.

	Study		Control		
	Mean	SD	Mean	SD	Significance
Maxillary skeletal					
ANS-PNS, absolute (mm)	56.8	3.75	58.2	3.96	NS
PP-SN7 (deg)	0.4	2.96	−1.2	2.22	NS
Maxillary dental					
Mx1-SN7 (deg)	113.1	6.51	102.8	7.48	***
Mandibular skeletal					
Ar-Pg, absolute (mm)	110.6	7.01	114.5	6.04	NS
MP-SN7 (deg)	24.9	7.43	26.1	4.69	NS
Mandibular dental					
Mn1-APg (mm)	2	1.43	1.4	2.71	NS
Mn1-MP (deg)	95.7	4.87	95.9	8.71	NS
General skeletal					
N-ANS y (mm)	54.6	3.83	58.5	3.76	**
ANS-Me y (mm)	67.3	5.74	68.6	5.29	NS
LFH(100)/TFH (%)	55.2	1.74	53.9	1.78	*
N-A-Pg (deg)	10.9	4.89	4.5	4.26	***
A-B(OP) (mm)	4.9	2.49	0.2	2.85	***
General dental					
OJ (mm)	6	1.88	4.1	1.33	***
Molar (mm)	3.2	1.2	0.4	0.95	***
OP-SN7 (deg)	9.5	9.53	11.4	4.13	NS
Inter-Inc (deg)	125.3	7.34	134.6	12.95	**
Soft tissue					
Inc-Stm (mm)	3.9	1.86	4.4	2.38	NS
UL-SnPg (mm)	5.3	1.83	3.6	3.55	NS
LL-SnPg (mm)	4.1	1.22	1.6	2.88	**
NL (deg)	125	9.4	114.2	12.26	**

Control measurements are normalized for size. *** $p<0.001$, ** $p<0.01$, * $p<0.05$.

moved inferiorly 2.1 mm compared to a 0.3 mm extrusion of the controls.

Incisors The maxillary incisors proclined 4.9° in the treatment group compared to 0.2° in the controls. The nature of the movement in the treatment group was uncontrolled tipping with 1 mm of coronal anterior movement and 0.6 mm posterior apical root movement.

Significant changes were observed in the lower incisor inclination with reduction of the proclination in the treatment group. This is reflected in the mean changes for Mn1-APG (−1.3 mm for the study and 0.1 mm for the control group) and IMPA (−4.1° in the treated group and 0° in the control group).

Overjet and Molar Discrepancy Overjet and molar discrepancy showed a significant difference between experimental and control groups. Overjet and molar discrepancy increased 2.5 mm and 1.2 mm respectively in the treated group. No change was seen in the controls.

Dentoalveolar Findings

The occlusal plane relapsed −2.2° in a counterclockwise direction in the experimental group compared to −0.2° rotation of the controls. This occlusal plane change contributed to the relapse in the A-B/OP discrepancy of 1.5 mm seen in the experimental group compared to the −0.1 mm change in the controls.

Table 13.3. Experimental T1–T2 TFBC changes.

	Study		Control		
	Mean	**SD**	**Mean**	**SD**	**Significance**
Maxillary skeletal					
ANS-PNS, absolute (mm)	0.4	1.25	0.1	0.38	NS
PP-SN7 (deg)	0.5	0.57	0.1	0.23	*
A Point *x* (mm)	−0.5	0.7	0.1	0.14	**
A Point *y* (mm)	1.7	1.45	0.4	0.32	***
ANS *x* (mm)	0	0.97	0.1	0.19	NS
ANS *y* (mm)	0.4	0.47	0.2	0.25	NS
Maxillary dental					
Mx1-SN7 (deg)	−7.4	3.45	0.1	0.54	***
Mx1 crown *x* (mm)	−1.8	0.92	0.1	0.13	***
Mx1 crown *y* (mm)	1	0.46	0.1	0.11	***
Mx1 root *x* (mm)	0.6	0.71	0.1	0.12	**
Mx1 root *y* (mm)	0	0.71	0.1	0.13	NS
Mx 6 crown *x* (mm)	−0.8	0.74	0.2	0.3	***
Mx 6 crown *y* (mm)	−1.1	0.5	0.2	0.2	***
Mx 6 MBroot *x* (mm)	−0.3	0.86	0.2	0.2	*
Mx 6 MBroot *y* (mm)	−1.1	0.53	0.2	0.22	***
Mandibular skeletal					
Ar-Pg, absolute (mm)	2.1	1.43	0.7	0.45	***
MP-SN7 (deg)	−0.2	1.29	0	0.19	NS
Pg *x* (mm)	0.2	1	0.2	0.2	NS
Me *y* (mm)	1.6	1.09	0.7	0.56	**
B pt *x* (mm)	0.2	0.97	0.1	0.16	NS
B pt *y* (mm)	2.6	2.09	0.5	0.55	***
Mandibular dental					
Mn1-APg (mm)	2.7	0.79	0	0.16	***
IMPA (deg)	7.7	3.06	0	0.7	***
Mn 1 crown *x* (mm)	2.4	1.06	0	0.1	***
Mn 1 crown *y* (mm)	2.5	1.21	−0.1	0.23	***
Mn 1 root *x* (mm)	0	0.81	0	0.18	NS
Mn 1 root *y* (mm)	1.2	0.7	−0.1	0.19	***
Mn 6 crown *x* (mm)	1.9	0.97	0.2	0.2	***
Mn 6 crown *y* (mm)	−1.2	1.01	−0.1	0.23	***
Mn 6 root *x* (mm)	0.7	1.15	0.2	0.3	NS
Mn 6 root *y* (mm)	−1.4	0.96	−0.1	0.21	***
General skeletal					
N-ANS *y* (mm)	0.5	0.59	0.2	0.52	NS
ANS-Me *y* (mm)	1.2	1.45	0.4	0.38	**
LFH(100)/TFH (%)	0.2	0.53	0.2	0.62	NS
N-A-Pg (deg)	−1.7	1.75	−0.3	0.41	**
A-B(OP) (mm)	−5	1.45	0	0.5	***

(cont'd)

Table 13.3. Experimental T1–T2 TFBC changes (*cont'd*).

	Study		Control		
	Mean	**SD**	**Mean**	**SD**	**Significance**
General dental					
OJ (mm)	−5.6	1.69	−0.1	0.09	***
Molar (mm)	−3.9	1.18	0	0.12	***
OP-SN7 (deg)	4.8	2.05	−0.1	0.61	***
Inter-Inc (deg)	−1	3.82	0.2	0.92	NS
Soft tissue					
Inc-Stm (mm)	0.4	1.11	0.1	0.33	NS
UL-SnPg (mm)	−0.7	1.42	0.1	0.53	*
LL-SnPg (mm)	0.8	1.75	0.2	0.51	NS
NL (deg)	2.1	3.06	0.1	1.9	*

*** $p<0.001$, ** $p<0.01$, * $p<0.05$.

Skeletal Findings

Skeletal convexity was reduced significantly in the experimental group compared to the controls (−2.1° and 0.6° respectively).

Maxilla and Mandible A significant change was observed in the vertical position of A point which moved superiorly 0.2 mm compared to 0.8 mm of inferior movement in the control group. B point showed a significant difference in the anteroposterior and vertical displacement between groups. The treated group showed a 1 mm anterior and 0.7 mm superior change compared to a 0.2 mm anterior and 1.3 mm inferior movement of the control group. Horizontally pogonion and vertically menton did not show significant differences between groups.

Mandibular length measured at Ar-Pg showed a significant difference with a greater mean average increase in length in the control of 1.8 mm compared to 0.3 mm in the experimental group.

Vertical Dimension Vertical heights significantly decreased in the experimental group compared to the controls. Lower facial height decreased on average by 0.2 mm in the experimental group compared to 1 mm increase in the controls. The LFH/TFH ratio also decreased by 0.4% compared to a 0.2% increase in the controls. In contrast, the MPA significantly increased by 1.9° in the experimental compared to no change in the control group.

Soft Tissue

Table 13.4 shows the small significant changes for Inc-Stm, LL-SnPg, and NL angle. All these measurements were reduced in the treatment group.

T1–T3

Results for the total treatment are summarized in Table 13.5.

Dental Findings

Molars A significant change was observed between experimental and control groups in the upper molar position. A 0.8 mm posterior and 1 mm superior molar movement at the coronal and apical level was evident in the treatment group in comparison to a 0.8 mm anterior and 0.7 mm inferior molar movement in the control group. The apical changes in the experimental group were 0.4 mm posterior and 0.9 mm intrusive movements compared to 0.6 mm anterior and 0.8 inferior molar movements in the control group.

Mandibular molar changes were significantly different between both groups. The experimental group showed an anterior and inferior movement of the crown of the lower first molar of 2.1 mm and 1 mm respectively. The control group had a 0.7 mm anterior and −0.5 mm superior movement.

Incisors Significant differences were found between both groups in terms of the upper incisal inclination. The upper incisor crown moved 0.7 mm posteriorly and 1.3 mm inferiorly. This tooth in the control group moved 0.4 mm anteriorly and 0.3 mm inferiorly.

Mandibular incisors flared during treatment. Measurement of incisor proclination (Mn1-APg) was 1.5 mm in the experimental compared to −0.1 mm in the controls. The IMPA increased 3.1° in the experimental compared to no increase in the controls. Mean vertical and horizontal lower incisor coronal changes in the treated group were 2.4 mm and 2.2 mm respectively.

Table 13.4. Experimental T2–T3 TFBC changes.

	Study		Control		
	Mean	**SD**	**Mean**	**SD**	**Significance**
Maxillary skeletal					
ANS-PNS, absolute (mm)	−0.1	1.66	0.3	0.87	NS
PP-SN7 (deg)	−0.6	1.89	0.2	0.52	NS
A Point *x* (mm)	0.1	0.95	0.2	0.29	NS
A Point *y* (mm)	−0.2	1.71	0.8	0.76	*
ANS *x* (mm)	0.1	1.33	0.3	0.44	NS
ANS *y* (mm)	0.6	0.79	0.5	0.58	NS
Maxillary dental					
Mx1-SN7 (deg)	4.9	3.59	0.2	1.25	***
Mx1 crown *x* (mm)	1	0.91	0.3	0.3	**
Mx1 crown *y* (mm)	0.3	1.18	0.2	0.27	NS
Mx1 root *x* (mm)	−0.6	1.23	0.2	0.31	**
Mx1 root *y* (mm)	1	0.81	0.3	0.35	**
Mx 6 crown *x* (mm)	0	0.12	0.6	0.71	***
Mx 6 crown *y* (mm)	0.1	0.49	0.5	0.48	*
Mx 6 MBroot *x* (mm)	−0.1	0.39	0.4	0.47	***
Mx 6 MBroot *y* (mm)	0.1	0.44	0.5	0.52	*
Mandibular skeletal					
Ar-Pg, absolute (mm)	0.3	1.83	1.8	1.22	**
MP-SN7 (deg)	1.9	2.18	0	0.41	***
Pg *x* (mm)	1.1	1.37	0.5	0.48	NS
Me *y* (mm)	0.9	1.37	1.5	1.31	NS
B pt *x* (mm)	1	1.25	0.2	0.38	**
B pt *y* (mm)	−0.7	2.4	1.3	1.29	**
Mandibular dental					
Mn1-APg (mm)	−1.3	1.13	−0.1	0.35	***
IMPA (deg)	−4.1	3.66	0	1.62	***
Mn 1 crown *x* (mm)	−0.2	1.62	0.1	0.22	NS
Mn 1 crown *y* (mm)	−0.1	1.48	−0.2	0.54	NS
Mn 1 root *x* (mm)	0.2	1.66	0.1	0.42	NS
Mn 1 root *y* (mm)	0.6	1.26	−0.2	0.45	*
Mn 6 crown *x* (mm)	0.2	1.74	0.5	0.46	NS
Mn 6 crown *y* (mm)	2.1	1.84	−0.3	0.52	***
Mn 6 root *x* (mm)	0.9	1.91	0.4	0.7	NS
Mn 6 root *y* (mm)	2.8	1.6	−0.3	0.51	***
General skeletal					
N-ANS *y* (mm)	0.6	0.82	0.5	1.23	NS
ANS-Me *y* (mm)	−0.2	2.14	1	0.91	*
LFH(100)/TFH (%)	−0.4	0.97	0.2	0.43	*
N-A-Pg (deg)	−2.1	1.59	−0.6	0.96	***
A-B(OP) (mm)	1.5	1.59	−0.1	1.19	***

(cont'd)

Table 13.4. Experimental T2–T3 TFBC changes (*cont'd*).

| | Study | | Control | | |
	Mean	SD	Mean	SD	Significance
General dental					
OJ (mm)	2.5	1.25	−0.1	0.2	***
Molar (mm)	1.2	1.39	0	0.29	***
OP-SN7 (deg)	−2.2	2.23	−0.2	1.43	**
Inter-Inc (deg)	−2.2	5.65	0.4	2.16	NS
Soft tissue					
Inc-Stm (mm)	−0.7	1.27	0.1	0.79	*
UL-SnPg (mm)	−0.2	1.43	0	1.37	NS
LL-SnPg (mm)	−0.9	1.78	0.3	1.27	*
NL (deg)	−5.2	8.7	0.4	4.6	*

*** $p < 0.001$, ** $p < 0.01$, * $p < 0.05$.

Overjet and Molar Discrepancy Overjet and molar discrepancy were significantly reduced in the experimental group (3.2 mm and 2.7 mm respectively) compared to the controls (0.2 mm and 0 mm respectively).

Dentoalveolar Findings

Rotation of the occlusal plane for the experimental group was 2.7° which was statistically significant compared to controls (−0.3°). This contributed to the significant A-B/OP reduction of 3.1 mm compared to 0.1 mm in the controls.

Skeletal Convexity

A significant reduction in the skeletal convexity of 3.7° in the experimental group compared to 0.8° in the control group was mostly attributed to posterior movement of A point (0.4 mm) and anterior movement of Pg (1.3 mm).

Maxilla and Mandible Position and Length

The only significant change in the position of the maxilla was measured at A point. This landmark was positioned −0.4 mm more posteriorly in the experimental group compared to a 0.3 mm anterior position in the controls.

The only significant difference in the anteroposterior position of the mandible was found at B point. A mean 1.2 mm anterior displacement in the treated group occurred compared to a 0.4 mm movement in the controls.

No significant difference in maxillary and mandibular length was found between groups.

Vertical Dimension

The only significant change in the vertical dimension was the 1.8° increase in the experimental group in the mandibular plane angle compared to no change in the control group.

Soft Tissue

The only small significant soft tissue change was the lip protrusion reduction of −1 mm measured at UL-SnPg in the experimental group. For the control group this distance increased 0.1 mm.

Figure 13.42 shows a composite of the average skeletal and dental changes between the time periods with the TFBC.

Finally, to assess the difference in skeletal, dental, and soft tissue changes related to skeletal maturity, the experimental sample was subdivided into patients with a skeletal maturation stage CVMS II and patients in stage CVMS I or III.[18] The only significant difference between these two groups was found in the absolute mandibular length. Patients in skeletal maturation CVMS II had significantly more mandibular length change (2.85 mm) compared to patients in stages CVMS I or III (0.76 mm).

Discussion

The Twin Force Bite Corrector is a fixed, intermaxillary, mandibular protrusive appliance, delivered through a piston system with a spring. The appliance can be classified as a fixed functional type of appliance for the correction of Class II malocclusions. Similar types of appliances called hybrid Herbsts[21] are currently used but few prospective clinical trials have been done for many of these.

The data in this study were evaluated in comparison to controls from the Bolton Growth Study, comprising patients with Class

Table 13.5. Experimental T1–T3 TFBC changes.

	Study		Control		
	Mean	**SD**	**Mean**	**SD**	**Significance**
Maxillary skeletal					
ANS-PNS, absolute (mm)	0.3	1.43	0.4	1.27	NS
PP-SN7 (deg)	−0.1	1.64	0.4	0.78	NS
A Point x (mm)	−0.4	0.96	0.3	0.46	**
A Point y (mm)	1.5	1.58	1.2	1.08	NS
ANS x (mm)	0.1	0.99	0.4	0.64	NS
ANS y (mm)	1.1	1.04	0.8	0.84	NS
Maxillary dental					
Mx1-SN7 (deg)	−1.9	4.8	0.3	1.88	NS
Mx1 crown x (mm)	−0.7	1.1	0.4	0.43	***
Mx1 crown y (mm)	1.3	1.27	0.3	0.37	**
Mx1 root x (mm)	0	1.24	0.3	0.42	NS
Mx1 root y (mm)	1	0.68	0.4	0.44	**
Mx 6 crown x (mm)	−0.8	0.77	0.8	1.01	***
Mx 6 crown y (mm)	−1	0.8	0.7	0.66	***
Mx 6 MBroot x (mm)	−0.4	0.89	0.6	0.69	***
Mx 6 MBroot y (mm)	−0.9	0.81	0.8	0.74	***
Mandibular skeletal					
Ar-Pg, absolute (mm)	2.4	1.68	2.3	1.52	NS
MP-SN7 (deg)	1.8	1.71	0	0.65	***
Pg x (mm)	1.3	1.29	0.7	0.68	NS
Me y (mm)	2.5	1.64	2.2	1.9	NS
B pt x (mm)	1.2	1.16	0.4	0.55	**
B pt y (mm)	2	1.77	1.8	1.87	NS
Mandibular dental					
Mn1-APg (mm)	1.5	1.02	−0.1	0.53	***
IMPA (deg)	3.1	4.39	0.1	2.35	*
Mn 1 crown x (mm)	2.2	1.27	0.1	0.32	***
Mn 1 crown x (mm)	2.4	1.53	−0.3	0.78	***
Mn 1 root x (mm)	0.2	1.56	0.1	0.61	NS
Mn 1 root y (mm)	1.8	1.24	−0.3	0.65	***
Mn 6 crown x (mm)	2.1	1.55	0.7	0.67	***
Mn 6 crown y (mm)	1	1.34	−0.5	0.76	***
Mn 6 root x (mm)	1.6	1.51	0.6	1.01	*
Mn 6 root y (mm)	1.4	1.28	−0.5	0.72	***
General skeletal					
N-ANS y (mm)	1.1	1.19	0.8	1.75	NS
ANS-Me y (mm)	0.9	2.01	1.5	1.29	NS
LFH(100)/TFH (%)	−0.2	0.88	0.2	0.62	NS
N-A-Pg (deg)	−3.7	1.8	−0.8	1.36	***
A-B(OP) (mm)	−3.5	1.61	−0.1	1.69	***

(cont'd)

Table 13.5. Experimental T1–T3 TFBC changes (*cont'd*).

	Study		Control		
	Mean	**SD**	**Mean**	**SD**	**Significance**
General dental					
OJ (mm)	−3.2	1.98	−0.2	0.29	***
Molar (mm)	−2.7	1.41	0	0.4	***
OP-SN7 (deg)	2.7	1.49	−0.3	2.05	***
Inter-Inc (deg)	−3.1	5.78	0.6	3.1	*
Soft tissue					
Inc-Stm (mm)	−0.3	1.52	0.2	1.13	NS
UL-SnPg (mm)	−1	1.03	0.1	1.94	*
LL-SnPg (mm)	−0.1	1.51	0.4	1.82	NS
NL (deg)	−3.1	8.68	0.6	6.59	NS

*** $p<0.001$, ** $p<0.01$, * $p<0.05$.

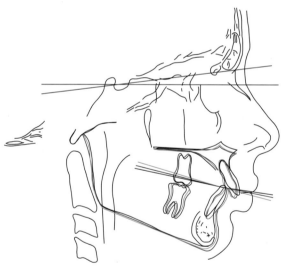

Figure 13.42 Composite depicting average skeletal and dental treatment changes from T1 to T3 with the TFBC.

and Class II malocclusions. Class I skeletal patterns have been shown to exhibit similar growth patterns to Class II patients.[22]

The results of this study are presented in two distinct phases and a summary of the total treatment. In the first phase of active appliance wear (average 3 months), the changes obtained were significant for the reduction of skeletal convexity compared to controls, which is in agreement with other studies using similar functional appliances.[23,24] This convexity was further reduced in the second phase of treatment by seating elastics with a Class II vector. Contributing to this reduction was a backward positioning of A point during the appliance phase. This agrees with the suggested small headgear effect found with the Herbst appliance.[7,25,26]

Interestingly, the absolute distance of the mandible measured at Ar-Pg was significantly different from controls in the first stage (T1–T2) but not significantly different in the second phase (T2–T3). Moreover, in the total treatment period (T1–T3) there were no differences between experimentals and controls in mandibular length. This differs from findings with the Herbst where an overall significant increase in mandibular length compared to Class II controls has been found.[25–27] However, there seems to be a deceleration of growth after the appliance removal.[26]

In the vertical dimension, results were conflicting. The lower facial height was increased in the first phase but reduced in the second phase. On the other hand, the mandibular plane angle was decreased in the first phase and significantly increased in the second phase. For the total treatment time, only the mandibular plane angle was significantly increased. These findings are in contrast to those on the Herbst appliance where the mandibular plane angle does not seem to increase.[7] However, they are in accordance with other studies where mandibular plane angle increases with Class II elastic wear.[11]

The dentoalveolar changes reflected a correction of the Class II malocclusion in all the cases. This was achieved through occlusal plane changes as well as dental movements. The occlusal plane steepened in the first phase significantly but rotated back almost half the distance of the initial change after the second phase. Reports on the Herbst appliance show a slightly less occlusal plane rotation (1.1°) after 6 months of treatment.[7] This difference may be accounted for by the appliance design. In the Herbst appliance the upper incisors are not engaged to the appliance, therefore the occlusal plane (measured from the first molar to the upper incisor edge) is not that much affected.

Occlusal plane changes at the end of treatment, once the occlusal plane is leveled, could yield a similar result to the TFBC. This is corroborated by the fact that the upper incisor extrusion at the end of treatment with the TFBC is very similar to the incisor extrusion with the Herbst at the end of fixed appliance treatment, 1.1 mm and 1.3 mm respectively.[28] It is also corroborated by the negligible vertical movement of the lower incisor during the initial Herbst therapy and the significant intrusion of the incisor (2.1 mm) at the end of treatment, a very similar value to the TFBC.[28] Moreover, the treatment effects after 3 months of TFBC and 6 months of Herbst therapy were very similar and in the range of 1 mm of lower intrusion. At the end of treatment both maintained this same amount of intrusion.[23]

The lower molar tends to extrude with Herbst therapy and through the end of treatment. Initially, 1 mm of lower molar extrusion is reported with the appliance and a total of 2 mm at the end of treatment. This differs with this TFBC protocol where there is a similar effect to the Herbst initially but after appliance removal, the amount of extrusion relapses to return to baseline measures. The upper molar intruded with both the Herbst and TFBC therapy, both having at the end of treatment approximately 1 mm of intrusion.[23,28,29]

Sagittal changes are the most often reported for all the jump-biting appliances. At the dentoalveolar level, the lingual movement of the upper incisor crown at the end of treatment was similar to that reported with other functional appliances.[25,30] Initially, with the TFBC appliance insertion, more retroclined incisors were achieved. This was reduced eventually after the TFBC removal.

The lower incisors flared significantly with the TFBC. After appliance removal, the incisors relapsed significantly to comparable levels of incisor flare obtained with the Herbst, which is approximately 2 mm. The overjet was reduced to normal values on every patient at the end of treatment, with an average of 3.2 mm, which is consistent with other functional appliances.[24,25,30] It is important to note that after TFBC therapy, the relapse tendencies in the incisors do not result in a reestablishment of increased overjet since the patient is treated to an anterior edge-to-edge relationship with the appliance.

The upper molar moved distally in a translatory manner approximately 1 mm with the TFBC which was maintained through the end of treatment. This differs with the Herbst appliance where some degree of relapse has been observed.[24] The explanation might be due to the appliance design in that forces applied with the Herbst are directly applied to the upper molar instead of the denture base, as occurs with the TFBC.

The 2 mm anterior movement of the lower molar is consistent with the Herbst appliance. The fast mesial movement can be appreciated in a patient with 1 month of TFBC treatment after inadvertently not cinching the lower archwire. Note the amount of space achieved distal to the lower 4 in 4 weeks (Fig. 13.43).

Finally, to evaluate the influence of skeletal maturation on the orthopedic effects, the experimental group was separated into CVMS stages. Upon appliance insertion, three patients represented CVMS I, 11 were CVMS II, and six patients CVMS III. Two groups were compared based on the skeletal maturity. One group had

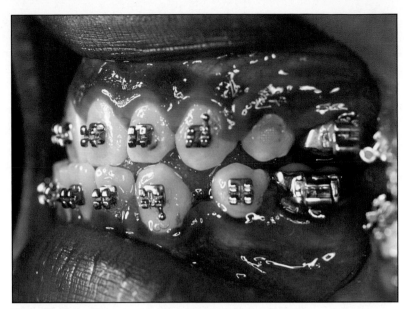

Figure 13.43 Significant space opening distal to the lower left canine over 1-month period after inadvertently not cinching the lower archwire.

patients in CVMS II and the other group had patients in CVMS I and CVMS III. The only significant difference between the groups was at the level of mandibular length. Patients at CVMS II had on average 2 mm more distance in the Ar-Pg measurement at T3. This is consistent with findings by Pancherz with the Herbst appliance where he states that greater skeletal changes can be achieved during peak height velocity when compared to pre and post peaks.[31,32]

Advantages of the TFBC

This appliance introduces a series of advantages over other types of fixed functional appliances. It allows mandibular freedom for lateral movements for patient comfort. Additionally, from the mechanical point of view, it introduces an oscillating force through the incorporation of a coil spring within the cylinder/plunger system. Mao has stated that the use of cyclic forces as opposed to static forces induces more sutural growth when comparing peak magnitude and duration.[33]

Another advantage of the TFBC over the Herbst is that it allows alteration of the vector of the intermaxillary force to a certain degree. The force vector can be altered within the interbracket distance between the first molar and second premolar in the upper arch and the canine and the first premolar in the lower arch.

Breakage is another important point. Since the appliance was changed to a titanium hex nut, no appliance breakage was observed in the treatment group. However, if the titanium screw is not tightened properly, the appliance can slip and become loose. This is

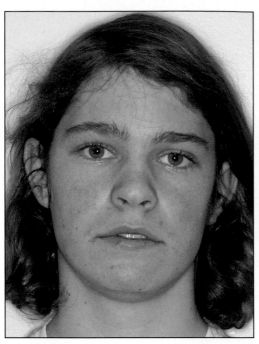

Figures 13.44–13.51 One-year follow-up after fixed appliance removal of patient presented in Figs 13.10–13.39.

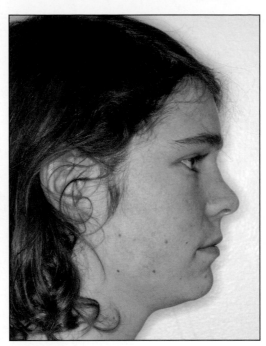

Figure 13.45

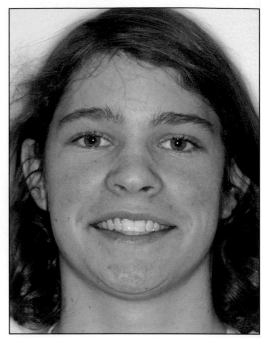

Figure 13.46

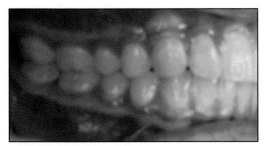

Figure 13.47

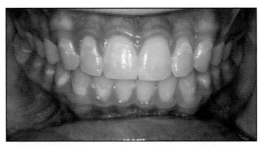

Figure 13.48

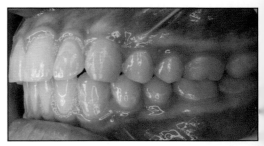

Figure 13.49

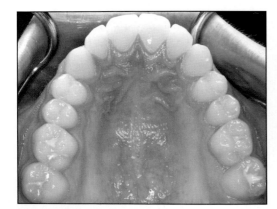

Figure 13.50

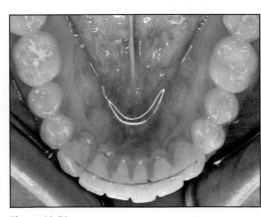

Figure 13.51

in contrast with the Herbst appliance where significant breakage and loosening have been reported.[34]

One final point worth mentioning in the study is in relation to the temporomandibular joint (TMJ). Although this study was not intended to directly measure the effects on the TMJ, it is important to note that none of the study patients experienced any symptoms of adverse effects on the joints. This has been studied by Ruff and Pancherz who found no adverse effects in the TMJ with the Herbst appliance.[35]

Conclusion

Great controversy exists about the magnitude of the skeletal effects achieved with functional appliance therapy. The TFBC showed very similar effects to other functional appliances in terms of mandibular growth. It is important to note that the mandibular length was measured from articulare. The use of this landmark for mandibular length changes has been shown to have limitations in differentiating a true increase in length from a postural change.[36] Additionally, it is important to note that after the removal of the TFBC, there was almost no increase in mandibular length reflected in the total treatment where there was no significant difference with controls.

Data are being collected at this point to evaluate the long-term stability of treatment. Preliminary data show that treatment effects are maintained after 1 year (Figs 13.44–13.51). This is in agreement with the long-term follow-up on the Herbst appliance.

Bite-jumping appliances have gained popularity in recent years with the advent of nonextraction therapies. This chapter describes the effects of a push-type intermaxillary appliance. Class II correction measured at the occlusal level was obtained with the appliance in an average of 3 months. Correction was maintained through intermaxillary elastics for an additional 3 months. The changes found were mainly dental in nature with some contribution attributed to orthopedic effect and normal growth. The shorter time of active appliance wear responsible for the occlusal change leads us to question how long a period of active bite-jumping appliance wear is needed for a Class II correction. More studies should address this question in the future.

Greater orthopedic changes were found in patients close to peak puberty than before or after peak. The TFBC as evaluated by this study appears to be a viable solution for the correction of the Class II malocclusion in growing children.

References

1. Rossouw PE, Preston CB, Lombard C. A longitudinal evaluation of extraction versus nonextraction treatment with special reference to the posttreatment irregularity of the lower incisors. Semin Orthod 1999;5:160–170.

2. Case C. The question of extraction in orthodontia. Am J Orthod 1963;50:656–691.

3. Sadowsky C. Objectives-driven orthodontics: effectiveness of mechanotherapy. Semin Orthod 2000;6:1–2.

4. Uribe F, Nanda R. Individualized orthodontic treatment planning. In: Nanda R, ed. Biomechanics and esthetic strategies in clinical orthodontics. St Louis: Elsevier; 2005.

5. Huang GJ. Making the case for evidence-based orthodontics. Am J Orthod Dentofacial Orthop 2004;125:405–406.

6. Burstone CJ. Contemporary management of Class II malocclusions: fact and fiction in Class II correction. In: Nanda R, ed. Biomechanics in clinical orthodontics. Philadelphia: W.B. Saunders; 1997: 246–256.

7. Pancherz H. The mechanism of Class II correction in Herbst appliance treatment. A cephalometric investigation. Am J Orthod 1982;82:104–113.

8. Graber TM. Functional appliances. In: Graber TM, ed. Orthodontics: current principles and techniques, 2nd edn. St Louis: Mosby; 1994: 383–436.

9. Angle EH. Anchorage. In: Angle EH, ed. Treatment of malocclusion of teeth, 7th edn. Philadelphia: S.S. White Dental Manufacturing Company; 1907: 224–235.

10. Nelson B, Hansen K, Hagg U. Overjet reduction and molar correction in fixed appliance treatment of class II, division 1, malocclusions: sagittal and vertical components. Am J Orthod Dentofacial Orthop 1999;115:13–23.

11. Nelson B, Hansen K, Hagg U. Class II correction in patients treated with class II elastics and with fixed functional appliances: a comparative study. Am J Orthod Dentofacial Orthop 2000;118: 142–149.

12. Rankin TH. Correction of Class II malocclusions with a fixed functional appliance. Masters thesis. Farmington: University of Connecticut; 1990.

13. Nalbantgil D, Arun T, Sayinsu K, Isik F. Skeletal, dental, and soft-tissue changes induced by the Jasper Jumper appliance in late adolescence. Angle Orthod 2005;75:382–392.

14. Pancherz H. Treatment of class II malocclusions by jumping the bite with the Herbst appliance. A cephalometric investigation. Am J Orthod 1979;76:423–442.

15. Schaefer AT, McNamara JA Jr, Franchi L, Baccetti T. A cephalometric comparison of treatment with the Twin-block and stainless steel crown Herbst appliances followed by fixed appliance therapy. Am J Orthod Dentofacial Orthop 2004;126:7–15.

16. O'Brien K, Wright J, Conboy F, et al. Effectiveness of treatment for Class II malocclusion with the Herbst or twin-block appliances: a randomized, controlled trial. Am J Orthod Dentofacial Orthop 2003;124:128–137.

17. Rothenberg J, Campbell ES, Nanda R. Class II correction with the Twin Force Bite Corrector. J Clin Orthod 2004;38:232–240.

18. Baccetti T, Franchi L, McNamara JA Jr. An improved version of the cervical vertebral maturation (CVM) method for the assessment of mandibular growth. Angle Orthod 2002;72:316–323.

19. Bjork A, Skieller V. Normal and abnormal growth of the mandible. A synthesis of longitudinal cephalometric implant studies over a period of 25 years. Eur J Orthod 1983;5:1–46.

20. Rothenberg J. A prospective clinical analysis of a push-type fixed intermaxillary Class II correction appliance with a stability analysis six months posttreatment. Farmington: University of Connecticut; 2004.

21. Pancherz H. History of the Herbst appliance. Semin Orthod 2003;9:3–11.

22. Bishara SE. Mandibular changes in persons with untreated and treated Class II division 1 malocclusion. Am J Orthod Dentofacial Orthop 1998; 113:661–673.

23. Pangrazio-Kulbersh V, Berger JL, Chermak DS, Kaczynski R, Simon ES, Haerian A. Treatment effects of the mandibular anterior repositioning appliance on patients with Class II malocclusion. Am J Orthod Dentofacial Orthop 2003; 123:286–295.

24. Franchi L, Baccetti T, McNamara JA Jr. Treatment and posttreatment effects of acrylic splint Herbst appliance therapy. Am J Orthod Dentofacial Orthop 1999;115:429–438.

25. Burkhardt D, Huge, S. The Herbst Appliance. In: McNamara JA Jr, ed. Orthodontics and dentofacial orthopedics. Ann Arbor: Needham Press Inc.; 2001: 285–318.

26. Lai M, McNamara JA Jr. An evaluation of two-phase treatment with the Herbst appliance and preadjusted edgewise therapy. Semin Orthod 1998;4:46–58.

27. Pancherz H, Fackel U. The skeletofacial growth pattern pre- and post-dentofacial orthopaedics. A long-term study of Class II malocclusions treated with the Herbst appliance. Eur J Orthod 1990;12:209–218.

28. Hagg U, Du X, Rabie BM, Bendeus M. What does headgear add to Herbst treatment and to retention? Semin Orthod 2003;9:57–66.

29. Pancherz H. The Herbst appliance: a powerful Class II corrector. In: Nanda R, ed. Biomechanics in clinical orthodontics. Philadelphia: W.B. Saunders; 1997: 265–280.

30. Toth LR, McNamara JA Jr. Treatment effects produced by the twin-block appliance and the FR-2 appliance of Frankel compared with an untreated Class II sample. Am J Orthod Dentofacial Orthop 1999; 116:597–609.

31. Pancherz H, Hagg U. Dentofacial orthopedics in relation to somatic maturation. An analysis of 70 consecutive cases treated with the Herbst appliance. Am J Orthod 1985;88:273–287.

32. Ruf S, Pancherz, H. When I choose the ideal period for Herbst therapy – early or late. Semin Orthod 2003;9:47–56.

33. Mao JJ, Wang X, Kopher RA. Biomechanics of craniofacial sutures: orthopedic implications. Angle Orthod 2003;73:128–135.

34. Sanden E, Pancherz H, Hansen K. Complications during Herbst appliance treatment. J Clin Orthod 2004;38:130–133.

35. Ruf S. Short- and long-term effects of the Herbst appliance on temporomandibular joint function. Semin Orthod 2003;9:74–86.

36. Aelbers CM, Dermaut LR. Orthopedics in orthodontics: Part I, Fiction or reality – a review of the literature. Am J Orthod Dentofacial Orthop 1996;110:513–519.

CHAPTER 14

The Sabbagh Universal Spring (SUS)

Aladin Sabbagh

Introduction

Orthodontic treatment of Class II malocclusions using removable functional orthopedic appliances has a long history. Various functional orthopedic devices have been developed since Kingsley presented the first jumping device in 1877. Given good cooperation and early commencement of treatment, removable appliances can yield excellent results. Difficulties arise, however, in the late treatment of adolescents when the main growth period has passed and the remaining growth is insufficient for treatment using classic functional orthopedic appliances.

Similarly, the classic solutions are not suited to patients whose cooperation is questionable or who cannot wear conventional functional devices, e.g. due to resin allergies or mouth breathing.

In 1905 Emil Herbst introduced his device which allowed one-step anterior repositioning of the mandible.[1,2] The new position is maintained during rest and function (chewing, speaking, and swallowing) for 6–9 months on average. Many patients have been successfully treated with various modifications of the Herbst appliance.[3–6] However, some orthodontists still have reservations about the Herbst appliance because of the following perceived disadvantages:

- it requires a great deal of lab work
- it requires extensive chair time
- it provides rigid forces
- it limits simultaneous treatment with multibracket systems
- it is susceptible to breakage in the anchorage unit (bands, crowns, splint, etc.).

Currently orthodontics is undergoing a period of radical change characterized by new materials, computer-based diagnostics and treatment planning, and new developments allowing an expanded scope of treatment and increased effectiveness. One of these new developments is the Sabbagh Universal Spring (SUS) (US patent 5944518, German patent 19809324) which enables orthodontic treatment of Class II patients and especially of problem cases such as:

- noncompliant patients
- limited growth potential (delayed treatment)
- retarded tissue reaction
- patients with temporomandibular disorders (TMD)
- handicapped patients
- when headgear or removable appliances are contraindicated or cannot be used.

The SUS is a combination of the Herbst appliance (as a telescope) (Dentaurum, Ispringen, Germany) and the Jasper Jumper™ (as a spring) (American Orthodontics, Sheboygan, WI), aiming to increase the efficacy of the treatment and to minimize their disadvantages (Fig. 14.1). This fixed functional appliance can save both time and trouble. It is effective 24 hours a day without being dependent on

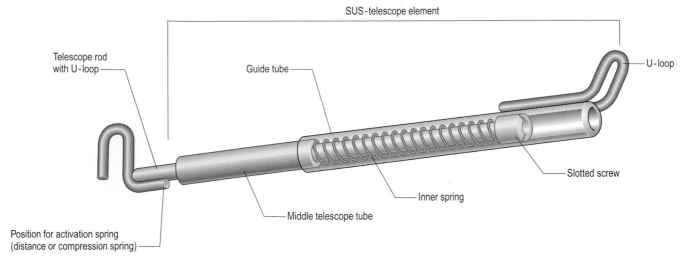

SUS-telescope element

Telescope rod
with U-loop

Guide tube

U-loop

Slotted screw

Inner spring

Middle telescope tube

Position for activation spring
(distance or compression spring)

Figure 14.1 The components of the SUS.

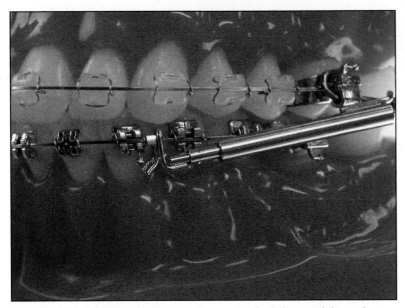

Figure 14.2 The brackets anchorage system. As a spring, the SUS can easily be used simultaneously with fixed appliances.

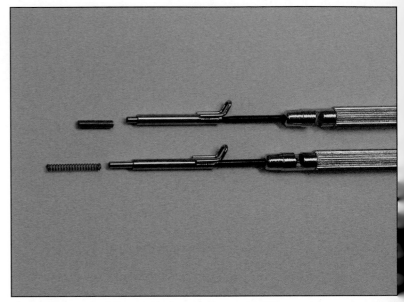

Figure 14.3 Top: the SUS as a rigid telescope. Bottom: the SUS as a spring.

patient compliance; it has just one universal size and can be fixed between the upper and lower jaws (in a way similar to the Jasper Jumper) (Fig. 14.2).

Rigid Telescope

The SUS can be used like the Herbst appliance. To obtain a rigid telescope effect, minimize the spring force by inserting and turning the middle telescope tube into the guide tube (unscrew the slotted screw anticlockwise with the activation screw). This deactivation of the spring force allows the SUS to work similarly to the Herbst appliances (Fig. 14.3).

Spring

The SUS can replace the headgear or class II elastics (dentoalveolar compensations). In this case, activate the spring force by turning the middle telescope tube outside the guide tube (screw the slotted screw clockwise with the activation key).

Anchorage

The SUS has one size, two different modes (a rigid telescope or a flexible spring), and can be fixed on three different anchorage systems:

- bands
- brackets
- splints.

The choice of the appropriate anchorage system depends on the desired effect (orthodontic, orthopedic) and on patient age.

Bands Anchorage System

The banded anchorage system resembles the conventional Herbst anchorage system (but requires less welding and lab work; technical details will be described later) and is the system of choice to achieve orthopedic changes/profile improvement using the rigid SUS (Fig. 14.4).

Bracket Anchorage System

To achieve dentoalveolar compensation without using a headgear and Class II elastics, especially in the noncompliant patient, the middle telescope spring of the SUS must be activated (screw out). Then the SUS can be fixed similar to the Jasper Jumper, employing the currently used bracket system (see Fig. 14.2).

Splint Anchorage System

This kind of anchorage is recommended in early Class II mixed dentition cases (Figs 14.5–14.7) and for treatment of TMD patients, especially those with some kind of disk displacement and a dorsal condyle position. Furthermore, in some snoring cases it may help achieve good results in cooperation with a sleep laboratory.

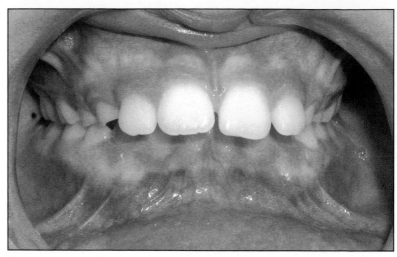

Figures 14.5, 14.6 The removable splint anchorage system, using 2 mm hard splints, with slight retrusion elastics. The treatment can be started in the early mixed dentition if necessary, as an alternative to the traditional functional appliance.

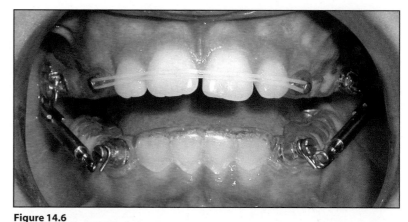

Figure 14.6

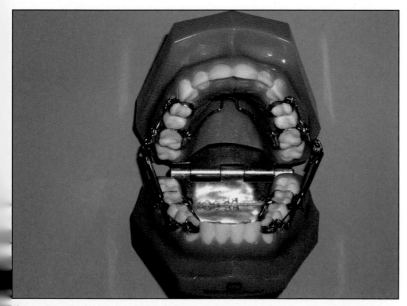

Figure 14.4 The banded anchorage system analogous to the conventional Herbst appliance.

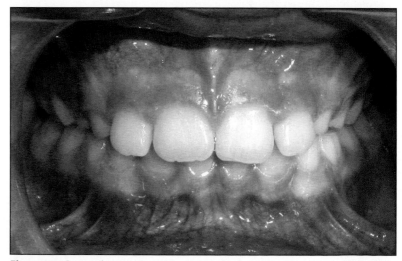

Figure 14.7 Patient shown in Figs 14.5 and 14.6 after 6 months of treatment with the SUS splint.

Indications and Contraindications

Indications

- Class II correction including skeletal changes (rigid telescope effect/Herbst effect)
- Class II correction with dentoalveolar compensation of the occlusion (spring effect/Class II elastics effect)
- Unilateral correction of Class II/laterognathism
- Distalizing/anchorage of the upper posterior teeth (headgear substitute)
- Closing the lower jaw spaces with maximum anchorage (aplasia)
- Temporomandibular joint therapy (reposition effect)

Contraindications

- Marked protrusion of the lower anterior teeth
- Marked crowding of the lower anterior teeth
- Severe gummy smile
- Poor oral hygiene

Theoretical Considerations of Functional Bite Jumping

In principle, treatment may be confined in some cases to exclusive dentoalveolar compensation, i.e. without changing the bite. However, mandible advancement (Herbst effect) is recommended for profile improvement. This kind of correction is a result of dentoalveolar and skeletal changes: growth stimulation and/or temporomandibular joint (TMJ) remodeling.

The ability to modify growth using functional orthopedics appliances is a controversial topic in scientific literature. However, studies have shown that improvements in sagittal incisor and molar relationships were achieved by dental changes rather than by skeletal ones. The amount of skeletal change contributing to overjet and molar correction was smaller in the young adult group (22% and 25%, respectively) than in the early adolescent group (39% and 41%, respectively).[7] These effects depend on age, treatment duration, sex, maturity, and facial growth patterns. Skeletal changes contributing to overjet and molar correction were larger in the hyperdivergent group (37% and 44%, respectively) than in the hypodivergent group (25% and 25%, respectively). Dental and skeletal changes contributing to Class II correction were found to be independent of the vertical jaw base relationship. Thus, a hyperdivergent jaw base relationship did not affect treatment response unfavorably.[8]

In view of the results of magnetic resonance imaging (MRI) studies on Herbst treatment, the debate about the skeletal effect of the mandible advancement has become less controversial among clinicians. The MR images confirm bone remodeling in the TMJ (which can be considered as a skeletal change), being a combination of condylar capping, glenoid fossa shift, and anterior condylar movement.[9] Such TMJ remodeling occurs also in adult patients. This revolutionary new finding means that treatment with a fixed functional appliance may be an alternative to orthognathic surgery in borderline Class II cases (Figs 14.8 and 14.9). Apparently, mandible advancement may stimulate the remarkable and unique process of TMJ adaptation and remodeling not only in young but also in adult

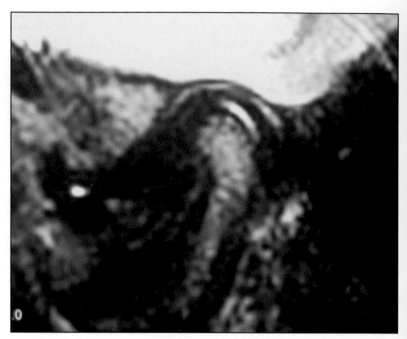

Figure 14.8 The MR images show a combination of condylar capping and glenoid fossa shifting. After 3 months of mandible advancement with the SUS.

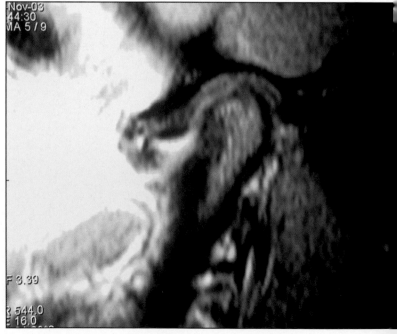

Figure 14.9 After 6 months of mandible advancement with the SUS.

patients. Treatment of adult Class II cases with a Herbst/multibracket appliance shows that both overjet and Class II molar relation were normalized. Overjet correction amounted to 6.75 mm on average, due to dental (87%) and skeletal changes (13%). Class II molar correction averaged 4.11 mm, resulting from 78% dental and 22% skeletal changes.[10]

Also, morphologic studies show that bite jumping of the mandible in adult rats affects the length of the condylar process, which increased significantly on day 30 and remained stable until day 60 in the experimental group. The angulations of the condylar process were significantly affected due to increased apposition of bone in the middle and especially the posterior parts of the condyle.

Bite-jumping appliances can improve proliferation of mesenchymal cells in the condylar cartilage in young rats.[11] The same mechanism may also exist in adult species. When more mesenchymal cells transform into chondrocytes, there will be more bone formation in the condyle. Thus, mandibular advancement could also stimulate the adaptive growth of the condyle in adult rats.[12] This finding does not support previous experimental results reporting that adult monkeys lost the ability for condylar remodeling.[13,14] This new finding attaches more significance to the TMJ diagnosis. Observations and studies from our practice show that TMJ remodeling depends not just on age, timing and duration of treatment, sex, maturity, and facial growth pattern, but also on the condition of the TMJ, especially its bands and ligaments. Therefore, a practical method of TMJ diagnosis is very important not only for preventive but also for prognostic purposes.

Class II Correction Including Skeletal Changes (Rigid Telescope Effect/ Herbst Effect)

The SUS can be used like the Herbst appliance. Deactivation of the spring force will change the SUS from a spring into a rigid telescope (with a small spring force acting as a shock absorber), and lets it work similarly to the Herbst appliance (see Fig. 14.3). In comparison to the conventional Herbst appliance, the advantages of the SUS system are as follows.

- The anchorage system requires less welding and lab work, the currently used band can be fitted, and there is no need to remove the band attachment, which will be left in place to receive the SUS.
- Two-step advancement of the mandible instead of one (maximal jumping) compared to the Herbst appliance, reduced load and breakage of the anchorage unit, larger skeletal contribution to the overjet correction, improved TMJ response with the mandible being repositioned forward in a stepwise manner compared to larger one-step protrusion.[15]

Practical Considerations

- First, a comprehensive diagnosis of the functional, dental, and skeletal aspects is required. This Class II correction including skeletal changes is especially recommended for patients who need profile improvement, particularly if extractions and/or surgery have to be avoided.
- The transverse dimension must be corrected (if necessary) just before bite jumping. Two to three weeks after insertion of the rapid palatal expansion (RPE) device, the mandible has to be advanced by means of two rigid SUS telescopes fixed to the mandible anchorage unit.
- The mandible anchorage system consists of a 0.9 mm lingual arch connecting the bands of the first molars and cuspids (see Fig. 14.4). Buccally, a thick sectional rectangular stainless steel archwire must be inserted and turned off between the band attachments. In the maxilla, the best results are obtained using the RPE device. If RPE is not required, sufficient anchorage is provided by a banded first upper molar and premolar with a thick rectangular stainless steel archwire in between, and a transpalatal archwire (TPA).
- To achieve a skeletal effect, the spring force has to be minimized by inserting and turning the inner telescope tube. By deactivation of the spring force, the SUS will change from a spring into a rigid telescope so as to work similarly to the Herbst appliances. Thus, the lower jaw is placed in a ventral position and cannot move back during function (eating, speaking, swallowing, etc.) for the next 6–9 months. Such stable advancement cannot be achieved with springs or flexible appliances (Figs 14.10–14.15).
- The SUS has one universal size which fits almost 80% of patients (this helps to decrease the inventory). The length of the SUS can be extended (if necessary) or activated by a piece of closed coil spring (Fig. 14.16).
- The first step forward usually does not exceed about 5 mm. The next steps follow within 8–10 week intervals and they also do not exceed 5 mm until the edge-to-edge position is achieved (overcorrection).

After minimizing the spring force to obtain a rigid telescope, the SUS will work similarly to the Herbst appliance. The first step is fixing the SUS in the maxilla. Insert the pin through the distal end of the headgear tube, leave about 4–5 mm distally and bend the mesial end of the pin 90° gingivally (see Fig. 14.2), then 90° distally, to fit it between the tooth and the hook, which is important to avoid rotation. Finally, bend the distal end of the pin 20–30°. Buccally, in the mandible, a slide hook has to be fixed distally of the canine brackets on the rectangular archwire which will later stabilize the U-loop (see Fig. 14.2).

Turn the U-loop of the telescope rod 90° to the right or left, depending on which side you want to start with, insert the rod into the telescope already placed in the maxilla, and hang the U-loop distally from the slide hook. Close the U-loop with an Adams plier and tie it with a chain or ligature to the slide hook to avoid rotation and biting on the appliance (see Fig. 14.2).

The SUS has a ready-to-fit size providing on average the 5 mm advancement needed. The advancement (and later the activation) can be assessed and monitored by measuring the rest of the sagittal

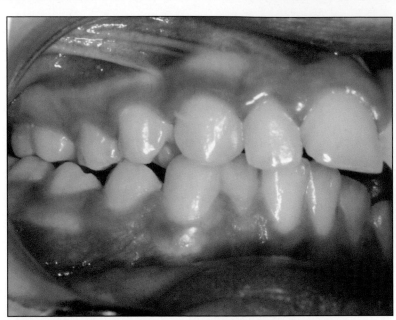

Figure 14.10 Female patient, 11 years and 6 months old, at the beginning of SUS treatment with an 8 mm sagittal step and a transverse deficiency.

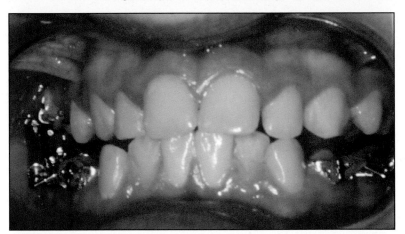

Figure 14.11 Because of the severe crowding a premolar band was used (exceptionally) instead of a canine band for the mandible anchorage unit. Bite jumping using the SUS as a rigid telescope (analogous to the Herbst appliance) lasts about 6 months.

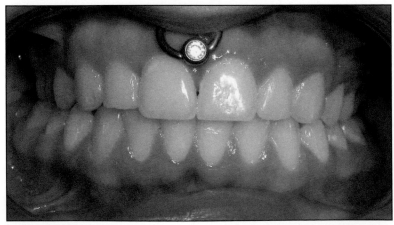

Figure 14.12 The patient after 3 years.

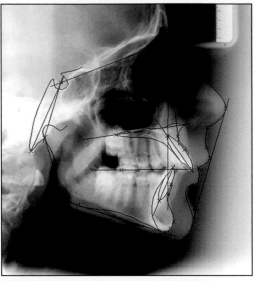

Figures 14.13–14.15 The skeletal and dental changes which occurred assessed by the superimposition of the lateral cephalograms on the nasion-sella line (NSL).

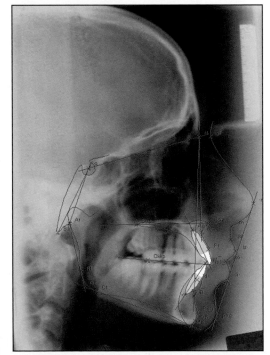

Figure 14.14

step. See the patient every 4 weeks. If necessary, the SUS can be activated or extended by a piece of closed coil spring, with steps not exceeding 5 mm every 8 weeks until the edge-to-edge overcorrection is achieved, and can be maintained for about 8–10 weeks. Check the SUS during opening and closing. If the patient reports any soft tissue discomfort or bites on the appliance, adjust it by changing the position of the distal end of the pin.

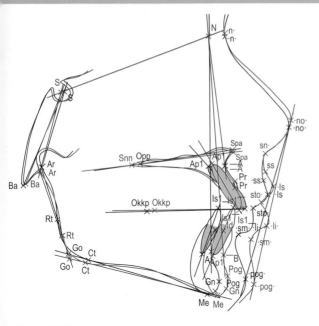

Figure 14.15

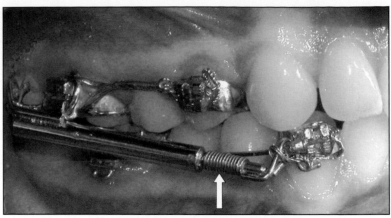

Figure 14.16 The length of the SUS can be extended (if necessary) or it can be activated by a piece of closed coil spring.

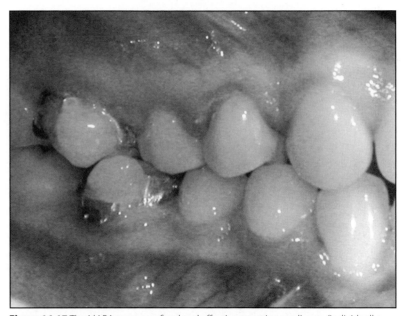

Figure 14.17 The MARA stops as a fixed and effective retention appliance. (Individually constructed passive modification of the MARA appliance.)

Treatment lasts approximately 6–9 months. If a case does not need to be finished using a multibracket system, a bimaxillary appliance such as an activator or Bionator has to be used to stabilize the results. A fixed retention is recommended, especially in severe noncompliance cases, retarded TMJ reaction or adult cases. The MARA stops (individually constructed, passive modification of the MARA appliance, Ormco, Orange, CA) have proved to be very appropriate for effective retention (Fig. 14.17).

However, most of the bite-jumping cases have to be finished using a multibracket system. In these cases, the previously mentioned anchorage system must be removed. The first molar bands in the mandible and the maxilla can be left and they are provided temporarily with MARA stops to maintain the sagittal relationship, similar to treatment with the multibracket system. Class II elastics rarely provide sufficient retention after the jumping phase.

Given the correct indications, we can confidently say that bite jumping with the rigid SUS is an effective way to treat adolescent and adult patients and helps to reduce extraction and surgery, especially in problem cases.

Class II Correction with Dentoalveolar Compensation of the Occlusion (Spring Effect/Class II Elastics Effect)

To achieve a dentoalveolar effect without changing the jaw position (e.g. distalizing the upper molars, mesializing the lower posterior teeth), the spring force must be maximized and activated by turning the middle telescope tube outside the guide tube (screw the slotted screw clockwise with the activation key). The SUS resembles the Herbst appliance but in this configuration it has been designed to provide a spring force (similar to the Jasper Jumper) with the lower jaw not being forced to adopt a ventral position (in contrast to the rigid SUS telescope). While the patient is able to bite in their previous Class II position, the compression of the spring will apply force on the teeth, thus causing orthodontic movement (Figs 14.18–14.21).

Probably due to the unchanged position of the condyles, the MR images showed almost no TMJ remodeling activity. Using this spring variation of the SUS, mainly dentoalveolar changes can be achieved:

- distal movement of the upper molars
- retrusion of the upper incisors
- mesial movement of the lower molars
- protrusion of the lower incisors
- rotation of the occlusal plane in clockwise direction.

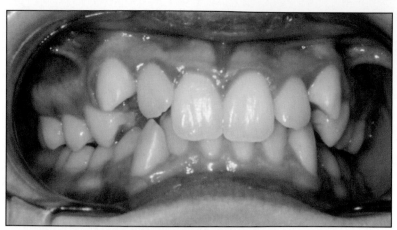

Figure 14.18 Male patient, 13 years and 7 months old, before treatment; Class II division 2, deep bite, anterior crowding.

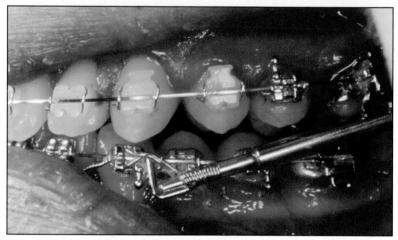

Figure 14.19 The SUS treatment phase lasts about 5 months.

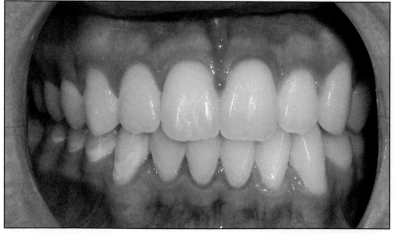

Figure 14.20 The patient at the end of the Bionator retention period (10 months).

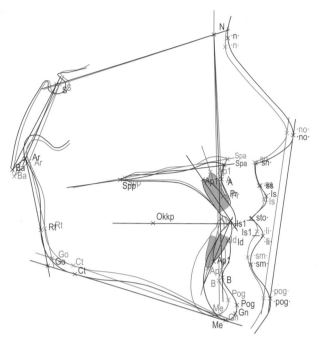

Figure 14.21 The skeletal and dental changes which occurred, assessed by superimposition of the lateral cephalograms on the nasion-sella line (NSL).

In contrast to intermaxillary elastics, the SUS produces pressure forces along the growth direction of the facial skeleton (*y*-axis), while avoiding extrusion which is undesired in most cases.

Practical Considerations

- The spring variation of the SUS can be used to treat moderate Class II cases, simultaneously to the fixed appliances, to replace headgear and Class II elastics and to avoid extraction, especially in noncompliant patients. The profile improvement is usually poor compared to the rigid SUS telescope method.

- Before the SUS is inserted, the transverse dimension must be corrected and the arches developed and leveled.

- The anchorage system consists of a multibracket system with banded first upper and lower molars and a thick rectangular stainless steel archwire for both dental arches. In the maxilla, a TPA must be placed. If larger distalization is desired, the end of the archwire must not be bent and the TPAs have to be passive.

- The lower archwire must be cinched back and tied as a unit; a molar-to-molar chain will help to avoid spacing. A lingual crown torque of the lower incisors is recommended to minimize protrusion.

- See the patient every 4 weeks. The SUS can be activated (if needed) by a piece of open coil spring. The force is adjustable and measurable individually and provides approximately 1 mm movement per month.

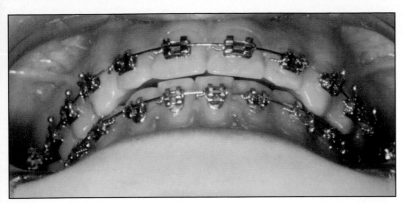

Figures 14.22, 14.23 Female patient, 14 years and 9 months old. Correction of unilateral Class II malocclusion. Situation before the SUS phase.

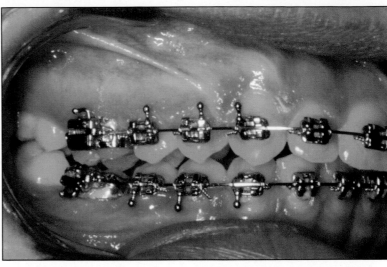

Figure 14.23

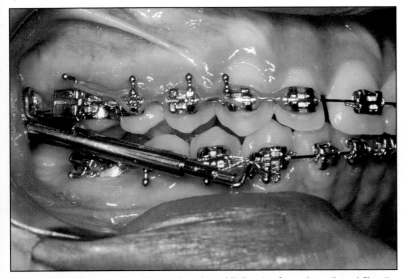

Figure 14.24 After 4 months with gentle unilateral SUS spring force, the unilateral Class II is almost corrected. The slightly open bite on the right side will close spontaneously during the finishing phase.

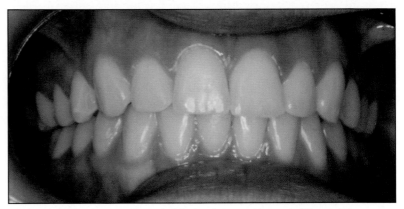

Figure 14.25 The patient at the end of the bionator retention period (9 months).

Setting of the SUS (spring variation) is very similar to fitting the rigid variation as described above, except for the following differences.

- While the rigid telescope variation needs a banded anchorage system with lingual arch, the common multibracket system is sufficient in the spring variation.
- The spring force must be minimized in the rigid variation, but maximized in the spring one.
- To avoid rotation and biting on the appliance, the U-loop must be closed with an Adams plier and tied with a chain or ligature to the slide hook fixed distally of the canine. In the multibracket system, a ligature between the hooks of the canine and the first premolar (over the U-loop) can be used as an alternative to fixation with the slide hook.
- In the rigid variation, activation/extension is achieved by a closed coil spring, whereas in the spring variation activation is done using a piece of open coil spring.

- In the spring variation, the patient is able to bite in their previous Class II position and the compression of the spring will apply force on the teeth, thus causing orthodontic movement, while in the rigid variation the mandible is forced to adopt a ventral position to induce orthopedic changes.

Unilateral Correction of Class II/ Laterognathism

The SUS may also be applied on one side only for correction of unilateral Class II relationships. Tilting of the frontal occlusal plane and a unilateral anterior open bite, frequently seen using the Jasper Jumper,[16] are largely avoided with the SUS due to a moderate and almost horizontal force application.

Application of the spring variation of the SUS enables dentoalveolar correction of unilateral Class II malocclusion (Figs 14.22–14.25) but with almost no profile changes. If improvement of facial symmetry is desired in the treatment of laterognathism, the rigid variation of the SUS including the band anchorage system has to be inserted in the following way. The distal side is repositioned ventrally in 2 mm steps until the mandibular midline is overcorrected by 1 mm. On the Class I side, the SUS is used passively to prevent dorsal compression forces upon the bilaminary zone. However, compared to the SUS treatment, enhanced facial symmetry and profile improvement can be achieved by surgical correction of the laterognathism.

Distalizing/Anchorage of Upper Posterior Teeth (Headgear Substitute)

To replace headgear and Class II elastics, especially in noncompliant patients, the spring force must be maximized and activated by turning the middle telescope tube outside the guide tube (screw the slotted screw clockwise with the activation key). Then the SUS can be fixed like the Jasper Jumper, employing the currently used bracket system (Figs 14.26–14.28).

In contrast to the headgear effect, the SUS produces pressure forces along the growth direction of the facial skeleton (y-axis), while avoiding extrusion, which is undesired in most patients. If greater distalization is needed, the end of the archwire must not be bent and the TPAs have to be passive or removed.

Closing the Lower Jaw Spaces with Maximum Anchorage (Aplasia)

The SUS maintains the upper molars and lower canines and incisors in their position, and helps to mesialize the posterior teeth in the mandible without loss of anchorage. Undesired retrusion of the lower anterior teeth is avoided. This application of the SUS is suitable in aplasia of the second premolars or after extractions in the lower posterior area in order to mesialize molars and premolars (Fig. 14.29).

TMJ Repositioning Effect

The SUS can be used to treat TMJ dysfunction such as dorsal joint compression and displacement of the articular disk. Successful and stable repositioning of the disk crucially depends upon the following prerequisites.[17–19]

- Class II relationship (no Class I or III).
- Evidence of a partial disk displacement with repositioning proved by manual functional diagnosis, dynamic compression, and translation.[20]
- Diagnostic exclusion of articular disk wear (especially of the posterior parts) by means of imaging techniques (MRI).

Advantages of disk repositioning with fixed functional appliances include:

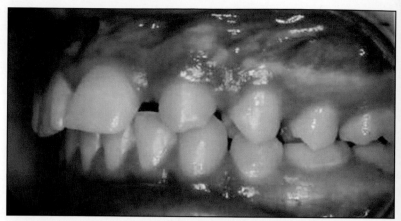

Figure 14.26 Female patient, 13 years and 4 months old, aplasia 12,22.35.

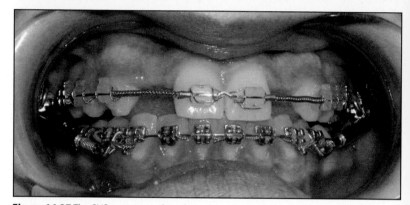

Figure 14.27 The SUS treatment phase lasts about 5 months.

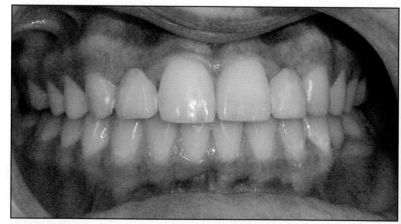

Figure 14.28 A 7.5 mm space was achieved by 12,22, for an appropriate prosthetic reconstruction.

- stable repositioning of the displaced disks (no break relapse), enabling all functions such as eating, speaking, etc. in the new therapeutic click-free TMJ position and thus preventing repeated trauma to the TMJ, in contrast to the traditional removable repositioning splint

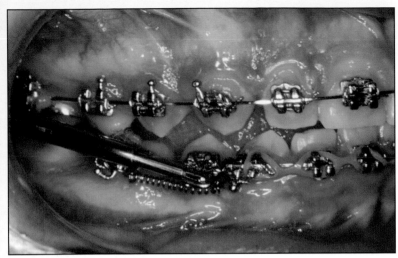

Figure 14.29 A pull coil mesializes the first and second molars; the SUS keeps the canine in its position to avoid loss of anchorage and the undesired retrusion of the lower anterior teeth.

- simultaneous occlusal rehabilitation, which is possible using the multibracket system.

Functional Considerations, TMJ, and Bite Jumping

Functional diagnostics in orthodontics has become an undisputed professional and forensic essential. Early recognition of problem cases helps to avoid treatment errors and functional disorders. Furthermore, manual examination (Fig. 14.30) ensures better prediction of treatment course and provides valuable hints on unfavorable tissue response and jeopardized joint structures. Treatment planning is improved, while relapse and disorders can be avoided or treated. In many cases, a TMJ dysfunction recognized before or during orthodontic therapy is amenable to orthodontic rehabilitation.

Analysis of manual functional diagnostics conducted in our patients before, during, and after treatment showed that the state of the articular capsule and the ligaments was particularly related to the effectiveness and stability of bite jumping. A lax capsule or ligament (soft end-feel by the joint play technique; Fig. 14.31) required longer treatment until bite correction was completed and proved less stable, requiring larger overcorrection and a longer retention period in contrast to a normal (physiologic) articular capsule (hard ligamentary end-feel). The same phenomenon was also observed in treatment using removable functional orthopedic devices.

Hence we think that orthopedic bite jumping is influenced not only by growth direction and potential, type, duration of treatment, and elongation of muscle fibers and tendons, but also by tightening of the healthy capsule and ligaments which have to exert sufficient tensile force to trigger the desired remodeling responses. Obviously, weak or lax capsules/ligaments are unable to build up sufficient tension to stimulate greater bone remodeling. Anterior advance-

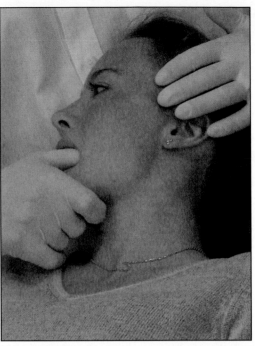

Figure 14.30 One of the important movements in the TMJ manual diagnostic is the passive compression upon the bilaminary zone, which can provide valuable information about possible risks or difficulties during orthodontic treatment.

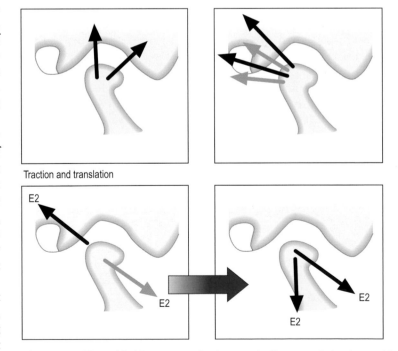

Traction and translation

Figure 14.31 The end feel E2 means weak or lax capsules/ligaments during the caudal traction examination. This joint play technique is part of the functional diagnostics of the TMJ and can easily provide valuable information for better orthodontic planning and treatment.

ment of the condyle appears to compare to a tooth movement which cannot be moved sufficiently and permanently in cases of weakened periodontium.

Naturally, physiologic differences will be observed upon manual examination of the articular capsule and interpretation of the findings. For instance, both capsule and ligaments are physiologically softer in youth and cannot be compared to those of an adult, and are physiologically softer in females than in male patients of the same age. This may be an additional factor accounting for the smaller skeletal effects of the Herbst appliance in female patients observed in several studies.[7]

Patients with TMJ hypermobility (hereditary or traumatic due to frequent surgery) display, in addition to the soft end-feel of capsule and ligaments, an above-average mouth opening and frequently a general connective tissue weakness with several hypermobile joints.

Management of Hypermobility

If hypermobility of the joint exists, a retarded reaction is fairly likely upon bite jumping, especially using removable functional orthopedic appliances. Nevertheless, successful bite correction can be achieved by prolongation of daily wearing time, the whole treatment time, and the retention period in order to compensate for the delayed reaction. However, a fixed bite-jumping appliance exerting a permanent effect would be desirable. Without daily relapse or dependence on patient cooperation, the chances of successful and stable treatment are markedly better despite unfavorable reactions. Nevertheless, the slight yet existing probability of extracting two upper premolars in case of insufficient reaction should be pointed out to the patient.

Studies have shown that the 6-month period of treatment with the Herbst appliance is sufficient to allow reestablishment of a physiologic joint space, while no harmful effects to the TMJ have been described in the literature. Most MRI studies on the Herbst effect, as well as reports from clinicians, showed no deleterious effects.[21] Furthermore, EMG analyses show that the Class II muscle contraction pattern was normalized during Herbst treatment; however, the muscles are likely to need a longer period for permanent adaptation.[22]

Short- and Long-Term Effects

To study the effect of bite jumping using the SUS appliance, 36 patients were selected from our practice (21 females, 15 males). All 36 patients studied displayed a skeletal distal bite with a bilateral dental Class II and were treated using the SUS device. Patient age at insertion averaged 13.2 years, with a range from 12.3 to 15.5 years.[23] Complete diagnostic records were obtained and analyzed at baseline and 6, 12, and 24 months into treatment to document the skeletal and dental changes. The appliance was checked once a month and activated when necessary. Moreover, the patients were interviewed monthly regarding pain, wearing comfort and possible difficulties with chewing, speaking, and brushing.

The skeletal and dental changes which occurred during treatment were assessed by superimposition of the lateral cephalograms on the nasion–sella line (NSL). The lateral cephalograms were analyzed by one person at two different time points. The longitudinal differences in the metric variables were tested for statistical significance at $\alpha=0.05$ using the Wilcoxon test. Cast analysis included measurements of the anterior and posterior widths of the upper and lower dental arches, overjet, overbite, and the occlusion of first molars and canines.

The normalization of the sagittal discrepancy using the SUS was achieved through skeletal and (prevailing) dentoalveolar changes. Both the ANB angle and the Wits variable changed significantly, while the SNA angle remained largely stable during treatment. This indicates an indirect growth inhibition of the maxilla when considering the increase of the SNA angle shown in Class II children without orthodontic treatment.[24] Only a slight increase was observed in the vertical dimension. The mandibular plane angle (ML-NSL), the maxillo-mandibular base angle (ML-NL), and the nasal plane angle (NL-NSL) did not change significantly. However, striking changes were observed in the occlusal planes which displayed a rotation towards bite opening. Also, marked dental changes were seen, particularly distalization and intrusion of the first upper molars, intrusion of the first premolars, and slight protrusion of the lower anterior teeth. These dental effects partly account for the bite-opening effect.

Cast analysis showed that the frequently reported expansion of the upper and lower arches scarcely ever occurred, due to the stabilization by the TPA or the RPE device.

Despite the numerous studies available, fixed functional orthodontic appliances do not lend themselves to an easy comparison, since the varying results are caused by many different factors such as patient age and gender, number of subjects, duration of treatment and retention, heterogeneous measurements and analyses, and the difficulty in reproducing measuring points. Not forgetting the individual reaction pattern, growth potential, and direction of the patient.[2,25,26] However, the above-mentioned findings clearly show greater agreement with studies with the Herbst appliance than with the Jasper Jumper, especially regarding changes of the SNB angle, tilting of the occlusal plane, and protrusion of the lower anterior teeth. Remarkably, tilting of the occlusal planes and protrusion of the upper front were more marked with the Jasper Jumper.[4,6,22,27–31]

The long-term cephalometric records obtained during retention showed that the maxilla partly resumed growth, which led to an increase of the SNA angle. Some patients displayed a slight retrusion of the lower incisors leading to an increase of overbite and overjet. These changes were smaller in cases stabilized with MARA stops and 3-3 retainers.

This fixed functional treatment can provide (in some adult borderline distal bite cases) sufficient dentoalveolar compensation and TMJ adaptation to manage treatment without surgical correction. Comparison of the outcomes and different effects between surgical and functional correction of borderline cases shows good results in both methods. However, skeletal changes and improvement in the soft tissues and profile are more marked in the surgery cases, i.e. we have to choose surgery if profound profile improvement is needed.

Retention, Stability and Relapse, Problem Solving

Like treatment with many other orthodontic appliances, the use of the SUS device is not relapse free. Stable intercuspation is the best guarantee of long-term outcome stability. Therefore, fixed appliance treatment is strongly recommended following therapy with the SUS. The SUS allows simultaneous multibracket treatment and mandibular protrusion (Herbst effect). Thus, maximum stabilization is achieved during multibracket treatment, leading to optimum retention and less relapse. A functional orthodontic device might serve as a retention device following treatment with fixed appliances. However, the previously described MARA stops have been proved to be most suitable.

For these reasons, treatment with fixed functional orthodontic appliances is not recommended in the mixed dentition except for special cases. Sometimes, recessions may form in the lower anterior teeth area, particularly if gingival attachment is low. A mucosal graft is recommended in such patients. Careful pretreatment, including correction of TMJ dysfunctions, habits and occlusal interference, has been proved to be very conducive to treatment stability.

If the lower anterior teeth are already protruded, the SUS device may cause undesired further protrusion. A large anchorage unit (bands and lingual arch) or a mandibular splint can reduce protrusion. In cases of complete mandibular banding, the following measures can minimize this side effect:

- use and sufficient bending of the thickest possible steel archwire
- lingual crown torque for the lower incisors
- lower archwire must be cinched back and tied as a unit
- molar-to-molar chain will help to avoid spacing and protrusion.

In contrast to other appliances, construction of the SUS relies neither on plastic parts nor on closed tubes for hygienic reasons and in order to avoid halitosis. The SUS is entirely open, so the salivary flow contributes to good hygienic conditions. However, calculus may accumulate on the inside of the telescope, especially in predisposed patients. In these cases, squirting Vaseline into the telescope may be helpful.

Technical difficulties may arise through disregard of the manufacturer's instructions, especially if securing of the pin in the maxilla or the U-loop in the mandible is omitted or insufficient (see Practical considerations, above).

Unlike most similar devices, the SUS consists of pieces which can be ordered separately. Should one piece of the SUS fail to function properly, it can easily and rapidly be replaced without removal of the entire appliance.

Limited mouth opening, especially while yawning, which was reported during treatment with the Jasper Jumper and similar appliances,[16,32] was not mentioned by the SUS patients. Owing to its telescopic construction, the SUS cannot restrict mouth opening. However, the telescope rod may slip out of the middle telescope in patients with TMJ hypermobility and mouth opening exceeding 60 mm (25% above average). The routine manual TMJ examination preceding any treatment should alert the clinician to this rare problem; the patient should be informed and instructed how to reassemble the SUS which in most cases is easier than inserting a headgear. If necessary, physiotherapeutic muscle building (rotation exercises) can counteract hypermobility and may also be indicated for TMJ preventive reasons.[17–19]

Conclusion

Most of the fixed functional appliances yield good improvement of sagittal discrepancy. Using telescopic appliances such as the Herbst and SUS devices, more marked skeletal changes and profile improvement can be achieved.

The SUS combines the advantages of telescopic and flexible fixed appliances, minimizes their complications, reduces chair time and thus provides an alternative appliance to treat Class II malocclusions.

References

1. Herbst E. Atlas und Grundriss der Zahnärztlichen Orthopädie. Munich: J. F. Lehmann Verlag; 1910.
2. Aelbers CMF, Dermaut LR. Orthopädie in der Orthodontie – Ein Literaturüberblick. Inf Orthod Kieferorthop 1999;31:65–79.
3. Pancherz H. Treatment of Class II malocclusions by jumping the bite with the Herbst appliance. A cephalometric investigation. Am J Orthod 1979; 76:423–442.
4. Pancherz H. The effect of continuous bite jumping on the dentofacial complex: a follow-up study after Herbst appliance treatment of Class II malocclusions. Eur J Orthod 1981;3:49–60.
5. Wieslander L. Intensive treatment of severe Class II malocclusions with a headgear-Herbst appliance in the early mixed dentition. Am J Orthod 1984; 861:1–13.
6. Wong GW, So LL, Hagg U. A comparative study of sagittal correction with the Herbst appliance in two different ethnic groups. Eur J Orthod 1997;19: 195–204.
7. Ruf S, Pancherz H. Dentoskeletal effects and facial profile changes in young adults treated with the Herbst appliance. Angle Orthod 1999;69: 239–246.
8. Ruf S, Pancherz H. The mechanism of Class II correction during Herbst therapy in relation to the vertical jaw base relationship: a cephalometric roentgenographic study. Angle Orthod 1997;67: 271–276.
9. Pancherz H, Ruf S, Kohlhas P. "Effective condylar growth" and chin position changes in Herbst treatment: a cephalometric roentgenographic long-term study. Am J Orthod Dentofacial Orthop 1998;114:437–446.
10. Schindler S. Dentoskelettale und faziale Veränderungen bei der Distalbissbehandlung (Klasse II-1) von Erwachsenen mit der Herbst-/Multibracket-Apparatur: eine roentgen-kephalometrische Untersuchung. Doctorate degree thesis. Giessen, Germany: University of Giessen; 2004. Available online at: http://geb.uni-giessen.de/geb/volltexte/2004/1392/
11. Rabie AB, Wong L, Tsai M. Replicating mesenchymal cells in the condyle and the glenoid fossa during

mandibular forward positioning. Am J Orthod Dentofacial Orthop 2003;123:49–57.

12. Xiong H, Hagg U, Tang GH, Rabie AB, Robinson W. The effect of continuous bite-jumping in adult rats: a morphological study. Angle Orthod 2004;74:86–92.

13. McNamara JA Jr. Neuromuscular and skeletal adaptations to altered function in the orofacial region. Am J Orthod 1973;64:578–606.

14. McNamara JA Jr, Hinton RJ, Hoffman DL. Histologic analysis of temporomandibular joint adaptation to protrusive function in young adult rhesus monkeys (Macaca mulatta). Am J Orthod 1982;82:288–298.

15. Du X, Hagg U, Rabie AB. Effects of headgear Herbst and mandibular step-by-step advancement versus conventional Herbst appliance and maximal jumping of the mandible. Eur J Orthod 2002; 24:167–174.

16. Schwindling F-P. Jasper Jumper™ Bildatlas. Merzig: Edition Schwindling; 1995: 75–82.

17. Sabbagh A. Kiefergelenkdysfunktion. Teil I, ZMK Nr. 3. Nuremberg: Spitta Verlag; 2000: 130,133.

18. Sabbagh A. Kiefergelenkdysfunktion. Teil II, ZMK Nr. 4. Nuremberg: Spitta Verlag; 2000: 210–212.

19. Sabbagh A. Kiefergelenkdysfunktion. Teil III, ZMK Nr. 5. Nuremberg: Spitta Verlag; 2000: 294–298.

20. Bumann A, Lotzmann U. Funktionsdiagnostik und Therapieprinzipien. Stuttgart, Germany: Thieme Verlag; 2000: 98–121.

21. Richter U, Richter F. An MRI-monitored investigation of condyle-fossa relationship during Herbst appliance treatment. Orthodontics 2004;1:43–51.

22. Pancherz H. The Herbst appliance – its biologic effects and clinical use. Am J Orthod 1985;87: 1–20.

23. Sabbagh A. Die Korrektur der Distalbisslage durch eine vereinfachte Herbstapparatur – die SUS Apparatur. Proceedings of the 76th Annual meeting of the German Orthodontic Society, September 10–14, 2003. Munich: German Orthodontic Society; 2003: 5 (Abstr. #4).

24. Gesch D. A longitudinal study on growth in untreated children with Angle Class II, division 1 malocclusion. J Orofac Orthop 2000;61:20–33.

25. Ehmer U, Tulloch CJ, Proffit WR, Phillips C. An international comparison of early treatment of angle Class-II/1 cases. Skeletal effects of the first phase of a prospective clinical trial. J Orofac Orthop 1999;60:392–408.

26. McNamara JA Jr, Howe RP, Dischinger TG. A comparison of the Herbst and Frankel appliances in the treatment of Class II malocclusion. Am J Orthod Dentofacial Orthop 1990;98:134–144.

27. Pancherz H. The mechanism of Class II correction in Herbst appliance treatment. A cephalometric investigation. Am J Orthod 1982;82:104–113.

28. Pancherz H, Hansen K. Occlusal changes during and after Herbst treatment: a cephalometric investigation. Eur J Orthod 1986;8:215–228.

29. Covell DA Jr, Trammell DW, Boero RP, West R. A cephalometric study of Class II division 1 malocclusions treated with the Jasper Jumper appliance. Angle Orthod 1999;69:311–320.

30. Stucki N, Ingervall B. The use of the Jasper Jumper for the correction of Class II malocclusion in the young permanent dentition. Eur J Orthod 1998;20:271–281.

31. Weiland FJ, Ingervall B, Bantleon HP, Droschl H. Initial effects of treatment of Class II malocclusion with the Herren activator, activator-headgear combination, and Jasper Jumper. Am J Orthod Dentofacial Orthop 1997;112:19–27.

32. Blackwood HO. Clinical management of the Jasper Jumper. J Clin Orthod 1991;25:755–760.

SECTION THREE

INTRAMAXILLARY DISTALIZATION APPLIANCES USED FOR THE MANAGEMENT OF CLASS II NONCOMPLIANT PATIENTS

This section includes chapters on the following:

Overview of the intramaxillary noncompliance distalization appliances

Moschos A. Papadopoulos

Appliances with a Flexible Distalization Force System Palatally Positioned

The main noncompliance appliances that use a flexible molar distalization force system which is palatally positioned are the Pendulum Appliance[1] and the Distal Jet Appliance[2] (see Table 2.2). Other appliances of the same category include the Intraoral Bodily Molar Distalizer,[3] the Simplified Molar Distalizer,[4] the Keles Slider,[5] Nance Appliances in conjunction with nickel-titanium (NiTi) open coil springs as proposed by Reiner[6] and Bondemark,[7] and the Fast Back Appliance.[8]

Pendulum Appliance

The Pendulum Appliance was first introduced by Hilgers[1] and consists of a large acrylic Nance button, that covers the midportion of the palate for anchorage, and two 0.032″ TMA springs (Ormco Corporation, Orange, CA) that are the active elements for molar distalization, delivering a light, continuous, and pendulum-like force from the midline of the palate to the upper molars.[1,9]

The Nance button usually extends from the maxillary first molars anteriorly to just posterior to the lingual papilla[10] and is stabilized with four retaining wires that extend bilaterally and are bonded as occlusal rests to the upper first and second premolars or to the first and second deciduous molars[11] (see Fig. 16.1). Alternatively, the two posterior wires can be soldered to first premolars or first deciduous molar bands, thus adding to the stability of the appliance.

Each of the two TMA springs consists of a recurved molar insertion wire, a small horizontal adjustment loop, a closed helix, and a loop for retention in the acrylic button.[1] These springs are mounted as close as possible to the center and distal aspects of the Nance button and when in a passive state, they extend posteriorly, almost parallel to the midpalatal raphe. When activated, each of the spring is inserted into a 0.036″ lingual sheath on bands cemented on the maxillary first molars, which produces almost 60° of activation, delivering a distalizing force of approximately 230 g that moves the molars distally and medially (see Fig. 16.4).[1,9,10]

After the initial activation of the springs, the patients should be seen usually every 3–4 weeks in order to check the spring pressure and to perform appropriate adjustments if needed.[1,9,10] According to Hilgers,[1] approximately 5 mm of distal molar movement can be achieved in a period of 3–4 months.

Modifications of the Pendulum Appliance

Pendex Appliance

The design of the Pendex Appliance is essentially the same as the pendulum appliance except for the addition of a midpalatal jackscrew into the center of the Nance button[1] (see Fig. 16.3). Therefore, it can be used when expansion of the maxillary arch is needed or to avoid the tendency toward transverse maxillary constriction during distalization. According to Hilgers,[1] the screw should be activated one-quarter turn every 3 days, after a week for patient adjustment, to produce a slow and stable expansion. Byloff & Darendeliler[12] have used this design but, in contrast to the recommendation of Hilgers,[1] they activated the pendulum springs by 45° instead of 60° with an initial force varying between 200 and 250 g, resulting in the need to reactivate them once ore twice during treatment. Further, in order to avoid distal tipping of the molars, Byloff et al used uprighting bends of 10–15° at the recurved end of the springs, which can be performed intraorally following the distal crown movement.[13]

Hilgers Palatal Expander

One year before the introduction of the Pendex Appliance, Hilgers introduced the Palatal Expander, a noncompliance device for maxillary molar distalization and expansion.[14] The appliance consists of two molar bands with soldered horizontal helices made from a 0.036″ stainless steel wire and an acrylic plate with an embedded jackscrew. Two anterior extensions of the wire are bonded occlusally on the first premolars or the first deciduous molars. The helices serve to rotate and distalize the first maxillary molars, using the soft tissue palate as anchorage in almost the same way as a large Nance button, while the jackscrew produces an orthopedic midpalatal dysjunction.

Penguin Pendulum Appliance (Mayes' Penguin Design)

This appliance is different from the pendulum appliance in three different aspects (see Fig. 17.1).[15] First, there is no expansion screw. If expansion is needed, this occurs prior to insertion of the appliance with a Hyrax Appliance. Second, the springs are fabricated with the distalizing arm as close to parallel to the molar root as possible in order to prevent buccal or lingual movement while allowing rotation of the tooth if required (see Fig. 17.3).[15] Third, the appliance is much thinner (2–3 mm) to avoid creating an iatrogenic tongue thrust and to allow easy patient adaptation. The Mayes Penguin Appliance in its latest version uses TMA removable springs, which can be activated without violating the TMA loop (see Fig. 17.2). The springs are activated at about a 45° angle to the distal. Reactivations follow at 7–8 week intervals.

Hilgers PhD Appliance

In contrast to the standard pendulum design, the PhD Appliance uses an occlusally bonded Hyrax Expander without any palatal acrylic, "locking wires" soldered to the molar bands allowing the appliance to act as an expander prior to molar distalization, and 0.027″ TMA pendulum springs seated into sheaths which have been laser welded to the palatal side of the screw body.[16] The PhD Appliance is fixed to the dentition by first premolar bands, when possible, and bondable occlusal rests on the second premolars or second deciduous molars. Alternatively, occlusal rests on the first premolars can be used. Expansion of the maxillary arch is performed before molar distalization, while the upper arch is stabilized by means of full bracketing and sectional archwires that extend from the second premolar to the midline, allowing the maxilla to unlock. Before appliance cementation, the springs are preactivated to the midline and placed into the lingual sheaths of the molars to deliver a distalizing force of approximately 175 g. After the expansion has been completed, the "locking wires" are cut off, allowing the molars to move distally. The appliance is used until the first maxillary molars have been distalized to a slightly overcorrected Class I occlusion.[17]

GrumRax Appliance

The GrumRax Appliance was developed by Grummons[18] and it is very similar to the Hilgers PhD Appliance. However, in the GrumRax Appliance, there are always occlusal rests on the first maxillary premolars, the design of the TMA spring includes horizontal adjustment loops, and there are no "locking wires." The appliance can act simultaneously in all three planes of space by widening the palate, distalizing the molars, and controlling the vertical dimension at the molars.

T-Rex Appliance

The T-Rex Appliance is a fixed rapid palatal expander that incorporates the rotation and distalization parts of the Pendulum Appliance.[19] Actually, the only difference between the T-Rex and the Pendex appliances is that the expansion screw is soldered mesial to the molar tubes to make the appliance rigid enough for rapid palatal expansion, while neutralizing the effect of the pendulum springs during the initial expansion phase. The acrylic part of the appliance, including a large Nance button, is connected to the dentition in the same way as the Pendex Appliance. The TMA springs should be preactivated 8–10 mm distally, but with a distance of 5–6 mm from the palatal tissue.

Tracey/Hilgers MDA Expander (Mini-Distalizing Appliance)

This appliance consists of a compact expansion screw, the compact rapid palatal expander (RPE) (Ormco Corporation, Orange, CA), which is soldered to bands on the maxillary first premolars and can expand up to 11 mm, and two 0.032″ TMA pendulum springs which deliver a constant force for reliable molar distalization.[20] The TMA springs are secured into sheaths that have been laser welded to the palatal side of the compact RPE. After the appliance is cemented, the lingual arms can be bonded to the palatal aspects of the second premolars or deciduous molars in order to enhance anchorage, especially for maxillary expansion. Fixed appliances on the maxillary arch and sectional wires extending from the second premolars to the midline can also be used to increase anchorage. To add rigidity to the appliance while allowing for expansion, stainless steel ligatures can be used to tie back the TMA springs to the RPE screw legs or locking wires soldered from the appliance at the premolar bands to the molar bands. Once expansion is achieved, the expansion screw can be sealed with light cure acrylic and the ligature wires can be released or the locking wires cut to allow molar distalization. In addition, the bond on the palatal aspect of the second premolars can be removed to allow these teeth to drift distally along with the maxillary first molars.

M-Pendulum Appliance

The M-Pendulum presents the following differences in comparison to the Pendulum or Pendex appliances.[21] The adjustment loops of the TMA springs are not distally oriented but are reversed to the mesial to provide bodily movement of the maxillary molars, rather than distal tipping and rotation. The TMA springs are activated initially by 40–45°, exerting a force of 125 g per side, and they can be removable. Further, in cases of excessive overjet or when anchorage is very important, as in patients with reduced periodontal support or excessive lower anterior facial height, four removable springs can be used bilaterally instead of two, for both first and second maxillary molars.[22] In this case the molars are distalized sequentially rather than simultaneously to decrease the pressure exerted by the appliance.

Once the second molars have been distalized, it is suggested that the corresponding springs are left passively in place for anchorage and the first molar springs are activated.[22] Following molar distalization, the appliance can be replaced by a Nance button and the treatment can be continued with comprehensive fixed appliances.

The M-Pendulum can produce a molar distalization of about 5 mm in 3–4 months. When removable springs are used, the distalization can reach a rate of 1.5 mm per month.[23]

K-Pendulum Appliance

The K-Pendulum differs from the Pendex Appliance in that it is fitted with a distal (sagittal) screw and integrated uprighting activation for the molars[24] (see Fig. 16.2). The distal screw divides the Nance button in two parts, the anterior part which provides anchorage and the posterior part including the repositioned pendulum springs. The springs are placed close to the palatal midline, while their helices are positioned as dorsal as possible to the maxillary first molars.[24] The activation of the distal screw can vary, depending on the requirements of each individual case. When the screw is activated, the sagittal center of rotation is repositioned and further molar distalization takes place due to the repositioning of the arc and the resulting automatic activation of the pendulum springs. In this way, the pendulum-like arc movement of the molars is altered and the tendency to posterior crossbites is minimized, while there is no need to activate the adjustment loop, which can result in extrusion forces.[24] Finally, one activation of the TMA springs is enough and there is no need for further reactivations during distalization.

Bipendulum and Quad Pendulum Appliances

Both appliances were introduced by Kinzinger et al[25] and consist of a Nance button and two removable Pendulum TMA springs placed unilaterally (bipendulum) or four removable springs placed bilaterally (quad pendulum), which allow distalization of the second and first maxillary molars in sequence. The appliance is fixed to the dentition in a similar way to the standard Pendulum Appliance. The springs are seated in palatal sheaths, originally provided for the molar bands, integrated into the acrylic button.

When starting with the distalization of the second molars, the first molars should be excluded from the anchorage block, if possible, to allow them to drift distally. After the second molars are sufficiently distalized, their corresponding springs are deactivated to increase the

anchorage for the distalization of the first molars that follows. During treatment, the TMA springs can be replaced with other springs with appropriately longer retention components, to achieve a shift in the horizontal and sagittal centers of molar rotation, in a similar way to the K-Pendulum.

Intraoral Bodily Molar Distalizer (IBMD)

The Intraoral Bodily Molar Distalizer (IBMD) was introduced by Keles & Sayinsu.[3] The appliance consists of two parts: an anchorage unit which includes a wide Nance acrylic button and an active unit with the distalizing 0.032 × 0.032″ TMA springs made of square sectioned wire to achieve improved control in the transverse plane. In addition, bands are placed on the maxillary first molars and premolars, 0.045″ stainless steel retaining wires are attached to the premolar bands and 0.032 × 0.032″ slot size cap palatal attachments are welded on the palatal side of the first molar bands.

The springs consist of two sections, the distalizing section which exerts a crown tipping force and the uprighting section which applies a root uprighting force to the first molars.[3] In contrast to the Pendulum Appliance, the springs distalize the upper first molars towards the direction in which the springs are inactive, exerting a distalizing force of Approximately 230 g. The Nance acrylic button is very wide, covering the palatal surfaces of the incisors as much as possible, to obtain support from a wider palatal tissue to increase the anterior anchorage. Thus, it functions as an anterior bite plane to help deep bite correction and to enhance molar distalization by discluding the posterior teeth.[3]

Class I molar relationship can be accomplished in an average period of 7.5 months. Then, the molars are stabilized for almost 2 months with a conventional Nance Appliance attached to the hinge caps, thus providing easy removal of the appliance in case of soft tissue irritation and for cleaning. Following the stabilization period, full fixed appliances are used as the second phase of the overall treatment.[3]

Simplified Molar Distalizer

The Simplified Molar Distalizer (SMD) (TP Orthodontics Inc., LaPorte, IN) consists of a Nance button, TMA pendulum springs, and a distal screw.[4] The springs of the SMD are removable and positioned through their middle segment into a slot on the distal side of the screw, and they are constructed from 032″ TMA or stainless steel wire. Further, they do not include helices but only horizontal adjustment loops mesially directed.[4] According to Walde, the appliance can distalize the maxillary first molars at a rate of 1–2 mm per month.[4] The activation of the screw requires minimal chair time and is performed intraorally, while each 360° turn of the screw can open the appliance 0.5 mm. The patient should be followed up every 4–8 weeks, depending on the amount of activation, and when the desired distalization has been achieved, the appliance screw should be stabilized with composite resin or acrylic to avoid back-up. Then the appliance can be disconnected from the premolars and is maintained in position for anchorage while the premolars and canines are distalized.

Distal Jet™

The Distal Jet™ Appliance (American Orthodontics, Sheboygan, WI) was introduced by Carano & Testa in 1996.[2] It consists mainly of two bayonet wires inserted in two bilateral tubes embedded in a modified acrylic Nance button (see Figs 18.1 and 18.2). The Nance button acts as an anchorage unit, while the active part of the appliance consists of a telescopic unit incorporating two NiTi or stainless steel springs with screw clamps, sliding through two 0.036″ internal diameter tubes attached bilaterally to the Nance button.[2] A wire, which ends in a bayonet bend, is inserted in the lingual sheath of the first molar bands and the free end is inserted like a piston into the bilateral tubes.[2,26–28] The telescopic unit and presumably the line of action of the distal jet should be parallel to the occlusal plane and located approximately 4–5 mm apical from the maxillary molars centroid, so that the force produced passes as close as possible to the centers of resistance of the molars.[2,29]

In the standard design of the distal jet, the Nance button should be constructed as large as possible to increase stability, extending about 5 mm from the teeth.[2] Usually, the Nance button is retained with wires extending bilaterally and soldered to bands on the first premolars,[28] the second premolars or the second deciduous molars.[2,26,27] Alternatively, the retaining wires can be bonded as occlusal rests to the maxillary first or second premolars.[2,28]

To activate the appliance, the screw clamp is moved distally, thus compressing the coil spring and creating a distalization force which is applied to the molar band for a period of 3–10.5 months,[2,26–28,30] until correction of Class II malocclusion[27] or a super Class I relationship has been achieved.[31] During this period the patient should be monitored every 4–6 weeks for further adjustments.[2,26,27,31]

Modifications of the Distal Jet

Modified Distal Jet Appliance

This modification of the distal jet, proposed by Quick & Harris,[32] is based on a rear entry of the sliding part into the lingual sheath, which allows the molars to be pulled distally. In this way, the double-back wire is inserted into the lingual sheath from the distal, allowing easier insertion and reactivation of the appliance, and is tied back with an elastomeric or stainless steel ligature. The appliance is activated by compressing the coil spring into the distal end of the supporting tube and a stop is soldered to the sliding wire. To reactivate the appliance, the safety ligature is cut, the sliding wire is pulled out distally, and a new, longer coil spring is inserted. Therefore, there is no need for set-screws to be used. According to Quick & Harris,[32] 4 mm of distal molar movement can be achieved in 3.5 months.

Keles Slider

The Keles Slider (US Patent No. 6, 626, 665 B1) was developed by Keles in 2001 for unilateral or bilateral noncompliance molar distalization.[5] It consists of a Nance button with an anterior bite plane, tubes soldered palatally to the maxillary first molars, 0.036″ wire rods for sliding of the first molars, 0.036″ heavy NiTi open coil springs, and screws to activate the spring[5,33,34] (see Fig. 19.1). In detail, the anchorage unit of the Keles Slider consists of a wide Nance button to minimize anchorage loss, including an anterior bite plane to disclude the posterior teeth, enhance the distal molar movement and correct the anterior deep bite. The acrylic Nance button is usually stabilized with retaining wires attached to bands on the maxillary first premolars, allowing the second premolars to drift distally with the help of transseptal fibers.[5,34]

The active unit of the appliance consists of several parts (see Fig. 19.2).[5,33,34] Tubes 1.1 mm in diameter are soldered palatally on the first molar bands and a 0.9 mm stainless steel wire is inserted in the acrylic about 5 mm apical to the first molar gingival margin, passing through the tube and parallel to the occlusal plane. A helix is placed at the distal end of the steel rod to control the amount of the distal molar movement and prevent any disconnection of the tube from the rod. NiTi coil springs are positioned between the screw on the wire and the tube in full compression, thus producing approximately 200 g of distalizing force to the molars. To inactivate the appliance before cementing it, another screw is placed at the distal side of the tube, which is then removed to activate the appliance. After placement of the appliance, the patient is monitored once a month and the screws can be reactivated if necessary.

According to Keles,[5] this biomechanical design aims to apply a consistent distal force at the level of the center of resistance of the first molar, thus producing a more bodily distal molar movement.

Nance Appliance with NiTi Coil Springs

The use of a Nance Appliance in conjunction with NiTi Coil Springs for unilateral maxillary molar distalization was first introduced by Reiner,[6] while a similar appliance for bilateral distalization of the maxillary first molars was introduced by Bondemark.[7]

The appliance developed by Reiner[6] is a modification of the traditional Nance holding arch and consists of an active Class II side, where molar distalization takes place, and an inactive Class I side. The inactive Class I side consists of a 0.036″ stainless steel wire framework ending in an anteriorly projecting arm like that of a quad-helix, to resist the horizontal moment which can cause distal molar rotation and expansion in the premolar area. The active Class II side, where molar distalization takes place, consist also of an arm bend like the quad-helix with the anterior end soldered to the first premolar band. An omega loop is soldered to the anterior end of the framework to allow the distal sliding of the loop when it is opened for activation. A 0.036″ open coil spring 10 mm long is positioned between the omega loop and the first molar band assembly. A 0.045″ tube is soldered on the lingual side of the first molar band and connected to the wire arm with the framework moving through the tube, thus allowing sliding of the band assembly. Following the appliance cementation, the omega loop is opened to compress the coil spring to a length of 7 mm, which delivers a distalization force of approximately 150 g. The patients are then monitored at 2-week intervals for further adjustments and reactivations until Class I molar relationship has been achieved.

The intraarch NiTi coil appliance proposed by Bondemark[7] for bilateral distalization of both first and second molars also consists of an anchorage unit and an active unit. The anchorage unit includes a modified Nance Appliance and a 0.9 mm lingual archwire soldered to bands on the maxillary second premolars. This lingual archwire has two distal pistons that pass through the palatal tubes of the first molars, which are parallel to the pistons both occlusally and sagittally. The active unit consists of a 10–14 mm long NiTi Coil Spring (GAC International Inc., Islandia, NY), 0.012″ in diameter with a lumen of 0.045″, which is inserted into the distal piston. The spring is compressed to half its length when the tube of the molar band is adapted to the distal piston of the lingual archwire, thus activating the spring and producing an initial distalization force of approximately 200 g, which falls to 180 g as the molars are distalized. No further activation is required during the distalization phase of the treatment.

Fast Back Appliance

The Fast Back Appliance (Leone SpA, Firenze, Italy) consists of a Nance acrylic button for anchorage, two palatally positioned sagittal screws, and superelastic open Memoria® Coil Springs (Leone SpA, Firenze, Italy).[8] The Nance button is stabilized with extension wires soldered on the first premolar bands and includes also the mesial parts of the screws. Each screw incorporates two wire arms. The mesial one is soldered on the first premolars, while the distal one passes through the palatal first molar tube and incorporates also an open Memoria Coil Spring that delivers a distalization force of approximately 200–300 g on the maxillary first molars. A self-locking terminal stop with a hole is added at the distal end of this arm for safety reasons. After the first molars are distalized 1.5–2 mm, the screws can be activated to compress the coil springs, thus maintaining the distalization force. Once the required distalization has been accomplished, the first molars can be maintained in position by tying a stainless steel ligature between the molar tubes and the hole of the self-locking terminal stop.

Appliances with a Flexible Distalization Force System Buccally Positioned

Among the appliances that use a flexible distalization force system which is buccally positioned, the Jones Jig[35] is one of the most commonly used in noncompliance Class II orthodontic treatment (see Table 2.2). Modifications of the Jones Jig include the Lokar Molar Distalizing Appliance[36] and the Sectional Jig Assembly.[37] Nickel-titanium coil springs in conjunction mainly with Nance buttons,[38,39] repelling magnets,[7,40–45] and NiTi wires[46–49] also belong to this category. The last group of appliances in this category are the various distalizing arches, including among others the Bimetric

Distalizing Arch introduced by Wilson[50] and the Molar Distalization Bow of Jeckel & Rakosi,[51] the acrylic distalization splints,[52,53] and the Carriere Distalizer.[54] It should be noted, however, that these latter devices require some patient compliance, since they can be removable, or they have to be used in conjunction with Class II elastics.

Jones Jig™

The Jones Jig™ (American Orthodontics, Sheboygan, WI) was introduced by Jones & White[35] and includes an active unit positioned buccally consisting of active arms or jig assemblies incorporating NiTi Open Coil Springs and an anchorage unit consisting of a modified Nance Appliance.

The modified Nance is stabilized with 0.036″ stainless steel wires that extend bilaterally and are soldered to bands on the maxillary first or second premolars or to deciduous second molars[35,55,56] (see Fig. 20.2). The jig assembly consists of a 0.036″ wire, which holds the NiTi Open Coil Spring and a sliding eyelet tube.[55] Further, an additional stabilizing wire is attached along with a hook to the distal portion of the main wire (see Fig. 20.1). Thus the jig assembly includes in its distal end two arms, which are used to stabilize the appliance.

After cementation of the modified Nance Appliance, the main arm of the Jones Jig is inserted into the headgear tube and the stabilizing arm is inserted into the archwire slot of the maxillary first molar buccal attachment.[55–58] In addition, the distal hook of the Jones Jig is tied with a stainless steel ligature to the hook of the buccal molar tube to further increase stability. The appliance is activated by tying back the sliding hook to the anchor teeth (first or second premolars), with a stainless steel ligature, thus compressing the open coil spring 1–5 mm (see Fig. 20.3). The activated open coil spring can produce approximately 70–75 g of continuous distalizing force to the maxillary first molars for a period of 2.5–9 months.[35,55–59] The patient is monitored every 4–5 weeks for further adjustments[35,55–57] and the maxillary molars are distalized until a Class I relationship has been achieved.[35,56,57]

Modifications of the Jones Jig

Lokar Appliance

The Lokar Appliance (Ormco Corporation, Orange, CA) consists of a nickel-titanium coil spring activated by a mesial sliding sleeve (mesial component) and an appropriately sized rectangular wire (distal component) which is inserted into the archwire tube of the first molar.[36] For anchorage, a Nance acrylic button can be used, which is stabilized to the second maxillary premolars with a 0.040″ stainless steel wire. Alternatively, fixed appliances can also be used. In addition, extraoral and lip bumper forces may be applied at the same time because the molar tubes are not used. After cementation of the molar bands and the Nance button, the Lokar Appliance is inserted into the archwire tube of the first molar and activated by tying back the mesial component by a ligature wire to the second premolars, thus compressing the spring.

Modified Sectional Jig Assembly

The Modified Sectional Jig Assembly consists of an active unit and an anchorage unit.[37,60] The anchorage unit is a modified Nance Appliance attached to the maxillary second premolar bands with a 0.032″ stainless steel wire (see Fig. 20.5). Thus all teeth mesial to the molars are indirectly utilized. Bands with headgear tubes and hooks placed gingivally are cemented to the first molars. The active unit consists of an active arm which is fabricated by a round 0.028″ stainless steel wire 30–35 mm long (see Fig. 20.4). A 3 mm long open loop constructed at a distance of 8 mm from the wire end divides the wire arm into two sections, a small distal and a larger mesial one. A NiTi open coil spring (25–30 mm long, with a wire cross-section of 0.010″ and a helix diameter of 0.030″) is inserted through the mesial end of the sectional wire. Two sliding tubes are used for positional stabilization of the spring. The distal tube is placed close to the loop of the sectional wire and stabilizes the coil spring, preventing its sliding into the loop. The mesial tube is provided with a hook and is placed close to the mesial end of the sectional wire, which is subsequently bent gingivally. This bend prevents the coil spring from sliding away from the wire and ensures that there is no soft tissue impingement.

After cementation of the modified Nance button and the first maxillary molar bands, the distal end of the Sectional Jig Assembly is inserted into the headgear tube of the first molar band. A stainless steel ligature is then tied between the open loop of the active arm and the gingival hook of the molar band, thus adding stability to the system and preventing rotation of the sectional archwire. The spring is activated by ligating the hook of the second (mesial) sliding tube to the bracket of the second premolar band (see Fig. 20.6). Optimal activation of the coil spring will deliver 80 g per side. The patient is monitored at 4-week intervals for further adjustments and reactivation of the appliance.

NiTi Coil Springs Used for Molar Distalization

NiTi Coil Springs are usually an integral part of the active units of distalization appliances.[38,39,61] Most commonly, the anchorage unit of these appliances consists of a modified Nance button retained through extension wires soldered to the maxillary first premolar bands or the maxillary second deciduous molars.[38,61] According to Erverdi et al,[38] the active unit consists of a 0.014 × 0.037″ NiTi Open Coil Spring placed buccally onto a stainless steel sectional wire connecting the first premolar and first molar bands. An appropriate length of spring is selected in order to produce approximately 225 g of force when the springs are compressed. Gianelly et al used NiTi Superelastic Coils which exerted a distalization force of 100 g by a compression of 8–10 mm.[61] These coils were placed onto 0.016 × 0.022″ sectional or continuous archwires between the first molars and the first premolars in conjunction with a vertical slotted fixed appliance.

Gianelly proposed another method of activation, by placement of a sliding lock in front of the coils and compressing the coils by moving the lock 10 mm posteriorly before fixing in position.[62] Pieringer et al used Sentalloy Red Coil Springs (GAC, Islandia, NY), which delivered 150–200 g of distalization force and were attached between the first molars and first premolars in conjunction with a preadjusted edgewise appliance or sectional archwires.[39]

Magnets Used for Molar Distalization

The development of permanent rare magnets has allowed the clinical application of magnetic forces in orthodontics. However, there has been speculation on the possible biologic effects of static magnetic fields on the mechanism of orthodontic tooth movement.[43,44,63,64]

Blechman was the first to develop an intraoral magnetic appliance in conjunction with fixed appliances and sectional archwires to distalize the maxillary first molars.[40] Later, Gianelly et al[41,42] introduced the Molar Distalizing System (MDS, Medical Magnetics, Ramsey, NJ) while Bondemark et al[65] used a prefabricated magnetic device (Modular Magnetic Inc., New City, NY) to distalize maxillary molars. Currently, commercially available magnets that are specially designed for molar distalization include the Magneforce (Ormco Corporation, Orange, CA) and the Magnet Force System (Ortho Organizers Inc., San Marcos, CA).

To reinforce anchorage, a modified Nance acrylic button is used, which is fabricated to contact the palatal surfaces of the incisors and is stabilized to the maxillary first or second premolar bands or maxillary first deciduous molar bands (see Fig. 21.1).[7,41,42,66–69] Bondemark et al suggested the incorporation of an anterior bite plane to the Nance button to disclude the posterior teeth.[65]

The active unit consists of a pair of repelling magnets attached to a sectional wire, the surfaces of which are brought into contact to deliver a distalization force (see Fig. 21.2).[41] The mesial magnet is mounted so that it can move freely along the sectional wire.[41,67] To activate the appliance, the repelling surfaces of the magnets are brought into contact by passing a 0.014″ ligature wire through the loop on the auxiliary wire and then tying back a washer anterior to the magnets (see Figs 21.3 and 21.4).[38,42] Thus, a continuous distalization force of 200–225 g can be produced.[7,38,41,69] As the distance between the magnets increases, this force decreases to a minimum of 60–100 g, when the magnets are at a distance of 1–1.5 mm, below which the magnets should be reactivated approximately every 1–4 weeks.[7,38,41,45,67–69]

NiTi Wires for Molar Distalization

The use of superelastic nickel-titanium wires for maxillary molar distalization was first introduced by Locatelli et al in conjunction with fixed appliances.[46] Later, other authors also proposed designs incorporating NiTi wires. Locatelli et al used a 100 g Neosentalloy wire with a curve which passes above the second premolar bracket, i placed through the first premolar brackets and first molar tubes, and maintained in position with stops.[46] The appliance can achieve a molar distalization rate of 1 mm per month.

The K-loop molar distalizer is fabricated from a 0.017 × 0.025″ TMA wire comprising two loops (in "K" shape) approximately 8 mm long and 1.5 mm wide.[48] The legs of the K-loop are bent down 20° to counteract the tipping moments of the loop, and the wire is inserted in the first premolar bracket and in the first molar tube. Following an initial activation of 2 mm, the loop is reactivated after 6–8 weeks.

The nickel-titanium double loop system consists of an 80 g Neosentalloy archwire, which is placed on the bonded maxillary dental arch equipped with stops positioned on marks distal to the first premolar bracket and about 5 mm distal to the first molar tube, and sectional NiTi archwires, one for each side, which are prepared with crimping stops distal and mesial to the second premolar brackets and about 5 mm distal to each second molar tube.[47] This design allows simultaneous distalization of both first and second maxillary molars. Class II elastics should be used in order to reinforce anchorage.

The U-shaped vertical loop consists of 0.018 × 0.025″ rectangular nitinol wire and incorporates a U-shaped vertical loop at the distal to fit in the molar band tubes.[49] The wire extends 5–6 mm anteriorly of the premolar tubes to allow reactivation when required. An archwire lock is incorporated on the wire near the vertical loop before insertion. The activation of the appliance is performed by sliding the lock forward to the premolar tube and securing it, thus compressing the wire 2–3 mm. The patient is monitored at 1-month intervals for necessary adjustments.

Distalizing Arches, Acrylic Distalization Splints and the Carriere Distalizer

Several other appliances have been proposed for maxillary molar distalization, including distalizing arches (such as the Bimetric Distalizing Arch (RMO, Denver, CO),[50] the Multi-Distalizing Arch (Ortho Organizers Inc., San Marcos, CA), the Molar Distalization Bow,[51] and the Korn Lip Bumper (American Orthodontics, Sheboygan, WI)), acrylic distalization splints (such as the Acrylic Splint with NiTi Coils[52] and the Removable Molar Distalization Splint[53]), and the Carriere Distalizer (ClassOne Orthodontics, Lubbock, TX).[54] However, almost all of these devices require some form of patient cooperation either because they are removable or because they have to be used in conjunction with intermaxillary elastics.

Appliances with a Double Flexible Distalization Force System Positioned Both Palatally and Buccally

Two appliances are included in this category (see Table 2.2). These are the Piston Appliance (in other words, the Greenfield Molar

Distalizer),[70] and the Nance Appliance in conjunction with NiTi Open Coil Springs and an edgewise appliance as proposed by Puente.[71]

Piston Appliance (Greenfield Molar Distalizer)

The Piston Appliance (nX Orthodontic Services, Coral Springs, FL) was introduced by Greenfield[70] and includes an active unit positioned both palatally and buccally, which consists of superelastic NiTi Open Coil Springs and an anchorage unit incorporating an enlarged modified Nance button. The modified Nance acrylic palatal button is stabilized with 0.040″ stainless steel wires which are soldered to the first premolar bands. The active unit consists of 0.055″ superelastic NiTi Open Coil Springs positioned around the piston assemblies. The piston assemblies are fabricated with 0.030″ stainless steel wires soldered buccally and palatally to the first molar bands and 0.036″ tubes soldered on the maxillary first premolar bands. To activate the appliance, 2 mm ring stops are added to the mesial of the buccal and palatal tubes in each piston every 6–8 weeks, thus delivering 25 g of distalizing force to each piston assembly and, subsequently, 50 g of distalization force for each molar. The molars are distalized with a monthly rate of 1 mm.

Nance Appliance with NiTi Coil Springs

Puente[71] developed a combined edgewise and modified Nance Appliance to be used in Class II treatment. The extension wire of the modified Nance Appliance includes a helical loop bilaterally, which passes through the palatal tubes of the first maxillary molar bands and is soldered on the first premolar bands. The mesial end of an additional omega loop is also soldered on the first premolar bands while the distal end can slide on the extension wire. Full fixed appliances and continuous archwires are used and nickel-titanium open coil springs are placed palatally between the omega loop and the first molar tubes and labially between the molar tubes and the first premolar brackets. The omega loops of the Nance Appliance are activated, thus delivering a distalization force which also compresses the coil springs. Consequently, both the Nance and the fixed appliance exert a distalization force through the coils to the maxillary first molars. The monthly rate of distal molar movement can reach 1 mm.

Appliances with a Rigid Distalization Force System Palatally Positioned

Appliances that use expansion screws as a rigid distalization force system which is positioned palatally include the Veltri's distalizer,[72] the New Distalizer,[73] and the P-Rax Molar Distalizer[74] (see Table 2.2).

Veltri's Distalizer

The Veltri's Distalizer (Leone SpA, Firenze, Italy) consists of a Veltri sagittal expansion screw palatally positioned incorporating four extension arms, which are soldered bilaterally to the first and second maxillary molar bands in a similar way to the Hyrax expansion screw.[72] The appliance is used for maxillary second molar distalization incorporating as anchorage all the teeth anterior to the second molars, including the first molars. The appliance is activated by turning the screw half a turn twice every week until the second molars are completely distalized. Then, the distalization of the first molars follows by means of nickel-titanium coil springs. To reinforce anchorage during the distalization of the first molars, a palatal bar with Nance button attached to the second molars, full fixed appliances incorporating an archwire with stops mesial to the second premolars, and Class II elastics can be used. Therefore, during this phase of treatment some form of patient compliance is required. When the first maxillary molars are in Class I relationship, the retraction of the anterior teeth can be initiated.

New Distalizer

The New Distalizer (Leone SpA, Firenze, Italy) was introduced by Baccetti & Franchi[73] and can be regarded as a modification of the Veltri's Distalizer. The appliance consists of a Veltri palatal sagittal screw for bilateral molar distalization (Leone SpA, Firenze, Italy), which is soldered by means of extension arms to bands on the maxillary first molars and second premolars (or second deciduous molars). A Nance button connected to the body of the screw by means of two soldered extension wires adds more anchorage. The appliance is activated at the rate of two quarters of a turn every week. When the distalization of the maxillary first molars has been accomplished, the screw is blocked and the arms connecting the screw with the second premolar bands are cut off. Thus the first molar position can be maintained and a second phase of treatment with full fixed appliances can follow.

P-Rax Molar Distalizer

The P-RAX Appliance (AOA/Pro Orthodontic Appliances, Sturtevant, WI) was developed by Paz.[74] It can be used to treat patients requiring molar distalization and can accommodate midpalatal expansion when indicated.

The appliance consists of a Nance button, used as anchorage when expansion is not required, or a compact rapid palatal expansion (RPE) screw (Ormco Corporation, Orange, CA), when expansion is needed. The extension wires of the Nance button or the stainless steel arms of the compact RPE can be bonded on the occlusal surfaces of the maxillary first or second premolars. The active unit includes two compact RPEs positioned bilaterally in sagittal direction, which are connected either to the Nance button or to the midpalatal compact RPE and are soldered to the maxillary first or second molar bands. The precise amount of molar distalization can be achieved through manual control of the turns of the compact RPEs. Slow distalization is recommended to prevent anchorage loss, molar distal tipping, and debonding of the occlusal arm.

Hybrid Appliances

The only hybrid appliance that uses a combination of a rigid distalization force system which is buccally positioned and a flexible one which is palatally positioned is the First Class Appliance[75,76] (see Table 2.2).

First Class Appliance

The First Class Appliance (FCA) (Leone SpA, Firenze, Italy) consists of a vestibular side, a palatal side, and four bands. The active unit of the appliance includes bilaterally a screw which is buccally positioned and a spring which is palatally positioned (see Fig. 22.10). On the buccal side of the first molar bands, 10 mm long vestibular screws are soldered occlusally to the 0.022 × 0.028″ single tubes, in which the base arches can be positioned after molar distalization.[75–77] The vestibular screws are seated into closed rings that are welded to the bands of the second deciduous molars or the second premolars. Each vestibular screw is activated by a quarter turn once per day for bilateral distalization.

The anchorage unit of the appliance consists of a large palatal Nance button having a "butterfly" shape with 0.045″ wires embedded in the acrylic. Anteriorly, these extension wires are soldered lingual to the second deciduous molar or premolar bands and posteriorly they are inserted into 0.045″ tubes welded to the palatal sides of the first molar bands.[75–77] The molar tubes act as a guide during distalization, to enhance bodily tooth movement. Between the solder joint on the second deciduous molar or premolar band and the tube on the molar band, 10 mm long NiTi Open Coil Springs are positioned in full compression. The continuous force produced by the springs compensates the action of the vestibular screws, so the distal molar movement takes place in a "double-track" system, preventing rotations or the development of posterior crossbites.[75,77]

Transpalatal Arches for Molar Rotation and/or Distalization

Transpalatal arches (TPA) can be an effective adjunct for gaining space in the maxillary dental arch in terms of molar derotation or distalization. They are especially useful when the need for derotation is the same on both sides of the dental arch. Since the introduction of the transpalatal bar by Goshgarian,[78] several designs, soldered (fixed) or removable, have become available (see Table 2.2).

Dahlquist et al[79] used a *prefabricated transpalatal arch* for maxillary molar derotation (GAC International Inc., Islandia, NY). The TPA was made of 0.036″ stainless steel round wire and was bent back at the ends to fit in the prefabricated rectangular tubes placed on the palatal surfaces of the maxillary molar bands. In addition, a mesially directed loop was included in the middle of the arch. The TPA was activated for derotation by changing the angle between the double-ended section and the main arch so that when the arch was inserted in one tube, the other end was positioned 8 mm distal of the other tube. The same activation was repeated for the other side to produce bilateral derotation and it was checked for symmetry by alternately inserting the arms in the tubes on both sides. The TPA was checked and reactivated every 6 weeks and the duration of the maxillary molar derotation varied between 60 and 198 days.

The Zachrisson-type Transpalatal Bar (ZTPB) consists of three loops and is fabricated from 0.036″ blue Elgiloy wire.[80,81] The central loop is longer and larger than the single loop of the Goshgarian Transpalatal Bar. The two distally oriented smaller loops are symmetrically positioned on either side of the central loop. These two small distal-directed loops add flexibility to the bar, thus making engagement into the sheaths easier with less activation loss. During derotation, while the central loop is closing, the small loops open approximately 0.5–1 mm, which allows the production of less contractive forces by the ZTPB. Further, the ends of the ZTPB are also longer to secure improved engagement to the lingual sheaths and make safe ligations possible.

The Palatal Rotation Arch is fabricated from 0.8 mm stainless steel wire and incorporates a large palatal loop which is distally oriented.[82] The ends of the arch are doubled over and inserted into 1.8 mm palatal, horizontal, universal sheaths welded to the palatal surfaces of the maxillary molar bands. During derotation, the activated palatal central loop moves upwards and therefore a 5 mm minimum distance must be left on the working model between the palatal loop and the palate to prevent tissue impingement.

Both the *Nitanium Molar Rotator2 (NMR2)* and *Nitanium Palatal Expander2 (NPE2)* (Ortho Organizers Inc., San Marcos, CA) are fabricated from shape memory and thermally activated NiTi wire.[83,84] Below the transition temperature of 35°C, the metal is flexible enough for activation. After insertion in the mouth, both versions tend to return to their original shape, exerting a light and continuous force to the molars. Both types are removable and their ends are inserted into the specially designed lingual sheaths of the maxillary molar bands. The NMR2 was developed mainly to correct molar rotations, also providing anchorage control and stabilization, torque control, expansion or contraction, molar distalization, and vertical control, while the NPE2 is mainly used for maxillary expansion and arch development, providing simultaneously the possibility of molar rotation and distalization.[83]

The 3D (Wilson) Palatal Appliance (RMO Inc., Denver, CO), is a dynamic three-dimensional appliance which can deliver predictable forces in all directions. It incorporates five separate angles, which can all be activated. The appliance is inserted in specially designed vertical tubes on the lingual aspects of the first molar bands. It has additional distal extensions made of 0.025″ stainless steel wire that act as occlusal rests on the second molar distal marginal ridges to increase the resistance towards distal tipping.[85]

The TMA Transpalatal Arch is fabricated from 0.032″ TMA bars (Ormco Corporation, Orange, CA).[86] It is attached on maxillary molar bands and inserted from the distal into the lingual tube of the molar used as anchorage and from the mesial into the tube of the molar to be distalized. The central omega loop is not required as the TMA transpalatal arch is not used for palatal expansion. When the TMA transpalatal arch is activated, it applies a mesiobuccal rotation to the anchor molar, which should be counteracted with fixed orthodontic appliances using a rectangular wire or a passive stainless steel wire segment between the second molar and the canine on the anchor side. In addition, a distalization force is applied to the opposite molar. To reinforce anchorage, the TMA arch should be used in combination with extraoral appliances. The appliance can only distalize one molar at a time and therefore it is recommended for use in unilateral or slight bilateral Class II molar relationships.

The Keles TPA is constructed from the Burstone Lingual System (Ormco Corporation, Orange, CA), including two helices bilaterally just before the terminal ends.[87] The wire is made of 0.032 × 0.032″ TMA, which is attached from the distal to Precision lingual hinge cap attachments (Ormco Corporation, Orange, CA), which are welded on the palatal aspects of the maxillary first molar bands (see Figs 23.3–23.5). The Keles TPA produces two equal and opposite forces on both sides which can also increase the intermolar width between the mesial cusp tips of the maxillary first molars (see Fig. 23.8).

The Distalix is based on the quad helix appliance, using the four helices as well as a distalization pendulum spring. The Distalix is fabricated from 0.032″ blue Elgiloy wire and can be either welded on maxillary molar and/or premolar bands or completely removable (or semi-removable), attached to palatal tubes on the molar bands.[88] The Distalix is, according to Langlade,[88] a frictionless automatic system that delivers a slow and continuous force, which varies between 200 and 350 g.

References

1. Hilgers JJ. The pendulum appliance for Class II noncompliance therapy. J Clin Orthod 1992;26:706–714.
2. Carano A, Testa M. The distal jet for upper molar distalization. J Clin Orthod 1996;30:374–380.
3. Keles A, Sayinsu K. A new approach in maxillary molar distalization: intraoral bodily molar distalizer. Am J Orthod Dentofacial Orthop 2000;117:39–48.
4. Walde KC. The simplified molar distalizer. J Clin Orthod 2003;37:616–619.
5. Keles A. Maxillary unilateral molar distalization with sliding mechanics: a preliminary investigation. Eur J Orthod 2001;23:507–515.
6. Reiner TJ. Modified Nance appliance for unilateral molar distalization. J Clin Orthod 1992;26:402–404.
7. Bondemark L. A comparative analysis of distal maxillary molar movement produced by a new lingual intra-arch NiTi coil appliance and a magnetic appliance. Eur J Orthod 2000;22:683–695.
8. Lanteri C, Francolini F, Lanteri V. Distalization using the Fast Back. Leone Boll Int 2002; Feb:1–3.
9. Ghosh J, Nanda RS. Evaluation of an intraoral maxillary molar distalization technique. Am J Orthod Dentofacial Orthop 1996;110:639–646.
10. Bussick TJ, McNamara JA Jr. Dentoalveolar and skeletal changes associated with the pendulum appliance. Am J Orthod Dentofacial Orthop 2000;117:333–343.
11. Hilgers JJ. The pendulum appliance: an update. Clin Impressions 1993;2:15–17.
12. Byloff FK, Darendeliler MA. Distal molar movement using the pendulum appliance. Part 1: Clinical and radiological evaluation. Angle Orthod 1997;67:249–260.
13. Byloff FK, Darendeliler MA, Clar E, Darendeliler A. Distal molar movement using the pendulum appliance. Part 2: The effects of maxillary molar root uprighting bands. Angle Orthod 1997;67:261–270.

14. Hilgers JJ. A palatal expansion appliance for noncompliance therapy. J Clin Orthod 1991;25:491–497.

15. Mayes JH. The Texas Penguin... a new approach to pendulum therapy. AOA Orthodontic Appliances 1999;3:1–2. Available online at: www.aoalab.com/learning/publications/aoaVol/ aoaVol3N1.pdf

16. Hilgers JJ. The Hilgers PhD. AOA Orthodontic Appliances 1998;2:5. Available online at: www.aoalab.com/learning/publications/aoaVol/aoaVol2N1.pdf

17. Hilgers JJ, Tracey S. Hyperefficient orthodontic treatment employing bioprogressive principles. Clin Impressions 2000;9:18–27.

18. Grummons D. Maxillary asymmetry and frontal analysis. Clin Impressions 1999;8:2–16, 23.

19. Snodgrass DJ. A fixed appliance for maxillary expansion, molar rotation, and molar distalization. J Clin Orthod 1996;30:156–159.

20. Hilgers JJ, Tracey S. Hilgers/Tracey MDA Expander. The Mini-Distalizing Appliance featuring the Ormco Compact RPE. AOA Orthodontic Appliances 2001;5:2. Available online at: www.aoalab.com/learning/publications/aoaVol/aoaVol5N1.pdf

21. Scuzzo G, Pisani F, Takemoto K. Maxillary molar distalization with a modified pendulum appliance. J Clin Orthod 1999;33:645–650.

22. Echarri P, Scuzzo G, Cirulli N. A modified pendulum appliance for anterior anchorage control. J Clin Orthod 2003;37:352–359.

23. Scuzzo G, Takemoto K, Pisani F, Della Vecchia S. The modified pendulum appliance with removable arms. J Clin Orthod 2000;34:244–246.

24. Kinzinger G, Fuhrmann R, Gross U, Diedrich P. Modified pendulum appliance including distal screw and uprighting activation for noncompliance therapy of Class II malocclusion in children and adolescents. J Orofac Orthop 2000;61:175–190.

25. Kinzinger G, Fritz U, Diedrich P. Bipendulum and quad pendulum for noncompliance molar distalization in adult patients. J Orofac Orthop 2002;63:154–162.

26. Carano A, Testa M. Clinical applications of the Distal Jet in Class II malocclusion nonextraction treatment. Hell Orthod Rev 2001;4:47–71.

27. Ngantung V, Nanda RS, Bowman, SJ. Postreatment evaluation of the distal jet appliance. Am J Orthod Dentofacial Orthop 2001;120:178–185.

28. Bolla E, Muratore F, Carano A, Bowman SJ. Evaluation of maxillary molar distalization with the distal jet: a comparison with other contemporary methods. Angle Orthod 2002;72:481–494.

29. Carano A, Testa M. Distal jet designed to be used alone. Am J Orthod Dentofacial Orthop 2001;120:13A–15A.

30. Nishii Y, Katada H, Yamaguchi H. Three-dimensional evaluation of the distal jet appliance. World J Orthod 2002;3:321–327.

31. Bowman SJ. Class II combination therapy (distal jet and Jasper Jumpers): a case report. J Orthod 2000;27:213–218.

32. Quick AN, Harris AM. Molar distalization with a modified distal jet appliance. J Clin Orthod 2000;34:419–423.

33. Keles A. Unilateral distalization of a maxillary molar with sliding mechanics: a case report. J Orthod 2002;29:97–100.

34. Keles A, Pamukcu B, Tokmak EC. Bilateral molar distalization with sliding mechanics: Keles Slider. World J Orthod 2002;3:57–66.

35. Jones RD, White MJ. Rapid Class II molar correction with an open-coil jig. J Clin Orthod 1992;26:661–664.

36. Scott MW. Molar distalization: more ammunition for your operatory. Clin Impressions 1996;5:16–27.

37. Papadopoulos MA. Simultaneous distalization of maxillary first and second molars by means of superelastic NiTi coils. Hell Orthod Rev 1998;1:71–76.

38. Erverdi N, Koyuturk O, Kucukkeles N. Nickel-titanium coil springs and repelling magnets: a comparison of two different intra-oral molar distalization techniques. Br J Orthod 1997;24:47–53.

39. Pieringer M, Droschl H, Permann R. Distalization with a Nance appliance and coil springs. J Clin Orthod 1997;31:321–326.

40. Blechman AM. Magnetic force systems in orthodontics: clinical results of a pilot study. Am J Orthod 1985;87:201–210.

41. Gianelly AA, Vaitas AS, Thomas WM, Berger DG. Distalization of molars with repelling magnets. J Clin Orthod 1988;22:40–44.

42. Gianelly AA, Vaitas AS, Thomas WM. The use of magnets to move molars distally. Am J Orthod Dentofacial Orthop 1989;96:161–167.

43. Papadopoulos MA. Clinical applications of magnets in orthodontics. Hell Orthod Rev 1999;1:31–42.

44. Papadopoulos MA. A study of the biomechanical characteristics of magnetic force systems used in orthodontics. Hell Orthod Rev 1999;2:89–97.

45. Blechman AM, Alexander C. New miniaturized magnets for molar distalization. Clin Impressions 1995;4:14–19.

46. Locatelli R, Bednar J, Dietz VS, Gianelly AA. Molar distalization with superelastic NiTi wire. J Clin Orthod 1992;26:277–279.

47. Giancotti A, Cozza P. Nickel titanium double-loop system for simultaneous distalization of first and second molars. J Clin Orthod 1998;32:255–260.

48. Kalra V. The K-loop molar distalizing appliance. J Clin Orthod 1995;29:298–301.

49. Vlock R. A fixed appliance for rapid distalization of upper molars. Orthodontic CYBERjournal 1998;3. Available online at: www.oc-j.com/issue7/vlock.htm

50. Wilson WL. Modular orthodontic systems. Part 2. J Clin Orthod 1978;12:358–375.

51. Jeckel N, Rakosi T. Molar distalization by intra-oral force application. Eur J Orthod 1991;3:43–46.

52. Manhartsberger C. [Headgear-free molar distalization.] Fortschr Kieferorthop 1994;55:330–336.

53. Ritto AK. Removable distalization splint. Orthodontic CYBERjournal 1997;2. Available online at: www.oc-j.com/issue6/ritto.htm & http://www.oc-j.com/issue2/ritto.htm

54. Carriere L. Syllabus on the Carriere distalizer and its use. ClassOne Orthodontics. Available online at: www.classoneorthodontics.com/customer_files/Class_One_Carriere.pdf

55. Runge ME, Martin JT, Bukai F. Analysis of rapid maxillary molar distal movement without patient cooperation. Am J Orthod Dentofacial Orthop 1999;115:153–157.

56. Brickman CD, Sinha PK, Nanda RS. Evaluation of the Jones jig appliance for distal molar movement. Am J Orthod Dentofacial Orthop 2000;118:526–534.

57. Gulati S, Kharbanda OP, Parkash H. Dental and skeletal changes after intraoral molar distalization with sectional jig assembly. Am J Orthod Dentofacial Orthop 1998;114:319–327.

58. Paul LD, O'Brien KD, Mandall NA. Upper removable appliance or Jones Jig for distalizing first molars? A randomized clinical trial. Orthod Craniofac Res 2002;5:238–242.

59. Haydar S, Uner O. Comparison of Jones jig molar distalization appliance with extraoral traction. Am J Orthod Dentofacial Orthop 2000;117:49–53.

60. Papadopoulos MA, Mavropoulos A, Karamouzos A. Cephalometric changes following simultaneous first and second maxillary molar distalization using a noncompliance intraoral appliance. J Orofac Orthop 2004;65:123–136.

61. Gianelly AA, Bednar J, Dietz VS. Japanese NiTi coils used to move molars distally. Am J Orthod Dentofacial Orthop 1991;99:564–566.

62. Gianelly AA. Distal movement of the maxillary molars. Am J Orthod Dentofacial Orthop 1998;114:66–72.

63. Papadopoulos MA, Hoerler I, Gerber H, Rahn B, Rakosi T. [The effect of static magnetic fields on osteoblast activity: an in-vitro study.] Fortschr Kieferorthop 1992;53:218–222.

64. Papadopoulos MA. Biological aspects of the use of permanent magnets and static magnetic fields in orthodontics. Hell Orthod Rev 1998;1:145–157.

65. Bondemark L, Kurol J, Bernhold M. Repelling magnets versus superelastic nickel-titanium coils in simultaneous distal movement of maxillary first and second molars. Angle Orthod 1994;64:189–198.

66. Cozzani M, Thomas WM, Gianelly AA. [Asymmetrical distalization of upper molars with magnets. A clinical case.] Mondo Orthod 1989;14:687–692.

67. Itoh T, Tokuda T, Kiyosue S, Hirose T, Matsumoto M, Chaconas SJ. Molar distalization with repelling magnets. J Clin Orthod 1991;25:611–617.

68. Steger ER, Blechman AM. Case reports: molar distalization with static repelling magnets. Part II. Am J Orthod Dentofacial Orthop 1995;108:547–555.

69. Bondemark L, Kurol J. Distalization of maxillary first and second molars simultaneously with repelling magnets. Eur J Orthod 1992;14:264–272.

70. Greenfield RL. Fixed piston appliance for rapid Class II correction. J Clin Orthod 1995;29:174–183.

71. Puente M. Class II correction with an edgewise-modified Nance appliance. J Clin Orthod 1997 31:178–182.

72. Veltri N, Baldini A. Slow sagittal and bilateral palatal expansion for the treatment of class II malocclusions. Leone Boll Int 2001;3:5–9.

73. Baccetti T, Franchi L. A new appliance for molar distalization. Leone Boll Int 2000;2:3–7.

74. Paz ME. Nonextraction therapy benefits from small expansion appliance. Clin Impressions 2001;10:12–15.

75. Fortini A, Lupoli M, Parri M. The First Class Appliance for rapid molar distalization. J Clin Orthod 1999;33:322–328.

76. Fortini A, Lupoli M, Giuntoli F, Franchi L. Dentoskeletal effects induced by rapid molar distalization with the first class appliance. Am J Orthod Dentofacial Orthop 2004;125:697–705.

77. Fortini A, Lupoli M. First Class: a new appliance for rapid molar distalization. Leone Boll Int 2000;1:5–13.

78. Goshgarian RA. Orthodontic palatal archwires. Washington DC: United States Government Patent Office; 1972.

79. Dahlquist A, Gebauer U, Ingervall B. The effect of a transpalatal arch for the correction of first molar rotation. Eur J Orthod 1996;18:257–267.

80. Gunduz E, Zachrisson BU, Honigl KD, Crismani AG, Bantleon HP. An improved transpalatal bar design. Part I. Comparison of moments and force

delivered by two bar designs for symmetrical molar derotation. Angle Orthod 2003;73:239–243.

81. Gunduz E, Crismani AG, Bantleon HP, Honigl KD, Zachrisson BU. An improved transpalatal bar design. Part II. Clinical upper molar derotation – case report. Angle Orthod 2003;73:244–248.

82. Cooke MS, Wreakes G. Molar derotation with a modified palatal arch: an improved technique. Br J Orthod 1978;5:201–203.

83. Corbett MC. Molar rotation and beyond. J Clin Orthod 1996;30:272–275.

84. Corbett MC. Slow and continuous maxillary expansion, molar rotation, and molar distalization. J Clin Orthod 1997;31:253–263.

85. Young DR. Orthodontic products update. Removable quadhelices and transpalatal arches. Br J Orthod 1997;24:248–256.

86. Mandurino M, Balducci L. Asymmetric distalization with a TMA transpalatal arch. J Clin Orthod 2001;35:174–178.

87. Keles A, Impram S. An effective and precise method for rapid molar derotation: Keles TPA. World J Orthod 2003;4:229–236.

88. Langlade M. Clinical distalization with the Distalix. World J Orthod 2003;4:215–228.

CHAPTER 16

The Pendulum Appliance

M. Ali Darendeliler, Gang Shen, Friedrich K. Byloff

Introduction

Nonextraction treatment of Class II malocclusion frequently requires upper molar distalization into a final Class I relationship. With extraoral mechanisms implementing molar distalization, the success of the treatment will decisively rely on the patient's compliance. An increasing need has been recognized in modem orthodontics for courses of treatment and devices that do not depend on patient cooperation. Since the early 1980s, therapeutic approaches and devices have been focused increasingly on options for correcting malocclusions in which patient compliance could be almost ignored.

Various molar distalizing systems have been developed aiming to minimize patient compliance. As a main approach of noncompliance appliances, intraarch devices for molar distalization have been introduced since the 1980s. Clinical application of repelling magnets,[1,2] acrylic cervical occipital (ACCO),[3] Wilson Biometric Distalizing Arch (BDA),[4] Jones Jig,[5] and Herbst or Forsus[6] appliances has demonstrated promising results. A modified Nance appliance has often been employed in conjunction with these force delivery systems to increase anchorage during distal movement or to keep the molars in position following distal movement.

It has been widely accepted that clinical management of intraarch devices is simple and efficient. As an important part of this intraarch system, the Pendulum Appliance (PA) was first introduced by Hilgers in 1992.[7] Since then, many variations have emerged and the clinical application of the PA has had great success, demonstrated by the many clinical studies and documented cases aimed at scientific evaluation of this therapeutic device.[8–10]

The Primary Design and Variations

Since its introduction in 1992 as a noncompliance approach, the PA has been implemented for correction of Class II malocclusion by achieving molar distalization. The primary design consists of a Nance button that incorporates four occlusal rests that are bonded either to the deciduous molars or to the first and second bicuspids. Two TMA 0.032" springs (Ormco, Orange, CA) inserted into a 0.036" lingual sheath on the maxillary molar bands are used as active elements for molar distalization. The springs are mounted as close to the center and distal edge of the Nance button as possible to produce a broad, swinging arc (or pendulum) of force. Each spring consists of a closed helix and an omega-shaped adjustable horizontal loop for molar expansion and prevention of the crossbite following the palatal movement of the molar (Fig. 16.1).[11]

Based on and inspired by the original design, many modifications or variations have emerged to improve treatment efficiency.[12–18] They can be categorized into two groups according to their improved functions.

Variations with Emphasis on Molar Control

Because the spring force is applied occlusally relative to the center of resistance of the molar, the molars are not distalized in a bodily fashion; instead, a crown distal tipping is expected. Furthermore, due to the swinging arc of the force, the molar distalization is not a linear movement; rather, a mesial-buccal rotation is inevitable. Also, because the depth of the maxillary vault and the position of Nance button, together with the helix mechanism attached to it, is higher than that of the molar and the lingual sheath, the helix springs therefore exert intrusive forces against the molars, causing them to intrude when they are moving distally. This points to the situation where the favorable molar distalization is accompanied, to some extent, by unfavorable movements which are manifested in the three dimensions of space.

Innovations of appliance design have been attempted to address the above side effects and have resulted in many PA variations. Byloff & Darendeliler have attempted to correct the molar tipping by

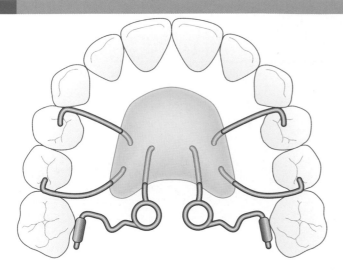

Figure 16.1 The primary design of pendulum appliance. The Nance button accommodates four occlusal rests that are bonded to the premolars, and two springs with closed helices which are activated by inserting them into the lingual sheath.

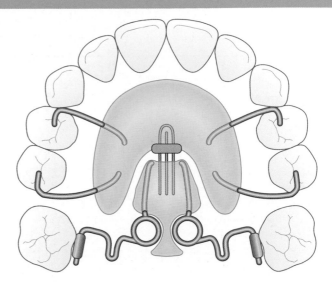

Figure 16.2 The modified PA (K-Pendulum) with a distal screw dividing the Nance button into two components. The anterior part bearing the occlusal rests serves as anchorage, whilst the posterior one bearing spring mechanics acts to generate molar distalization.

incorporating an uprighting bend (10–15° in the sagittal plane) in the pendulum spring after distalization and achievement of a super Class I molar relationship.[8] However, this has resulted in reduced molar tipping, more anchorage loss, and 64.1% increased treatment time.[8]

To maintain molar distalization along a linear course, Kinzinger et al presented a modified design named the K-Pendulum.[18] The appliance includes a distal screw dividing the Nance button into two sections. The anterior section provides anchorage and the posterior section accommodates the pendulum springs. The pendulum springs are additionally incorporated with a built-in straightening activation and toe-in bending, to allow for an elimination of molar rotation. The appliance is activated intraorally by the therapist at the check-up appointments by adjusting the distal screw; there is no need for the pendulum springs to be disengaged from the lingual sheaths.[18]

Variations with Emphasis on Anchorage Enforcement

The helix force acting to distalize the molars will generate reciprocal force acting against the Nance button, through which some degree of the force is transferred into the upper front teeth, resulting in proclination of the upper labial segment teeth and an increase of overjet. Sfondrini et al report that a future improvement to the current noncompliance distalizing devices will be the use of palatal implants or mini-screws connected to the Nance button for reinforcing the anchorage and avoiding side effects in the anterior region.[11]

As mentioned earlier, the K-Pendulum Appliance divides the Nance button into two sections. The anterior section provides anchorage and the posterior section accommodates the pendulum springs. By designating the two functions (anchorage and distalization) to be implemented by two separate components, the reciprocal force acting against the labial segment might be reduced (Fig. 16.2). Contrary to

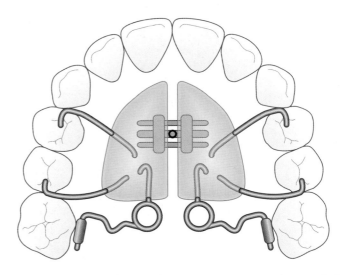

Figure 16.3 The modified PA with transverse expansion mechanism, which is intended to prevent maxillary constriction and reinforce anchorage.

this distal screw design, a transverse expansion mechanism is also incorporated into the Nance button, not only to correct the constricted upper dental arch but, more importantly, to reduce the anchorage burden in the labial segment by transforming part of the reciprocal force into the buccal segment[8] (Fig. 16.3).

Working Mechanisms

The PA consists of a large acrylic Nance button resting on the anterior palate. This is used for anchorage and serves as an attachment for two posteriorly extending 0.036″ TMA wire arms. In the passive state, these arms extend posteriorly, parallel to the midpalatal suture

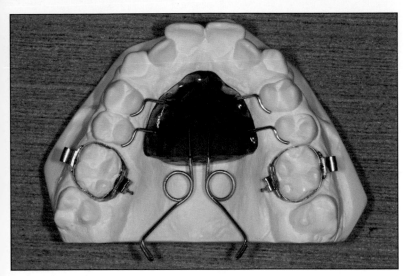

Figure 16.4 The retention wires are bonded on the lingual surface of the premolars to minimize occlusion interference.

The springs are activated by attaching their free ends into lingual sheaths on the molars and a distalizing component of force is thus created.

In the original design these ends are recurved, which could create more molar intrusion and better control of molar movement and could avoid molar rotation. In the design by Byloff & Darendeliler,[8] the PA does not have the omega-shaped adjustment loop, which also contributes to the above-mentioned advantages. To avoid occlusion interference, the retention wires could be bonded so as to avoid occlusal contacts, e.g. on the lingual surface of the premolars (Fig. 16.4).

The magnitude of this force varies, depending on the passive location of the arms. As this force is exerted against the sheaths, it tends to move the maxillary molars in a distopalatal arc. To compensate for this opening, loops are bent into the pendulum arms and adjustments in these loops are made as needed by the clinician.[19] Distalization generated by the PA is rapid and a 1–2 mm space mesial to the first molar can be expected within 6 weeks of insertion. The PA can provide 4–5 mm of arch length on each side.[19]

The modified K-Pendulum Appliance (see Fig. 16.2) is characterized by a modified location of the 0.032″ TMA spring, a distal screw, uprighting activation, and a toe-in bend.[16] As the centers of rotation, the pendulum loops are located distally to the centers of resistance of the molars, and the toe-in bends are also applied at the end of the pendulum arms. Therefore, the molars are initially derotated and distalized in the horizontal plane. The intraoral reactivation of the sagittal screw causes a dorsal displacement of the horizontal center of rotation, resulting in modification or readjustment of the arc on which the tooth is moved.[18] Due to the pendulum-like, occlusally directed pathway, bodily molar distalization is achieved in the sagittal plane. No tendency towards crossbite is induced in the horizontal plane and the U-loops of the pendulum springs need no intraoral reactivation. The uprighting activation at the end of distalization with the PA induces root uprighting and an intrusive force. Since the moments and vertical forces largely neutralize each other, the overall molar movement is almost a translatory distalization.[18]

Byloff et al describe the working mechanism of their modified appliance with a two-phase theory.[12]

Distal Molar Crown Movement (Phase 1)

During this first phase, the springs are activated 45° in the center of the helices on the sagittal plane until an overcorrected Class I relationship is obtained. One or two intraoral reactivations are generally necessary. To facilitate intraoral reinsertion of the spring, the lingual sheath should have an inset of 8° (GAC, Islandia, NY).

Molar Root Uprighting (Phase 2)

When the necessary sagittal correction and amount of space are obtained, the appliance is modified by adding a bend to the spring design to upright the molars by moving the roots distally. In order to make the uprighting bends, the angle between the recurved end of the spring, which is engaged into the palatal molar sheaths, and the long arm of the spring is increased intraorally in the sagittal plan 10–15°. The moment created is expected to upright the molars. The springs are still slightly active in the sagittal plane to maintain the position of the molar crowns. The appliance is left in place until the molar crown seems to be sufficiently uprighted.

As an alternative, uprighting bends can also be incorporated at the beginning of the distalization. In this situation, the restriction of crown tipping is implemented through the whole process of molar distalization.

Clinical Management

Force Magnitude and Activation

The forces generated by a pendulum arm are in the range of 3.5 g/degree and the normal amount of activation results in 100–200 g of force on a molar.[19] The generation of force could be managed in two ways.

Stepwise Activation

Some authors suggest that, in contrast to the recommendation of Hilgers, the PA springs are activated 45° (instead of 60°) in the center of the helices on the sagittal plane with an initial force of 200–250 g. Depending on the molar movement required, activation is repeated intraorally once or twice during treatment.[8] With the expansion mechanism, patients are instructed to turn the expansion screw once every 3 days for a period of 4 weeks. As a general principle, patients with molar crossbite tendencies or complete crossbites are asked to continue the activation for up to 12 weeks, depending on how much expansion is needed. The PA is worn until a super Class I relation is obtained.[8]

Single Activation

Joseph & Butchart recommend that the PA should be activated only once by bending the springs 90° to the base of the appliance, and should be maintained in the mouth until all the molars are overcorrected to a super Class I relationship.[10]

Considerations of Eruption Status of the Second and Third Molars

Influence of the Fully Erupted Second Molars

A controversy exists concerning the influence of the second and/or third molars on the distal movement of the first molars. The presence of second molars has been considered to be a hindrance to traditional means of distalization, such as the use of the headgear. However, this is not the case with the PA. Distalization seems to be successfully achieved regardless of the status of the second molar teeth, patient's age or molar calcification.[10] Patients who have second molars erupted achieve a correction as quickly as those who do not.[20] The noninfluence hypothesis is further echoed by a study in which no statistically significant differences in linear or angular changes were found among three groups of eruption stages of second molars.[12]

However, some authors contend that erupted second molars create resistance to the distalizing first molar. Worms et al describe how the second molar being in contact with the first molar represents a resistance to distal movement.[21] When the first molars move to the distal, the second molars move with them, whether or not they have already erupted. Second and third molars are impacted in the same way, moving distally when the first (or second) molars move towards them. Remodeling processes in the area of the tuberosity enable molar distalization. Bondemark & Kurol, on the other hand, have found that the first molar and unbanded second molar are mesiobuccally rotated during PA therapy, apparently confirming the influence of the second molar.[2]

Influences of the Budding of the Second and Third Molars

Regarding the influence of the second or third molar at budding stage, a majority of the studies on the PA agree that there is no connection between second molar budding stages, linear-angular changes, magnitude of molar distalization or loss of anchorage, and duration of therapy.[9,20]

On application of headgear for first molar distalization, Graber concluded that, when the second molar has not yet erupted, distalization is by tipping rather than by bodily movement.[22] Bondemark et al state that the presence of the second molar impacts tipping and distal movement of the first molars.[23] According to

Gianelly et al, the duration of therapeutic treatment increases if patients have their second molars.[24] In addition, Ten Hoeve,[25] Jeckel & Rakosi,[26] and Gianelly[27] concluded that distalization of the first molars is impacted by the degree of breakthrough of the second molars and recommend distalization before second molar eruption. Hilgers, in the article that introduced the PA, also claimed that the most opportune time for distalization of the first molars is before eruption of the second molars.[7] However, these recommendations were not evidence based.

A study by Kinzinger et al supports the hypothesis that the eruption stages of the second molar have a qualitative and quantitative impact on the distalization of the first molars.[28] In the study, the patients are divided into three groups (PG 1–3) according to the stage of eruption of their second and third molars. In PG 1, eruption of the second molars has either not yet taken place or is not complete. In PG 2, the second molars have already developed as far as the occlusal plane, with the third molars at the budding stage. In PG 3, germectomy of the wisdom teeth has been carried out, and the first and second molars on both sides have completely erupted. It has been reckoned that in the direction of distalization, a tooth bud acts on the mesial neighboring tooth like a fulcrum and that tipping of the first molars in patients in whom the second molar is still at the budding stage is thus greater. In patients whose second molars have erupted completely, the degree of tipping is greater again when a third molar bud is located in the direction of movement. In patients in whom germectomy of the wisdom teeth has been conducted, bodily distalization of both molars is evident. However, if the PA distalizes the first and second molars simultaneously, the duration of therapy will lengthen, greater forces will be needed, and more anchorage will be lost.[28]

The above phenomenon may be explained by reference to the individual developmental stage of the second molars. If they are still at the germ stage, they provide less resistance, functioning as a fulcrum for the distalizing first molar, which is tipped across the germ of the second molar. With increasing root development and eruption of the second molars, the contact point of the molars is moved continuously in a coronal direction. The consequence is increased resistance against the first molar and a reduced tendency for the tooth to tip, so that there is less distalization but more mesial movement of the incisors. Overall, the proportion of molar distalization in the total movement is thus comparably high in patients in the early mixed dentition (78.7% vs 63.8%).[18]

Anchorage Reinforcement

It has been concluded that the cost of more space opening and distal molar crown movement, and especially more root movement and reduced final tipping of the molars, is increased total treatment time and more anchorage loss at the premolars and at the incisor edge level.[12] Anterior anchorage loss has also been a constant finding of several other studies which claim a significant amount of incisor labial tipping, producing an anterior anchorage loss which represents

24–29% of the space opened between molars and premolars. Consequently, distal molar movement represents 71–76% of that space.[9,11]

The following measures might be considered in order to obtain a solid anchorage with PA distalizing treatment.

Transverse Expansion and Split Distal Screw

As mentioned earlier with the K-Pendulum, a split distal screw separates the Nance button into two parts, with the anterior part specifically serving to reinforce anchorage. On the other hand, slow expansion incorporated into the Nance button may also lead to an improved anchorage. However, the study by Byloff et al found that there is no significant difference in anchorage loss between patients with slow rates of expansion and patients without expansion.[12] This finding shows that the lateral forces exerted by the expansion screw to the palate and premolars might not substantially help to maintain anterior anchorage.

Increased Coverage of Nance Button

An increased area of the Nance button could include as much anterior palatal tissue as possible into the anchorage system to resist reciprocal force coming from molar distalization. The even, accurate and intimate coverage of the Nance button with the maxillary palate will also contribute to the wide distribution of the resistant force, leading to an effective anchorage. This, however, necessitates taking a careful impression and a delicate appliance fabrication.

Careful Case Selection

There appears to be some correlation between the amount of distalization and the extent of side effects, e.g. incisor proclination. It has been found that a distalization of 3.7 mm produces 4.9° of incisal proclination.[10] The PA may be detrimental for patients who cannot tolerate maxillary incisor advancement. Examples of such patients would be those with thin labial bone, deficient gingival height, severe incisor proclination or in combinations with a flatter palatal vault and buccally tipped upper incisors.

Implant-Supportive Anchorage

Implantation is the most solid and reliable approach for anchorage enforcement. Due to its invasive procedure, difficult clinical handling and sometimes frequent rate of loss, implantation has not become a routine to be incorporated into, or combined with, the PA for anchorage purposes. However, even the rare reports of its clinical application are quite convincing. Based on the philosophy of the PA, Byloff et al have presented a nonintegrated implant-supported device, the Graz Implant-Supported Pendulum (GISP).[13] It consists of two parts: the anchorage plate, which is fixed to the palatal bone via four mini-screws (Fig. 16.5), and the removable part, which is a

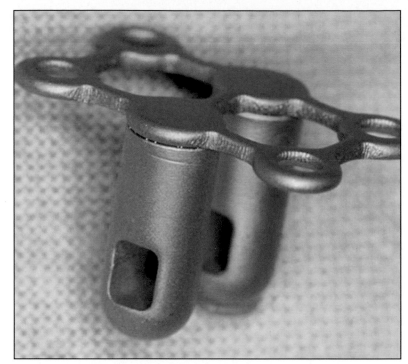

Figure 16.5 The Graz Implant-Supported Pendulum (GISP) is designed to secure anchorage enforcement. The anchorage plate is fixed to the palatal bone via four mini-screws.

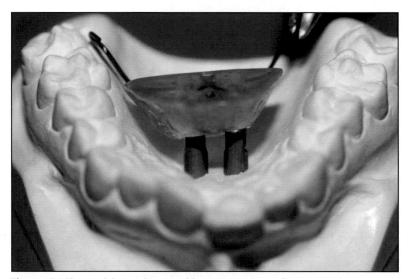

Figure 16.6 The pendulum-style removable part is incorporated into the implant.

pendulum-type appliance (Fig. 16.6). The PA system can be loaded 2 weeks after surgical placement and can actively distalize maxillary molars consecutively (Fig. 16.7). The implant component serves as an active anchor unit and provides stability against rotational movements.[13]

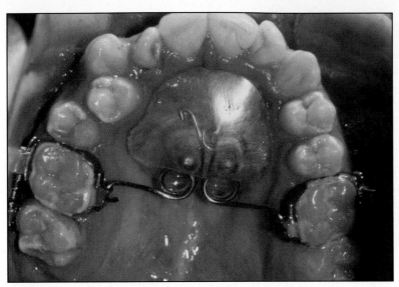

Figure 16.7 The whole system in place.

Case Implications

Dentoalveolar Patterns

Suitable Class II patients for the PA are those in whom the cusp-to-cusp Class II molar relationship is mainly caused by mesial drifting of the upper buccal segment teeth, rather than a retrusive mandible. The mesial drifting of the upper molars could be due to a protrusive maxilla and/or proclined upper anteriors. Under these circumstances, distalization of the buccal segment rearranges the molar relationship by bringing the upper molars back to the position they should be in. The degree of proclination and severity of crowding of upper anteriors should be moderate, otherwise extraction might be indicated. The PA could also be a solution for regaining the space lost by premature exfoliation of the deciduous second molar where considerable amounts of upper crowding can be relieved by the PA without extraction.

Skeletal Patterns

Conventional molar distalization is not always indicated for Class II correction. It is contraindicated in open-bite patients and in the presence of a severe protrusive profile. In open-bite patients molar distalization would determine a clockwise mandibular rotation, thus increasing the lower face height and worsening the facial appearance.[11] However, due to the intrusive action of the PA with recurved ends, moderate open-bite patients with crowding can be treated with this PA type. In patients with a severe protrusive facial profile, the anterior anchorage loss, which occurs during molar distalization, would worsen the inclination of front teeth and, consequently, the profile itself. Molar distalization is recommended for the correction of Class II malocclusions in deep-bite patients and in the presence of a concave or normal facial profile.[11] In borderline patients, the choice between extraction or distalization must be made by taking into account the expense of a longer treatment time, especially the possible compromise of the soft tissue profile, when a nonextraction approach is preferred.

In patients with more severe skeletal Class II problems, the PA might resolve upper arch crowding, with the skeletal problem being corrected, e.g. by an activator in the case of a retrusive mandible. The PA is particularly indicated in skeletal Class III tendency cases with upper arch crowding, where space has to be created and anchorage maintenance for the molars is not as critical as in Class II cases.

Treatment Timing

For young patients, the best time to start therapy with a PA is before the eruption of the second molars, in which situation the molar could be moving efficiently and the assumption of anchorage is limited, however, at the cost of molar tipping. If distalization of the first and second molars is to be carried out simultaneously (in which case the banded first molars are pushing the second molars along during distalization), prior germectomy of the third molar is strongly recommended.[28] In this circumstance, greater loss of anchorage and vestibular drift of the second molar should be expected.

The follow-up treatment with fixed appliances after removal of the PA should also be taken into consideration when treatment timing for the PA is decided. Most patients treated with the PA in the early mixed dentition must have a follow-up treatment with fixed appliances once all permanent teeth have erupted. Because one of the positive outcomes achieved by the PA is a well-developed dental arch, especially in the sagittal plane, the eruption of the canines and premolars will encounter little disruption, if predecessor deciduous molars are removed in timely fashion. In this circumstance, an intriguing phenomenon has been observed, in that the germs of canines and premolars spontaneously drift towards a distal orientation, leading to a spontaneous retraction of the anteriors with little consumption of anchorage.[18,29,30]

On the other hand, if PA treatment is postponed until the permanent dentition is complete, the teeth will have already erupted in a crowded position. In this case, the molars must first be distalized and stabilized to allow for a subsequent distalization of the premolars and cuspids. During this phase the molars serve as an anchorage unit, largely relying on the Nance button that rests against the palate. However, there is a potential risk of anchorage loss. In this situation the follow-up treatment time is prolonged and anchorage support becomes more challenging.[18]

Integral Coordination with Lower Dental Arch

Although the PA is is working only in the upper arch, one should not isolate it therapeutically from the lower dental arch, especially when the catching up of the lower arch to the changes in the upper is essential for overall correction of the malocclusion.

Kinzinger et al report on a lower lingual arch design specially used in conjunction with the PA.[18] The lingual arch appliance consists of two molar bands with a soldered 0.040″ stainless steel wire. Mesially to the solder joints at the molar bands, the lingual arch runs on both sides by an occlusally directed U-loop into a lingual arm. This arm is designed to run distally to the contralateral lateral incisor and to fit against the teeth halfway up the clinical crown. The activation of this lingual arch appliance will facilitate slight arch expansion, anterior protrusion and molar uprighting, allowing for a harmonious correction of sagittal arch length deficiencies through the distalization and uprighting of upper and lower first permanent molars. Slight incisor protrusion has to be accepted as a side effect in the early mixed dentition when this combined approach is adopted.[18]

Distalization Maintenance and Consolidation

The net effect of PA distalization passing to the follow-up treatment stage is most likely a certain loss of its original gain. It has been reported that during the fixed-appliance phase of treatment, there is considerable rebound in the position of the maxillary molars and premolars. After comprehensive treatment, the maxillary first molar is only 0.8 mm distal to its original position (the PA originally created 5.9 mm distalization), and the first premolar had returned to the anteroposterior position in which it began.[6] This points to the extreme importance of distalization maintenance in the aftermath of PA treatment. It is critical that, after active distalization with the PA, the molars must be held where they have been repositioned, not only providing the spaces for future retraction of the anteriors but, more challengingly, preparing themselves well as anchorage for this retraction. This is especially the case when PA treatment commences in the permanent dentition stage. The following approaches might be beneficial to keep distally positioned molars from rebounding.

Bodily Molar Distalization

The distalization achieved by a bodily movement of the molars might be more likely to be maintained than that achieved by crown tipping. Based on clinical experience, some authors hypothesize that, by incorporating uprighting bends into the spring design of the PA, one can facilitate fixed-appliance treatment in a more efficient way. In so doing, the more bodily the molars are moved distally (as opposed to tipping), the less anchorage loss one would expect.[12]

Sufficient Retention

A sufficient retention after PA distalization is crucial for the consolidation of the new molar position, by giving sufficient time for the remodeling of periodontal ligament and alveolar bone tissue. For this purpose, the PA could stay for a length of time without activation. Or a new Nance button is made to aid in molar stabilization, while the premolars and anterior teeth are retracted using the newly positioned molars as anchorage. In this way the undesirable side effects, in particular the premolar mesialization and incisor tipping, will undergo a beneficial relapse. The wires which hold the acrylic Nance button should ideally be soldered to the molar bands to provide maximum anchorage. To further prevent loss of molar anchorage, extraoral force may be considered as the patient matures and compliance improves.

Sequential Anchorage Organization

A sequential and progressive involvement of the buccal segment teeth in the anchorage system must be well organized to secure a safe retraction of the anterior teeth. After a sufficient retention, both the first and second molars are serving as the anchorage for the gentle distalization of, individually, first and second premolars. The first and second premolars then could be included in the anchorage system together with the molars, which in turn finally provide support for retraction of the whole labial segment teeth.

Favorable Growth Pattern

It has been found that, although up to 87% of the molar distalization achieved during the PA phase of treatment can be lost during the follow-up phase, the Class I molar relationship can still be maintained and overjet can be corrected.[6]

Maintenance of the Class I molar relationship and improvement in overjet in adolescent patients can be explained by a favorable growth pattern (skeletal changes) and dentoalveolar compensation (e.g. intercuspation).[31] Lande found that the mandible outgrows the maxilla and becomes more prognathic relative to the cranial base during normal growth.[32] Johnston has shown that 9/10 Class II patients have a favorable growth pattern in which the mandible outgrows the maxilla.[33] After the Class I molar relationship is established during the first phase of treatment, the mandible outgrows the maxilla in most patients. Thus, the maxillary first molars must move anteriorly to the same extent that the mandibular first molars move anteriorly. If the maxillary first molars do not compensate, a Class III molar relationship would result. Because of dentoalveolar compensation and the practice of overcorrecting the molar relationship during the PA treatment, it is not surprising that only 0.8 mm of the original 5.9 mm remained at the end of comprehensive treatment in a growing patient.[6]

Treatment Effects

In principle, treatment of any sagittal arch length discrepancy is possible with a Pendulum Appliance but because few skeletal effects can be expected during PA therapy, the exclusive focus of application has been and remains restricted to distalization in the dentoalveolar region.

Dentoalveolar Effects

The Pendulum Appliance, principally a dentoalveolar treatment device, achieves Class II correction largely by tooth movement rather than by growth alteration. Several studies have reported that the PA causes the maxillary first molar to distalize with significant distal crown tipping and intrusion.[10,20] As for the premolars under PA treatment, it has been observed that the first premolars are moving mesially with mesial tipping and extrusion.[34] The eruption of the maxillary second molars has some effect on distalization of the first molars. When the first molars are being distalized, the maxillary second molars are also posteriorly displaced, tipped distally, and moved buccally.[20] A significant correlation between the amount of distalization and the degree of distal molar tipping has been found.[10] As mentioned earlier, Byloff et al have attempted to correct the molar tipping by incorporating an uprighting bend in the pendulum spring after achievement of a super Class I molar relationship.[12] The addition of an uprighting bend, however, leads to more anchorage loss and longer treatment time.

The data obtained in a study by Byloff & Darendeliler suggest that the PA is effective in moving the maxillary first molars distally at a mean monthly rate of 1.02 mm (±0.68 mm), using an initial force of 200–250 g in a mean period of 4 months.[8] Compared with other intraarch distalizing mechanisms, the treatment efficiency of PA is satisfactory. Kurol & Bjerklin advocate the use of 250 g of cervical force on each side and move molars distally in 9–12 months.[35] Hubbard et al used records of treatment with the traditional Kloehn-type of cervical headgear delivering 680–770 g on each side for a mean of 6 months, depending on patient cooperation.[36] When combined high-pull and cervical traction were used, the total force level is 1135–1360 g per side, and molars moved distally an average of 2.4 mm in a mean of 4 months.[37] On the other hand, treatment with a combination of cervical headgear and activator or high-pull headgear and activator producing 400 g of extraoral force per side requires a period of about 1 year to obtain a Class I molar relationship.[38]

Skeletal Effects

The skeletal changes during PA therapy are relatively unimportant. PA therapy alone seems to indicate that little impact is to be expected on the patient's skeletal skull development.[9]

Evaluation of the effects of the PA on the lower anterior facial height has shown conflicting results. Bussick & McNamara have reported statistically significant increases in lower anterior facial height in all their patients, regardless of original facial type.[9] Byloff & Darendeliler have reported that there is no tendency to bite opening with PA treatment, and there is an increase of the y-axis angle of 0.81° and PP/MP angle of 0.89°, whose clinical relevance seems to be negligible.[8] In the study by Ghosh & Nanda, a small backward rotation of the mandible (mean 1.09°) was observed.[20] They divide their patients into three groups based on the Frankfort mandibular plane angle and claim that there is a trend after PA treatment toward an increase in the mandibular plane angle, which, however, is not statistically significant.

It should be noted that when molars are distalized with a significant proportion of crown distal tipping, an increased mandibular angle, and subsequently an increased lower facial height or even creation of open bite, is expected.[27] This phenomenon does not happen during PA treatment, possibly due to the fact that the appliance appears to tip the molars back in an arc with tipping occurring near the apex of the roots. This is especially advantageous in the treatment of high angle Class II and/or dentally crowded patients.

References

1. Gianelly AA, Vaitas AS, Thomas WM. The use of magnets to move molars distally. Am J Orthod Dentofacial Orthop 1989;96:161–167.
2. Bondemark L, Kurol J. Distalization of maxillary first and second molars simultaneously with repelling magnets. Eur J Orthod 1992;14:264–272.
3. Ferro F, Monsurro A, Perillo L. Sagittal and vertical changes after treatment of Class II division I malocclusion according to the Cetlin method. Am J Orthod Dentofacial Orthop 2000;118:150–158.
4. Rana R, Becher MK. Class II correction using the Bimetric Distalizing Arch. Semin Orthod 2000;6:106–118.
5. Brickman CD, Sinha PK, Nanda RS. Evaluation of the Jones jig appliance for distal molar movement. Am J Orthod Dentofacial Orthop 2000;118:526–534.
6. Burkhardt DR, McNamara JA Jr, Baccetti T. Maxillary molar distalization or mandibular enhancement: a cephalometric comparison of comprehensive orthodontic treatment including the pendulum and the Herbst appliances. Am J Orthod Dentofacial Orthop 2003;123:108–116.
7. Hilgers JJ. The pendulum appliance for Class II non-compliance therapy. J Clin Orthod 1992;26:706–714.
8. Byloff FK, Darendeliler MA. Distal molar movement using the pendulum appliance. Part 1: Clinical and radiological evaluation. Angle Orthod 1997;67:249–260.
9. Bussick TJ, McNamara JA Jr. Dentoalveolar and skeletal changes associated with the pendulum appliance. Am J Orthod Dentofacial Orthop 2000;117:333–343.
10. Joseph AA, Butchart CJ. An evaluation of the pendulum distalizing appliance. Semin Orthod 2000;6:129–135.
11. Sfondrini MF, Cacciafesta V, Sfondrini G. Upper molar distalization: a critical analysis. Orthod Craniofac Res 2002;5:114–126.
12. Byloff FK, Darendeliler MA, Clar E, Darendeliler A. Distal molar movement using the pendulum appliance. Part 2: The effects of maxillary molar root uprighting bands. Angle Orthod 1997;67:261–270.
13. Byloff FK, Karcher H, Clar E, Stoff F. An implant to eliminate anchorage loss during molar distalization: a case report involving the Graz implant-supported pendulum. Int J Adult Orthod Orthognath Surg 2000;15:129–137.
14. Grummons D. Nonextraction emphasis: space-gaining efficiencies, Part 1. World J Orthod 2001;2:21–32.
15. Scuzzo G, Takemoto K, Pisani F, Della Vecchia S. The modified pendulum appliance with removable arms. J Clin Orthod 2000;34:244–246.
16. Kinzinger G, Fuhrmann R, Gross U, Diedrich P. Modified pendulum appliance including distal screw and uprighting activation for non-compliance therapy of Class II malocclusion in children and adolescents. J Orofac Orthop 2000;61:175–190.
17. Kinzinger G, Fritz U, Diedrich P. Bipendulum and quad pendulum for non-compliance molar distalization in adult patients. J Orofac Orthop 2002;63:154–162.
18. Kinzinger G, Fritz U, Stenmans A, Diedrich P. Pendulum K-group: pendulum appliances for non-compliance molar distalization in children and adolescents. Kieferorthop 2003;7:11–24.
19. DeVincenzo DJ. Treatment options for sagittal corrections in noncompliant patients. In: Graber TM, Vanarsdall RL Jr, eds. Orthodontics: current principles and techniques, 3rd edn. St Louis: Mosby; 2000: 779–800.
20. Ghosh J, Nanda RS. Evaluation of an intraoral maxillary molar distalization technique. Am J Orthod Dentofacial Orthop 1996;110:639–646.
21. Worms FW, Isaacson RJ, Speidel TM. A concept and classification of centers of rotation and extraoral force systems. Angle Orthod 1973;43:384–401.
22. Graber TM. Extraoral forces – facts and fallacies. Am J Orthod 1955;41:490–505.
23. Bondemark L, Kurol J, Bemhold M. Repelling magnets versus superelastic nickel titanium coils in the simultaneous distal movement of maxillary first and second molars. Angle Orthod 1994;64:189–198.
24. Gianelly AA, Vaitas AS, Thomas WM, Berger OG. Distalization of molars with repelling magnets. Case report. J Clin Orthod 1988;22:40–44.

25. Ten Hoeve A. Palatal bar and lip bumper in nonextraction treatment. J Clin Orthod 1985; 19:272–291.

26. Jeckel N, Rakosi T. Molar distalization by intra-oral force application. Eur J Orthod 1991;3:43–46.

27. Gianelly AA. Distal movement of the maxillary molars. Am J Orthod Dentofacial Orthop 1998; 114:66–72.

28. Kinzinger GS, Fritz UB, Sander FG, Diedrich PR. Efficiency of a pendulum appliance for molar distalization related to second and third molar eruption stage. Am J Orthod Dentofacial Orthop 2004;125:8–23.

29. Hotz RP. Zahnmedizin bei Kindern und jugendlichen. Stuttgart: Thieme; 1976.

30. Korn M, Schnabel S. Flexible upper and lower lip bumpers in mixed dentition therapy. Kieferorthop 1994;8:81–88.

31. Solow B. The dentoalveolar compensatory mechanism: background and clinical implications. Br J Orthod 1980;7:145–161.

32. Lande MJ. Growth behavior of the human bony facial profile as revealed by serial cephalometric roentgenology. Angle Orthod 1952;22:78–90.

33. Johnston LE Jr. Growth and the Class II patient: rendering unto Caesar. Semin Orthod 1998;4:59–62.

34. Toroglu MS, Uzel I, Cam OY, Hancioglu ZB. Cephalometric evaluation of the effects of pendulum appliance on various vertical growth patterns and of the changes during short-term stabilization. Clin Orthod Res 2001;4:15–27.

35. Kurol J, Bjerklin K. Treatment of children with ectopic eruption of the maxillary first permanent molar by cervical traction. Am J Orthod 1984;86:483–492.

36. Hubbard GW, Nanda RS, Currier GF. A cephalometric evaluation of nonextraction cervical headgear treatment in Class II malocclusions. Angle Orthod 1994;64:359–370.

37. Badell MC. An evaluation of extraoral combined high-pull traction and cervical traction to the maxilla. Am J Orthod 1976;69:431–446.

38. Ngan P, Scheick J, Florman M. A tensor analysis to evaluate the effect of high-pull headgear on Class II malocclusions. Am J Orthod Dentofacial Orthop 1993;103:267–279.

CHAPTER 17

The Penguin Pendulum

Joe H. Mayes

CONTENTS

Introduction

This unique molar distalizing appliance was developed in the mid 1990s to alleviate the problems I was experiencing with other distalizing appliances: A point and upper incisors moving forward as a result of the pressure to move the molars back.[1]

There are several things that are different about this appliance when compared to other distalizing appliances (Fig. 17.1). There is no expansion screw in it as this would waste the best palatal anchorage area and the only place in the palate where a 1–1.5 mm vertical component of cortical bone is present. Unlike all other molar distalizers, this appliance uses the palate for anchorage. All other appliances use a combination of palatal support and/or tooth support and have reciprocal movement of upper bicuspids and molars. This appliance is only as thick as a Hawley retainer and has a smooth swallowing trough for comfort. The distalizing springs are as close to parallel to the long axis of the molar as possible and are removable for easy adjustment (Figs 17.2 and 17.3). There is a single bonded attachment on each side to hold the appliance in place and slightly open the bite to allow more rapid molar distalizing.[2]

The second bicuspids are free to move distal on their own, being pulled by transseptal fibers from the molars. The appliance uses the forces of occlusion to help distalize the molars. The pressure forces in the palate to move the molars distally are as close to parallel to the trabecular pattern in the palate as possible (Fig. 17.4). Finally, due to the combination of bodily/tipping movement of the molars distally, a "Tweed tent stake" type of anchorage is achieved.

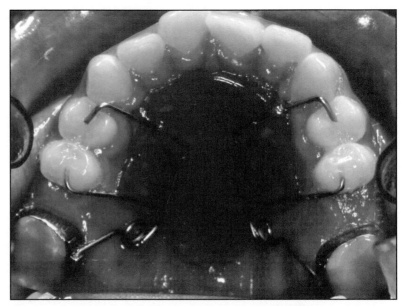

Figure 17.1 The original Penguin Pendulum. Note the bonding material off the occlusal of the first bicuspids. This occurred due to rocking over the occlusal attachment to the second bicuspid and is the reason only one attachment is needed.

Clinical Study

The Penguin Pendulum clinically did not appear to advance A point or the upper incisors. Since anecdotal data or clinical experiences are not scientific, a study was developed to test the efficacy of all molar distalizing appliances available at the time. Four things were to be tracked for evaluation: treatment time in minutes of chair time and total treatment time in months; compare actual treatment times to estimated treatment times, measure comfort levels; and compare different appliances' abilities to distalize upper molars. Six appliances were evaluated in this study: the Hilgers Pendulum,[3] T-Rex and Pendex, PHD and MDA,[4] Nance with braces and springs, Distal Jet, and Penguin Pendulum. The groups consisted of 20 consecutively treated patients each.

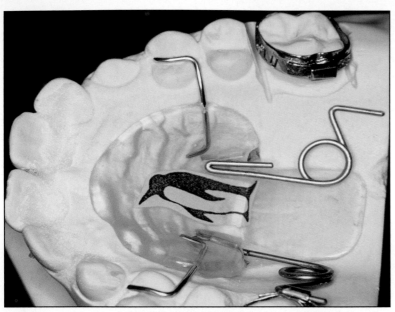

Figure 17.2 The distalizing springs are removable for easy activation before delivery of the appliance and during molar distalization. Observe the smooth swallowing trough; the second bicuspids are free to distalize following the molars.

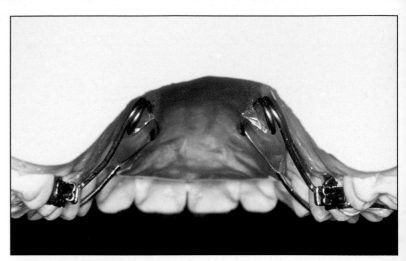

Figure 17.3 From the distal of the palate, it can be seen that the lever arms of the distalizing springs are as close to parallel to the long axis of the molar as possible. This is the major difference between this appliance and other molar distalizing appliances.

A letter was given to each patient to share with their spouse/parents explaining what the study was trying to accomplish. In the letter it was noted that the appliance currently being used was probably the best for moving their teeth distally and the study was being performed to verify this. This was emphasized to reassure patients that they were being treated with the best appliance available. Headfilms were measured before treatment and compared to posttreatment appliance headfilms to measure advancement of A point and upper incisors. An electronic caliper was used to measure from the most anterior-inferior portion of the sella turcica to both A point and the incisal edge of the upper incisor. All appliances satisfactorily moved the upper molars distally in two visits (9–10 week intervals or 4.5–5 months) of active treatment (Table 17.1).

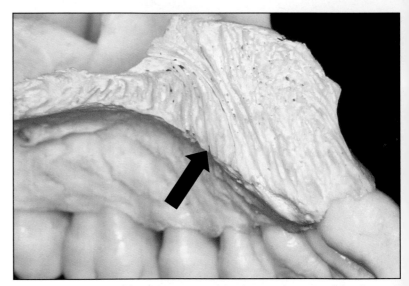

Figure 17.4 The center of the pressure against the palate is as close to parallel to the trabecular pattern as possible. The Penguin Pendulum creates the molar distalizing force by pressing against the palate and is not a tooth-borne appliance trading tooth movement for tooth movement.

Table 17.1. The results of the in-office clinical study: averages of each appliance group.

Appliance	Comfort (scale 1–40)	A point change (mm)	Upper incisor change (mm)
Pendulum (Hilgers)	6.85	0.24	0.33
T-Rex, Pendex	4.3	0.45	1.37
PHD, MDA	5.9	0.16	0.9
Nance with braces	6.45	0.18	0.85
Distal Jet	6.6	0.42	1.07
Penguin Pendulum	7.55	0.05	0.1

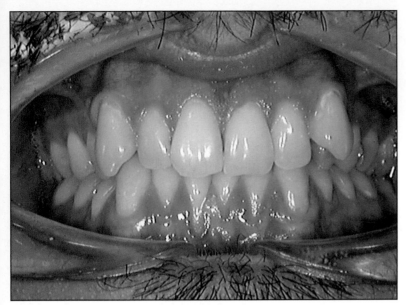
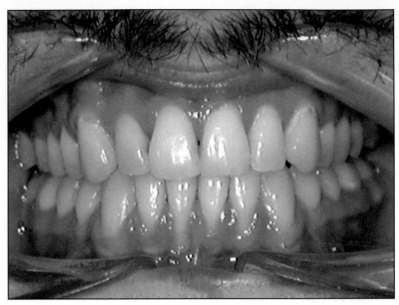

Figures 17.5, 17.6 Anterior view and tracing before treatment.

Figures 17.7,17.8 Anterior view and tracing after treatment. Note the tracings show no advancement of the upper anteriors while marked torque was effected.

Name:
ID:
DOB: 02/17/71
X-Ray: 04/10/00
Age: 29 yrs 1 mos
Desc: 04/10/2000

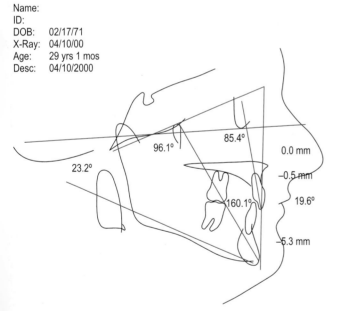

Figure 17.6

Name:
ID:
DOB: 02/17/71
X-Ray: 10/02/02
Age: 31 yrs 7 mos
Desc: 10/02/02

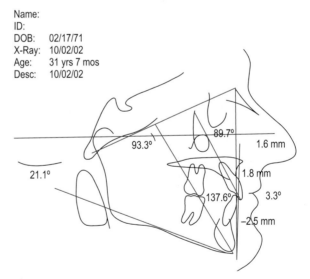

Figure 17.8

Sample Case

A 32-year-old male patient presented for orthodontic evaluation and treatment. He was diagnosed as skeletal Class I with dental Class II molar and cuspid relationships. Both upper cuspids were blocked labially. His upper midline was approximately 3 mm to the left of the center of his face. He had minimal crowding of the lower arch with a dehiscence of the lower right central, moderately deep anterior bite and a small labial area of enamel missing on his upper left cuspid. The agreed treatment plan was to distalize his upper molars to create room to unravel the maxillary crowding without the need for tooth structure removal. Braces would be placed on the lower arch first and bite turbos would be used to open his bite. Progressive anterior bonding of his upper buccal segments would be done and space closure would be accomplished without upper archwires and using elastic chains and a Nance holding arch

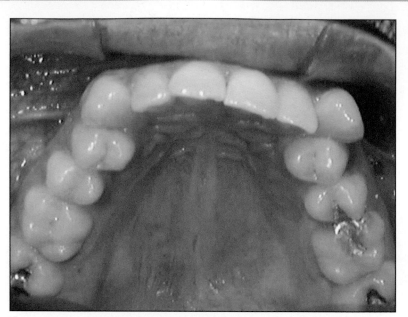

Figure 17.9 Maxillary occlusal view before treatment.

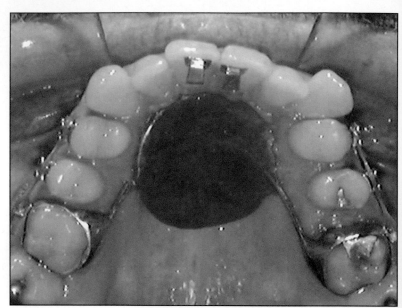

Figure 17.10 Partial retraction of upper buccal segments.

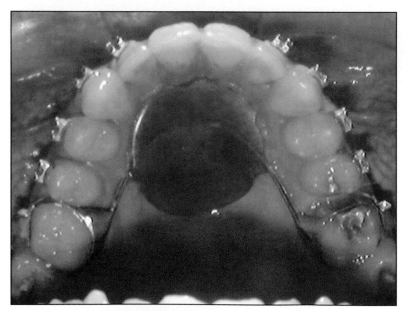

Figure 17.11 Progressive bonding anteriorly.

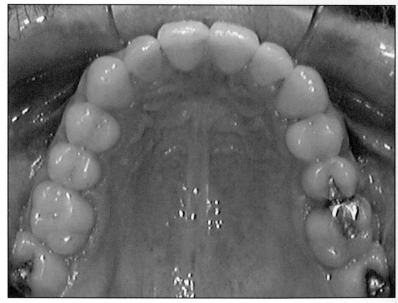

Figure 17.12 Upper arch after treatment.

for anchorage after molar distalization. Treatment involved 21 months of active therapy and 14 visits, from new patient exam to retainer delivery (Figs 17.5–17.23).

Troubleshooting

The three most common problems with the Penguin Pendulum are all due to inappropriate adjustments of the distalizing springs. The most common problem is to leave the bend in the 0.032″ TMA wire (Ormco, Orange, CA) too long and embed the distal of the swallowing trough into the palate. The second most common problem is to make the same bend too short and embed the anterior part of the appliance into the palate. The third most common error is to overactivate the distalizing spring. The spring should only be activated 45°. Remember that the spring is removable and can be reactivated as needed without removing the appliance.

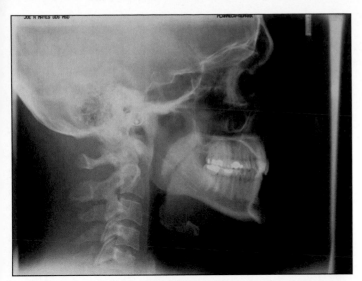

Figure 17.13 Head film before treatment.

Conclusion

Whenever the force to move the molars distally was horizontal, the appliance tended to be tooth borne and advance and extrude the bicuspids. It would also trade reciprocal movement of the anchorage teeth for movement of the molars. Whether the horizontal force was in the palate (Hilgers' Pendulum), part way down the palate (Distal Jet) or near the occlusal plane (Nance with braces), a horizontal force tended to open the bite and advance upper bicuspids. The reciprocal movement of the molars was a result of moving bicuspids forward and/or palatal anchorage that was allowing the palatal button to slip forward and down. The Penguin Pendulum worked just as well with

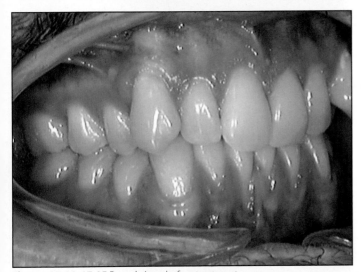

Figures 17.14, 17.15 Buccal views before treatment.

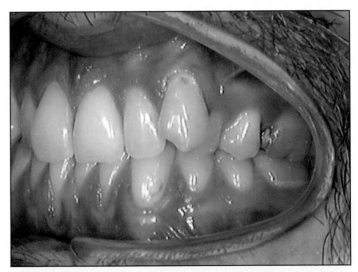

Figure 17.15

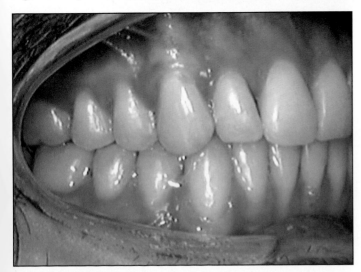

Figures 17.16, 17.17 Buccal views after treatment.

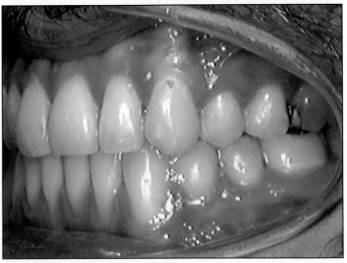

Figure 17.17

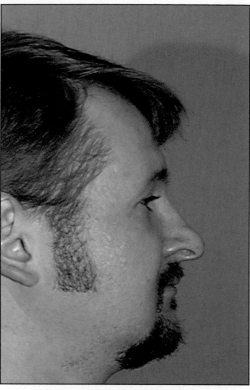

Figure 17.18 Profile view before treatment.

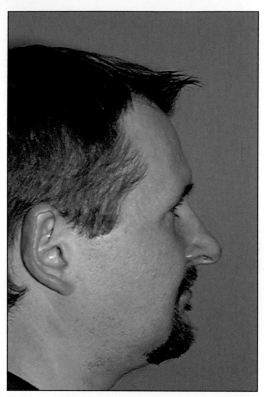

Figure 17.19 Profile view after treatment.

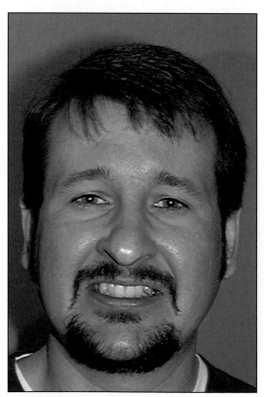

Figure 17.20 Frontal smiling view before treatment.

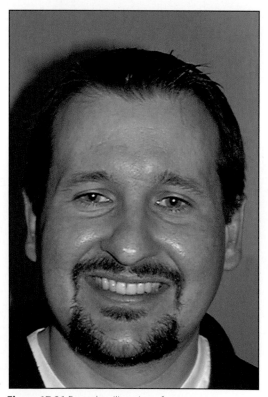

Figure 17.21 Frontal smiling view after treatment.

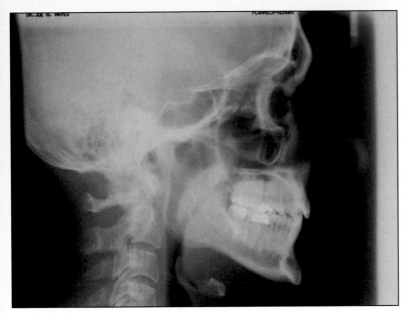

Figure 17.22 Head film after treatment.

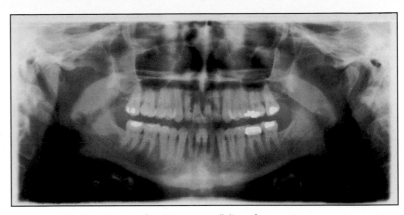

Figure 17.23 Panoramic view showing root parallelism after treatment.

unilateral corrections as with bilateral corrections. The single drawback with the Penguin Pendulum is in treating open bites. Due to the fact that it uses occlusal forces to help distalize the upper molars; open-bite cases should probably be treated with upper bicuspid extractions.

References

1. Mayes JH. The Texas Penguin... new approach to pendulum therapy. AOA Orthodontic Appliances 1999;3:1–2.

2. Mayes JH, Clark J, Paz M, Tracey S. Fixed molar distalizing appliances. Clin Impressions 2003;12: 18–21.

3. Hilgers JJ. The Pendulum appliance...an update. Clin Impressions 1993;2:15–17.

4. Hilgers JJ, Bennet RK. The pendulum appliance: creating the gain. Clin Impressions 1994;3:14–23.

CHAPTER 18

Noncompliance Class II treatment with the Distal Jet™

†Aldo Carano, Steven Jay Bowman

CONTENTS

Introduction

One of the most commonly treated orthodontic problems is the Class II malocclusion. It is prevalent in 15–20% of the American population and seen mostly in Caucasians of northern European descent.[1] Since the turn of the 20th century many articles have delved into the etiology and correction of this dental and skeletal problem. Many researchers have developed numerous treatment modalities for Class II correction from compliance-oriented headgear treatment to noncompliance treatment using intraoral devices to distalize the maxillary molars into a Class I occlusion. Although most of these methods have been shown to be effective, some of them may be subject to failure due to lack of patient cooperation. Headgear must be worn for 12–14 hours a day with constant force placed on the dentition in order to be effective. In today's lifestyle, with children involved in many activities, finding an extended period of time to wear the appliance is usually problematic. Unfortunately, the success of orthodontic care is often dependent upon compliance, a commodity that is unpredictable and unfortunately declining.

Over the past decade, nonextraction treatments with noncompliance therapies have become very popular in treating Class II malocclusions. While some therapies are designed to advance the mandible,[2–4] others are designed to distalize the maxillary molars into a Class I position.[5,6] One of the exciting developments in orthodontics is the use of maxillary molar distalization devices for the correction of Class II malocclusions. The number of different fixed and removable appliances available to practitioners is extensive and they range from complicated devices that are cemented[7] and are activated by the orthodontist to the simple use of compressed open coil springs to translate molars distally. Magnets have also been incorporated into appliances with a Nance button framework and have been used with success.[8] Nickel-titanium (NiTi) coil springs have become popular due to the constant forces they exert rather than the dissipating forces of the magnets.[6] Nickel-titanium coil springs have been incorporated into many devices such as the Jones Jig[9] and Wilson's Bimetric Distalizing Arch,[10] and the springs have been used alone.[6]

The deflection of wires also has been used to produce distal molar movement. For example, the Pendulum Appliance uses a large acrylic Nance button that covers the midportion of the palate for anchorage, while helical springs (made of 0.032″ TMA wire) exert the distalizing force.[11,12] Another option for distal molar movement is to use a 100 g NiTi wire, compressed between the maxillary first premolars and maxillary first molars with crimpable stops.[13] Most of these therapies utilize some variation of palatal coverage to provide anchorage in an attempt to reduce unwanted incisor flaring.

In 1995, Carano & Testa introduced a new "distalizer" with the purpose of improving the control of molars during distal movement.[14–16] Over the past several years, the Distal Jet™ has become the molar distalizing appliance of choice in many practices worldwide. Consistently reliable results together with the esthetic and noncompliance aspects of the appliance are the features that initially generated interest in the Distal Jet and are responsible for its continuing rise in popularity and acceptance as an established method of treatment.

Since the introduction of the Distal Jet, several modifications of the initial design have been suggested. In 1998, dual control (palatal and buccal) for upper molar distalization was suggested by Fortini et al using a buccal screw, turned once a day, to obtain the distalization.[17] Celestino suggested inverting the telescopic units of the original design with two adjustable locks, one for activation and the other connected to the lingual sheath of the molar band.[18] Both locks were free to slide upon a 1.2 mm wire that functioned as a guide for molar distalization. A nickel-titanium open coil spring was positioned between the two locking clamps and activated by the movement of the mesial clamp towards the distal one. A similar design concept was introduced by Bowman when developing a reuseable distalizing appliance for use by students in typodont training at the University of Michigan.[19]

The Distal Jet

With respect to the aforementioned appliances, the Distal Jet, a palatally positioned distalization appliance, is said to feature several distinct advantages: the maxillary molars are distalized with less distal tipping and without the lingual constriction of molars that can occur with the other noncompliance "distalizers" (e.g. Pendulum, Jones Jig, Greenfield Appliance), and it can be easily converted into a Nance holding arch to maintain the distalized molar position.[5,16] Consequently, this device serves two purposes with one laboratory fabrication.

Fabrication of the Distal Jet

The Distal Jet is constructed with two bilateral tubes embedded in a modified acrylic Nance palatal button according to the recommendations of the inventors (Figs 18.1 and 18.2).[14–16] The position of these tubes is critical for proper functioning and will be discussed later. The Nance button is typically anchored by supporting wires to the first premolars but in some applications the second premolars or deciduous molars could also be used. A bayonet wire is inserted into the lingual sheath of each first molar band and the free end is inserted into the tubes, much like a piston. A nickel-titanium open coil spring and an activation collar (i.e. screw clamp) are placed on each tube. A distally directed force is generated by compressing the coil spring: the activation collar is retracted and the mesial set-screw in each collar is locked onto the tube to maintain the force (Figs 18.3 and 18.4).

The activation collar plays the major role in both the distalization and retention phases of molar correction with the Distal Jet. Because the Distal Jet is encompassed entirely within the palatal vault, space availability and patient comfort were primary considerations in its original design. As such, the set-screw within the activation collar and its wrench are small, which generated some concerns:

- inability to adequately visualize the screw location (hex head opening)
- difficult access to the screw head
- stripping of the hex portion of the screw, the thin activation wrench, or both
- inability to obtain positive engagement of the lock on the tube (bayonet director) to fully compress the spring
- a subjective feeling of "looseness" (lack of rigidity) of the appliance in the retention phase.

Comparing the old design of the locking mechanism with the new one,[20] the following changes have been made:

- the lock has been totally redesigned for better functionality and efficiency
- the manufacturing of the lock has been changed from a machining process to a casting process using MIM (Metal Injection Molding) technology. This has allowed new design options that the original part would not
- the screw and activation wrench are much more substantial in size and fabricated with small tolerances to each other for greater durability and security, and to minimize any potential stripping that might occur (see Fig. 18.3).

The changes to the activation collar are readily evident (see Fig. 18.4). Of particular note is the return to a single screw design from the dual screw design in the original lock.

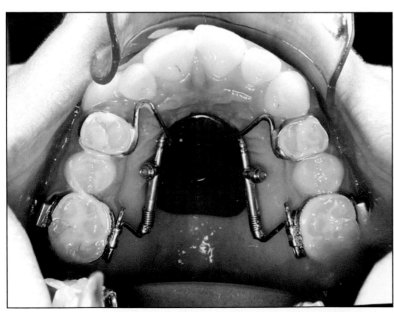

Figure 18.1 The Distal Jet before distalization.

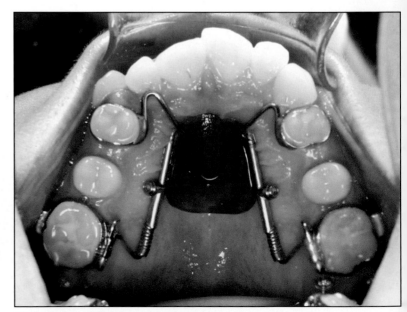

Figure 18.2 The Distal Jet after distalization.

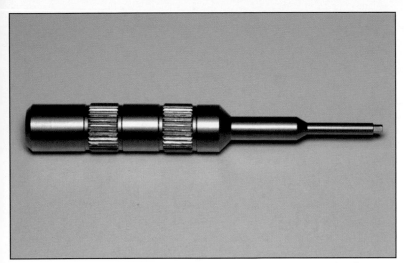

Figures 18.3, 18.4 The activation collar is retracted and the set-screw in each collar is locked with a wrench onto the tube to maintain the force.

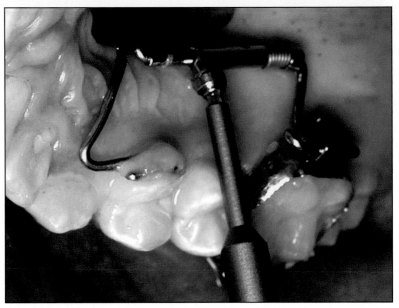

Figure 18.4 The nickel-titanium open-coil spring is totally compressed and delivers a distalizing force passing through a couple close to the center of resistance of the molars.

- The single screw design simplifies chairside management of the Distal Jet by eliminating any potential confusion as to which screw(s) to activate during distalization and conversion to retaining Nance space maintainer.

- In conjunction with the single screw, the barrel (horizontal portion) of the lock has been extended by 7 mm, thereby extending the working range of the appliance and simplifying the activation. The screw is more mesial than the previous lock, thus facilitating access to the screw.

- The extension of the lock simplifies the conversion process, as will be explained shortly.

- The barrel has also seen considerable reduction in its diameter; not only for increased patient comfort but also to allow more precise positioning of the tube (bayonet director) and the piston (bayonet) as well as making fabrication easier, especially in patients with smaller, narrow palates.

- The vertical component of the lock serves a dual purpose: it not only orients the screw in a more accessible position with easier visualization (mesially and occlusally), but it also can be used as a tie-back post for appliance delivery and stabilization of the Distal Jet when converting from active appliance to molar retainer.

A seemingly minor but important change is the introduction of a matching posterior stop. This tiny part prevents the coil spring from migrating up the bayonet wire. The new stop is fabricated from stainless steel tubing and, when compared to the previous plastic ball stop, it will not deform under pressure. It provides better resistance for more consistent and positive spring compression and force delivery during distalization. The diameter and profile of the stop also match with the new lock to give a seamless junction, continuity of parts, and improved hygiene upon appliance conversion to a retainer. Both activation and conversion of the Distal Jet have been simplified for easier clinical management and more effective treatment results.

With respect to appliance construction, the orientation of the distalizing force, the anatomy of the palate, and the position of the germs of the maxillary second molars are all variables that appear to influence molar tipping during distalization. For example, the position of the tube/piston telescopic unit is critical for proper functioning of the Distal Jet. The tube/piston should be oriented parallel, but 4–5 mm superior, to the occlusal plane. The intent of this construction is to direct the line of action to the level of the center of resistance of the maxillary first molars to limit molar tipping.

The depth of the palate also plays an important role in determining the position of this line of action and also the dimensions of the Nance palatal button. A shallow palate may prevent construction of a piston wire with sufficient vertical length from the first molar to the bayonet bend, thereby producing a line of action that is occlusal to the molar's center of resistance. This could, in turn, create more tipping of the molar during distalization. Originally, the telescopic units were not fabricated absolutely parallel to the occlusal plane, but rather with the posterior portion of the device inclined 3° superiorly, towards the cranial base. This small difference in inclination may have reduced molar extrusion and prevented increases in the vertical dimension, but perhaps contributed to more molar tipping.

Altering the construction design can modulate the amount of maxillary first molar expansion from the Distal Jet. Typically, the Distal Jet is fabricated with the telescopic unit positioned parallel to a line passing through the contact points of the posterior teeth (Fig. 18.5). With this geometry, distalization should produce divergence of the right and left molars along the natural shape of

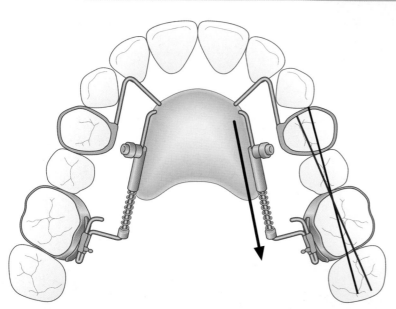

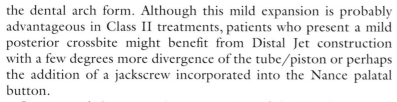

Figure 18.5 The Distal Jet is fabricated with the telescopic unit positioned parallel to a line passing through the contact points of the posterior teeth (black line). It is not parallel to the line passing through the center of the occlusal tables.

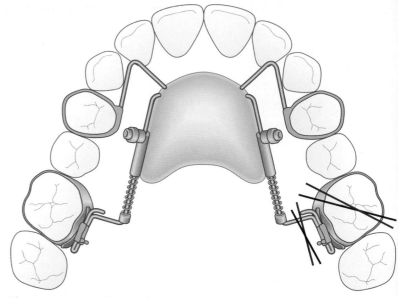

Figure 18.6 In cases where the first molars are mesially rotated (profile in black), a simple modification to the design of the Distal Jet (a compensating bend placed in the double-back portion of the bayonet wire just prior to seating the Distal Jet) may derotate the molars (profile in red).

the dental arch form. Although this mild expansion is probably advantageous in Class II treatments, patients who present a mild posterior crossbite might benefit from Distal Jet construction with a few degrees more divergence of the tube/piston or perhaps the addition of a jackscrew incorporated into the Nance palatal button.

Large angulation errors in construction of the Distal Jet could result in more dramatic clinical concerns such as increased lower anterior face height resulting from extruded molars or the development of posterior open bites from intruded molars. Consequently, attention to detail during the construction of this appliance is critical to its clinical performance.

Since the distal force of the Distal Jet Appliance is delivered to the lingual of the molars, it is not unreasonable to expect some adverse mesial rotation of the buccal cusps of the maxillary first molar around the palatal root. A simple modification of the Distal Jet (i.e. a compensating bend is placed in the double-back portion of the bayonet wire that inserts into the lingual sheath on the molar tube) is made just prior to seating the appliance to help to prevent adverse rotation of the molar or, in fact, to create a distal rotation of the molar around the palatal root.[5] This type of rotation has been advocated as favorable to the correction of many Class II molar relationships (Fig. 18.6).

Once the first molars have been moved into a Class I or super Class III overcorrected relationship, the Distal Jet is converted into a modified Nance holding arch by sealing the clamp-spring assemblies with cold-cure acrylic or by locking the set-screws of the activation collars onto the tube and piston. Subsequently, the coil spring and supporting wires to the first premolars are cut and removed.[5]

Appliance Activation

After trial fit and subsequent cementation of the Distal Jet, the lingual sheath should be squeezed with a utility plier to secure the double-back bayonet wire. This firms up the connection of the molar to the bayonet wire for more precise control during distalization. Alternatively, either a steel ligature or separating elastic may be used to tie the sheath and wire together. The separating elastics have the advantage of providing a "cushion effect" for increased patient comfort. They must be checked at each appointment and replaced when necessary.

The activation wrench is then positioned into the recess in the screw head (0.050 hex head). Using the wrench as a guide, the activation collar or lock is directed distally to compress the spring. The screw is then tightened onto the tube to maintain the force (see Figs 18.3 and 18.4). The Distal Jet is typically reactivated every 4–6 weeks during a 5–6 month period of treatment.

Derotation of the Molars Before Distalization

A unique feature of the Distal Jet is its ability to correct and control rotated molars. Rotational bends are easily placed in the double-back wire sections of the double-back portion of the bayonet wires, just as they would be with a transpalatal bar (see Fig. 18.6).[5]

- These corrective bends should be made *before* the appliance is cemented in the mouth. This can be done in the lab, during appliance construction, or at the chairside, when the appliance is delivered.

- Rotations should be corrected *before* activating the appliance to distalize the molars.

Lengthening the barrel of the new locks has greatly facilitated these adjustments.

Converting to a Retainer

After distalization of the molar(s) has been completed, the Distal Jet is now converted to a passive appliance (modified Nance holding arch) to retain the molar(s) in their new positions. The conversion steps are quite simple.

- Loosen the set-screw in each activation collar to decompress the coil spring (Fig. 18.7).
- Peel the spring from the bayonet wire (piston) by grabbing the mesial end with a slim-nosed Weingart utility or other appropriate pliers and pull the spring away in one continuous motion (Fig. 18.8).

- Slide the activation collar distally against the steel stop and tighten the screw (Fig. 18.9). The lock/screw combination has been designed to accommodate up to 7.5 mm of distalization (i.e. the mesiodistal width of a premolar).
- Squeeze the terminal end of the activation collar tube tightly onto the bayonet wire using a utility pliers or wire cutter. This step locks the unit together and prevents potential movement of the acrylic button out of the palate (Figs 18.10 and 18.11).
- Alternatively, a steel or elastic tie may be placed from the vertical leg of the bayonet wire to the vertical arm of the activation lock, thus accomplishing the same result. Of course, both techniques may be used together, if desired (Fig. 18.12).
- Cut the arms that connect the resin button of the palate to the premolars (Fig. 18.13).

Implants for Absolute Anchorage

All the previous studies on molar distalization have shown some degree of reciprocal (anterior) anchorage loss. A skeletal anchorage system (i.e. implant-based anchorage) may help as an adjunct to or substitute for dental anchorage. The ideal implant site, based on the flexibility of the anchorage application, would seem to be the palate even though it requires an invasive procedure to place the implant and another to remove it. As a result, when considering the procedures required to insert, integrate and remove a palatal, osseointegrated implant for orthodontic anchorage, many will deem this procedure as too excessive, expensive or invasive, despite the advantages.

The use of a mini-screw anchorage system (e.g. palatal implants) combined with the Distal Jet may represent an easier solution as

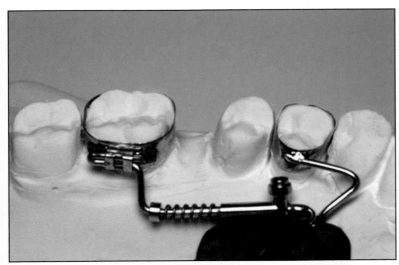

Figures 18.7–18.13 The conversion steps to a retainer. Loosen the set-screw to decompress the coil spring.

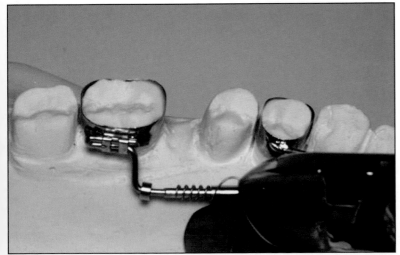

Figure 18.8 Peel the spring from the bayonet wire.

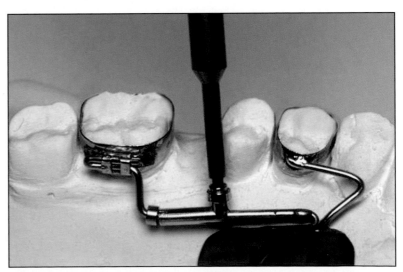

Figure 18.9 Slide the activation collar distally against the steel stop and tighten the screw.

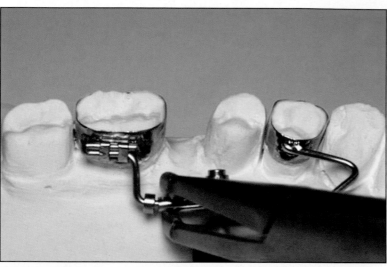

Figures 18.10, 18.11 Squeeze the terminal end of the activation collar tube.

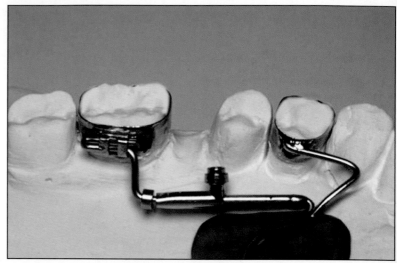

Figure 18.11

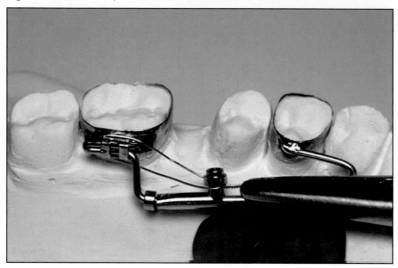

Figure 18.12 Place a steel tie from the vertical leg of the bayonet wire to the vertical arm of the activation lock.

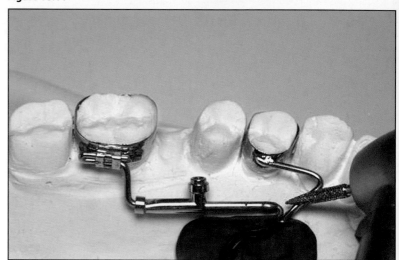

Figure 18.13 Cut the arms that connect the resin button of the palate to the premolars.

these types of implants are typically not osseointegrated (Fig. 18.14), thereby precluding the need for a trephination procedure for their removal. As a consequence, mini-screws are cheaper and easier to place and to remove.

An ideal site for the placement of a micro- or mini-screw implant is the maxillary alveolar process and, more precisely, the site in between the root of the first and second premolars. After the molar distalization appliance (Distal Jet) has been positioned and activated, the mini-screws are positioned bilaterally, just mesial to the activation lock (Figs 18.15–18.18). The mini-screw will block the mesial movement of the appliance during the distalization and consequently, the loss of anterior anchorage will be prevented. During the distalization, further compression of the coil spring of the Distal Jet will move the lock more distally and far from the head of the mini-screw. In this phase, the loss of anchorage can be prevented by placing

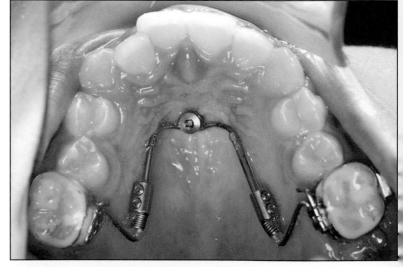

Figure 18.14 The use of a mini-screw anchorage system (e.g. palatal implants) combined with the Distal Jet may represent an easier solution to the risk of anchorage loss.

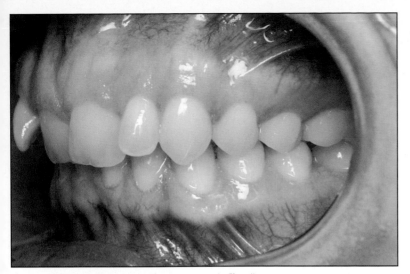

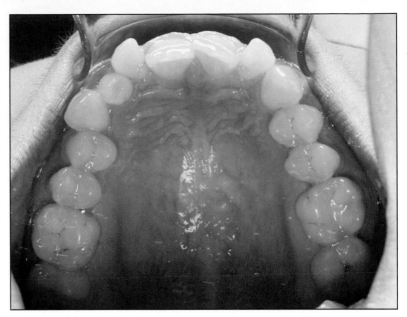

Figures 18.15–18.22 Patient with an asymmetric Class II.

Figure 18.16

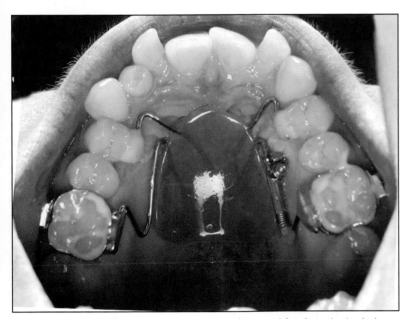

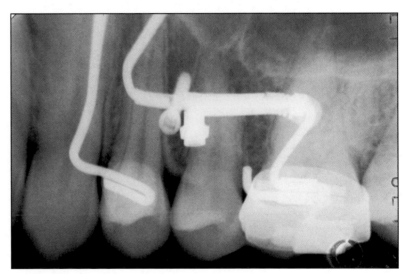

Figures 18.17, 18.18 The mini-screw was positioned just mesial to the activation lock.

Figure 18.18

some light-cure composite in between the head of the mini-screw anchorage system and the lock (Figs 18.19 and 18.20).

After molar distalization is complete, the Distal Jet is converted into a retainer and full-fixed appliances are bonded on the remaining teeth to complete treatment. After 4–5 months, or after residual spaces are closed, the Distal Jet retainer can be removed (Fig. 18.21). Another option is to remove the mini-screws that are mesial to the activation collar and place them just mesial to the distalized molar to prevent mesial molar anchorage loss during retraction of the remaining maxillary dentition (Fig. 18.22). Currently, this protocol (Distal Jet + mini-screw) is considered only for patients in the permanent dentition as these screws may jeopardize the developing permanent teeth.

An alternative site for mini-screw anchorage would be adjacent to the midpalatal suture in the anterior maxillary vault. A simplified version of the Distal Jet (i.e. without supporting wires to the premolars or an acrylic button) is abutted to the implant during both molar distalization and as support for subsequent retraction.[21]

Clinical Effects

A summary of the clinical effects of the Distal Jet is given in Figure 18.23.

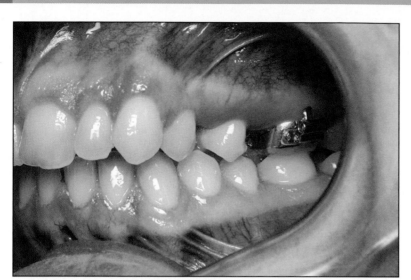

Figures 18.19, 18.20 During the distalization some light cure composite is placed in between the head of the screw and the lock.

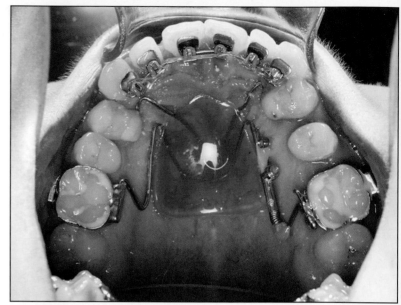

Figure 18.20

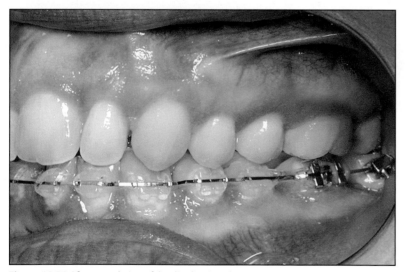

Figure 18.21 After completion of the distalization phase.

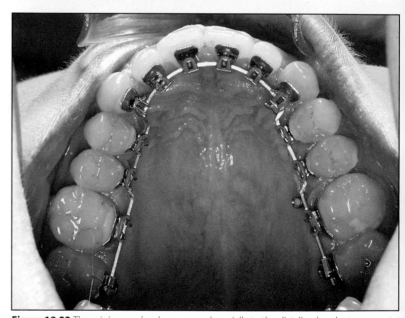

Figure 18.22 The mini-screw has been moved mesially to the distalized molar to prevent mesial molar anchorage loss during retraction of the remaining maxillary dentition.

Molar Distalization and Tipping

During a 5–6 month period, the Distal Jet moves the crowns of the maxillary first molars distally on average 3.2 mm/side into a Class I relationship.[22] In 20 consecutive patients treated with only the Distal Jet, the maxillary first molars were also tipped distally by an average of 3.1°,[22] a lesser effect than reported by Guiterrez[23] (7.3°) but comparable to that seen by Chiu et al[24] in similar evaluation of the Distal Jet without concurrent use of orthodontic brackets (3.8°) (Fig. 18.24).

Molar Distalization and Creation of Spaces

During molar distalization with the Distal Jet, space is created between the maxillary first molar and first premolar; however, this space is not due solely to bodily movement of the molars. The reciprocal forces result in a loss of anterior anchorage that is responsible for some of the space that appears. In a recent study,[22] distal movement of the molar crown contributed 71% of the 4.5 mm of space created on each side during distalization, the remaining 29% resulted from mesial movement of the anchoring premolars. In a comparable study of patients treated with only the Distal Jet,[24] molar distalization contributed 85% of the 5.4 mm of space created on each side versus 15% from anchorage loss. Both of these reports demonstrate slightly less anchorage loss when the Distal Jet is used alone compared to its use combined with full-fixed brackets.[25–27]

In a series of studies, the Distal Jet is reported to have generated 1.9–3.7 mm/side of distal molar movement[23,26] and 0.4–3.0 mm of anchorage loss per side.[24,26] Therefore, the total amount of space created during distalization ranged from 2.3 to 6.7 mm (average 5.65 mm). These estimates of space are somewhat less than those reported for the Pendulum (average 7.5 mm)[28,29] but the Pendulum produced significantly more tipping of the molars and premolars.

Anchorage Loss and Tipping of the Premolars

During distalization with the Distal Jet, the first premolars did not tend to tip mesially, as has been found in many investigations of other intraoral "distalizing" devices. Rather, the premolars exhibited 2.8° of distal tipping. In comparison, Chiu et al[24] are the only investigators who have described distal tipping of the first premolar (−1.7°) with the pendulum appliance. As a result, there appears to be no consensus on the direction that premolars tip during the process of molar distalization.

It has also been hypothesized that distal tipping of premolars with the Distal Jet is due to the geometry of the appliance.[26,30] Specifically, the line of action of the distal force is directed by a couple from the tube/piston and coil spring assembly that is constructed superiorly to the crown of the first molar. The intention of this arrangement is to direct the forces parallel to the level of the center of resistance of the first molars to reduce molar tipping. As the molars are distalized, these forces tend to cause some inferior rotation of the Nance palatal button, thereby tipping the first premolars distally.

In comparison to the Distal Jet, the Pendulum Appliance has demonstrated 1.3–2.6 mm/side of first premolar anchorage loss and from 1.7° of distal to 4.8° of *mesial* tipping (Fig. 18.25).[24,28,29] The Jones Jig exhibited similar amounts of second premolar anchorage loss (2.2–2.4 mm/side) but it also produced the most mesial tipping of the premolars (5.9–9.5°) of any of the appliances presently under discussion (Fig. 18.26).[31,32] In conclusion, it appears likely that, for the current methods of molar distalization involving reciprocal anchorage, some degree of anterior arch loss appears to be the "cost" of achieving a Class I molar relationship. The use of mini-screw anchorage may alleviate that concern in some cases.

Anchorage from First or Second Premolars

The Pendulum typically has been constructed with support arms to the Nance button from the first premolars and the Jones Jig from the second premolars. It has been proposed that there are two more teeth to serve as anchorage when the Distal Jet is constructed with support derived from the second premolars. When the results for Distal Jets constructed using the first premolars are compared to those in which the second premolars were used, there appears to be no significant difference in anchorage loss.[23,25–27,33] Perhaps it may be more efficient to use the first premolars and permit the second premolars to drift distally, along with the molars, due to the forces of the transseptal fibers.

Rate of Distalization

After accounting for the contributions of reciprocal movements during distalization, it has been inferred that the average "distalizing" velocity of the Distal Jet for each first molar was 0.6 mm per month, somewhat less than that of both the Jones Jig and Pendulum.[24] The degree of tipping of the molars and premolars nonetheless plays a conspicuous role in the net amount of space created during distalization. If more distal tipping of molars and simultaneous mesial tipping of premolars is produced by an appliance (e.g. Pendulum, Jones Jig), then more net space is created when producing a Class I molar relationship when compared to an appliance that produces less molar tipping and some distal tipping of the premolar (e.g. Distal Jet). Because all patients in the reports of the effects of the various "distalizing" devices were corrected to a Class I molar relationship in 5–7 months, the question arises "How much distalization do you need?" "Enough to correct the Class II." Perhaps the relative rate of space opening versus tipping of the teeth adjacent to that space is of more importance clinically.

If the recovery from tipping of both molars and premolars (i.e. uprighting to pretreatment angulations) is subtracted from the total space generated by distalization, the "effective space" for the Pendulum, Distal Jet with brackets, and Distal Jet alone was estimated to be about the same (4 mm/side), while the Jones Jig is the least effective (Table 18.1). It seems reasonable to assume that appliances that produce more tipping (e.g. Jones Jig, Pendulum) may introduce more inefficiency into the system.

Effects of Second Molar Eruption

From recent studies it appears that greater tipping of the maxillary first molars (4.3°) was found in patients whose second molars were unerupted (positioned at the apical third of the maxillary first molars). When the second molars were partially or totally erupted, there was significantly less tipping of the first molar (2°).[22] Normally, the center of resistance of the maxillary first molar is close to the trifurcation of the roots, but when the germ of the second molar is an obstacle to distal movement, the center of resistance tends to move superiorly and may lead to greater tipping. These findings confirm Graber's observations of tipping of the first molar when distalizing with a cervical headgear prior to the eruption of the second molar.[34]

There was also significantly less anchorage loss (1.7 mm vs 0.9 mm) and extrusion (1.7 mm vs 0.5 mm) measured at the first premolars for

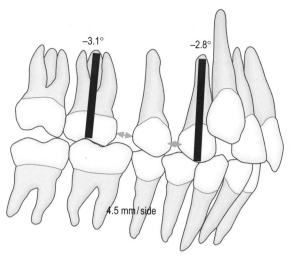

Figure 18.23 Clinical effects of the Distal Jet as described by Bolla et al.[22]

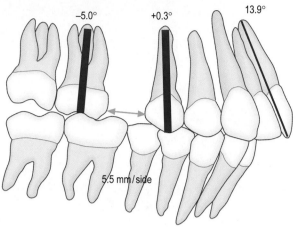

Figure 18.24 Clinical effects of the Distal Jet with concurrent use of orthodontic brackets as described by Chiu et al.[24] It appears evident that the higher amount of anchorage loss occurs when the Distal Jet is used with brackets. Therefore, the Distal Jet should be used alone.

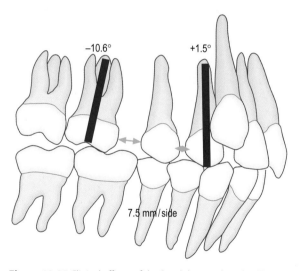

Figure 18.25 Clinical effects of the Pendulum as described by Bussik & McNamara.[43]

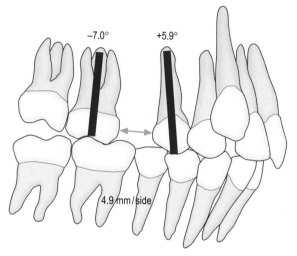

Figure 18.26 Clinical effects of the Jones Jig as described by Brickman et al.[32]

Table 18.1. Effects of popular methods of maxillary molar distalization.

Report	Device	Molar crown distalization	Anchorage loss	Total space	Distance 6 to 4	"Effective" space
Brickman et al (2000)[32]	Jones Jig	2.5	2.4	4.9	11	1.6
Bussick & McNamara (2000)[43]	Pendulum	5.7	1.8	7.5	14	4.3
Chiu et al (2005)[24]*	Distal Jet	3.0	2.5	5.5	12	4.1
Bolla et al (2002)[22]	Distal Jet	3.2	1.3	4.5	11	4.4

*Results represent effects of the Distal Jet and full-fixed preadjusted brackets.

those patients whose second molars were erupted as compared to those with unerupted second molars when using the Distal Jet. As noted by other workers, there was also no statistically significant difference in the amount of space created when second molars were unerupted or erupted.[24,25,28,32,35,36] These findings do not support the recommendation that distalization is always preferable prior to eruption of the second molars.

Originally, there was a Distal Jet design difference for those patients with erupted second molars and those without. Coil springs, calibrated to produce 240 g of force, were typically selected for patients with second molars erupted and lighter springs were used for patients in the mixed dentition. It was assumed that more force was necessary to move the first molars when the second molars were erupted. The effect of heavy versus lighter forces was tested as a sample of 26 patients, treated with Distal Jets constructed with 180 g springs, was compared to 19 patients who were treated with Distal Jets constructed with 240 g springs.[37] Although all the patients were in the permanent dentition, no differentiation of second molar eruption status was made in selecting the sample. The lighter springs demonstrated no advantage as the time for distalization was similar, but heavier forces produced about 1 mm more distalization, 3° less molar tipping, and 0.7 mm less anchorage loss at the premolars. Therefore, there appears to be no reason to use lighter forces with the Distal Jet, at least for adolescent patients. There also appears to be some advantage in treating patients with second molars partially or fully erupted; therefore, early treatment can be successful but often requires a two-phase approach.

Vertical Effects

It has been theorized that "clockwise" mandibular rotation may be produced when molars are distalized into the "wedge." According to this simplified view of the relationship between the maxilla and mandible, the backwards movement of the molars would prop open the anterior dentition. Consequently, molar distalization often is not recommended as a treatment strategy for hyperdivergent patients (i.e. those with open bites or high mandibular plane angles).[7] In reality, other elements such as the cant of the occlusal plane, the condyle-to-molar distance,[38–40] and occlusal forces[41,42] may be more important risk factors for molar distalization if opening the vertical dimension is a concern.

The extrusion of the molars during distalization can induce a backward rotation of the mandible. The maxillary first molars do not undergo any significant vertical changes during the molar distalization phase of treatment with the Distal Jet and, as a result, the mandibular plane remains virtually unchanged (−0.3°).[22] Similar results have been reported in other investigations of the Distal Jet.[23,25,33] In contrast, other noncompliance intraoral devices for molar distalization seem to produce a small increase in the mandibular plane angle.[24,31,35,36,43] With the Distal Jet there were no significant changes in lower anterior face height among patients with high, neutral or low pretreatment mandibular planes.

Molar Width and Rotational Changes

Some maxillary expansion is often a prerequisite for Class II correction. On average, the patients treated with the Distal Jet demonstrated some transverse changes during molar distalization. Specifically, the intermolar width was increased an average of 2.9 mm. This increase in width is necessary to maintain a proper transverse relationship of the maxillary to mandibular molars during distalization.

Lemons & Holmes reported that the majority of patients with Class II malocclusion exhibit maxillary first molars that are rotated mesially around the palatal root.[44] As a result, a variety of methods to correct this molar rotation have been advocated.[11,12,45] With the Distal Jet the first molars developed a mild but adverse distal rotation of the lingual cusps during distalization. Favorable molar expansion (3.7–4.4 mm) but undesirable rotations were found in all studies of the Distal Jet. In comparison, the Pendulum, Jones Jig, Greenfield Appliance, and sagittal appliance have been reported to produce a favorable distal rotation around the palatal roots; however, these appliances also delivered some undesirable constriction of the first molars.[24,27,29,31,33,43]

A Comparison with Other Distalization Devices

A number of noncompliance fixed appliances have been developed to apply a distal force to the maxillary molars. Ghosh & Nanda evaluated 41 patients treated with such a device, the Pendulum Appliance, and found that 57% of the maxillary space created was from molar distalization.[28,46] The remaining 43% resulted from anchorage loss (mesial movement) measured at the maxillary first premolars and anteriors. They also reported an average of 8.4° of first molar distal tipping. This report stands in contrast to the 10.7° of tipping but only 19% anchorage loss described by Chiu et al.[24] Other studies have reported even more molar tipping (13.1–15.7°) with the Pendulum.[29,35]

On balance, it might be concluded that the Pendulum produces 8–16° of molar tipping and 19–43% of anchorage loss. This substantial distal tipping and concern about undesirable bite opening led Bussick & McNamara to suggest that the Pendulum Appliance is used most effectively when constructed with anchorage support from maxillary second deciduous molars and when maxillary permanent second molars are unerupted.[43]

Brickman et al examined the results of 72 consecutive patients treated with another distalizing device, the Jones Jig.[32] They found that 55% of the space created between the molar and premolar was from distal movement of the first molar crown, an amount similar to that reported by Ghosh & Nanda for the Pendulum Appliance.[28] Haydar & Uner reported that the Jones Jig produced distalization much like a cervical headgear, but with a 55% anchorage loss.[47] Runge et al[31] found 50% of the space was generated from mesial premolar movement while Gulati and co-workers[48] described only 26% anchorage loss with the Jones Jig. It appears, therefore, that treatment with the Jones Jig produces from 26% to 55% anchorage loss, an amount similar to that found with the Pendulum.

The total distance from the molars to the first premolars (the sum of the space created plus the width of the second premolars) for four popular distalization methods (Pendulum, Jones Jig, Distal Jet, Distal Jet with brackets) averaged 11 mm/side for the Distal Jet and Jones Jig, 12 mm/side for the Distal Jet with brackets, and 14 mm/side for the Pendulum. However, the Distal Jet produced significantly less tipping than that typically seen with other distalizing mechanics, such as the Wilson modular technique,[10] repelling magnets,[8,49,50] Jones Jig,[32,48] and the Pendulum.[28,43]

Each of these methods resolves the Class II molar relationship but in the process there are some differences in the amount of space generated to achieve this correction. The total space created during distalization is defined as the sum of the molar distal movement plus the anchorage loss. Each appliance produces some degree of tipping of both molars and premolars. If the adverse tipping produced by each appliance is corrected to pretreatment angulations by molar or premolar uprighting (as though the appliance had generated pure bodily movement), then some decrease in the space that was created during distalization would be expected. The recovery of this tipping would, therefore, result in some degree of subsequent anchorage loss as the molars and premolars are tipped toward that space to parallel their roots.

The space remaining after the recovery of the tipping might be considered to be the "effective space" that each appliance created. The effective space was determined for each appliance by subtracting the anticipated space loss (from uprighting molars and premolars) from the total space that had been originally generated during the distalization process. From this examination, the Jones Jig appeared to be the least effective as only 1.6 mm/side of space would be expected after uprighting the molars and especially the significantly tipped premolars. The Pendulum, Distal Jet alone, and Distal Jet with fixed brackets all generated about 4 mm/side of effective space (see Table 18.1).

Although the Pendulum produced the greatest amount of total space between molars and premolars, it also required more recovery of the tipped molars and premolars than the Distal Jet alone. The mechanics required to upright molars and premolars after distalization with the Pendulum may be assumed to increase the risk of further anchorage loss and introduce greater inefficiency into this system of Class II resolution compared to the Distal Jet.

Molar Distalization versus Herbst Mechanics

When the effects of maxillary molar distalization (a sample of patients treated with the Pendulum) were compared with the effects of mandibular protraction (patients treated with the Herbst appliance), there were no significant differences in total treatment time (combining phase I and II) or in the final skeletal, occlusal, and facial results.[51] Specifically, the amount of mandibular growth demonstrated in both samples was nearly identical, despite the fact that different jaws were being addressed by treatment in each sample. It appears from the results of the present examination that the Distal Jet performed favorably when compared to the Pendulum. Presumably, the Distal Jet would also be expected to compare favorably to Herbst-type mechanics for the treatment of Class II.

Postdistalization Mechanics

Molar distalization is just the first step of Class II treatment as retraction of the remaining upper dentition is still required. Consequently, a variety of mechanics are available to complete the steps necessary to retract the remaining upper teeth. Essentially, postdistalization mechanics can be divided into two types, immediate active retraction or a passive phase of retraction, which are often chosen dependent upon the timing of treatment (i.e. distalization in mixed or permanent dentition).

Late Mixed Dentition: Active Postdistalization Mechanics

Upon completion of molar distalization in the mixed dentition, the overjet can be resolved by immediate and active retraction of the incisors. This is often accomplished using upper and lower utility archwires and Class II elastics. In this scenario, the incisors, deciduous canines, and deciduous molars are moved distally en masse (Figs 18.27–18.30). The subsequent eruption of permanent

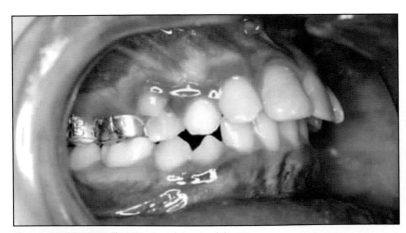

Figures 18.27, 18.28 Class II patient, late mixed dentition.

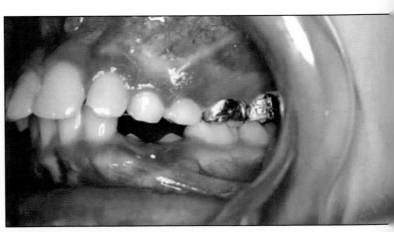

Figure 18.28

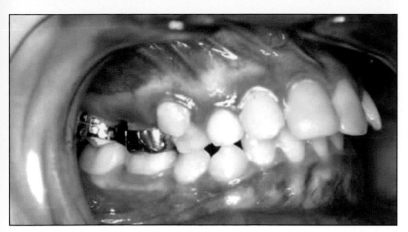

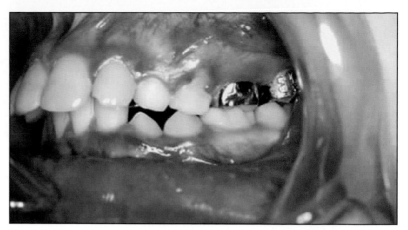

Figures 18.29, 18.30 After completion of molar distalization.

Figure 18.30

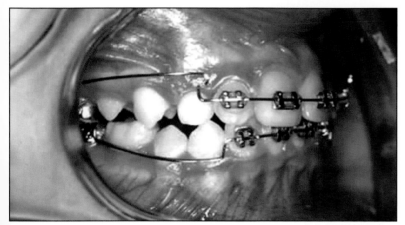

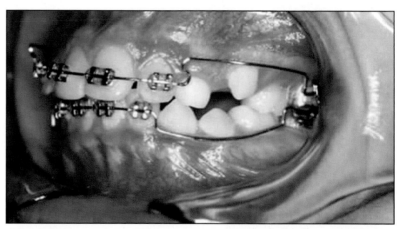

Figures 18.31, 18.32 Retraction of the incisors, accomplished using upper and lower utility archwires and Class II elastics.

Figure 18.32

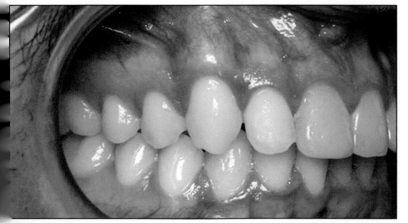

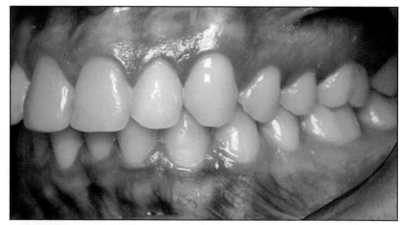

Figures 18.33, 18.34 The case was stable 6 years after the beginning of treatment.

Figure 18.34

teeth is typically into good intercuspation, with only limited treatment for final alignment required (Figs 18.31–18.34).

The drawback of this procedure is the need for patient compliance and some concerns over mandibular anchorage loss from Class II elastic reciprocal forces. If the patient is uncooperative, as happens

50% of the time, the gains from molar distalization may even be jeopardized. In those instances, an active or passive fixed functional appliance (e.g. Jasper Jumper, Flat Spring Jumpers, Gentle Jumpers), applied to a lip bumper (a so-called bumper jumper) to support the mesial forces and thereby prevent labial flaring of the lower incisors, might be an alternative.[7] The fixed functional appliance serves much like a cervical headgear, without the need for compliance, to support the molar position during active retraction of maxillary teeth.

Either active treatment with Class II elastics and utility arches or combination therapy (i.e. Distal Jet followed by a fixed functional) is indicated for patients in late mixed dentition. As the remaining permanent teeth erupt, they are immediately incorporated in the traditional edgewise mechanics, eliminating

a prolonged pause or transition period between treatment phases.

A different approach is suggested for patients in early mixed dentition.

Early Mixed Dentition Treatment: Passive Postdistalization Mechanics

For patients in the early mixed dentition, the Distal Jet is applied using the second deciduous molars as anchorage (Figs 18.35–18.37). The second deciduous molars are the last succedaneous teeth to exfoliate; therefore, they can provide solid anchorage during 5–6 months of distal molar movement.

After Class I molar position has been achieved, the Distal Jet is converted to a retainer as described previously (Figs 18.38–18.42). The converted appliance is maintained for 4–6 months and then may be replaced by a traditional Nance button if needed. The molars are held in Class I intercuspation until the complete eruption of the premolars, typically into normal intercuspation (Fig. 18.43). The following second phase of treatment requires a simple alignment with a limited use of intermaxillary elastics for finishing (Figs 18.44–18.47). This two-phase approach reduces the time with full-fixed appliances during the adolescent years when patient compliance, including oral hygiene, is unreliable.

Permanent Dentition Postdistalization Mechanics

Upon the completion of molar distal movement and conversion of the Distal Jet to a modified Nance holding arch to maintain the new molar position, there are a number of alternatives for the completion of treatment. As the difficult part of Class II correction has been achieved (i.e. moving the molars into Class I relationship), only a

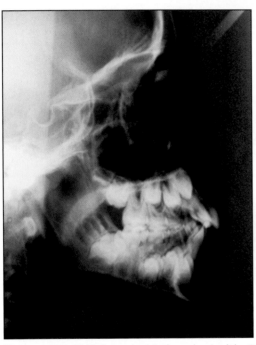

Figures 18.35–18.37 For patients in the early mixed dentition, the Distal Jet is applied using the second deciduous molars as anchorage.

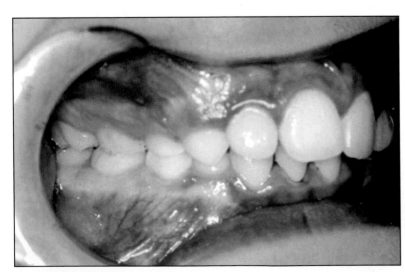

Figure 18.36

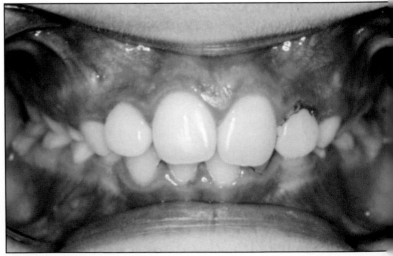

Figure 18.37

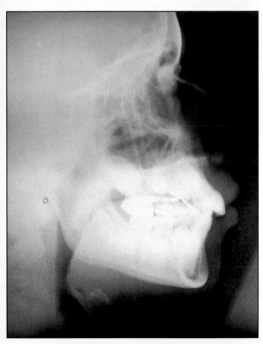

Figures 18.38–18.42 After Class I molar position has been achieved, the Distal Jet is converted to a retainer.

Class I spacing problem remains. Typical orthodontic biomechanics with preadjusted appliances (e.g. butterfly system) can be applied for case completion.[19,52,53]

En Masse Retraction with Class II Elastics

After Class I molar relationship is achieved, the distalization of the premolars and canines may be accomplished en masse and not in sequence (Figs 18.48–18.59). In this instance, the full-size lower arch once again acts as an anchorage for Class II elastics. To prevent maxillary molar anchorage loss, the Distal Jet has been converted to a Nance holding arch and a continuous archwire with a mesial stop is used. After correcting the canine relationship, the Nance button and the mesial stops should be removed and Class II elastics can be used to retract the incisors using sliding mechanics.

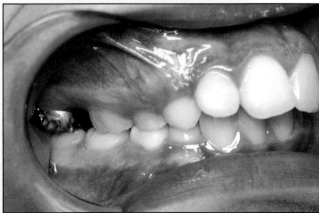

Figure 18.39

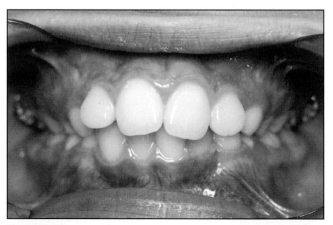

Figure 18.40

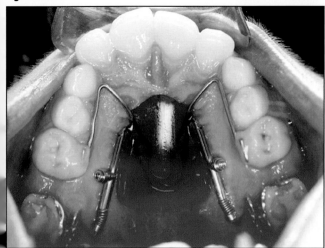

Figure 18.41

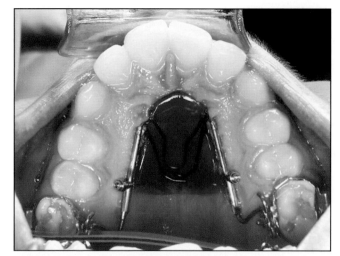

Figure 18.42

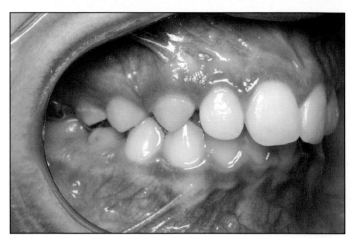

Figure 18.43 The molars are held in Class I intercuspation until the complete eruption of the premolars.

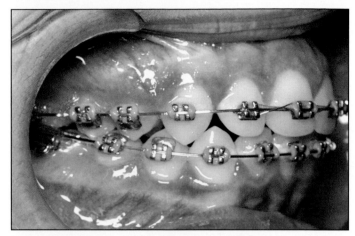

Figures 18.44–18.47 The following second phase of treatment requires a simple alignment with a limited use of intermaxillary elastics for finishing.

Figure 18.45

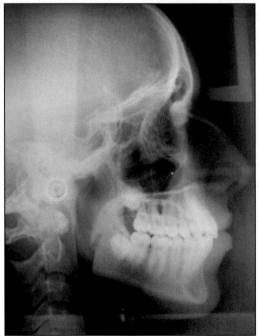

Sequential Asymmetric Retraction

Another method for completing Class II correction after molar distalization is by using so-called "tripod mechanics." After distalization, the Distal Jet is converted to a retainer only on one side (i.e. the premolar supporting wire is cut only on one side to permit distal movement of the buccal segment of teeth on that same side) (Figs 18.60–18.62). In this manner, two molars and one of the premolars have been stabilized for anchorage (tripod) support during the retraction of the premolars on the side where conversion of the Distal Jet was completed.

Elastic chain or compressed nickel-titanium coil springs can be used for continuous arch sliding retraction of these teeth. Once the retraction of this buccal segment is completed (see Fig. 18.62), the opposite side of the Distal Jet is converted. Retraction of the buccal segment on the same side is now supported by the modified Nance holding arch that is supported by the consolidated teeth of the buccal segment on the opposite side of

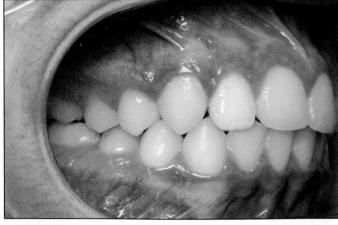

Figure 18.46

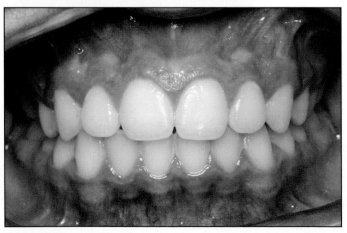

Figure 18.47

the arch (Fig. 18.63). This tripod of anchorage is sufficient in cases where a modest retraction of the premolars is required but it cannot be considered a stable anchorage method for severe Class II corrections.

Once asymmetric sequential retraction of the premolars is completed (see Fig. 18.63), then the canines and the incisors are retracted with a choice of different intraarch mechanics (e.g. sliding or loop mechanics). In the final phases of treatment, limited use of intermaxillary Class II elastics may be necessary to obtain optimal intercuspation.

Combination Therapy (Distal Jet Followed by Fixed Functional Appliance)

There are some indications for additional anchorage during post-distalization mechanics. If molar distal movement is insufficient with a fixed device, if significant overjet remains, if patient compliance has

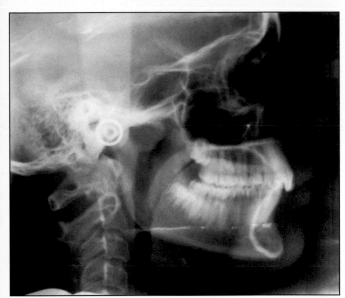

Figures 18.48–18.50 Class II hypodivergent patient.

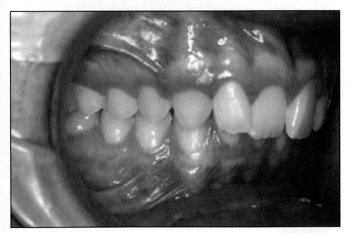

Figure 18.49

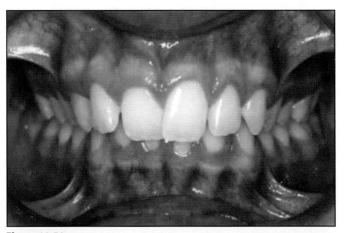

Figure 18.50

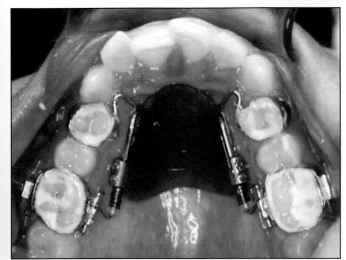

Figures 18.51–18.54 Class I molar relationship was achieved with the Distal Jet in 5 months.

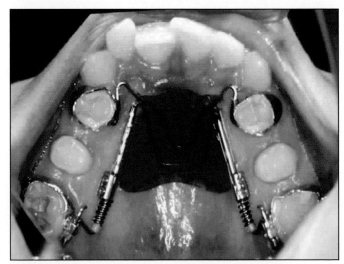

Figure 18.52

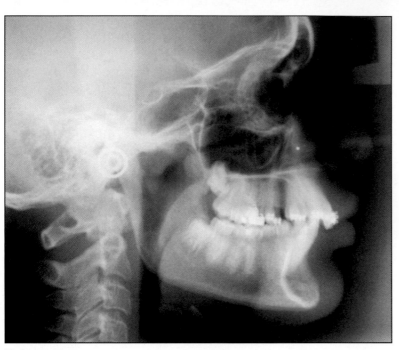

Figure 18.53

been poor and is not expected with elastic wear, or if loss of anchorage during subsequent retraction is intolerable, then the addition of a fixed functional appliance may be considered.[5,54]

Fixed functional appliances (e.g. Herbst, Jasper Jumper) can provide some additional maxillary molar distalization or at least support during retraction of the rest of the maxillary dentition. Unfortunately, flaring of the lower incisors and adverse facial esthetics are undesirable side effects. If the positive benefits of molar support can be harnessed while diminishing the side effects, then fixed functionals are useful in the resolution of Class II malocclusions. Lingual crown torque (either bent into the wire or part of a preadjusted prescription such as the Butterfly System)[19] applied to the mandibular anterior teeth using a full-sized archwire can help to prevent incisor flaring.[7,19,53]

Interestingly, Burkhardt et al have demonstrated that the final treatment results from fixed functionals or molar distalization (including the amount of mandibular growth) are essentially the same.[51] Consequently, the addition of a fixed functional may be required only on occasions when molar distalizers, such as the distal jet, are used.

If Class II combination therapy is selected,[54] then upon completion of distal molar movement, a fixed functional appliance is installed from the maxillary first molars extending to a supporting mandibular full-sized archwire (see Fig. 18.66). For example, devices such as the

Figure 18.54

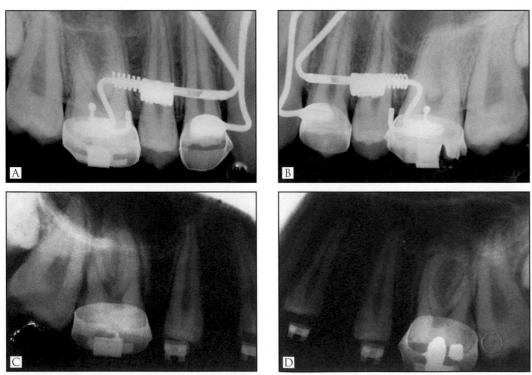

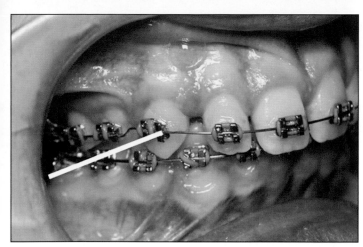

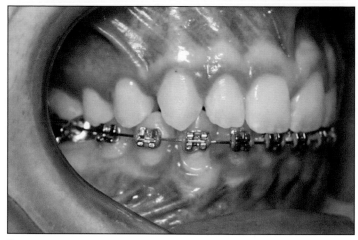

Figures 18.55, 18.56 The distalization of the premolars and canines was accomplished en masse with class II elastics.

Figure 18.56

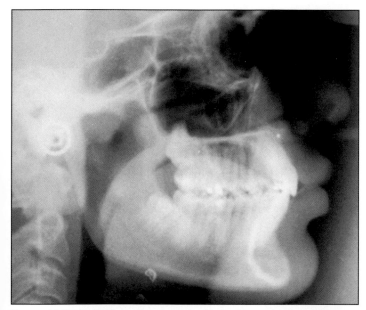

Figures 18.57–18.59 The case was completed after 22 months of treatment.

Jasper, Gentle, and Flat Spring Jumpers are retained by annealed ball pins inserted through the appropriate eyelet end of a jumper and the buccal headgear tube of the first maxillary molar band. The other eyelet end of the jumper is either applied directly to the mandibular base archwire (NB: the mandibular first premolar brackets are removed to permit sliding of this device along the wire) or to auxiliary jig or outrigger wires that are, in turn, attached to the base wire. In either alternative, the mandibular teeth must be consolidated by lacing them together with continuous steel ligation or the base wire must be "tied back" to prevent spaces from opening.

Immediate retraction of the remaining maxillary dentition can be accomplished using sliding mechanics on a continuous archwire or via "floating" mechanics in a segmental system. If a continuous archwire is used, then the maxillary incisors are ligated together and the teeth in the buccal segment are retracted using

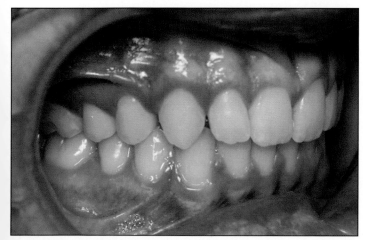

Figure 18.58

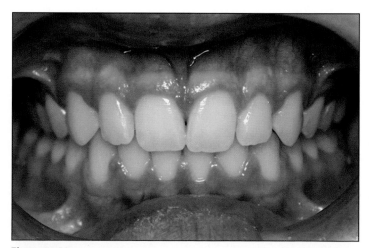

Figure 18.59

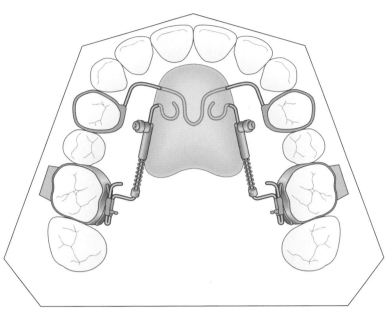

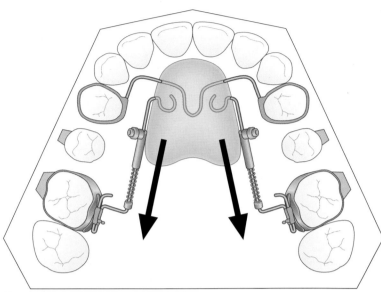

Figures 18.60–18.62 Illustrations of the "tripod mechanics." After distalization, the Distal Jet is converted to a retainer on one side only.

Figure 18.61

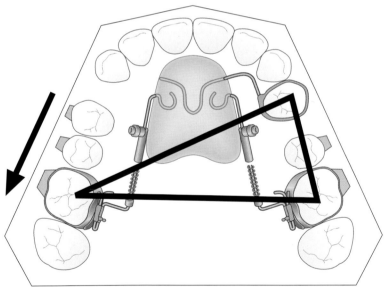

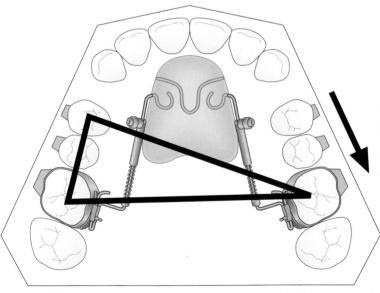

Figure 18.62

Figure 18.63 Once the retraction of this buccal segment is completed, the opposite side of the Distal Jet is converted.

elastic chain or coil springs (Figs 18.64–18.67). Each tooth (i.e. canine and the two premolars) is retracted together or sequentially as desired.

If segmental mechanics are used, once again the maxillary incisors are tied together or consolidated using an archwire that also bypasses the teeth in the buccal segment (i.e. a Ricketts' utility archwire). The teeth in the buccal segment are retracted

individually or together using elastic chain or thread extending from the first molar. Although these teeth move quickly due to the lack of sliding friction, they will also rotate and tip distally, necessitating some recovery with a light superelastic wire upon completion of the retraction.

The maxillary incisors are finally retracted using either sliding or closed-loop mechanics. A large-dimension stainless steel archwire is

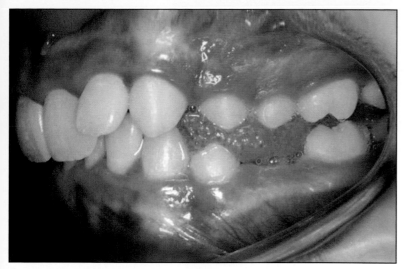

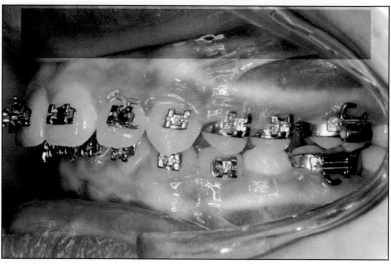

Figures 18.64–18.67 After molar distalization, immediate retraction of the remaining maxillary dentition can be accomplished using sliding mechanics while the Jasper Jumper holds the distalized molars in Class I relationship.

Figure 18.65

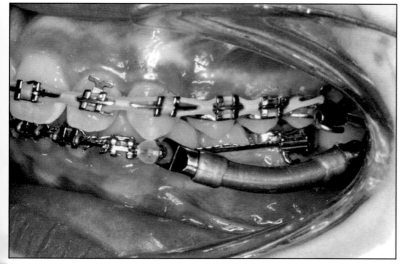

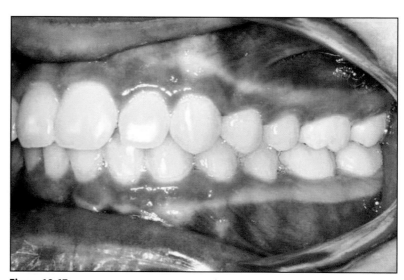

Figure 18.66

Figure 18.67

marked just distal to the lateral incisors. The wire is then acid reduced, using a wire polisher, distal to the lateral incisors. In this manner, the anterior portion of the wire will maintain appropriate torque for the incisors while the posterior portion slides more freely during retraction. Force for retraction can be applied by elastic chain, elastic modules or coil springs. Periodic visits are required to clip the distal portions of the archwire that extend out of the molar tubes as the wire translates posteriorly.

The use of a beta-titanium alloy rectangular archwire, bent into an asymmetric T-loop with accentuated curve of Spee (to assist in reduction of any residual overbite), is a closed-loop alternative for anterior retraction.[55] The rectangular wire helps to maintain anterior torque control and there is no friction when these T-loops are opened every 4–6 weeks. Although there are no distal wire ends to clip, these archwires are more complex to bend or may be purchased as a preformed product.

Upon complete space closure, the fixed functionals are removed along with the Nance holding arch. The mandibular premolar brackets are replaced if they had been removed for installation of the functional device. The dental arches are subsequently coordinated and intermaxillary elastics (e.g. "triangle") are used to refine intercuspation.

Conclusion

The Distal Jet is a fixed, lingual appliance designed to produce distalization of maxillary first molars. This device provides an effective and predictable method for the correction of a Class II malocclusion given that no patient cooperation is required. This consideration is particularly significant given that general patient compliance is said to be decreasing, is certainly unpredictable individually, and yet appears to be the most important factor in determining treatment success.

On the basis of recent clinical research, the following findings regarding the use of the Distal Jet for the distal movement of maxillary first molars during the correction of Class II have been reported.

- Class II molar relationship is corrected to a Class I in about 5–6 months.

- The typical age to begin treatment is 12–13 years old, an age that corresponds to the optimum amount of mandibular growth, which may also be useful in resolving the Class II relationship.

- The distalizing force on the maxillary molar results in 70% molar distalization and 30% reciprocal anchorage loss measured at the maxillary first premolar. This division is comparable to that reported for other types of intraoral methods of molar distalization.

- The maxillary first molars are moved distally an average of 3 mm/side, with 3° of distal crown tipping. Net distalization is less than that seen with the pendulum; however, the amount of molar tipping is significantly less than has been found with comparable intraoral distalizers, including the Pendulum.

- Anchorage loss, measured at the first premolars, is 1.3 mm/side, with 2.8° of distal crown tipping – results comparable clinically to other intraoral distalizers.

- Less molar tipping (2.3° vs 4.3°) and anchorage loss (0.9 mm/side vs 1.7 mm/side) are noted for patients whose maxillary second molars are partially or completely erupted when compared to those with second molars that are not erupted.

- No significant vertical changes are observed during distalization.

- If the recovery from tipping of both molars and premolars (i.e. uprighting to pretreatment angulations) is subtracted from the total space generated by distalization, the "effective space" for the Pendulum, Distal Jet with brackets, and Distal Jet alone was estimated to be about the same (4 mm/side). However, it seems reasonable to assume that appliances that produce more tipping (e.g. Jones Jig, Pendulum) may introduce more inefficiency into the system.

In conclusion, the Distal Jet Appliance compares favorably with other intraoral distalization devices[56] and also with mechanics featuring mandibular protraction (e.g. Herbst)[51] for the treatment of patients with Class II malocclusion, despite the fact that these appliances address different jaws.

References

1. Proffit WR. Contemporary orthodontics. St Louis, MO: Mosby; 1993.
2. Pancherz H. The Herbst appliance – its biological effects and clinical use. Am J Orthod Dentofacial Orthop 1985;87:1–20.
3. Pancherz H, Anehus-Pancherz M. The headgear effect of the Herbst appliance: a cephalometric long-term study. Am J Orthod Dentofacial Orthop 1993;103:510–520.
4. Jasper JJ, McNamara JA. The correction of interarch malocclusions using a fixed force module. Am J Orthod Dentofacial Orthop 1995;108:641–650.
5. Bowman SJ. Modifications of the distal jet. J Clin Orthod 1998;32:549–556.
6. Pieringer M, Droschl H, Permann R. Distalization with a Nance appliance and coil springs. J Clin Orthod 1997;31:321–326.
7. Bowman SJ. Class II combination therapy. J Clin Orthod 1998;32:611–620.
8. Gianelly AA, Vaitas AS, Thomas WM, Berger DG. Distalization of molars with repelling magnets. J Clin Orthod 1988;22:40–44.
9. Jones R, White JM. Rapid Class II molar correction with an open-coil jig. J Clin Orthod 1992;26:661–664.
10. Muse DS, Filhnan MJ, Emerson WJ, Mitchell RD. Molar and incisal changes with the Wilson rapid molar distalization. Am J Orthod Dentofacial Orthop 1993;104:556–565.
11. Hilgers JJ. Adjuncts to bioprogressive therapy: a palatal expansion appliance for noncompliance therapy. J Clin Orthod 1991;25:491–497.
12. Hilgers JJ. The pendulum appliance for Class II noncompliance therapy. J Clin Orthod 1992;26:706–714.
13. Locatelli R, Bednar J, Dietz VS, Gianelly AA. Molar distalization with superelastic NiTi wire. J Clin Orthod 1992;26:277–279.
14. Carano A, Testa M, Siciliani G. Una nuova metodica per la distalizzazione dei molari superiori. Ortognatodonzia Italiana 1995;4:525–533.
15. Carano A, Testa M, Siciliani G. The lingual distalizer system. Eur J Orthod 1996;18:445–448.
16. Carano A, Testa M. The distal jet for upper molar distalization. J Clin Orthod 1996;30:374–390.
17. Fortini A, Lupoli M, Parri M. The First Class appliance for rapid molar distalization. J Clin Orthod 1999;33:322–328.
18. Celestino E. Classe II non estrattive: il distalizzatore rapido. Mondo Ortodontico 1999;6:342–348.
19. Bowman SJ. Pre-adjusted typodont course manual. Ann Arbor: University of Michigan; 1999.
20. Carano A, Testa M, Bowman SJ. The distal jet simplified and updated. J Clin Orthod 2002;36:586–590.
21. Bowman SJ. Molar distalization: bad English, good practice. J Clin Orthod 2006 (in press).
22. Bolla E, Muratore F, Carano A, Bowman SJ. Evaluation of maxillary molar distalization with the distal jet: a comparison with other contemporary methods. Angle Orthod 2002;72:481–494.
23. Gutierrez VME. Treatment effects of the distal jet appliance with and without edgewise therapy. Masters degree thesis. St Louis, MO: Saint Louis University; 2001.
24. Chiu PP, McNamara JA Jr, Franchi L. A comparison of two intraoral molar distalization appliances: Distal Jet versus pendulum appliance. Am J Orthod Dentofac Orthop 2005;128:353–365.
25. Heurter G. A retrospective evaluation of maxillary molar distalization with the distal jet appliance. Masters degree thesis. St Louis, MO: Saint Louis University, Center for Advanced Dental Education; 2000.
26. Patel AN. Analysis of the distal jet appliance for maxillary molar distalization. Masters degree thesis. Oklahoma City, OK: University of Oklahoma Health Sciences Center; 1999.
27. Lee SH. Comparison of the treatment effects of two molar distalization appliances. Masters degree thesis. St Louis, MO: Saint Louis University; 2001.
28. Ghosh J, Nanda RS. Evaluation of an intraoral maxillary molar distalization technique. Am J Orthod Dentofacial Orthop 1996;110:639–646.
29. Chaques-Asensi J, Kalra V. Effects of the pendulum appliance on the dentofacial complex. J Clin Orthod 2001;35:254–257.
30. Ngantung V, Nanda RS, Bowman, SJ. Posttreatment evaluation of the distal jet appliance. Am J Orthod Dentofacial Orthop 2001;120:178–185.
31. Runge ME, Martin JT, Bukai F. Analysis of rapid maxillary molar distal movement without patient cooperation. Am J Orthod Dentofacial Orthop 1999;115:153–157.

32. Brickman CD, Sinha PK, Nanda RS. Evaluation of the Jones jig appliance for distal molar movement. Am J Orthod Dentofacial Orthop 2000;118: 526–534.

33. Davis EC. A comparison of two maxillary molar distalization appliances. Masters degree thesis. St Louis, MO: Saint Louis University; 2001.

34. Graber TM. Extra-oral force – facts and fallacies. Am J Orthod 1955;41:490–505.

35. Byloff FK, Darendeliler MA. Distal molar movement using the pendulum appliance. Part 1: Clinical and radiological evaluation. Angle Orthod 1997;67:249–260.

36. Byloff FK, Darendeliler NR, Clar E, Darendeliler A. Distal molar movement using the pendulum appliance. Part 2: The effects of maxillary molar root uprighting bends. Angle Orthod 1997;67: 261–270.

37. Maginnis JJ. Treatment effects of the distal jet with 180 gram and 240 gram springs. Masters degree thesis. St Louis, MO: Saint Louis University; 2002.

38. Osborn JW. Relationship between the mandibular condyle and the occlusal plane during hominid evolution: some of its effects on jaw mechanics. Am J Physic Anthrop 1987;73:193–207.

39. Baragar FA, Osborn JW. Efficiency as a predictor of human jaw design in the sagittal plane. J Biomech 1987;20:447–457.

40. Smith RJ. Etiology, diagnosis and treatment of excessive vertical dimension. Lecture, 90th Annual Session of the American Association of Orthodontists. Washington DC, 1990.

41. Proffit WR, Gamble JW, Christiansen RL. Generalized muscular weakness with severe anterior open bite. Am J Orthod 1968;54:104–110.

42. Proffit WR, Fields HW, Nixon WL. Occlusal forces in normal and long-face adults. J Dent Res 1983; 62:566–571.

43. Bussick TJ, McNamara JA. Dentoalveolar and skeletal changes associated with the pendulum appliance. Am J Orthod Dentofacial Orthop 2000; 177:333–343.

44. Lemons FF, Holmes CW. The problem of the rotated maxillary first permanent molar. Am J Orthod 1961;47:246–272.

45. Cetlin NM, Ten Hoeve A. Nonextraction treatment. J Clin Orthod 1983;17:396–413.

46. Ghosh J, Nanda RS. Class II, division 1 malocclusion treated with molar distalization therapy. Am J Orthod Dentofacial Orthop 1996;110:672–677.

47. Haydar S, Uner O. Comparison of Jones Jig molar distalization appliance with extraoral traction. Am J Orthod Dentofacial Orthop 2000;117: 49–53.

48. Gulati S, Kharbanda OP, Parkash H. Dental and skeletal changes after intraoral molar distalization with sectional jig assembly. Am J Orthod Dentofacial Orthop 1998;114:319–327.

49. Bondemark L, Kurol J. Distalization of maxillary first and second molars simultaneously with repelling magnets. Eur J Orthod 1992;14:264–272.

50. Bondemark L, Kurol J, Bernhold, M. Repelling magnets versus superelastic nickel-titanium coils in simultaneous distal movement of maxillary first and second molars. Angle Orthod 1994;64: 189–198.

51. Burkhardt DR, McNamara JA Jr, Baccetti T. Maxillary molar distalization or mandibular enhancement: a cephalometric comparison of comprehensive orthodontic treatment including the pendulum and the Herbst appliances. Am J Orthod Dentofacial Orthop 2003;123:108–116.

52. Bowman SJ. Alternatives after molar distalization. Good Pract 2000;1:2–3.

53. Bowman SJ, Carano A. The Butterfly system. J Clin Orthod 2004;38:274–287.

54. Bowman SJ. Class II combination therapy (Distal jet and Jasper jumpers): a case report. J Orthod 2000;27:213–218.

55. Hilgers JJ, Farzin-Nia F. The asymmetrical "T" archwire. J Clin Orthod 1992;26:81–86.

56. Ferguson DJ, Bowman SJ, Carano A. A comparison of two maxillary molar distalization appliances with the distal jet. World J Orthod 2005 (in press).

CHAPTER 19

The Keles Slider Appliance for bilateral and unilateral maxillary molar distalization

Ahmet Keles

CONTENTS

Introduction

Over the past decade, nonextraction treatment and noncompliance therapies have become more popular in correction of Class II malocclusions. Conventional treatment of Class II cases usually requires distal movement of maxillary molars in order to achieve a Class I molar and canine relationship. However, if the maxillary molars are not distalized bodily and adequate anchorage is not established to move premolars and canines distally, anchorage will be easily lost. The literature shows that various devices have been developed for molar distalization; headgear was used routinely for distal movement of maxillary molars.[1-3] However, headgear relies totally on patient cooperation, which could reduce treatment success and increase treatment duration.

The difficulties involved with headgear wear and dependence on patient cooperation stimulated many investigators to develop intraoral devices and techniques for distal movement of molars. Blechman & Smiley,[4] Gianelly et al,[5] and Bondemark & Kurol[6] used magnets for molar distalization. Gianelly et al[7] and Bondemark et al[8] used superelastic nickel-titanium (NiTi) coil springs for distal movement of maxillary molars.

In 1992, Hilgers developed the Pendulum Appliance for distal movement of molars.[9] The appliance consisted of beta-titanium alloy (TMA) springs and a button on the palate. Since 1996, numerous investigators have conducted studies on the Pendulum Appliance which demonstrated that the molars were distalized but that distal tipping also occurred.[10-13] The amount of tipping in

these Pendulum studies varied from 6.07° to 17.7°. Keles & Sayinsu developed the Intraoral Bodily Molar Distalizer (IBMD) for molar distalization.[14] The distalizing TMA (0.032 × 0.032″) spring design of the IBMD (Ormco, Orange, CA) was composed of two pieces that enabled bodily movement of molars. Their results showed that the molars distalized without tipping but anchorage loss also occurred.

The intraoral distalization appliances developed in the last decade of the 20th century eliminated the need for patient cooperation. However, distal tipping of molars and anchorage loss also occurred with most of these new devices.

In this chapter, the Keles Slider (US Patent No: 6,626,665 B1) appliance will be introduced and its effectiveness assessed.

Appliance Construction

The maxillary first molars and first premolars are banded. Tubes of 0.045″ diameter are soldered to the palatal side of the Class II first molar bands. First premolar bands are attached to an acrylic Nance Appliance with 0.040″ diameter stainless steel retaining wires (Fig. 19.1). The acrylic button also consists of an anterior bite plane. The purpose of creating an anterior bite plane is to disocclude the posterior teeth, enhance the molar distalization, and correct the anterior deep bite. On the palatal side of the molars, 0.040″ diameter stainless steel wires are embedded into the acrylic about 5 mm apical to the gingival margin of the first molars. These wires pass through the tube and are oriented parallel to the occlusal plane (Fig. 19.2). For molar distalization a heavy NiTi coil spring (2 cm long, 0.045″ diameter and 0.016″ thick) is placed between the lock on the wire and the tube, in full compression. The amount of force generated with the full compression of the 2 cm open coil is about 200 g. This force system allows consistent application of force at the level of the center of resistance of the first molars.

The biomechanics of the force system is presented in Figure 19.3. Patients are seen once a month and the screw is activated with the use of a special wrench. After the distalization, the appliance is removed and the molars are stabilized by a Nance Appliance for

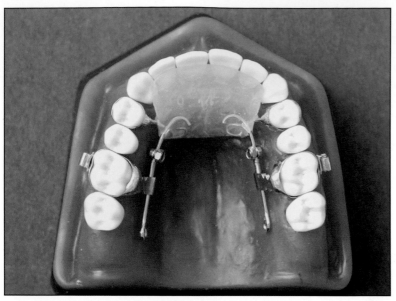

Figure 19.1 Occlusal view of the Keles Slider.

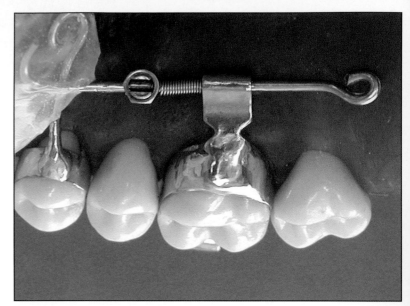

Figure 19.2 Palatal view of the Keles Slider.

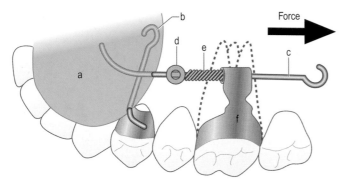

Figure 19.3 Biomechanics of the force system. Distal force is applied at the level of the center of resistance of the maxillary first molar. (a) Acrylic anterior bite plane. (b) Retaining wire for maxillary first premolar. (c) 0.040″ wire rod for distal sliding of maxillary first molar. (d) Adjustable screw for activation of the coil spring. (e) 0.040″ heavy NiTi open-coil spring. (f) Special tube soldered to the first molar band.

2 months before the second phase of orthodontic treatment and maintained until the end of canine distalization. Currently, instead of fabricating the Nance Appliance, the Keles Slider can be converted to a Nance Appliance by cutting the premolar retaining wires and removal of the anterior bite plane, which eliminates impression taking, model construction, and lab work. For better adaptation to the palate, the acrylic is relined at the chairside with light-cure acrylic Triad gel material (Dentsply, USA) (Figs 19.4–19.6).

Bilateral Distalization

The cephalometric results of a preliminary investigation on 10 patients showed that the maxillary first molars were distalized bodily by an average of 4.1 mm.[15] Distal tipping and molar extrusion were not observed during distalization. A Class I molar relationship was achieved on average in a period of 5.5 months. The maxillary first premolars moved forward 2.7 mm, the incisors protruded 2.05 mm and proclined 3.45°. The overjet was increased 2.2 mm and the overbite was reduced by 1.9 mm on average. Another report related to bilateral distalization with the Keles Slider with implant support showed that the molars moved distally with no anchorage loss. In fact, the first and second premolars drifted distally with the help of transseptal fibers. The molars moved distally without tipping in a bodily fashion.[16]

Patient 1

PA was a female 19 years and 2 months old diagnosed with Class II, division 1 malocclusion.[17] Her primary complaint involved the buccally positioned maxillary canines. Dentally, she had a full cusp Class II molar and canine relationship with 7 mm of maxillary crowding (Figs 19.7–19.10). There was 80% overbite and 3 mm overjet. She had large restorations and hypersensitivity of the maxillary second molars; maxillary third molars were unerupted.

The treatment plan included extraction of the maxillary second molars and distalization of the first molars. The Keles Slider was cemented in place (see Fig. 19.11). Following 7 months of treatment, the maxillary molars had distalized 5 mm on the right side and 6 mm on the left side, with each side achieving a super Class I molar relationship (Figs 19.12 and 19.13). There was 1 mm anchorage loss for the right first premolar and 2 mm anchorage loss for the left first premolar. The maxillary second premolars had drifted distally, with the help of the transseptal fibers. Maxillary incisors had slightly proclined. A Nance Appliance was cemented immediately after removal

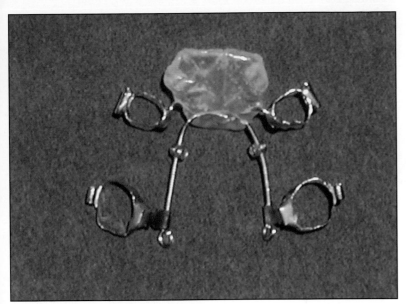

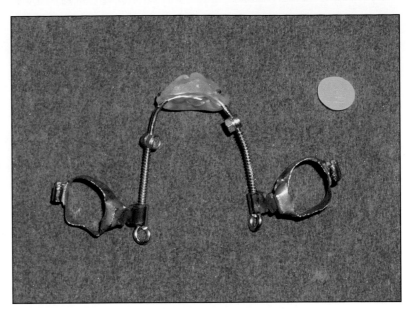

Figures 19.4–19.6 Chairside Nance construction from Keles Slider. Appliance is being removed after the distalization. *(From Keles et al 2002,[17] with kind permission of Quintessence Publishing Co. Inc.)*

Figure 19.5 Anterior bite plane and retaining wire are removed.

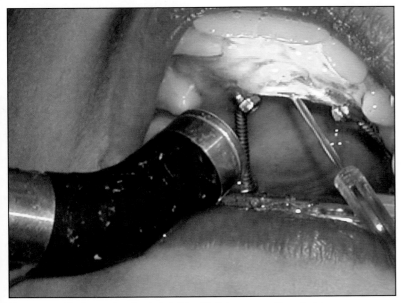

Figure 19.6 The button is relined chairside with light-cure acrylic material.

of the Keles Slider and was maintained for 2 months to prevent mesial relapse of molars.

Two months later, during the Nance stabilization period, the first premolars and the canines had drifted distally to their initial position (Figs 19.14 and 19.15). Therefore anterior crowding was relieved. The molars were distalized in a parallel fashion and the maxillary third molars were erupting without any difficulty (Fig. 19.16). Anterior deep bite was corrected with the help of the anterior bite plane. Class I molar and canine relationships were achieved on both sides at the end of orthodontic treatment, overbite was reduced to 20%, and overjet was reduced to 2 mm (Figs 19.17–19.20). The maxillary third molars erupted without any difficulty. The patient's smile was improved and her straight profile was maintained.

Unilateral Distalization

The cephalometric results of a preliminary investigation showed that the maxillary first molars were distalized bodily on average 4.9 mm.[18] Distal tipping and molar extrusion were not observed during distalization. A Class I molar relationship was achieved on average in a period of 6.1 months. The maxillary first premolars moved forward bodily 1.3 mm, the incisors protruded 1.8 mm and proclined 3.2°. The overjet was increased 2.1 mm and the overbite was reduced by 3.12 mm on average.

Patient 2

OY was a female, 14 years 7 months of age, diagnosed as Class II, division 1 subdivision right malocclusion.[19] Dentally, she had 10% overbite, 3 mm overjet, and 4 mm maxillary midline left deviation. The maxillary canines were out of the arch and 9 mm crowding was present. The maxillary third molars were congenitally missing (Figs 19.21–19.24). A unilateral Keles Slider was applied for the first phase of treatment to distalize the Class II molars into Class I (Fig. 19.25). Five months later we observed that the maxillary molars had distalized bodily 4 mm on the right side and a Class I molar relationship was maintained on the left side (Figs 19.26–19.29). The maxillary second premolars had drifted distally with the help of the transseptal fibers. No anchorage loss on the first premolars was observed but the maxillary incisors were proclined and overjet was

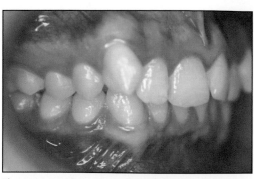

Figure 19.7 Right intraoral view. *(From Keles et al 2002,[17] with kind permission of Quintessence Publishing Co. Inc.)*

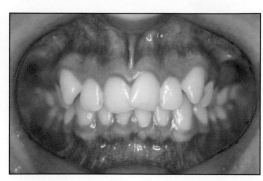

Figure 19.8 Frontal intraoral views of patient 1 before distalization. *(From Keles et al 2002,[17] with kind permission of Quintessence Publishing Co. Inc.)*

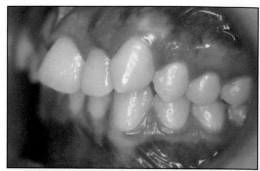

Figure 19.9 Left intraoral view. *(From Keles et al 2002,[17] with kind permission of Quintessence Publishing Co. Inc.)*

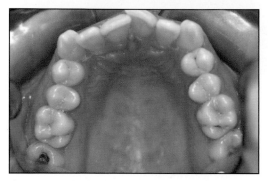

Figure 19.10 Occlusal intraoral view. *(From Keles et al 2002,[17] with kind permission of Quintessence Publishing Co. Inc.)*

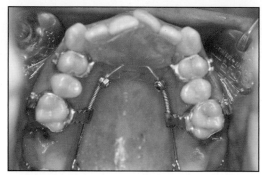

Figure 19.11 Occlusal view after cementation of the Keles Slider (maxillary second molars have been extracted). *(From Keles et al 2002,[17] with kind permission of Quintessence Publishing Co. Inc.)*

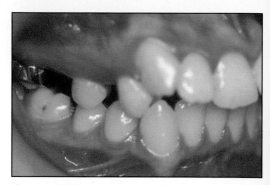

Figure 19.12 Right intraoral view of patient 1 after removal of the Keles Slider. *(From Keles et al 2002,[17] with kind permission of Quintessence Publishing Co. Inc.)*

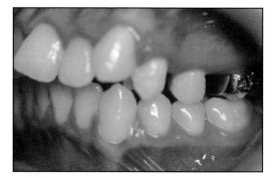

Figure 19.13 Left intraoral view. *(From Keles et al 2002,[17] with kind permission of Quintessence Publishing Co. Inc.)*

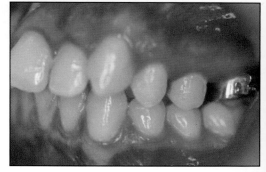

Figure 19.14 Right intraoral view of patient 1 at 2 months after removal of the Keles Slider. The Class I molar relationship was maintained and distal drift of the first premolars and canines, as well as reduction of the overjet, was achieved without any mechanotherapy. *(From Keles et al 2002,[17] with kind permission of Quintessence Publishing Co. Inc.)*

Figure 19.15 Left intraoral view. *(From Keles et al 2002,[17] with kind permission of Quintessence Publishing Co. Inc.)*

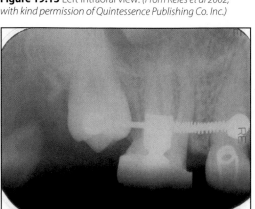

Figure 19.16 Periapical radiograph of patient 1 during distalization. Parallel distal migration of the first molars and the line of force application passing through the center of resistance of the first molars. *(From Keles et al 2002,[17] with kind permission of Quintessence Publishing Co. Inc.)*

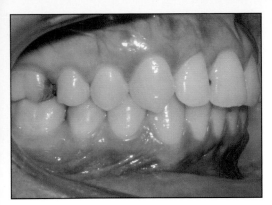

Figure 19.17 Right intraoral view.

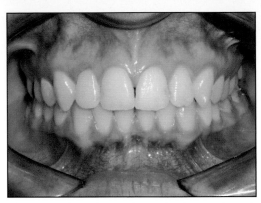

Figure 19.18 Frontal intraoral view of patient 1 at the end of fixed orthodontic treatment.

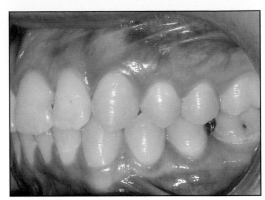

Figure 19.19 Left intraoral view.

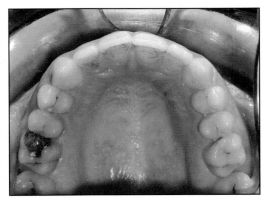

Figure 19.20 Occlusal intraoral view.

increased 2 mm. The molars were stabilized by a Nance button for 2 months before the fixed orthodontic treatment. Second-stage fixed bonded and banded treatment lasted 14 months and bands and brackets were removed at the end of fixed appliance therapy (Figs 19.30–19.33).

Keles Jig

To make clinical application of the appliance easier, a modification has been made. This jig design allows the clinician to fit the appliance at the chairside. The jig consists of a distalizing rod, 0.040″ stainless steel round wire with a ball tip, a lock (Rocky Mountain Orthodontics Co., USA) and 10 mm long NiTi heavy coil spring, and a 0.045″ tube with wire extension which attaches to the cleat on the first molar bands (patent pending: 10/816,714) (Fig. 19.34).

For the acrylic button construction, light-cure acrylic Triad gel material (Dentsply, USA) is applied at the chairside. The first premolars are attached with 0.040″ stainless steel round wire to the button. The steel rod of the jig is embedded into the acrylic about 5 mm apical to the gingival margin of the molars, passes through the tube and is oriented parallel to the occlusal plane.

This new method of application of the jig allows the chairside construction of a Keles Slider without the need for laboratory construction. The construction stages are presented in Figures 19.35–19.37. The progress pictures of the first-phase treatment are presented in Figures 19.38–19.41.

After distalization is complete, the Keles Slider is converted to a Nance holding appliance and distopalatal bends are made on the terminal ends of the wire connected to the tubes in order to derotate the molars if mesiobuccal rotations are needed (Figs 19.42–19.45).

Conclusion

Our results show that the Keles Slider is an effective appliance for the bodily distalization of molars. A Class I molar relationship can be established in a short period of time and there is little anchorage loss in comparison with other intraoral distalization mechanisms. The appliance is effective in deep bite correction with the help of the anterior bite plane accommodated to the Nance button. After the molar distalization is completed, the coil springs should be inactivated and the bite plane and the retaining wires for the first premolars

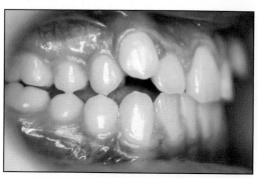

Figure 19.21 Right intraoral view.

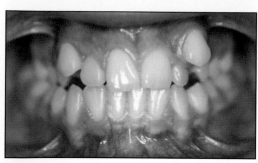

Figure 19.22 Frontal intraoral view of patient 2 before distalization.

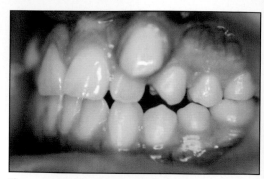

Figure 19.23 Left intraoral view.

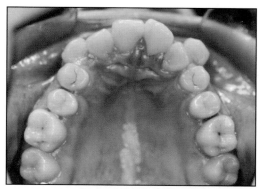

Figure 19.24 Occlusal intraoral view.

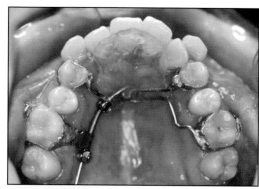

Figure 19.25 After the appliance has been cemented (to make the cementation, the lock is placed on the distal of the tube and will be removed after cementation).

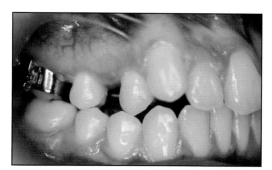

Figure 19.26 Right intraoral view.

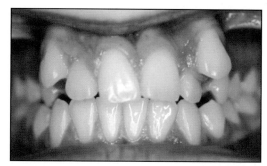

Figure 19.27 Frontal intraoral view of patient 2 after removal of the Keles Slider.

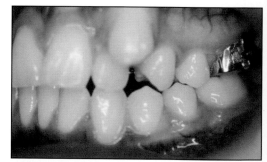

Figure 19.28 Left intraoral view.

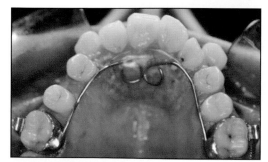

Figure 19.29 Occlusal intraoral view.

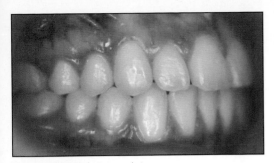

Figure 19.30 Right intraoral view.

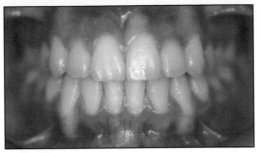

Figure 19.31 Frontal intraoral view of patient 2 at the end of fixed orthodontic treatment.

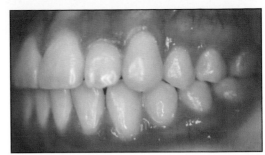

Figure 19.32 Left intraoral view.

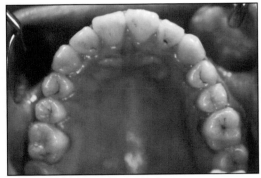

Figure 19.33 Occlusal intraoral view.

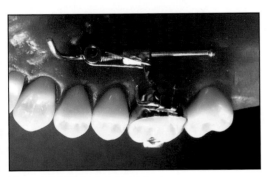

Figure 19.34 Keles jig (palatal view).

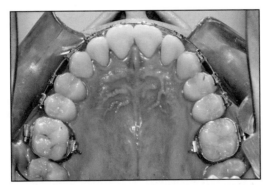

Figures 19.35–19.37 Stages in the chairside construction of the Keles Slider.

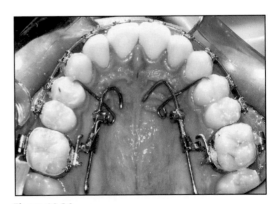

Figure 19.36

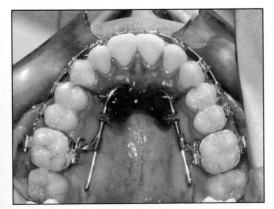

Figure 19.37

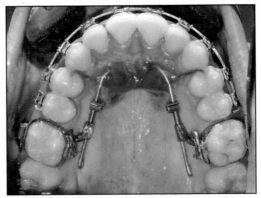

Figure 19.38 Patient 3: distal translation of first and second molars. Initial occlusal photographs.

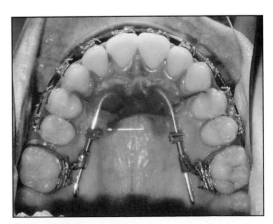

Figure 19.39 One month later.

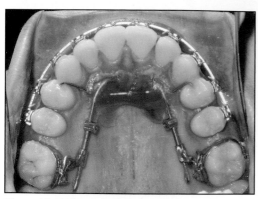

Figure 19.40 Three months later.

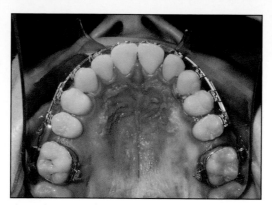

Figure 19.41 Four months later.

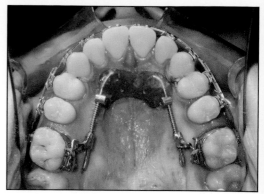

Figures 19.42–19.45 Conversion of Keles Slider to anchorage appliance with anti-rotation bends to derotate the molars if further rotations are needed.

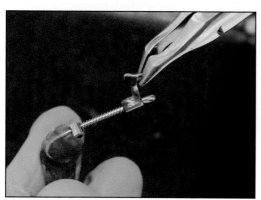

Figure 19.43

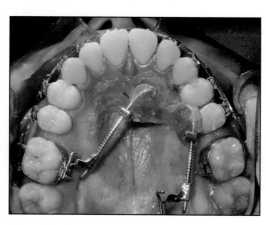

Figure 19.44

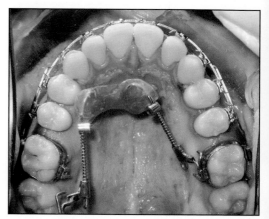

Figure 19.45

should be removed from the appliance and should be kept in the mouth for 2 months as a Nance Appliance. Overcorrection and stabilization of molars by converting the device into a passive holding appliance for 2 months would allow the first premolars to drift distally to their initial position and allow some time for the newly formed and remodeled bone around the roots of the first molars to mineralize. When second-stage orthodontic treatment starts, the molars would provide good anchorage for canine distalization and anterior retraction.

Another advantage of this appliance is the ease of activation; chair time for activation is very short. The latest version with the new jig design enables the appliance to be constructed at the chairside. Guided consistent distal force at the level of the center of resistance allows the molars to slide distally without the problems of tipping, excessive anchorage loss, and questionable patient cooperation.

Newton's third law of action and reaction (equal and opposite forces) is applicable in the design of the Keles Slider. A compressed coil spring applies distal force at the level of the center of resistance of the first molars which enables bodily distalization of molars (action principle). The reciprocal effect of the compressed coil spring applies mesial force at a higher level along the roots of the first premolars and anterior teeth. The support from the anterior aspect of the palate would reduce the mesial dental movement (reaction principle).

The Keles Slider is effective in distalizing molars with intraarch mechanics and should not be misused in the correction of skeletal Class II. It can be used on patients with dental Class II malocclusion underlying a Class I skeletal pattern with minimum or no mandibular crowding. Third molars should be addressed and removed surgically if the patient is older than 15 years.

References

1. Poulton DR. The influence of extraoral traction. Am J Orthod 1967;53:8–18.

2. Cangialosi TJ, Meistrell ME Jr, Leung MA, Ko JY. Cephalometric appraisal of edgewise Class II nonextraction treatment with extraoral force. Am J Orthod Dentofacial Orthop 1988;93: 315–324.

3. Arvystas MG. Nonextraction treatment of severe Class II, division 2 malocclusions. Part 2. Am J Orthod Dentofacial Orthop 1991;99:74–84.

4. Blechman AM, Smiley H. Magnetic force in orthodontics. Am J Orthod Dentofacial Orthop 1978;74:435–443.

5. Gianelly AA, Vaitas AS, Thomas WM, Berger DG. Distalization of molars with repelling magnets. J Clin Orthod 1988;22:40–44.

6. Bondemark L, Kurol J. Distalization of maxillary first and second molars simultaneously with repelling magnets. Eur J Orthod 1992;14:264–272.

7. Gianelly AA, Bednar J, Dietz VS. Japanese NiTi coils used to move molars distally. Am J Orthod Dentofacial Orthop 1991;99:564–566.

8. Bondemark L, Kurol J, Bernhold M. Repelling magnets versus superelastic nickel-titanium coils in simultaneous distal movement of maxillary first and second molars. Angle Orthod 1994;63: 189–198.

9. Hilgers JJ. The pendulum appliance for Class II non-compliance therapy. J Clin Orthod 1992;26: 706–714.

10. Ghosh J, Nanda RS. Evaluation of an intraoral maxillary molar distalization technique. Am J Orthod Dentofacial Orthop 1996;110: 639–646.

11. Byloff FK, Darendeliler MA, Clar E, Darendeliler A. Distal molar movement using the pendulum appliance. Part 2: The effect of maxillary molar root uprighting bends. Angle Orthod 1997;67: 261–270.

12. Bussick TJ, McNamara JA Jr. Dentoalveolar and skeletal changes associated with the pendulum appliance. Am J Orthod Dentofacial Orthop 2000;117:333–343.

13. Joseph A, Butchart C. An evaluation of the pendulum distalizing appliance Semin Orthod 2000; 6:129–135.

14. Keles A, Sayinsu K. A New approach in maxillary molar distalization: intraoral bodily molar distalizer. Am J Orthod Dentofacial Orthop 2000;117: 39–48.

15. Tahir A. Cephalometric evaluation of Keles Slider appliance. Masters degree thesis. Istanbul: Marmara University; 2002.

16. Keles A, Erverdi N, Sezen S. Bodily molar distalization with absolute anchorage. Angle Orthod 2003;73:471–482.

17. Keles A, Pamukcu B, Cetinkaya E. Bilateral maxillary molar distalization with sliding mechanics: Keles Slider. World J Orthod 2002;3:57–66.

18. Keles A. Maxillary unilateral molar distalization with sliding mechanics: a preliminary investigation. Eur J Orthod 2001;23:507–515.

19. Keles A, Isguden B. Unilateral molar distalization with molar slider (two case reports). Turkish J Orthod 1999;12:193–202.

CHAPTER 20

The Jones Jig™ and modifications

Moschos A. Papadopoulos

CONTENTS

Introduction

Class II malocclusion is one of the most common problems in orthodontics, with an estimated one-third of all orthodontic patients treated for this condition.[1] Many treatment options are available for the correction of Class II malocclusion, depending on what part of the craniofacial skeleton is affected. In general, treatment of Class II malocclusion can include growth modification in terms of mandibular advancement (to treat patients with mandibular skeletal retrusion), maxillary retraction (to treat patients with maxillary skeletal protrusion), and maxillary molar distalization (to treat patients with maxillary dentoalveolar protrusion).[2–4] Treatment approaches include the use of functional or removable appliances, extraoral traction by means of headgears, and fixed appliances combined with Class II elastics.[1]

Unfortunately, successful orthodontic treatment using these modalities often relies heavily on the patient's willingness to wear the suggested appliance. For example, regarding the wearing of headgear, apart from the discomfort and the extraoral appearance of the patient (factors that can reduce their cooperation), there is also a risk of the headgear causing eye and facial tissue damage.[5–13] In addition, the elastic cervical strap puts a nonphysiologic strain on the cervical spine and on the neck muscles and in some patients it causes irritation of the skin.[14,15] Furthermore, cephalometric evaluations have revealed that extraoral appliances can produce skeletal effects in addition to maxillary molar distalization,[3,4,16,17] which could be a drawback when there is no need for growth guidance.

For all the above reasons, nonextraction treatment as well as noncompliance approaches have became very popular for the correction of Class II malocclusions. Many treatment modalities, known as "noncompliance appliances," have been introduced which minimize or eliminate the need for patient compliance in order to activate the relevant force systems. A major category is the "noncompliance distalization appliances," which are used for the treatment of patients with maxillary dentoalveolar protrusion. These appliances derive their anchorage in an intramaxillary manner and act only in the maxillary arch in order to move the molars distally, e.g. the Pendulum Appliance,[18] the Distal Jet,[19] repelling magnets,[20–22] the Jones Jig,[23] the New Distalizer,[24] etc. The force system of these appliances can be flexible or rigid and can be positioned buccally or palatally.

Nickel-titanium coil springs have been used in conjunction with various noncompliance appliances to produce rapid maxillary molar movement[19,23,25–27] because it was found that they have greater springback and superelastic properties than stainless steel coils.[28] Furthermore, the most important reason for their implementation in noncompliance distalization devices is their ability to exert a very long range of constant, light and continuous forces.[29]

Among the distalization appliances that use nickel-titanium coil springs as a buccally positioned flexible force system, the Jones Jig is one of the most commonly used in noncompliance Class II orthodontic treatment.[23]

Jones Jig™

The Jones Jig™ (American Orthodontics, Sheboygan, WI) (Fig. 20.1) was introduced by Jones & White[23] and includes an active unit positioned buccally, consisting of active arms or jig assemblies incorporating nickel-titanium open coil springs and an anchorage unit consisting of a modified Nance Appliance.

The modified Nance Appliance includes an acrylic palatal button of at least 15 mm in diameter, which is stabilized with 0.036″ stainless steel wires that extend bilaterally and are soldered to bands on maxillary first or second premolars or to deciduous second molars (Fig. 20.2).[23,30,31] Gulati et al stabilized the Nance holding arch to both maxillary first and second premolars with 0.040″ stainless steel wire.[32] The Nance button should not be in contact with the anterior teeth and the incisal papilla, while it should resemble a modified

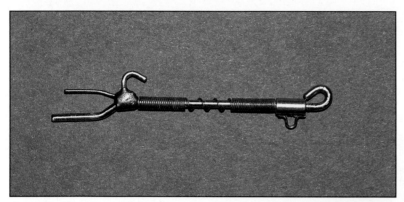

Figure 20.1 The Jones Jig Appliance.

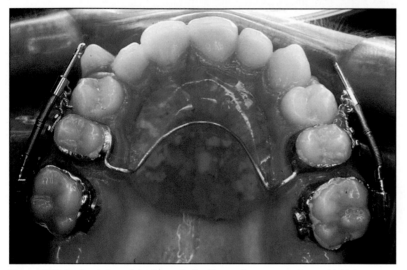

Figure 20.2 Occlusal view of the Jones Jig Appliance after cementation and initial distalization.

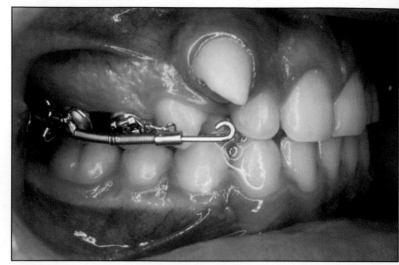

Figure 20.3 Lateral view of the Jones Jig Appliance after cementation and initial distalization.

"butterfly" extending from the mesial of the maxillary second premolars to the middle of the canines and laterally within 3.5 mm of the canine and the first premolar.

The jig assembly consists of a 0.036″ wire, which holds the nickel-titanium open coil spring or the superelastic Japanese nickel-titanium spring,[32] and a sliding eyelet tube.[30] An additional stabilizing wire is attached along with a hook to the distal portion of the main wire. Thus the jig assembly comprises in its distal end two arms, which are used to stabilize the appliance (see Fig. 20.1).

Clinical Management

After cementation of the modified Nance Appliance, the main arm of the Jones Jig is inserted into the headgear tube and the stabilizing arm is inserted into the archwire slot of the maxillary first molar buccal attachment.[30–33] In addition, the distal hook of the Jones Jig is tied with a stainless steel ligature to the hook of the buccal molar tube to further increase the stability of the appliance (Fig. 20.3).

Gulati et al recommend the use of bands with gingivally positioned headgear tubes to allow the force vector to pass closer to the center of resistance of the first maxillary molar, thus reducing molar distal tipping.[32] Thus, the distalization spring can be positioned about 3 mm more gingival compared with the standard Jones Jig.

The appliance is activated by tying back the sliding hook to the anchor teeth (first or second premolars), with a 0.012″ or 0.010″ stainless steel ligature, thus compressing the open coil spring 1–5 mm.[23,30–33] The activated open coil spring can produce approximately 70–75 g of continuous distalizing force to the maxillary first molars for a period of 2.5–9 months.[23,30–34] Gulati et al used Sentalloy Open Coil Springs instead of nickel-titanium springs, which according to them can exert a distalizing force of 150 g.[32] The patients are monitored every 4–5 weeks for further adjustments.[23,30–32] When the anchoring teeth are the first premolars, the second premolars seem to follow the molar distal movement during distalization due to the pull of the transseptal fibers.[23]

The maxillary molars are distalized until a Class I relationship has been achieved.[23,31,32] Then, the molar position should be stabilized with a Nance holding arch appliance, a utility archwire or a stopped archwire mesial to molars, while the premolars drift distally due to the pull of transseptal fibers.[31] Further, alternative ways of maintaining the first molar position include the use of Korn maxillary lip bumpers, maxillary Hawley-type appliances with wire stops mesial to molars, transpalatal bars and passive Jasper Jumpers.

Indications and Contraindications

The Jones Jig Appliance is indicated for the noncompliance bilateral or unilateral distalization of the maxillary first molars in patients with Class II malocclusion and erupted or unerupted maxillary second molars, as well as in Class II patients with mild anterior crowding.[23,30–34] However, the Jones Jig is contraindicated in patients with an excessive vertical growth pattern because the extrusion of the maxillary first molars cannot be adequately controlled.[23,32]

Advantages and Disadvantages

The main advantages of the Jones Jig include minimal reliance on patient compliance, the lack of pain, the rapid distalization, better control of molar distal tipping and rotation, and the continuous force application.[23,31,32,34] In addition, the Jones Jig is quite comfortable for the patient.[34] However, the anchorage loss due to the mesial movement of the anterior teeth and the distal tipping of the molars are the main disadvantages of the Jones Jig.[30–34]

Treatment Effects

According to most investigators the Jones Jig was effective in distalizing the maxillary first molars with no dependence on patient cooperation, although some anchorage loss occurred at the same time. The Jones Jig influenced the maxillary dentition, while less pronounced effects were observed in the hard and soft tissues.

Sagittal Changes

Following treatment with the Jones Jig, the maxillary first molars were distalized between 1.17 mm and 2.8 mm, with a monthly rate of 0.83 mm.[30–34] However, the distal movement of the first molars was in most cases accompanied with unfavorable distal tipping that varied between 3.50° and 7.85°.[30–34] The maxillary second molars were also influenced due to the first molar distal movement. They were distalized from 1.54 mm to 2.70 mm and tipped distally from 3.30° up to 7.89°.[30–32]

The anchor unit could not resist the reciprocal mesial forces of the Jones Jig and anterior anchorage loss was found in most of the studies. The maxillary first premolars moved mesially 1.10 mm and also tipped mesially 2.60°.[32] The second premolars, when they were used as anchor teeth, moved mesially about 2 mm and tipped mesially between 3.45° and 9.43°.[30,31,34]

In addition, anterior movement and proclination of the maxillary incisors were also found during the distalization phase with the Jones Jig. The maxillary incisors were found to move mesially between 0.25 mm and 0.55 mm and to procline between 1° and 2°.[30,31,34] The overjet was also affected during the distalization period and increased between 0.45 mm and 1.53 mm.[30–32]

Vertical Changes

The first molars demonstrated vertical changes during the distalization phase. Some investigators observed an extrusion between 0.90 mm and 2.08 mm,[30,32,34] while others found a nonsignificant extrusion of 0.14 mm.[31] Not only the maxillary first molars but also the maxillary second molars extruded by 2 mm.[30]

Further, the maxillary first premolars presented an extrusion of 3.23 mm.[30] The second premolars were extruded 1.88 mm according to Brickman et al,[31] while in contrast Haydar & Uner[34] found 1.85 mm of intrusion.

The maxillary incisors also presented a 3.08 mm extrusion[30] while Haydar & Uner[34] observed an intrusion of 0.95 mm. Further, the overbite was decreased between 0.23 mm and 1.28 mm.[30–32]

Skeletal changes concerning the vertical dimension were also found after distalization with the Jones Jig Appliance. The lower anterior facial height was increased from 1 mm to 1.46 mm.[30,31] The mandibular plane angle was also increased by 1.30°[32] whereas Runge et al[30] found this angle almost unchanged after treatment.

Soft Tissue Changes

The soft tissues were also affected by the anchorage loss of the anterior teeth. Brickman et al observed a 0.03 mm protrusion of the upper lip and a 0.68 mm protrusion of the lower lip, as measured from the E-plane.[31] Runge et al observed similar changes: 0.38 mm for the upper lip and 1.06 mm for the lower lip.[30]

Modifications of the Jones Jig

Since the initial introduction of the Jones Jig, two modifications have been developed. In 1996 Scott proposed the Lokar Appliance,[35] while in 1998 Papadopoulos introduced the Modified Sectional Jig Assembly for simultaneous first and second molar distalization.[36]

Lokar Appliance

The Lokar Appliance (Ormco, Orange, CA) consists of a nickel-titanium coil spring activated by a mesial sliding sleeve (mesial component) and an appropriately sized rectangular wire (distal component) which is inserted into the archwire tube of the first molar.[35] For anchorage, a Nance acrylic button 2–3 mm thick can be used which is stabilized to the maxillary second premolars with a 0.040″ stainless steel wire. Alternatively, fixed appliances can be used. In addition, extraoral and lip bumper forces may be applied at the same time because the molar tubes are not used.

After cementation of the molar bands and Nance button, the Lokar Appliance is inserted into the archwire tube of the first molar and adapted so that it is parallel to the occlusal plane and close to the teeth for maximum patient comfort. It is important to have both mesial and distal ends of the appliance adapted as close as possible to the teeth, so they will not irritate the cheek or the lip. In addition, bends should not be placed in the sliding components of the appliance because they could inhibit efficient molar distalization.

For activation of the Lokar Appliance, the mesial component is tied back by a ligature wire to the second premolars, thus compressing the spring. The optimal compression of the spring is about 1–2 mm. The patient is monitored every 5 weeks, at which points the appliance can be reactivated: the ligature is untied, the spring is compressed, and the ligature is tied again. Each reactivation can produce 1–3 mm of molar distal movement. The first molars are distalized until a Class III molar relationship has been achieved, which is needed to counteract the mesial movement of the maxillary premolars and the anchorage loss during retraction of the anterior teeth.

The appliance can be used alone or in combination with fixed appliances. After distalization of the molars is complete, the Nance holding arch and Lokar Appliance are removed and a new Nance is placed to maintain the molar position. Then, full-fixed appliances or 2 × 4 fixed appliances can be used as a second phase of the overall orthodontic treatment.

According to Scott,[35] the Lokar Appliance is indicated in patients with Class II malocclusion due to maxillary protrusion, canine impaction or ectopic eruption of the maxillary premolars and in any other situation in which first molar distalization is indicated. However, the appliance is contraindicated in Class II patients with mandibular retrognathism.

The main advantages of the Lokar Appliance include the production of persistent and predictable results, increased efficiency, easy insertion, ligation and use, as well as the short chair time required to initiate treatment and for reactivations.[35]

Modified Sectional Jig Assembly

The Modified Sectional Jig Assembly, a simple intraoral minimal-compliance fixed appliance, was introduced in 1998 for simultaneous distalization of first and second maxillary molars (Figs 20.4–20.6).[36] The appliance takes full advantage of the nickel-titanium coil springs, can be regarded as a modification of the Jones Jig, and can be used as an alternative or perhaps as a realistic compromise for patients who are unable or unwilling to wear the headgear.

The appliance can produce rapid simultaneous distalization of maxillary first and second molars, although some anchorage loss of the anterior dental unit can be observed. For the moment, the only approaches that are not associated with anchorage loss during distalization are the headgear and the use of orthodontic implants. The use of headgear requires maximum patient cooperation especially when both first and second molars are to be distalized simultaneously, while the use of orthodontic implants as absolute anchorage for molar distalization is a somewhat complicated procedure requiring advanced skills from the practitioner. In addition, it is associated with surgical procedures and high cost, factors that will influence the patients' decision to accept such treatment except in extreme cases.

Other appliances such as nickel-titanium wires, nickel-titanium coil springs, and repelling magnets require less patient cooperation but also present some disadvantages. For example, when continuous superelastic wires are used for distalization of the molars by means of wire deformations mesial to the first molar,[37] the leveling and alignment of the anterior teeth decrease the anchorage value of these teeth. Further, the disadvantages of magnets are related to the

proportionate and variable character of the force produced,[22] their high cost, the patient's discomfort, and the lack of complete knowledge concerning their biologic effects.[38,39]

The Modified Sectional Jig Assembly consists of an active and an anchorage unit (Figs 20.4–20.6).[36] The anchorage unit is a modified Nance Appliance attached to the maxillary second premolar bands (which are provided with brackets) with a 0.032″ stainless steel wire (Fig. 20.5). Thus all teeth mesial to molars are indirectly utilized. Bands with headgear tubes and hooks placed gingivally are cemented to the first molars.

The active unit consists of an active arm fabricated from a round 0.028″ stainless steel wire with a length of 30–35 mm. A 3 mm long open loop constructed at a distance of 8 mm from the wire end divides the wire arm into two sections, a small distal and a larger

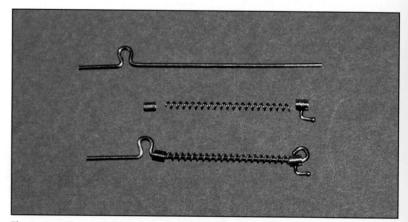

Figure 20.4 The parts of the sectional jig assembly: 0.028″ stainless steel wire with loop, sliding tubes, nickel-titanium open coil spring, and the whole distalization unit.

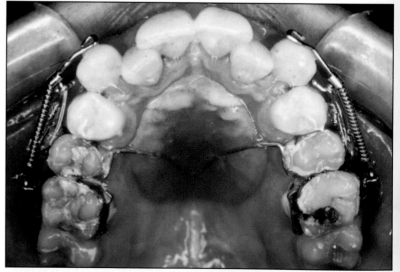

Figure 20.5 Occlusal view of the sectional jig assembly after cementation and initial activation. *(From Papadopoulos et al 2004,[40] by kind permission of Urban & Vogel Publishers, Munich)*

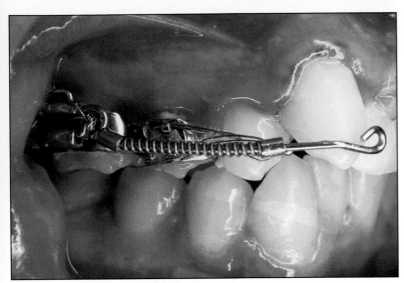

Figure 20.6 Lateral view of the sectional jig assembly after cementation and initial activation. *(From Papadopoulos et al 2004,⁴⁰ by kind permission of Urban & Vogel Publishers, Munich)*

mesial one (Fig. 20.4). A nickel-titanium open coil spring (25–30 mm long, with a wire cross section of 0.010″ and a helix diameter of 0.030″) is inserted through the mesial end of the sectional wire. Two sliding tubes are used for positional stabilization of the spring. The distal tube is placed close to the loop of the sectional wire and stabilizes the coil spring, preventing it sliding into the loop. The mesial tube, put in place after insertion of the spring, is provided with a hook and is placed close to the mesial end of the sectional wire, which is subsequently bent gingivally. This bend prevents the coil spring from sliding away from the wire and ensures that there is no soft tissue impingement.

Clinical Management

After cementation of the modified Nance button and the first maxillary molar bands, the distal end of the sectional jig assembly is inserted into the headgear tube of the first molar band. A stainless steel ligature is then tied between the open loop of the active arm and the gingival hook of the molar band, adding stability to the system and preventing rotation of the sectional archwire (Fig. 20.7).

The spring is activated by ligating the hook of the second (mesial) sliding tube to the bracket of the second premolar band. Optimal activation of the coil spring will deliver 80 g per side. The patient is monitored at 4-week intervals for further adjustments and reactivation of the appliance.

The first maxillary molars are distalized until a super Class I molar relationship has been achieved (Fig. 20.8). After distalization has been accomplished, the appliance is removed (Figs 20.9–20.12) and the first molars are retained in position by either a new Nance holding arch or a transpalatal arch for approximately 2 months. This allows a spontaneous distal drift of the first and second premolars via the pull of the transseptal fibers during the stabilization period. Additionally, a utility archwire or a stopped archwire mesial to molars can also be used to maintain the first molar position. After this stabilization period, a second phase of comprehensive orthodontic treatment with full-fixed appliances can follow in order to retract the anterior teeth and level and align the dental arches.

Indications and Contraindications

The Modified Sectional Jig Assembly is indicated in patients with Class II malocclusion presenting minimal compliance when a bilateral or unilateral distalization of the maxillary first and second molars is required.[36,40]

The use of this noncompliance distalization appliance presents some contraindications. These may take into consideration the crowding or spacing condition of the maxillary dental arch and the growth pattern of the craniofacial complex, as well as the anatomic characteristics of the palatal vault. Significant crowding or spacing in the maxillary dental arch can lead to disproportionate anchorage loss. Thus, patients with an extreme vertical growth pattern and the presence of or a tendency towards an anterior open bite as well as those with insufficient seating of the Nance button due to reduced

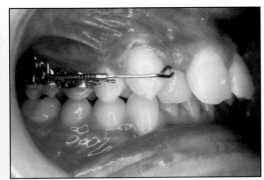

Figure 20.7 Patient SG, treated with the sectional jig assembly. Intraoral view before activation of the appliance. *(From Papadopoulos et al 2004,⁴⁰ by kind permission of Urban & Vogel Publishers, Munich)*

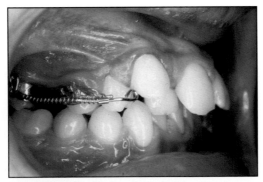

Figure 20.8 Patient SG. Intraoral view after molar distalization. *(From Papadopoulos et al 2004,⁴⁰ by kind permission of Urban & Vogel Publishers, Munich)*

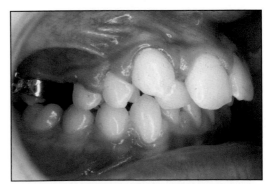

Figure 20.9 Patient SG. Intraoral view after appliance removal. *(From Papadopoulos et al 2004,⁴⁰ with kind permission of Urban & Vogel Publishers, Munich)*

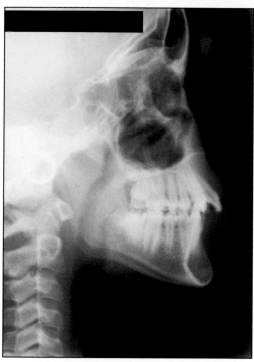

Figure 20.10 Patient SG. Lateral cephalometric radiograph before insertion of the appliance. *(From Papadopoulos 1998,[36] by kind permission of the Greek Orthodontic Society)*

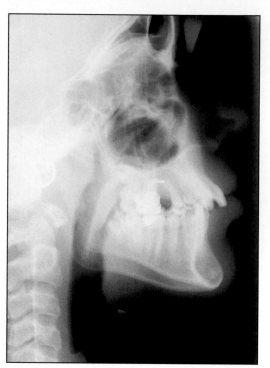

Figure 20.11 Patient SG. Lateral cephalometric radiograph after removal of the appliance. *(From Papadopoulos 1998,[36] by kind permission of the Greek Orthodontic Society)*

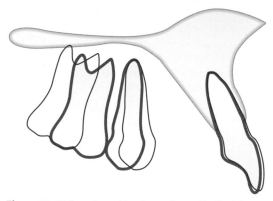

Figure 20.12 Superimposition (according to Björk) of the pretreatment (gray line) and posttreatment (red line) tracings of the maxilla. *(From Papadopoulos 1998,[36] by kind permission of the Greek Orthodontic Society)*

palatal vault inclination may be unsuitable candidates for simultaneous first and second maxillary molar distalization with this appliance. For all these reasons, case selection is a very important factor for successful treatment and is strongly recommended before performing simultaneous distalization of maxillary first and second molars with the Modified Sectional Jig Assembly.[36,40]

Advantages and Disadvantages

The main advantages of the Modified Sectional Jig Assembly are the following:[36]

- it requires minimal patient cooperation
- it can be easily fabricated by the clinician using simple components
- it is inexpensive in comparison to other prefabricated intraoral appliances
- it requires minimal chair time for reactivations
- it can be used unilaterally or bilaterally
- it is based on sound biologic and biomechanic principles.

Although the appliance can produce rapid simultaneous distalization of maxillary first and second molars, it presents some disadvantages such as anchorage loss in the anterior segment (in terms of incisor proclination or increased overjet) and distal tipping of the molars. Therefore, the mesial movement and slight protrusion of the anchorage unit during intraoral distalization have to be taken seriously into consideration before applying this treatment approach.[36,40,41]

Case Presentation

The patient (PS, male, 11 years 5 months) presented with a Class II, division 1 malocclusion characterized by an increased overjet of 12 mm and an overbite of 5.5 mm (Figs 20.13–20.16). The cephalometric analysis revealed a convex profile, Class II sagittal skeletal relationships between maxilla and mandible, and a great proclination of the upper incisors (Fig. 20.13).

The patient suffered from severe hypermobility and was unable to wear any removable appliances (such as extraoral or functional) or

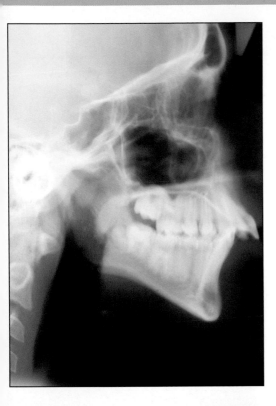

Figure 20.13 Patient PS. Pretreatment lateral cephalometric radiograph.

fixed functional appliances (such as the Herbst appliance). Further, his parents insisted on a treatment plan without extractions or surgical interventions. For these reasons, a nonextraction approach was proposed, including distalization of maxillary molars by means of a sectional jig assembly followed by comprehensive fixed orthodontic appliance treatment.

A sectional jig assembly was inserted (Figs 20.14–20.16) in order to distalize simultaneously the first and second maxillary molars. Following 2.5 months of treatment, the first molars were moved to a super Class I relationship (Figs 20.17–20.19). After removal of the distalization appliance, a transpalatal bar was inserted to retain the first maxillary molars in place and to allow distal drifting of the first and second premolars (Figs 20.20–20.22). The overjet observed immediately after treatment was 14 mm (increase of 2 mm), the overbite was 4 mm (decrease of 1.5 mm), and the inclination of the upper incisors to the SN line was slightly increased.

Following a stabilization period of 2 months, full-fixed orthodontic appliances were inserted to retract the maxillary anterior teeth and align the upper and lower dental arches. At the end of treatment (aged 13 years and 8 months), the patient presented a good occlusion,

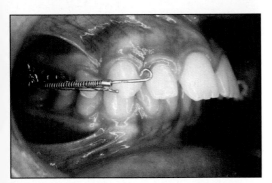
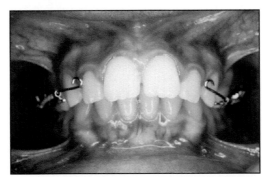
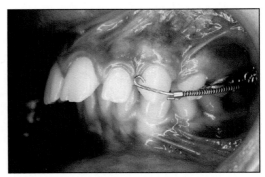

Figures 20.14–20.16 Patient PS. Intraoral photographs immediately after insertion of the sectional jig assembly. *(From Mavropoulos et al 2005,[41] with kind permission of The Angle Orthodontist, Allen Press)*

Figure 20.15

Figure 20.16

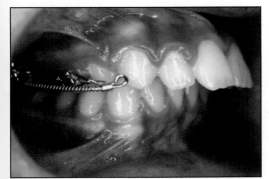
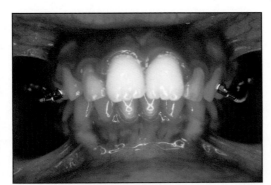
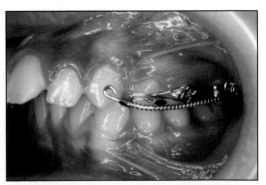

Figures 20.17–20.19 Patient PS. Intraoral photographs at end of distalization with sectional jig assembly still in place.

Figure 20.18

Figure 20.19

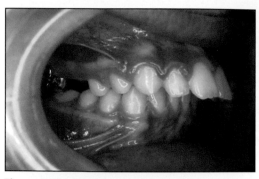
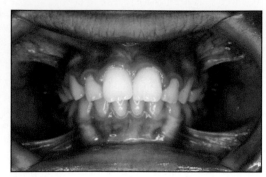
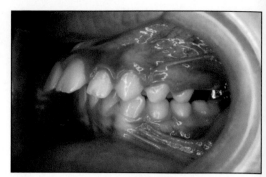

Figures 20.20–20.22 Patient PS. Intraoral photographs at the end of distalization immediately after removal of the sectional jig assembly. *(From Mavropoulos et al 2005,[41] with kind permission of The Angle Orthodontist, Allen Press)*

Figure 20.21

Figure 20.22

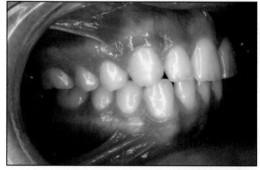
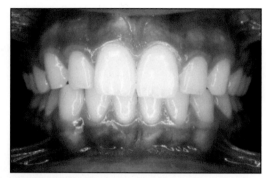
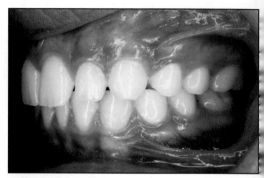

Figures 20.23–20.25 Patient PS. Intraoral photographs at the end of treatment following the removal of full fixed appliances. *(From Mavropoulos et al 2005,[41] with kind permission of The Angle Orthodontist, Allen Press)*

Figure 20.24

Figure 20.25

resulting in bilateral Class I molar and canine relationships. Overjet and overbite were also corrected (Figs 20.23–20.25), while the upper and lower incisors showed a good axial inclination (Fig. 20.26).

Treatment Effects

In order to evaluate the clinical effectiveness of this simple intraoral minimal-compliance fixed appliance, we have used the sectional jig assembly for simultaneous distalization of both first and second maxillary molars in patients presenting with Class II malocclusion. Two studies were performed, the first by means of cephalometric analysis on lateral cephalometric radiographs (Figs 20.27 and 20.28), taken before insertion and immediately after removal of the sectional jig assembly,[40] and the second by means of three-dimensional (3D) superimposition analysis on dental casts (Fig. 20.29) as well as cephalometric analysis on lateral cephalometric radiographs again taken before insertion and immediately after removal of the distalization appliance.[41]

The first study sample[40] consisted of 14 consecutive patients (six boys and eight girls with a mean age of 13.4 years), while the second study sample[41] consisted of 10 patients (five boys and five girls with a mean age of 13.2 years). All patients presented bilateral Class II molar relationships and maxillary second molars already erupted and were treated with the sectional jig assembly during the first phase of their overall orthodontic treatment by the author. No other molar distalization procedure was performed during the study period. After Class I molar relationship was accomplished, the sectional jig assembly was removed and the first molars were stabilized by means of a transpalatal bar for a period of 2 months prior to the final stage of orthodontic treatment with full-fixed appliances. The stabilization was to encourage the spontaneous distal drift of the first and second premolars, taking advantage of the transseptal fiber pull.

Distalization Effect

Distal movement of both first and second maxillary molars in full occlusion is considered extremely difficult to accomplish without patient cooperation or substantial anchorage loss. The intraoral appliance used was successful in the simultaneous distalization of maxillary first and second molars into a bilateral Class I molar relationship in all cases, which was achieved during an average

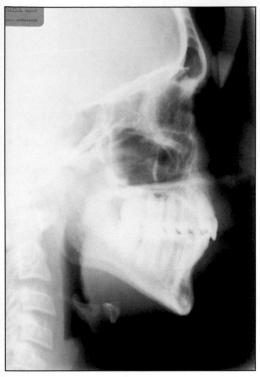

Figure 20.26 Patient PS. Posttreatment lateral cephalometric radiograph.

treatment period of 16.5 and 17.5 weeks, for the first and second studies respectively.[40,41]

The correction of the Class II relationship was achieved by a mean maxillary first molar distal movement of 1.4 mm, while the second molars were distalized by a mean of 1.2 mm.[40] These movements were accompanied by distal tipping of the maxillary first and second molars by a mean 6.8° and 8.3°, respectively. On the other hand, the 3D superimposition analysis on dental casts revealed that the first maxillary molars were distalized 2.8 mm.[41] However, first molar distalization was accompanied by distal tipping of 6.8° and distal rotation of 7.9°.

The space created between the maxillary first molars and second premolars averaged 6.1 mm (Fig. 20.30).[41] A part of this space was due to distal tipping of the first molars and part due to mesial tipping of the second premolars. Distal movement of the molar crown accounted for 46% of the total space created on each side. However, individual variations as well as differences between the right and the left side in the same patient were significant.

The rate of first molar distal movement was 0.37 mm[40] or 0.64 mm[41] per month, which was in accordance with the rates reported by other studies using similar noncompliance devices.[25,30,31,34,42] Further, molar distalization using magnets generally moves molar crowns at a similar[43] or slightly slower rate[42] than the appliance used in this study.

The effect of distalization on the maxillary third molars was extremely varied. In general, there was no distal movement but distal tipping by a mean 4.0° was observed, but this was not statistically significant. Despite their lack of statistical significance, these positional changes of the third molars can lead to their impaction,

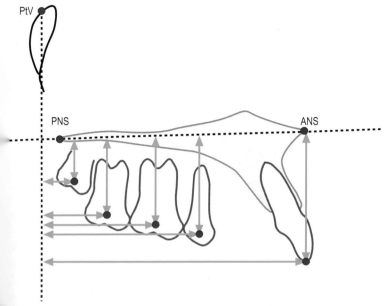

Figure 20.27 Cephalometric dental linear measurements used in the study. *(From Papadopoulos et al 2004,[40] by kind permission of Urban & Vogel Publishers, Munich)*

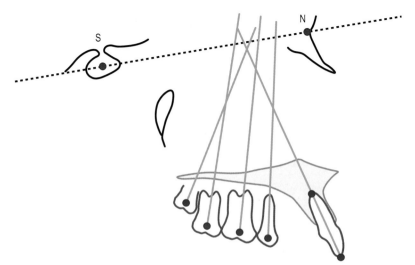

Figure 20.28 Cephalometric dental angular measurements used in the study. *(From Papadopoulos et al 2004,[40] by kind permission of Urban & Vogel Publishers, Munich)*

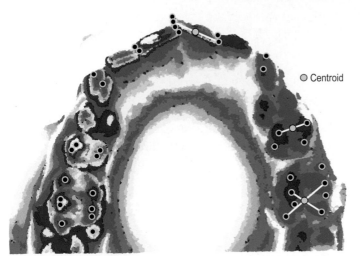

Figure 20.29 3D superimposition analysis on dental casts. The result of the fusion of the two holograms after their superimposition on the palate. Colors are used to facilitate the reading of the image. *(From Mavropoulos et al 2005,[41] with kind permission of The Angle Orthodontist, Allen Press)*

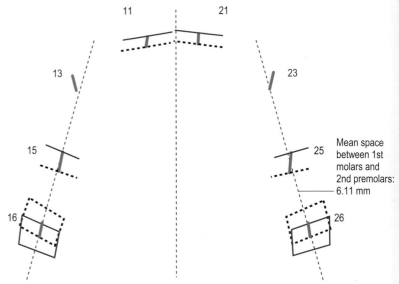

Figure 20.30 Mean tracing, where the mean positional changes of the teeth under investigation are shown in solid thick lines. Dashed and solid thin lines represent the position of the teeth before and after treatment, respectively. *(From Mavropoulos et al 2005,[41] with kind permission of The Angle Orthodontist, Allen Press)*

especially if the space available at the beginning of treatment is not adequate. Therefore, they often need to be extracted. The changes in the vertical position of all maxillary molars in relation to the palatal plane were statistically insignificant.

The above-mentioned findings following the use of the sectional jig assembly confirm the results of previous studies using similar noncompliance distalizing modalities, such as the Jones Jig,[23,30–32,34] the Distal Jet,[44] and Pendulum Appliance[45–48] (Table 20.1). In these studies, the samples consisted of patients with either unerupted or both erupted and unerupted second molars. The observed differences concerning the amount and type of molar distalization as well as the associated undesirable dentoalveolar side effects can be attributed to the different approaches and different treatment times used, as well as to the presence or absence of the second maxillary molars. However, the influence of the second molars on the distal movement of the first molars remains a matter of controversy.

It has been reported that the presence of second molars increases treatment time,[20,25] produces more tipping,[42] and more anchorage loss,[49] and that tipping of the second molar is greater when a third molar bud is present.[49] Germectomy of wisdom teeth has been recommended in order to achieve bodily distalization of both molars.[49] On the other hand, some authors have reported that the presence and position of second molars do not influence the amount and type of maxillary first molar distalization.[46,47,50]

Anchorage Loss

The anchorage unit was unable to completely resist the reciprocal mesial forces of the activated coil springs. Loss of anchorage was demonstrated mainly by mesial movement and tipping of the second premolars, and by proclination of central incisors.

According to the findings of the first study, the second premolars were moved mesially by a mean 2.6 mm and tipped by a mean 8.1°

without significant extrusion, while the maxillary central incisors were proclined by a mean 4.8°.[40] These results were similar to the findings of the second study,[41] which revealed that anchorage loss was manifested as mesial movement (3.3 mm), mesial tipping (7.5°), buccal displacement (0.7 mm) and slight mesial rotation of the second premolars (3.7 mm), as well as proclination of the maxillary central incisors (5.2°).

The mean increase in overjet was 0.9 mm and the mean decrease in overbite 1.0 mm. Taking the latter into consideration, it could be suggested that treatment with the sectional jig assembly should be avoided in cases with an extreme vertical growth pattern and the presence of or a tendency towards an anterior open bite.

The above findings were similar to those reported in earlier studies using closely related noncompliance distalization appliances. Runge et al reported 2.2 mm mesial movement, 9.5° tipping, and 3.8 mm extrusion of the second premolars, while the overjet increased by 1.53 mm.[30] Gulati et al reported 1.0 mm forward movement of the maxillary first premolar and an increase of 1.1 mm in overjet.[32] Haydar & Uner investigated the dentoalveolar and skeletal effects of the Jones Jig Appliance and compared them with the effects of extraoral cervical traction in patients in mixed dentition with unerupted second molars.[34] They concluded that the molars were distalized effectively by both treatment methods, but the main difference was the anchorage loss occurring in the Jones Jig treatment group. Brickman et al,[31] also using the Jones Jig Appliance, found that 45% of the space created between the molar and premolar was due to mesial premolar movement, an amount similar to that reported by Ghosh & Nanda[45] when evaluating the Pendulum Appliance. A comparable amount of anchorage loss was also reported in further studies using analogous noncompliance distalization approaches (Table 20.1).[46,47,51,52]

Table 20.1. Comparison of dentoalveolar changes induced by similar minimal-compliance distalization appliances.

Report	Appliance	First molar crown distalization (mm)	Molar tipping (degrees)	Anchorage loss (mm)	Premolar tipping (degrees)	Presence of second molars
Gulati et al (1998)[32]	Jones Jig	2.7	3.5	1.1	2.6	Yes
Runge et al (1999)[30]	Jones Jig	2.2	4.0	2.2	9.5	NA
Haydar & Uner (2000)[34]	Jones Jig	2.8	7.8	1.8	3.4	No
Brickman et al (2000)[31]	Jones Jig	2.5	7.5	2.0	4.8	In 44 of 72 cases
Bolla et al (2002)[44]	Distal Jet	3.2	3.1	1.3	2.8	In 6 of 20 cases
Ghosh & Nanda (1996)[45]	Pendulum	3.4	8.4	2.5	1.3	In 18 of 41 cases
Byloff & Darendeliler (1997)[46]	Pendulum	3.4	14.5	1.6	NA	In 4 of 13 cases
Bussick & McNamara (2000)[47]	Pendulum	5.7	10.6	1.8	1.5	In 57 of 101 cases
Bondemark et al (1994)[42]	NiTi coils	3.2	1.0	1.9	NA	Yes
	Magnets	2.2				
Papadopoulos et al (2004)[40]	Sectional Jig Assembly	1.4	6.8	2.6	8.1	Yes
Mavropoulos et al (2005)[41]	Sectional Jig Assembly	2.8	6.8	3.3	7.5	Yes

(NA: no data available)

However, it should be noted that there is marked interindividual variation in patient response. In three patients in our first study, the anchorage loss was found to be 0–0.5 mm, while in another three it was more than 4 mm.[40] This can be attributed, at least partially, to the anatomic characteristics of the palatal vault. Therefore, patients with insufficient seating of the Nance button due to reduced palatal vault inclination might not be suitable candidates for noncompliance maxillary molar distalization with this appliance. Further, the absence or irregularity of contact points between spaced or severely malaligned teeth probably diminished the capacity of the anchorage unit to resist forward movement.

The most interesting finding of the 3D superimposition analysis on dental casts was the asymmetric effect of the appliance on the second premolars and canines between right and left side, which amounted to more than 1.5 mm.[41] This observation could be attributed to the different states of leveling and alignment between the two sides of the dental arch. Individual variations and asymmetric effects were also apparent in the case of the anterior teeth, with the midline off to either direction almost 1 mm on average.

Skeletal and Soft Tissue Changes

According to the results of our first study, the sectional jig assembly mainly affects the maxillary dentition, with less marked effects on the craniofacial skeleton and the soft tissues.[40] With regard to skeletal changes concerning the maxilla, the SNA angle showed no statistically significant difference before and after treatment with the distalization appliance, confirming previous findings using similar noncompliance methods with nickel-titanium coil springs.[31,32,34] However, the distance from A point to PtV plane (A point–PtV) was significantly increased by a mean 1.4 mm.

On the other hand, the SNB angle showed a statistically significant increase during the same period, most probably due to mandibular growth. For this reason it is relevant to consider that the correction to a Class I molar relationship resulted not only from the distal movement of the upper first molars but also from the mesial repositioning of the lower first molars as the mandible grew forward. However, growth and development also result in a downward and forward movement of the maxilla, along with which the maxillary molars are carried forward, increasing their distance from the PtV.[53] In this respect, the distalizing effect of the appliance is probably slightly underestimated by measuring the various distances from the pterygoid vertical, since these distances increase with growth. For the same reason, the anchorage loss is probably somewhat overestimated when measured with the PtV as reference.

No significant changes were observed in lower anterior facial height (ANS–menton) and in the inclination of the palatal, mandibular, and functional occlusal planes in relation to the anterior cranial base (SN).

Finally, evaluation of the soft tissue changes revealed that the upper lip protruded by a mean of 0.7 mm relative to the esthetic line; this was, however, not statistically significant. This tendency can be explained by the proclination of the maxillary incisors and the forward movement of A point. Surprisingly, the lower lip also protruded by a mean 1.3 mm, probably as a consequence of mandibular growth.

Conclusion

Noncompliance approaches are an important option for the orthodontic treatment of patients with Class II malocclusion who present minimal or no cooperation, especially when nonextraction treatment protocols have to be utilized. Open coil springs usually constitute an integral part of most of these noncompliance appliances, delivering the appropriate force in order to distalize maxillary molars.

According to our findings, it can be concluded that the sectional jig assembly could be an efficient option for the correction of Class II molar relationship by distalizing first and second maxillary molars simultaneously, requiring minimal patient cooperation, since a bilateral Class I molar relationship was achieved in all cases. A Class I molar relationship was established in a mean treatment period of 16.5–17.5 weeks although second maxillary molars were present in all cases. However, distal movement of the first molar crown accounted only for 46% of the total space created on each side. The effects of the appliance were limited primarily to the dentoalveolar structures. In addition, a substantial variation among patients and an asymmetric mesiodistal effect were also observed.

However, although the appliance can produce rapid simultaneous distalization of maxillary first and second molars, it presents some disadvantages such as anchorage loss in the anterior segment (in terms of incisor proclination or increased overjet) and distal tipping of the molars, which can be observed in selected cases. Therefore, the mesial movement and slight protrusion of the anchorage unit during intraoral distalization have to be taken seriously into consideration before applying this treatment approach.

The use of this noncompliance distalization appliance also includes some contraindications. These may take into consideration the crowding or spacing condition of the maxillary dental arch and the growth pattern of the craniofacial complex, as well as the anatomic characteristics of the palatal vault. Significant crowding or spacing in the maxillary dental arch can lead to disproportionate anchorage loss. Thus, patients with an extreme vertical growth pattern and the presence of or a tendency towards an anterior open bite as well as those with insufficient seating of the Nance button due to reduced palatal vault inclination may be unsuitable candidates for simultaneous first and second maxillary molar distalization with this appliance.

For all these reasons, case selection is a very important factor for the success of treatment and is strongly recommended before performing simultaneous distalization of maxillary first and second molars with the sectional jig assembly.

References

1. Proffit WR. Contemporary orthodontics. St Louis, MI: Mosby; 2000.
2. Rakosi T. Funktionelle Therapie in der Kieferorthopädie. Munich: Carl Hanser Verlag; 1985.
3. Papadopoulos MA. Kieferorthopädische-therapeutische Beeinflussbarkeit der Wachstums-Vorgänge des Ober- und Unterkiefers bei skelettalen Anomalien der Klasse II. Doctorate degree thesis. Freiburg: University of Freiburg; 1988.
4. Papadopoulos MA, Rakosi T. Results of a comparative study of skeletal class II cases after activator, headgear and combined headgear-activator treatment. Hell Stomatol Annals 1990;34:87–96.
5. Holland GN, Wallace DA, Mondino BJ, Cole SH, Ryan SJ. Severe ocular injuries from orthodontic headgear. Arch Ophthalmol 1985;103:649–651.
6. Holland GN, Wallace DA, Mondino BJ, Cole SH, Ryan SJ. Severe ocular injuries from headgear. Am J Orthod 1986;89:173.
7. Booth-Mason S, Birnie D. Penetrating eye injury from orthodontic headgear – a case report. Eur J Orthod 1988;102:111–114.
8. Postlethwaite K. The range of effectiveness of safety headgear products. Eur J Orthod 1989;11:228–234.
9. Samuels RHA. A review of orthodontic facebow injuries and safety equipment. Am J Orthod Dentofacial Orthop 1996;110:269–272.
10. Samuels RH, Evans SM, Wigglesworth SW. Safety catch for a Kloehn facebow. J Clin Orthod 1993;27:138–141.
11. Samuels RH, Willner F, Knox J, Jones ML. A national survey of orthodontic facebow injuries in the UK and Eire. Br J Orthod 1996;23:11–20.
12. Samuels RH, Jones ML. Orthodontic facebow injuries and safety equipment. Eur J Orthod 1994;16:385–394.
13. Samuels RH, Brezniak N. Orthodontic facebows: safety issues and current management. J Orthod 2002;29:101–107.
14. Berg KK. Komplikationen bei Anwendung von Zervikalem Nackenzug. Inf Orthod Kieferorthop 1974;1:39–44.
15. Rebholz K, Rakosi T. Extraorale Kräfte und die Wirbelsäule. Fortschr Kieferorthop 1977;38:324–331.
16. Baumrind S, Korn EL, Isaacson RJ, West EE, Molthen R. Quantitative analysis of the orthodontic and orthopedic effects of maxillary traction. Am J Orthod 1983;84:284–298.
17. Firouz M, Zernik J, Nanda R. Dental and orthopedic effects of high-pull headgear in treatment of Class II, Division I malocclusion. Am J Orthod Dentofacial Orthop 1992;102:197–205.
18. Hilgers JJ. The pendulum appliance for Class II noncompliance therapy. J Clin Orthod 1992;26:706–714.
19. Carano A, Testa M. The distal jet for upper molar distalization. J Clin Orthod 1996;30:374–380.
20. Gianelly AA, Vaitas AS, Thomas WM. The use of magnets to move molars distally. Am J Orthod Dentofacial Orthop 1989;96:161–167.
21. Papadopoulos MA. Clinical applications of magnets in orthodontics. Hell Orthod Rev 1999;1:31–42.
22. Papadopoulos MA. A study of the biomechanical characteristics of magnetic force systems used in orthodontics. Hell Orthod Rev 1999;2:89–97.
23. Jones RD, White MJ. Rapid Class II molar correction with an open-coil jig. J Clin Orthod 1992;26:661–664.
24. Baccetti T, Franchi L. A new appliance for molar distalization. Leone Boll Int 2000;2:3–7.
25. Gianelly AA, Bednar J, Dietz VS. Japanese NiTi coils used to move molars distally. Am J Orthod Dentofacial Orthop 1991;99:564–566.
26. Puente M. Class II Correction with an edgewise-modified Nance appliance. J Clin Orthod 1997;31:178–182.
27. Reiner TJ. Modified Nance appliance for unilateral molar distalization. J Clin Orthod 1992;26:402–404.
28. Miura F, Mogi M, Ohura Y, Karibe M. The super-elastic Japanese NiTi alloy wire for use in orthodontics. Part III. Studies on the Japanese NiTi alloy coil springs. Am J Orthod Dentofacial Orthop 1988;94:89–96.
29. Bourauel C, Drescher D, Ebling J, Broome D, Kanarachos A. Superelastic nickel titanium alloy retraction springs: an experimental investigation of force systems. Eur J Orthod 1997;19:491–500.
30. Runge ME, Martin JT, Bukai F. Analysis of rapid maxillary molar distal movement without patient cooperation. Am J Orthod Dentofacial Orthop 1999;115:153–157.
31. Brickman CD, Sinha PK, Nanda RS. Evaluation of the Jones jig appliance for distal molar movement. Am J Orthod Dentofacial Orthop 2000;118:526–534.
32. Gulati S, Kharbanda OP, Parkash H. Dental and skeletal changes after intraoral molar distalization with sectional jig assembly. Am J Orthod Dentofacial Orthop 1998;114:319–327.
33. Paul LD, O'Brien KD, Mandall NA. Upper removable appliance or Jones jig for distalizing first molars? A randomized clinical trial. Orthod Craniofac Res 2002;5:238–242.
34. Haydar S, Uner O. Comparison of Jones jig molar distalization appliance with extraoral traction. Am J Orthod Dentofacial Orthop 2000;117:49–53.
35. Scott MW. Molar distalization: more ammunition for your operatory. Clin Impressions 1996;5:16–27.
36. Papadopoulos MA. Simultaneous distalization of maxillary first and second molars by means of superelastic NiTi coils. Hell Orthod Rev 1998;1:71–76.
37. Locatelli R, Bednar J, Dietz VS, Gianelly AA. Molar distalization with superelastic NiTi wire. J Clin Orthod 1992;26:277–279.

38. Papadopoulos M, Hoerler I, Gerber H, Rahn B, Rakosi T. [The effect of static magnetic fields on osteoblast activity: an in-vitro study.] Fortschr Kieferorthop 1992;53:218–222.

39. Papadopoulos MA. Biological aspects of the use of permanent magnets and static magnetic fields in orthodontics. Hell Orthod Rev 1998;1: 145–157.

40. Papadopoulos MA, Mavropoulos A, Karamouzos A. Cephalometric changes following simultaneous first and second maxillary molar distalization using a noncompliance intraoral appliance. J Orofac Orthop 2004;65:123–136.

41. Mavropoulos A, Karamouzos A, Kiliaridis S, Papadopoulos MA. Efficiency of noncompliance simultaneous first and second upper molar distalization: a 3D tooth movement analysis. Angle Orthod 2005;75:468–475.

42. Bondemark L, Kurol J, Bernhold M. Repelling magnets versus super-elastic nickel-titanium coils in simultaneous distal movement of maxillary first and second molars. Angle Orthod 1994;64:189–198.

43. Erverdi N, Koyuturk O, Kucukkeles N. Nickel-titanium coil springs and repelling magnets: a comparison of two different intra-oral molar distalization techniques. Br J Orthod 1997;24: 47–53.

44. Bolla E, Muratore F, Carano A, Bowman SJ. Evaluation of maxillary molar distalization with the distal jet: a comparison with other contemporary methods. Angle Orthod 2002;72:481–494.

45. Ghosh J, Nanda RS. Evaluation of an intraoral maxillary molar distalization technique. Am J Orthod Dentofacial Orthop 1996;110:639–646.

46. Byloff FK, Darendeliler MA. Distal molar movement using the pendulum appliance. Part 1: Clinical and radiological evaluation. Angle Orthod 1997;67:249–260.

47. Bussick TJ, McNamara JA Jr. Dentoalveolar and skeletal changes associated with the pendulum appliance. Am J Orthod Dentofacial Orthop 2000;117:333–343.

48. Toroglu MS, Uzel I, Cam OY, Hancioglu ZB. Cephalometric evaluation of the effects of pendulum appliance on various vertical growth patterns and of the changes during short-term stabilization. Clin Orthod Res 2001;4: 15–27.

49. Kinzinger GS, Fritz UB, Sander FG, Diedrich PR. Efficiency of a pendulum appliance for molar distalization related to second and third molar eruption stage. Am J Orthod Dentofacial Orthop 2004;125:8–23.

50. Muse DS, Fillman MJ, Emmerson WJ, Mitchell RD. Molar and incisor changes with Wilson rapid molar distalization. Am J Orthod Dentofacial Orthop 1993;104:556–565.

51. Bondemark L, Kurol J. Distalization of maxillary first and second molars simultaneously with repelling magnets. Eur J Orthod 1992;14: 264–272.

52. Gianelly AA. Distal movement of the maxillary molars. Am J Orthod Dentofacial Orthop 1998;114: 66–72.

53. Sinha P. Reply to "Letter to the Editor." Am J Orthod Dentofacial Orthop 2001;119:12A–13A.

CHAPTER 21

The use of magnets for maxillary molar distalization

Lars Bondemark

Introduction

One of the first practical uses of magnets in medicine was in about 1820 in Paris, when Abraham used magnets to retrieve iron splinters that had accidentally entered the eyes of needle sharpeners, blacksmiths, and other metal workers.[1] In dentistry, the use of magnets is quite recent. In 1960 Behrman[2] described the use of implanted magnets in the jaws to aid denture retention and the use of magnets for tooth movements was first described by Crefcoeur[3] and later on by Blechman & Smiley.[4]

During the 20th century, new magnetic materials were developed to meet the growing needs of power generation and telecommunications. Three notable material developments occurred during the 1960s: rare earth permanent magnets, chromium-cobalt-iron magnets and the high-induction grain-oriented soft magnetic silicon steels. In 1966, Hoffer and Strnat of the US Air Force Materials Laboratory reported on the extremely high magnetocrystalline anisotropy of rare earth cobalt and emphasized the potential of such components as permanent magnetic alloys. Thereafter, the development of rare earth magnets such as samarium-cobalt ($SmCo_5$, Sm_2Co_{17}) and neodymium-iron-boron ($Nd_2Fe_{14}B$) really took off.[5]

The exceptionally high maximum energy product values and high resistance to demagnetization of rare earth magnets permit their use in devices where small size and superior performance are desired. Moreover, through the use of rare earth magnets in automotive accessory motors, electronic wristwatches, earphones of portable radio and CD players, it has become possible to design these devices with an overall reduction in size and mass.

For orthodontic purposes, it is claimed that magnets and magnet forces provide predictable and high forces in either attraction or repulsion. In the literature, several studies in animals (Table 21.1) and humans (Table 21.2) have documented the reliability of using magnetic forces for different tooth movements. So far the most common use of magnets has been for distal molar movement of maxillary molars. In prosthetics, various types of paired magnets have been used to assemble multicomponent maxillofacial prostheses and obturators.[6–8] Furthermore, magnet-retained dentures have been

Table 21.1. Reported orthodontic treatment possibilities using magnetic forces in animals.

Treatment	Authors	Year	Material
Distal movement of cuspids	Blechman & Smiley	1978[4]	2 cats
Intrusion of posterior teeth with repelling magnets	Woods & Nanda	1988[45]	6 baboons
	Woods & Nanda	1991[46]	4 baboons
Repelling magnets for transverse expansion of the maxilla	Vardimon et al	1987[47]	4 monkeys
Attractive magnets in functional orthopedic appliances	Vardimon et al	1989[48]	13 monkeys
	Vardimon et al	1990[49]	6 monkeys
Attractive magnets for extrusion of impacted teeth	Vardimon et al	1991[50]	1 monkey
Attractive magnets for incisor root extrusion	Parlange & Sims	1993[51]	10 marmosets

Table 21.2. Reported orthodontic treatment possibilities using magnetic forces in humans.

Treatment	Authors	Year	Material
Intrusion of posterior teeth with repelling magnets in open bite cases	Crefcoeur	1953[3]	1
	Dellinger	1986[52]	3
	Kalra et al	1989[53]	10
	Kiliaridis et al	1990[54]	10
	Breunig & Rakosi	1992[55]	1
Attractive magnets for extrusion of impacted teeth	Sandler et al	1989[56]	1
	Sandler	1991[57]	2
	Vardimon et al	1991[50]	4
	Darendeliler & Friedli	1994[58]	1
	Cole et al	2003[59]	8
Intra- and intermaxillary forces with attractive and repelling magnets	Blechman	1985[60]	2
Attractive magnets in functional orthopedic appliances	Darendeliler & Joho	1993[61]	3
	Darendeliler et al	1993[62]	1
Molar distalization with repelling magnets	Gianelly et al	1989[14]	8
	Cozzani et al	1989[63]	1
	Cosentino & Amato	1990[64]	4
	Itoh et al	1991[15]	10
	Bondemark & Kurol	1992[13]	10
	Bondemark et al	1994[16]	18
	Steger & Blechman	1995[65]	2
	Bondemark	2000[22]	21
Repelling magnets for expansion of the maxilla	Darendeliler et al	1994[66]	6
Attractive magnets to close diastema or to achieve an ideal arch form	Muller	1984[67]	7
	Kawata et al	1987[68]	1
	Darendeliler & Joho	1992[69]	1
Attractive magnets for extrusion of crown–root fractured teeth	McCord & Harvie	1984[70]	1
	Bondemark et al	1997[71]	2
Attractive magnets for retention	Springate & Sandler	1991[72]	1

applied together with osseointegrated systems,[9,10] and attractive magnets have been used in splints for mandibular advancement in treatment of snoring and sleep apnea patients.[11]

Distal Movement of Maxillary Molars with Magnets

Design of the Intraarch Appliance

Usually, prefabricated repelling samarium-cobalt (SmCo) magnets are used in each quadrant of the maxilla and a Nance acrylic button provides anchorage (Fig. 21.1). The magnets (single size 4 × 5 × 2 mm) are encased in stainless steel without covering the pole faces and mounted so the mesial magnet is free to move along a sectional bar (1.5 × 0.5 × 22.0 mm) (Fig. 21.2). The buccally placed magnets are attached to the first maxillary molar band by a three-prong fork. The middle prong is sized for insertion into the headgear tube and

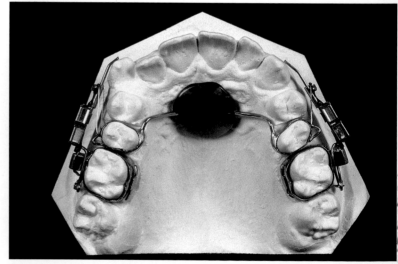

Figure 21.1 Occlusal view of the intraarch magnetic appliance.

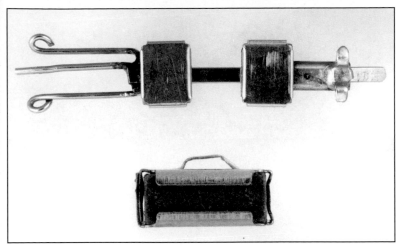

Figure 21.2 The two magnets are mounted on a section bar that ends distally with a three-prong fork for insertion into the headgear tube. A sliding yoke mesial to the magnets is used when the magnets are activated. Below: a single magnet that is removed from the bar. The magnet is encased in a stainless jacket without covering the pole face.

ligation around the two outer prongs secures the bar with magnets to the molar tube. The system is activated by a 0.25 mm ligature wire, ligated from a distobuccal vertical tube or an eyelet on the second premolar band to a sliding yoke mesial to the magnets (Figs 21.3 and 21.4).

When the repelling magnets are ligated together, two forces are produced, one distally directed to move the molars distally and one reciprocal mesially directed force. To provide anchorage against the reciprocal force, a Nance button is attached to a 0.9 mm lingual archwire which is usually soldered lingually to the second premolar band or, in the mixed dentition, to the second deciduous molar band (see Fig. 21.1). In patients with deep bite, the Nance button can be changed to a frontal acrylic bite plane extended to the palatal vault in order to produce bite opening and anchorage simultaneously.

Magnetic Force

Although high forces can be produced by even small magnets, the force diminishes to the square of the distance, which is characteristic for Coulomb's law of magnetic force ($F \sim 1/d^2$). Consequently, the magnetic forces are predominantly effective at pole face contact or

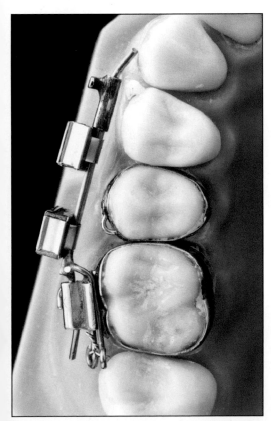

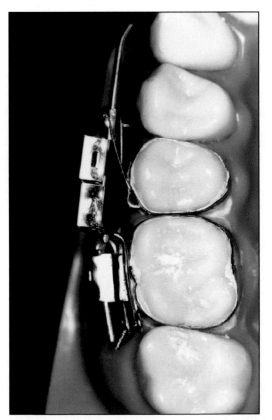

Figures 21.3, 21.4 Occlusal detail showing the buccally placed inactivated repelling magnets and the repelling magnets in maximal contact, i.e. maximal loading. The activation of the magnets is performed via a ligature wire ligated between a distobuccal eyelet on the second premolar and the sliding yoke mesial to the magnets.

Figure 21.4

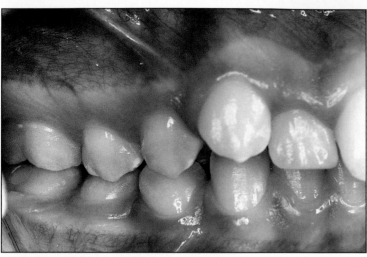

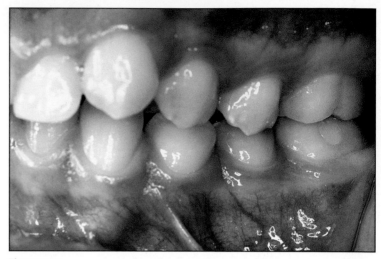

Figures 21.5, 21.6 A 13-year-old girl with Class II occlusion, first and second maxillary molars in occlusion and moderate space deficiency in the maxilla. Pretreatment.

Figure 21.6

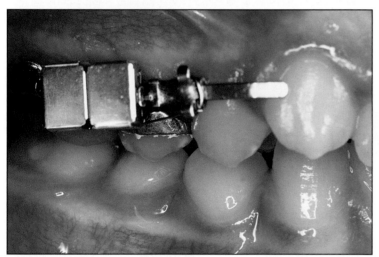

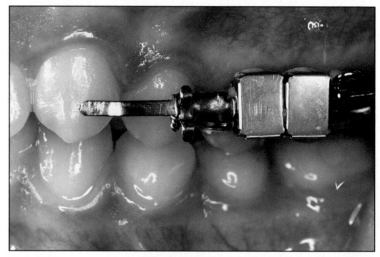

Figures 21.7, 21.8 With the magnets inserted.

Figure 21.8

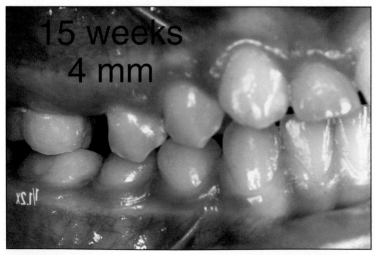

15 weeks
4 mm

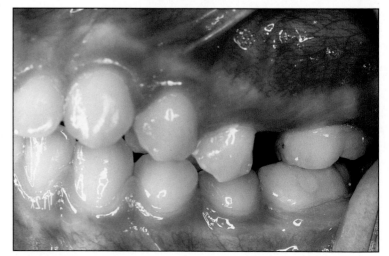

Figures 21.9, 21.10 A Class I molar relationship was achieved in 15 weeks with a molar movement of 4 mm. Note the anchorage loss, i.e. mesial movement of premolars and cuspids.

Figure 21.10

Table 21.3. Force variation with different pole face distances for repelling magnets.

Distance (mm)	Repelling force (cN)
0.25	215
0.5	170
1.0	115
2.0	60
3.0	30
4.0	20

with a short distance between them. A maximal force of approximately 225 g is provided when the magnets are ligated together[12] and as the pole face distance increases, the force rapidly decreases. This also means that after tooth movement, the forces will drop drastically.

In contrast to conventional mechanics, such as engaging an archwire in a bracket slot, where forces are usually difficult to estimate, the magnetic force level is easy to predict. Forces produced with different intermagnet distances are listed in Table 21.3. By means of the specific force–distance diagrams of the magnets, the force level can be calculated at any time by measuring the gap between the magnets and thus a proper force can be maintained throughout the treatment. It is recommended to reactivate and ligate the magnets in contact with each other every fourth week during the molar distalization period.[13] Since SmCo magnets possess extremely high resistance to demagnetization, the magnet forces, in contrast to other force systems, e.g. elastic or elastomeric elements, show no fatigue of force over time.[12]

The Efficiency of Magnets for Distal Molar Movement

Several studies have reported that maxillary molars, even in the presence of second maxillary molars, can be distalized with a movement rate of 0.75–1.0 mm per month.[13–16] Furthermore, the magnets are easy to insert and well tolerated and patient cooperation is not required during the treatment period. Using repelling magnets for simultaneous distal movement of maxillary first and second molars is illustrated in Figures 21.5–21.10. After the molar distalization, i.e. after a Class I molar relationship and sufficient space are achieved, the magnets and the Nance button are removed and the molars are held in place by a new Nance button attached to the first molars. In cases with a high risk of relapse, a transpalatal bar that unites the Nance button can be inserted. When the Nance button is removed, the palatal mucosa under the button often shows inflammation but this symptom usually disappears within a week.

After the first treatment phase is ended there is no need to immediately rush into the second phase with a multibracket appliance for retraction and alignment of the anterior teeth. Instead, it is advisable to wait for spontaneous distal movement of the maxillary bicuspids and cuspids (Figs 21.11 and 21.12).

Anchorage Loss

When intraarch appliances move the molars distally, the anterior teeth, premolars and the palatal vault via the Nance button are used for anchorage control. However, anchorage loss will still occur.[13,16–19] Due to the reciprocal mesially directed forces in the system, the anchorage loss results in forward movement of premolars, cuspids and incisors, and thus, increased overjet of 0.5–2 mm. To reduce the anchorage loss, the lightest force possible should be used and the Nance button has to be attached to the second instead of the first premolar. In the mixed dentition a stable deciduous second molar can be used but avoid the deciduous first molar since this tooth will provide poor anchorage.

In most instances, the problem of forward movement of the incisors can be controlled with modest intervention. Therefore, in order to correct or reverse the forward movement of the maxillary incisors, subsequent multibracket therapy with Class II elastics is recommended.[17,20] In a study by Bondemark & Kurol, it was shown that the forward movement of the maxillary incisors associated with the distal molar movement was totally reversed and eliminated by intermaxillary Class II elastics.[21] On the other hand, in cases with retroclined maxillary incisors, for example in patients with a Class II, division 2 malocclusion, the reciprocal effect of forces in an intraarch appliance can be utilized for proclination of the incisors.

Modification of the Appliance to Avoid Distal Molar Tipping

In the magnet force system, the main intention is to move the molars without a tipping movement. However, undesirable distal crown tipping is generally experienced, as with other force systems. Distal molar tipping of 7–14° has been reported during distal molar movement.[13,15,17–20] This means that nearly one-half of the distal molar movement can be related to tipping and so there is an obvious risk of relapse of the achieved molar distalization.

One way to overcome the problem of distal tipping is to over-correct the molars. However, even when a molar is overcorrected, a subsequent supplemental force system has to be used to provide a moment that uprights the molar root which leads to a significant risk of anchorage loss during the uprighting procedure.

To avoid undesirable distal crown tipping, a modified appliance has been introduced. The appliance consists of maxillary first molar and second premolar bands on the right and left sides. Lingually on the molar band, a tube, 1.1 mm in diameter and approximately 10 mm in length, is soldered (Figs 21.13 and 21.14). A 0.9 mm lingual archwire, which unites a Nance button or a fixed frontal acrylic bite plane, is soldered lingually to the second premolar band. The lingual archwire is provided with two distal pistons that pass bilaterally through the palatal tubes of the maxillary molar bands (see Figs 21.13 and 21.14). The tubes and pistons must be parallel in both the occlusal and sagittal views. Thus, the lingual arrangement of tubes and pistons permits bodily movement of the maxillary molars.

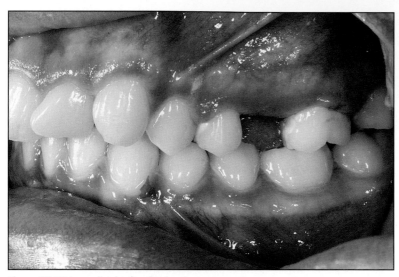

Figure 21.11 Immediately after distal molar movement.

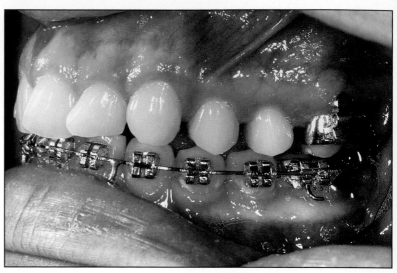

Figure 21.12 Four months later, when the stretched supracrestal fibers have moved the cuspids and premolars distally.

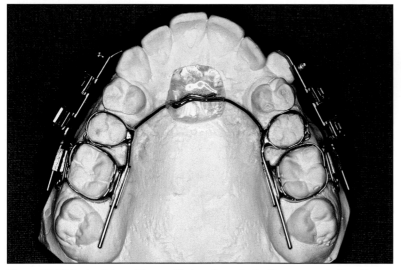

Figure 21.13 Occlusal view of the modified appliance for bodily movement of maxillary molars.

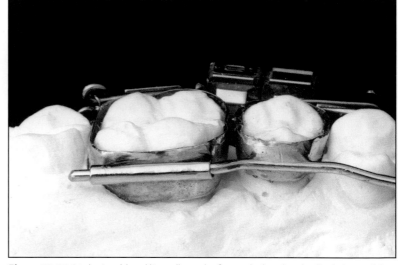

Figure 21.14 A tube is soldered lingually on the first molar band and a distal piston of the lingual archwire passes through the tube. When the buccally placed repelling magnets are activated, the molar will slide along the piston without distal tipping.

The repelling magnets are attached to the headgear tube of the first maxillary molar band and activated as usual. This modified appliance has proven to produce distal molar movement with minimal tipping (0–4°) and acceptable anchorage loss.[16,22] A patient treated with the modified appliance is illustrated in Figures 21.15–21.23.

Biologic Safety of the Magnet System

Dental materials and appliances often contain potentially toxic elements that may release harmful products, which can produce side effects at a local or systemic level. A complete biologic evaluation must include three levels of testing:[23]

- level 1: in vitro testing in order to establish the toxic, allergic or carcinogenic nature of the material
- level 2: in-use testing on animals
- level 3: clinical trials.

Corrosion and Cytotoxicity of Magnetic Material

A number of analyses have been performed to evaluate the biologic effects of the corrosion products of rare earth magnets. From these

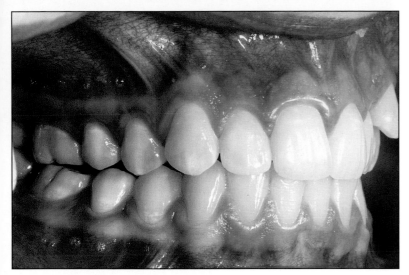

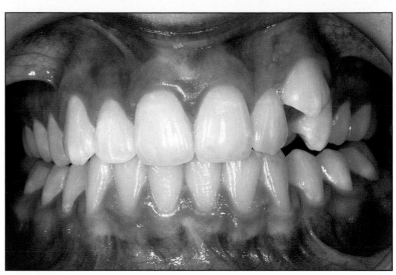

Figures 21.15–21.17 Pretreatment intraoral views of a 13.5-year-old girl. The molar relationship was Class II, midline shift to the left and space deficiency for the left cuspid. Both first and second maxillary molars were in occlusion.

Figure 21.16

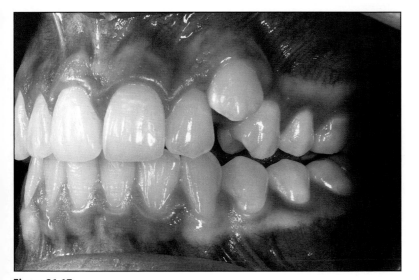

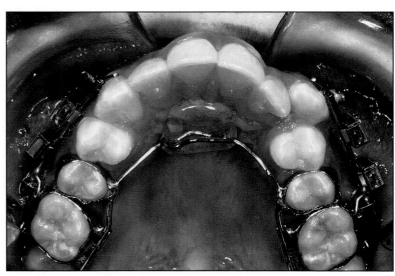

Figure 21.17

Figure 21.18 The modified magnetic appliance inserted.

studies, it can be concluded that the corrosion resistance of neodymium-iron-boron magnets is low,[24] while samarium-cobalt magnets corrode but their corrosion resistance is similar to that of normal dental casting alloys (Fig. 21.24).[25] Moreover, it has been demonstrated that uncoated samarium-cobalt magnets exhibit moderate cytotoxicity while uncoated neodymium-iron-boron magnets show low or negligible cytotoxicity.[26] The high content of cobalt is the main reason for the cytotoxicity.[27] However, if samarium-cobalt magnets are coated, the cytotoxicity is negligible.[26]

Although the cytotoxic effects of rare earth magnets can be considered moderate at worst, it is of paramount importance to prevent cytotoxicity and corrosion from occurring since corrosion in particular leads to substance loss and disturbs the physical properties of the magnets. Consequently, it is advisable before clinical use to seal or encase the magnets with an impervious and robust biocompatible material, e.g. stainless steel or titanium.

Effects of the Magnetic Field on Tissues and Cells

The use of rare earth magnets in medicine and dentistry has increased research interest in the biologic effects of magnets and magnetic fields. Numerous experimental in vitro studies, results of in-use testing on

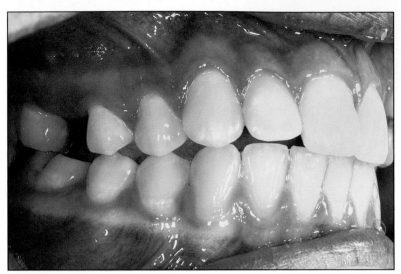

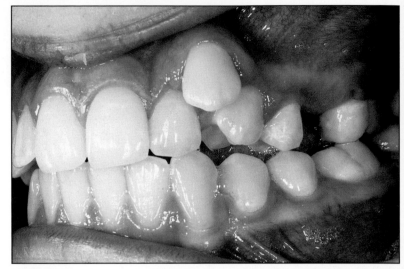

Figures 21.19, 21.20 After 14 weeks the distal molar movement was completed, i.e. when a Class I molar relation and bilateral distal molar movements of 3 mm have been achieved. In this patient, 12 months of subsequent straight-wire appliance wear in the maxilla was required to retract and align the anterior teeth after the distal molar movement.

Figure 21.20

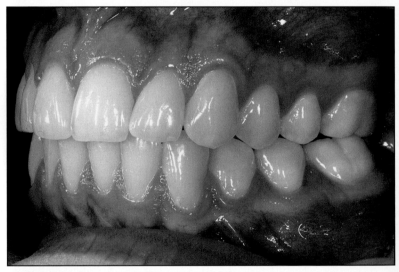

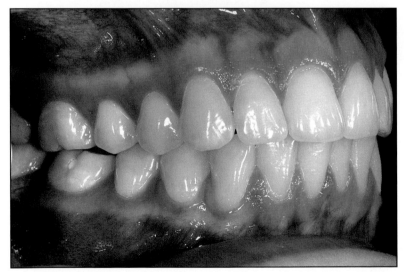

Figure 21.22

Figures 21.21–21.23 The 2-year posttreatment result.

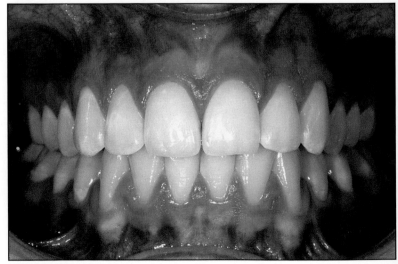

Figure 21.23

animals, and clinical studies in humans have been published. It must be remembered that magnetism is a physical phenomenon and that magnetic fields are part of the electromagnetic spectrum, existing in the vicinity of a magnetic body or formed around a conductor carrying a current. In principle, magnetic fields can be divided into static and time-varying fields and since permanent magnets are used in orthodontics, the static magnetic fields attract special interest. The static type of magnetic field is usually schematically reproduced and characterized by "lines." The magnetic field or, as more correctly designated, the magnetic flux density (B) is the magnetic

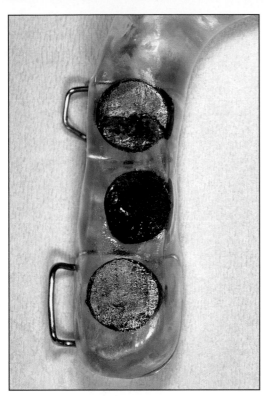

Figure 21.24 Wear and corrosion of two samarium-cobalt magnets and one neodymium-iron-boron magnet. The severely corroded and tarnished neodymium-iron-boron magnet between the two samarium-cobalt magnets. The magnets have been encased in an acrylic splint used for mandibular advancement of a patient treated for snoring and sleep apnea. Apparently the acrylic cover of the magnets was not sufficiently robust.

flux per unit area and can be measured by a Hall probe. The units of the flux density are Vs/m^2, Wb/m^2, tesla (T) or gauss (G), where $1 Vs/m^2 = 1 Wb/m^2 = 1T = 10\ 000$ G. In medical literature, gauss and tesla are frequently used as magnetic flux units.

It must be recognized that during normal daily life there are several sources of static magnetic energy. We are surrounded by a natural static magnetic field that varies from ~30 to 70 μT depending on the geographic location.[28] Under high direct current (DC) transmission lines, static magnetic fields of about 20 μT are produced and with new means of transportation, such as fast passenger trains based on magnetic levitation, flux densities of 10–100 mT can be generated. High-energy technologies using thermonuclear reactors also produce strong fields. The highest exposure for members of the general public occurs in patients undergoing diagnostic examination by magnetic resonance imaging (MRI). In the MRI device, the patient is exposed to stationary magnetic fields with flux densities between 0.5 and 2 T during examinations ranging from 15 minutes to 1 hour.[28] In medical or dental applications, such as devices holding various prostheses in place, colonic stoma, magnet-retained dentures and magnet-containing orthodontic appliances, local-body exposures up to 250 mT can occur.[29–31] Moreover, it has been shown that outside a sphere with a radius of up to 60 mm, the flux density of an orthodontic magnet is at the level of the natural

magnetic earth field.[31] Consequently, it can be concluded that the magnetic field exposure of surrounding tissues is low and limited when magnets are used for medical and dental purposes.

Theoretically, static magnetic fields can interact with living matter by electrodynamic interaction (moving electrolytes) and through magnetomechanical effects (rotation and torque of molecules). Furthermore, the field can influence the movement of dissolved oxygen, the orientation of cell membrane anisotropic phospholipids, and enzyme activity.[32–34] The breadth of static magnetic field studies on biologic phenomena has been considerable. It includes in vitro studies on cells and embryos, on DNA and DNA synthesis, effects on the movements of ions, changes in orientation of macromolecules, enzyme alterations, influence on microorganisms, effects on the nervous system, and in vivo experiments with laboratory animals evaluating developmental, behavioral, and physiologic parameters.

Most of the claimed biologic effects of static magnetic fields are the result of exposure to a particular magnetic flux value, field direction and duration, unique to that research team. Often the experiments are inconsistent because the field parameters are not always identical from experiment to experiment. The lack of robustness of experiments and their resultant inability to be readily transferable between laboratories has been a major stumbling block to the advancement of research in this area. However, available consistent knowledge indicates an absence of significant effects on developmental, behavioral, and physiologic parameters at static magnetic flux densities up to 2 T. Furthermore, there are negligible risks of harmful biologic effects of local exposure to static magnetic fields up to 300 mT.[32,34] When magnet-containing orthodontic appliances are used, local exposure up to 250 mT occurs,[31] which suggests low or negligible risks of harmful biologic effects. In particular, in one clinical, histologic, and immunohistochemical study no adverse long-term effects were found on human buccal mucosa which had been in contact with an acrylic-coated neodymium-iron-boron magnet and subjected to a static field.[35]

Beneficial Effects for Orthodontic Tooth Movement

Interdisciplinary research has tried to elucidate whether a beneficial synergistic effect exists between force application and static magnetic field during use of magnets for orthodontic tooth movement. Indirect evidence has demonstrated that certain static or time-varying fields enhance bone remodeling and accelerate cellular reactions in the periodontal ligament.[36–38] However, other studies have not found an association between static magnetic fields and bone remodeling or enhanced tooth movement.[33,39,40]

A general assumption in studies with magnetic fields may be that stronger fields have greater effects on biologic specimens, similar to assuming that higher doses of drugs exert more pronounced effects on cells and tissues. In fact, experimental results show that certain intermediate magnetic fields or flux densities are apparently more effective in altering development than either higher or lower fields.[41] Such unique combinations have been called "windows of sensitivity".[37,42] Thus, future biomagnetic research may perhaps determine whether beneficial synergistic effects exist between force application and static magnetic fields during use of magnets for orthodontic tooth movement.

Advantages and Disadvantages of Magnets

Advantages

- The repelling magnets give a rapid result in terms of distal molar movement.

- The magnet system affords a precise control over the forces by means of the specific force–distance diagrams and the force level can easily be calculated at any time by measuring the distance between the magnets.

- The properties of the magnets are such that they have constant power over time, which means that, in contrast to other force systems, e.g. elastics or elastomeric elements, there will be no risk of fatigue of forces over relevant clinical time.

- The magnetic forces and magnetic field can be exerted through mucosa and bone, which means that it is possible that orthodontic tooth movements may be increased by accelerated cellular reactions in the periodontal ligament and/or enhanced bone remodeling.

Disadvantages

- The magnet system requires frequent activation appointments, at least every third week, since the force drops dramatically with increased distance between the magnets.

- It is also well known that the magnets easily corrode which leads to substance loss and disturbed physical properties. To retain good physical properties, the magnets have to be encased in a robust biocompatible material to protect them clinically from corrosive assault.

- The magnets are expensive due to complicated fabrication processes. First, the material is reduced to a powder of suitable particle size and then it must be aligned by a strong magnetic field so that the easy axes of all the particles are made parallel. When magnetized, it must be compacted into dense form, which can be accomplished either by mechanical pressure or by a sintering process.

- The magnets are brittle, particularly the samarium-cobalt magnets, and suffer irreversible magnetic loss if heated. If the magnets are heated to even modest temperatures, above 60–70°, there is a significant and irreversible loss in flux or force.[43]

- Evidence exists to suggest that magnets for distal molar movement offer no advantages over other approaches such as, for example, intraarch appliances that use superelastic coils as a force system.[16,22,44]

References

1. Macklis RM. Magnetic healing, quackery, and the debate about the health effects of electromagnetic fields. Ann Int Med 1993;118:376–383.

2. Behrman SJ. The implantation of magnets in the jaw to aid denture retention. J Prosthetic Dent 1960;10:807–841.

3. Crefcoeur JM. Ferro-magnetisme als kaak orthopaedisch hulpmiddel. Ned Tijdschr Tandh 1953;60:1–2.

4. Blechman AM, Smiley H. Magnetic force in orthodontics. Am J Orthod 1978;74:435–443.

5. Chin GY. New magnetic alloys. Science 1980;208:888–894.

6. Javid N. The use of magnets in a maxillofacial prosthesis. J Prosthet Dent 1971;25:334–341.

7. Federick DR. A magnetically retained interim maxillary obturator. J Prosthet Dent 1976;36:671–675.

8. Gillings BRD. Magnetic retention for complete and partial over dentures. Part I. J Prosthet Dent 1981;45:484–491.

9. Sendax VI. Magnetic retention systems for implant prosthodontics. J Oral Implantol 1987;13:128–155.

10. Walmsley AD, Brady CL, Smith PL, Frame JW. Magnet retained overdentures using the Astra dental implant system. Br Dent J 1993;174:399–404.

11. Bernhold M, Bondemark L. A magnetic appliance for treatment of snoring patients with and without obstructive sleep apnea. Am J Orthod Dentofacial Orthop 1998;113:144–155.

12. Bondemark L, Kurol J. Force-distance relation and properties of repelling Sm-Co magnets in orthodontic clinical use: an experimental model. Scand J Dent Res 1992;100:228–231.

13. Bondemark L, Kurol J. Distalization of maxillary first and second molars simultaneously with repelling magnets. Eur J Orthod 1992;14:264–272.

14. Gianelly AA, Vaitas AS, Thomas WM. The use of magnets to move molars distally. Am J Orthod Dentofacial Orthop 1989;96:161–167.

15. Itoh T, Tokuda T, Kiyosue S, Hirose T, Matsumoto M, Chaconas S. Molar distalization with repelling magnets. J Clin Orthod 1991;25:611–617.

16. Bondemark L, Kurol J, Bernhold M. Repelling magnets versus superelastic nickel-titanium coils in simultaneous distal movement of maxillary first and second molars. Angle Orthod 1994;64:189–198.

17. Muse DS, Fillman MJ, Emmerson WJ, Mitchell RD. Molar and incisor changes with Wilson rapid molar distalization. Am J Orthod Dentofacial Orthop 1993;104:556–565.

18. Ghosh J, Nanda RS. Evaluation of an intraoral maxillary molar distalization technique. Am J Orthod Dentofacial Orthop 1996;110:639–646.

19. Byloff FK, Darendeliler MA. Distal molar movement using the pendulum appliance. Part 1: Clinical and radiological evaluation. Angle Orthod 1997;67:249–260.

20. Gianelly AA. Distal movement of the maxillary molars. Am J Orthod Dentofacial Orthop 1998;114:66–72.

21. Bondemark L, Kurol J. Class II correction with magnets and superelastic coils followed by straight-wire mechanotherapy. Occlusal changes during and after dental therapy. J Orofac Orthop 1998;59:127–138.

22. Bondemark L. A comparative analysis of distal maxillary molar movement produced by a new lingual intraarch Ni-Ti coil appliance and a magnetic appliance. Eur J Orthod 2000;22:683–695.

23. Bondemark L. Orthodontic magnets. A study of force and field pattern, biocompatibility and clinical effects. Thesis Odont Dr. Sw Dent J Suppl 1994;99:1–148.

24. Wilson M, Patel H, Kpendema M, Noar JH, Hunt NP, Mordan NJ. Corrosion of intra-oral magnets by multi-species biofilms in the presence and absence of sucrose. Biomaterials 1997;18:53–57.

25. Tsutsui H, Kinouchi Y, Sasaki H, Shiota M, Ushita T. Studies on the Sm-Co magnet as a dental material. J Dent Res 1979;58:1597–1606.

26. Bondemark L, Kurol J, Wennberg A. Orthodontic rare earth magnets – in vitro assessment of cytotoxicity. Br J Orthod 1994;21:335–341.

27. Mjör IA, Christensen GJ. Assessment of local side effects of casting alloys. Quintessence Int 1993;24: 343–351.

28. United Nations Environment Programme/World Health Organization/International Radiation Protection Association (UNEP/WHO/IRPA). Environmental Health Criteria No 69. Magnetic Fields. Geneva: UNEP; 1987.

29. Hennig G, Feustel H, Hennig K. Rare earth-cobalt magnets in modern medicine. Goldschmidt Informiert 1975;4:85–90.

30. Esformes I, Kummer F, Livelli T. Biologic effects of magnetic fields generated with CoSm magnets. Bull Hosp Jt Dis Orthop Inst 1981;41:81–87.

31. Bondemark L, Kurol J, Wisten Å. Extent and flux density of static magnetic fields generated by orthodontic samarium-cobalt magnets. Am J Orthod Dentofacial Orthop 1995;107:488–496.

32. Tenforde TS. Biologic effects of stationary magnetic fields. In: Grandolfo M, Michaelson SM, Rindi A, eds. Biologic effects and dosimetry of static and ELF electromagnetic fields. New York: Plenum Press; 1985: 93–127.

33. Camilleri S, McDonald F. Static magnetic field effects on the sagittal suture in Rattus Norvegicus. Am J Orthod Dentofacial Orthop 1993;103:240–246.

34. International Commision on Non-Ionizing Radiation Protection (ICNIRP). Guidelines on limits of exposure to static magnetic fields. Health Physics 1994;66:100–106.

35. Bondemark L, Kurol J, Larsson Å. Long-term effects of orthodontic magnets on human buccal mucosa – a clinical and immunohistochemical study. Eur J Orthod 1998;20:211–218.

36. Stark TM, Sinclair PM. Effects of pulsed electromagnetic fields on orthodontic tooth movement. Am J Orthod Dentofacial Orthop 1987;91:91–104.

37. Blechman AM, Steger E. A possible mechanism of action of repelling, molar distalizing magnets. Part I. Am J Orthod Dentofacial Orthop 1995;108: 428–431.

38. Darendeliler MA, Sinclair PM, Kusy RP. The effects of samarium cobalt and pulsed electromagnetic fields on tooth movement. Am J Orthod Dentofacial Orthop 1995;107:578–587.

39. Papadopoulos MA, Hörler I, Gerber H, Rahn BA, Rakosi T. Einfluss statischer magnetischer Felder auf die Aktivität von Osteoblasten: eine In-vitro-Untersuchung. Fortschr Kieferorthop 1992;53: 212–222.

40. Tengku BS, Joseph BK, Harbrow D, Taverne AAR, Symons AL. Effect of a static magnetic field on orthodontics tooth movement in the rat. Eur J Orthod 2000;22:475–487.

41. Koch W, Koch B, Martin A, Moses G. Examination of the development of chicken embryos following exposure to magnetic fields. Comp Biochem Physiol 1993;105A:617–624.

42. Morgan MG, Nair I. Alternative functional relationships between ELF field exposure and possible health effects: report on an expert workshop. Bioelectromag 1992;13:335–350.

43. Noar JH, Evans RD. Rare earth magnets in orthodontics: an overview. Br J Orthod 1999;26:29–37.

44. Erverdi N, Koyuturk O, Kucukkeles N. Nickel-titanium coil springs and repelling magnets: a comparison of two different intra-oral molar distalization techniques. Br J Orthod 1997;24: 47–53.

45. Woods MG, Nanda RS. Intrusion of posterior teeth with magnets. An experiment in growing baboons. Angle Orthod 1988;58:136–150.

46. Woods MG, Nanda RS. Intrusion of posterior teeth with magnets: an experiment in nongrowing baboons. Am J Orthod Dentofacial Orthop 1991;100:393–400.

47. Vardimon AD, Graber TM, Voss LR, Verrusio E. Magnetic versus mechanical expansion with different force thresholds and points of force application. Am J Orthod Dentofacial Orthop 1987;92:455–466.

48. Vardimon AD, Stutzmann JJ, Graber TM, Voss LR, Petrovic AG. Functional orthopedic magnetic appliance (FOMA) II – modus operandi. Am J Orthod Dentofacial Orthop 1989;95:371–387.

49. Vardimon AD, Graber TM, Voss LR, Muller TP. Functional orthopedic magnetic appliance (FOMA) III – modus operandi. Am J Orthod Dentofacial Orthop 1990;97:135–148.

50. Vardimon AD, Graber TM, Drescher D, Bourauel C. Rare earth magnets and impaction. Am J Orthod Dentofacial Orthop 1991;100:494–512.

51. Parlange LM, Sims MR. A T.E.M. stereological analysis of blood vessels and nerves in marmoset periodontal ligament following endodontics and magnetic incisor extrusion. Eur J Orthod 1993;15: 33–44.

52. Dellinger EL. A clinical assessment of the active vertical corrector – a nonsurgical alternative for skeletal open bite treatment. Am J Orthod 1986; 89:428–436.

53. Kalra V, Burstone CJ, Nanda R. Effects of a fixed magnetic appliance on the dentofacial complex. Am J Orthod Dentofacial Orthop 1989;95: 467–478.

54. Kiliaridis S, Egermark I, Thilander B. Anterior open bite treatment with magnets. Eur J Orthod 1990;12:447–457.

55. Breunig A, Rakosi T. Die Behandlung des offenen Bisses mit Magneten. Fortschr Kieferorthop 1992;53:179–186.

56. Sandler PJ, Meghji S, Murray AM, et al. Magnets and orthodontics. Br J Orthod 1989;16:243–249.

57. Sandler PJ. An attractive solution to unerupted teeth. Am J Orthod Dentofacial Orthop 1991;100: 489–493.

58. Darendeliler MA, Friedli JM. Case report. Treatment of an impacted canine with magnets. J Clin Orthod 1994;28:639–643.

59. Cole BO, Shaw AJ, Hobson RS, et al. The role of magnets in the management of unerupted teeth in children and adolescents. Int J Paediatr Dent 2003; 13:204–207.

60. Blechman AM. Magnetic force systems in orthodontics. Clinical results of a pilot study. Am J Orthod 1985;87:201–210.

61. Darendeliler MA, Joho JP. Magnetic activator device II (MAD) for correction of Class II, division 1 malocclusions. Am J Orthod Dentofacial Orthop 1993;103:223–239.

62. Darendeliler MA, Chiarini M, Joho JP. Case report: early Class III treatment with magnet appliances. J Clin Orthod 1993;27:563–569.

63. Cozzani M, Thomas WM, Gianelly AA. Distalizzazione asimmetrica di molare superiore con magneti: caso clinico. Mondo Ortodontico 1989; 14:687–692.

64. Cosentino S, Amato S. La distalizzazione con forze magnetiche dei molari superiori. Attualita Dentale 1990;6:12–25.

65. Steger ER, Blechman AM. Case reports: molar distalization with static repelling magnets. Part II. Am J Orthod Dentofacial Orthop 1995;108: 547–555.

66. Darendeliler MA, Strahm C, Joho JP. Light maxillary expansion forces with the magnetic expansion device. A preliminary investigation. Eur J Orthod 1994;16: 479–490.

67. Muller M. The use of magnets in orthodontics: an alternative means to produce tooth movement. Eur J Orthod 1984;6:247–253.

68. Kawata Y, Hirota K, Sumitani K, et al. A new orthodontic force system of magnetic brackets. Am J Orthod Dentofacial Orthop 1987;92:241–248.

69. Darendeliler MA, Joho JP. Class II bimaxillary protrusion treated with magnetic forces. J Clin Orthod 1992;26:361–368.

70. McCord JF, Harvie H. An alternative treatment of anterior teeth fractured beneath the gingival margin. Br Dent J 1984;157:320–322.

71. Bondemark L, Kurol J, Hallonsten AL, Andreasen JO. Attractive magnets for orthodontic extrusion of crown-root fractured teeth. Am J Orthod Dentofacial Orthop 1997;112:187–193.

72. Springate SD, Sandler PJ. Micro-magnetic retainers: an attractive solution to fixed retention. Br J Orthod 1991;18:139–141.

CHAPTER 22

The First Class Appliance

Arturo Fortini, Lorenzo Franchi

Introduction

The use of the so-called "distalizing appliances" for the nonextraction treatment of Class II malocclusion has become increasingly popular during recent years. Most traditional techniques for molar distalization, such as extraoral traction,[1-3] the Cetlin removable plate,[4,5] and the Wilson arches,[6-8] have been used widely in the past as efficient nonextraction approaches in the treatment of Class II malocclusion. However, all these distalizing appliances partially or totally relied on patient cooperation, which could endanger treatment success and increase treatment duration.

More recently, the problems related to patient compliance have led many clinicians to prefer intraoral distalizing systems that minimize reliance on the patient and that are under the control of the orthodontist. Most of the intraoral distalizing systems that have been proposed in the literature consist of an anchorage unit (usually comprising premolars or deciduous molars and an acrylic Nance button) and a force-generating unit. Different types of active force components include repelling magnets,[9-13] coil springs on continuous archwires,[14,15] superelastic nickel titanium archwires,[16] coil springs on a sectional archwire (the Jones Jig),[17-21] Distal Jet,[22-25] Keles Slider,[26,27] Fast Back,[28] beta-titanium alloy springs (Pendulum),[29-35] Pendulum with distal screw,[36,37] K-loop,[38] and Intraoral Bodily Molar Distalizer.[39] Although these intraoral devices require minimal patient collaboration, they have some unfavorable side effects including different degrees of anchorage loss, maxillary first molar tipping, posterior rotation of the mandibular plane, and lip protrusion.

Recently we presented a new intraoral device that allows rapid distal movement of the maxillary molars: the First Class Appliance (Leone SpA, Firenze, Italy).[40]

Distalization

The use of molar distalizing appliances for the treatment of tooth size/arch size discrepancies at the upper arch should be based on an accurate cephalometric evaluation of the individual dentoskeletal relationships. Molar distalization is indicated typically in those cases presenting with crowding at the upper arch associated with Class II molar relationship and Class I skeletal relationship. A precise cephalometric evaluation of the posterior limit of the dentition can be obtained with the method proposed by Ricketts[41] (Fig. 22.1).

The evaluation of the vertical skeletal relationships of the individual patient to be treated with distalizing appliances is only relatively important. A typical nonextraction approach for molar distalization (e.g. by means of a facebow) in hyperdivergent patients could result in clockwise mandibular rotation, increase in lower face height and worsening of the Class II relationships. These unfavorable effects may be ascribed mainly to distal movement of the maxillary molars that occurred by distal tipping associated with relative extrusion. Today, the appliances available to the clinician are able to produce molar distalization mainly by bodily movement with minimal distal tipping. Therefore, the possible adverse sequalae affecting the vertical skeletal relationships that typically were associated with distalization of the maxillary molars can be kept to a minimum.

Biomechanics of Distalization

Ideally the distalization of the upper molars should occur by bodily movement without distal tipping. The greater the distal tipping, the more unfavorable the consequences on the occlusion and on the stability of treatment results.

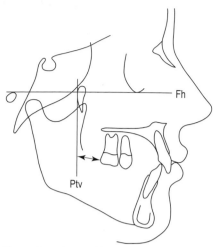

Figure 22.1 A vertical line perpendicular to the Frankfort plane is traced tangentially to the posterior border of the pterygomaxillary fissure. The linear distance from this vertical line to the most distal point on the crown of the maxillary first permanent molar is called PTV-6. The normal value is calculated on the basis of the following formula: age of the patient (reported in millimeters) + 3 mm. The standard deviation is ± 3 mm. The residual increment that will take place along with growth also has to be evaluated.

In order to produce pure translatory movement, the force vector should pass as close as possible to the center of resistance (CR) of the molar that is located approximately at the trifurcation of the root. When analyzing the biomechanics of distalization of the maxillary molars, the effects of the force vector in relation to the CR should be evaluated on both the sagittal and horizontal planes of space. Regarding effects on the sagittal plane, distal tipping of the molar can be minimized by placing the distal force close to the CR. This concept is utilized by appliances like the Distal Jet,[22] or the Keles Slider[27] in which a compressed coil spring is placed palatally at the level of the CR of the maxillary molar. An alternative for the control of distal tipping is to apply the distal force at the level of the crown of the molar in association with either a rigid guiding system (First Class Appliance,[40] Fast Back[28]) or a molar root uprighting system (K-loop[38], Intraoral Bodily Molar Distalizer,[39] or Pendulum with uprighting bends).[32,36]

On the horizontal plane, from an occlusal viewpoint the CR of the upper molar appears to be displaced toward the palatal side. The application of a distal force on the buccal or lingual surface of the maxillary molar creates a moment that tends to rotate the tooth in the horizontal plane. In order to counteract this tendency, the distalizing appliances are provided with either a guiding system (Distal Jet,[22] Intraoral Bodily Molar Distalizer,[39] Keles Slider,[27] Fast Back[28]) or a rigid wire associated with a compressed coil spring (First Class Appliance[40]) that prevents molar rotation.

Indications

The distalization is indicated in the following clinical situations.
- Tooth size/arch size discrepancy at the upper arch in presence of Class II molar relationship.
- Class II malocclusion with protrusion of the entire maxillary dental arch relative to the skeletal portion of the maxilla.
- Skeletal Class II relationships with prevalent maxillary skeletal protrusion in individuals at the end of growth.
- Skeletal Class II relationship when the lack of compliance limits the orthopedic therapy aimed at restraining the unfavorable growth of the maxilla.
- Class II malocclusions associated with skeletal and/or dentoalveolar deep bite (Class II, division 2 malocclusion).
- Opening of spaces due to agenesis or previous extractions.

Contraindications

There are no real contraindications to molar distalization provided that an appropriate diagnosis has been made by the clinician and that the most recent types of distalizing appliances are used. Distalization of the upper molars, however, should not be performed in cases showing severe maxillary protrusion, severe mandibular retrusion or mandibular skeletal deficiency.

Before starting treatment with a distalizing appliance, some fundamental issues or questions have to be considered, as suggested by Cisneros.[42]
- What are the specific side effects that can be expected when using a distalizing appliance?
- Are there specific patient types that would be better treated by one or another type of appliance?
- How much arch length can be created by a given distalizing appliance?
- When is the appropriate time to use these appliances?
- What type of cooperation is needed from the patient to use such appliances?

The First Class Appliance

History

The history of the First Class Appliance (FCA) is relatively recent and constantly developing. The FCA can be considered as a new interpretation of the "tooth-regulating device" proposed by Knapp in 1899, which incorporated two screws for molar distalization (Fig. 22.2). The new screw for molar distalization was first presented in 1996 at the 96th Annual Session of the American Association of Orthodontists in Denver. This device had been developed by an engineer as a possible system of distalization with the screw positioned on the palatal side. The prototype had not been clinically tested at that time, however.

Later, the initial version of a distalizing appliance (Fig. 22.3) that incorporated the screw was developed, even though neither the activation rate nor the force it could develop was known. The clinical

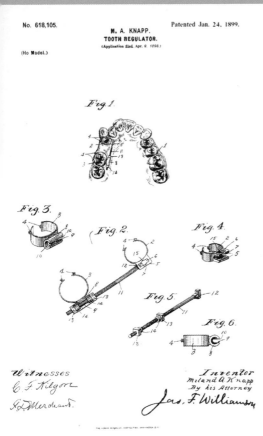

Figure 22.2 The "tooth regulating device" proposed by Knapp in 1899.

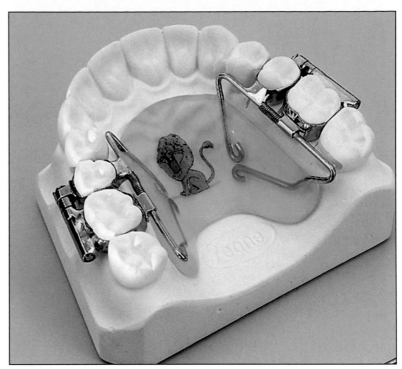

Figure 22.4 The latest version of the First Class Appliance.

latest version, that is completely different from its initial prototype, has been widely tested from a clinical point of view.

Appliance Design

The FCA can be used both in the mixed and permanent dentitions for bilateral or unilateral molar distalization. A particular feature of this appliance is that it can produce rapid molar distalization with minimal tipping, even in the presence of completely erupted second molars.

The First Class Appliance (Leone SpA, Firenze, Italy) consists of four bands, a vestibular side, and a palatal side (Fig. 22.5).

The Bands

Two bands are placed on the upper first molars and two bands either on the second premolars or on the second deciduous teeth.

Vestibular Side

On the buccal side of the first molar bands, vestibular screws (the active unit of the appliance) are soldered occlusally to the 0.022 × 0.028″ single tubes. The screws are 10 mm long with four holes for activation. The vestibular screws are seated into closed rings that are welded to the bands of the second deciduous molars or the second premolars.

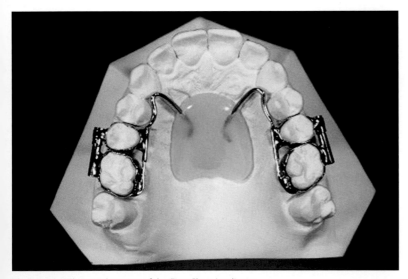

Figure 22.3 The initial version of the First Class Appliance.

results with this version of the FCA were encouraging. The major concerns regarded the usefulness of including the expansion screw in the Nance button and, above all, the consistent loss of anchorage. After several attempts, a satisfactory version of the FCA that incorporated a new screw of 10 mm was developed (Fig. 22.4). This

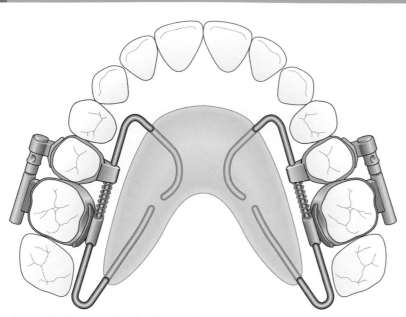

Figure 22.5 Drawing of the First Class Appliance.

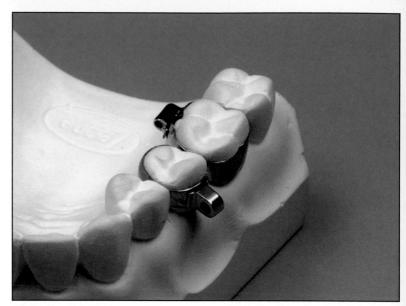

Figure 22.6 The closed ring and the palatal tube welded on the bands of the second premolar and first molar, respectively.

Palatal Side

The palatal aspect of the appliance has a "butterfly" shape and consists of a Nance button with 0.045″ wires embedded in the acrylic. The acrylic button is large to enhance anchorage control during both the active phase of treatment and the retention phase. The 0.045″ wires are shaped in a single piece, in order to avoid any breakage because of the presence of welded joints. These wires are soldered lingual of the second deciduous molar/premolar bands, while posteriorly they are inserted into 0.045″ tube sections welded to the palatal sides of the first molar bands. The tubes act as a guide during molar distalization to promote a bodily tooth movement. Ten millimeter long open nickel-titanium $0.010 \times 0.045″$ coil springs are fully compressed between the solder joint on the second deciduous molar/premolar band and the tube on the molar band. The continuous force delivered by the springs is able to counterbalance the action of the vestibular screws. The distal molar movement takes place in a "double-track" system that prevents rotations or contractions of the molars.

Clinical Management

Impression

The maxillary second premolars/second deciduous molars and first molars should have been separated at the previous appointment to create interproximally adequate space for the placement of bands. After band placement is completed, an alginate impression of the upper arch is made using a standard aluminum tray. It is fundamental to have an adequate reproduction not only of the teeth but also of the palatal region. The bands are removed from the teeth and placed in their appropriate positions in the impression. To avoid movement during pouring of the work model, the bands can be secured to the alginate with sticky wax.

Fabrication

- Before pouring the impression, a layer of wax should be placed on the inside surface of the bands.
- After the work model has been poured, check that the bands on the maxillary second premolars/second deciduous molars and the first molars are in their proper position.
- The 0.045″ tubes are welded on the palatal side molar bands and the closed rings are welded on the vestibular side of the second premolar/second deciduous molar bands (Fig. 22.6).
- A 0.045″ wire is bent by the first premolar and looped on the end for retention in the acrylic. It is then placed in the molar palatal tube.
- The screw is placed in the closed ring (Fig. 22.7).
- The screw and the palatal wire are parallelized by means of a specific device (Fig. 22.8).
- The device for parallelization of the screw and the palatal wire is stabilized on the dental cast with wax.
- The screw and the lingual wire are soldered to the molar band and to the premolar band, respectively.
- A piece of 10 mm nickel-titanium $0.010 \times 0.045″$ coil spring is placed on the palatal wires distal to the solder joint on the premolar band.

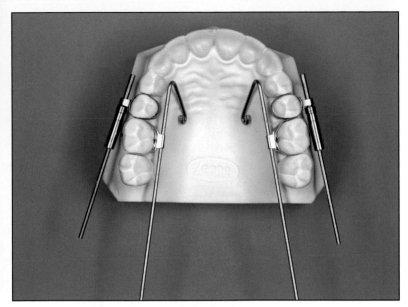

Figure 22.7 The screws are placed inside the closed rings.

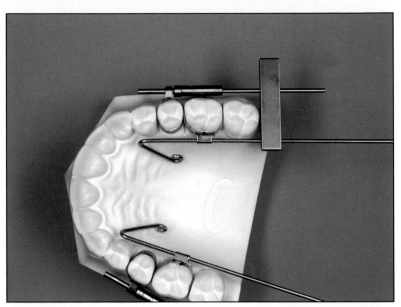

Figure 22.8 The screw and the palatal wire are parallelized with a specific device.

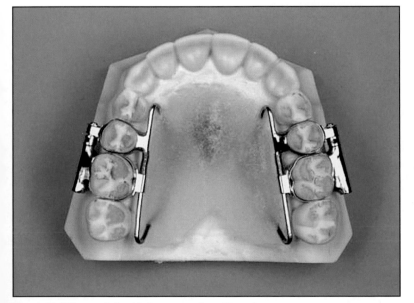

Figure 22.9 The acrylic is added to create a large Nance button.

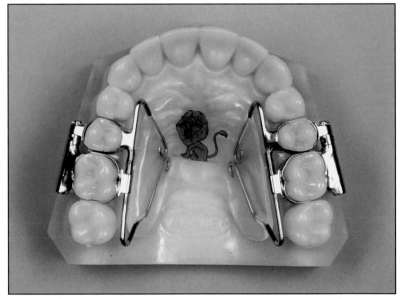

Figure 22.10 The acrylic of the Nance button is finished and polished.

- The distal end of the palatal wire is bent at an appropriate distalizing distance into the palatal area and looped for retention in the acrylic. The closed ring is crimped on the anterior portion of the screw.
- The acrylic is added on the palate to create the Nance button (Fig. 22.9).
- The Nance button is finished and polished (Fig. 22.10).

Delivery of the Appliance and Activation Instructions

The cementation of the FCA is accomplished using a glass ionomer cement (e.g. Transbond™ Plus light-cure band adhesive, 3M Unitek or Leone light-cure fluoride-releasing cement) with the following characteristics:

- a single-paste, no-mix cement. The elimination of mixing presents several advantages including reduced clean-up, more consistent adhesive performance, increased office efficiency, and less chair time

- light-curing cement with a rapid 30-s set time to reduce the risk of moisture contamination

- release of fluoride and the ability to reload its fluoride ion content when exposed to other fluoride-containing systems like fluoride-containing water or toothpaste

- a distinctive color that allows it to be easily detected during banding and to make clean-up of excess easy.

The patient is told to activate one or both of the two vestibular screws (for unilateral or bilateral distalization, respectively) one quarter of a turn (0.1 mm) in a counterclockwise direction (clockwise direction as viewed in the mirror) once per day for a prescribed period of time. The patient is seen at 2-week intervals until the desired distalization of the molars has been accomplished.

Clinical Effects of the First Class Appliance

Clinical Evaluation

At the end of molar distalization, the screws of the appliance may show either a partial or complete activation. In both instances the appliance still maintains the typical features of solidity and stability. The precise amount of force developed on the maxillary first molars by the screw is very difficult to quantify clinically. The force level achieved by the activation of the screws, however, does not produce any unfavorable reaction on the tooth (e.g. root resorption) or on the periodontal structures (e.g. pockets or recessions) as revealed by the clinical and radiographic examinations (intraoral X-rays) that were performed before and after completion of distalization on a large sample of patients (Figs 22.11–22.13).[40]

The clinical results show that the FCA is able to produce an efficient distalization of the maxillary molars. A more complete analysis of both favorable and unfavorable effects produced by the FCA can be performed by means of a cephalometric evaluation of the dentoskeletal changes induced at the completion of molar distalization.

Cephalometric Evaluation

In a recent study,[43] we analyzed the dentoskeletal effects induced by rapid molar distalization with the FCA. The sample consisted of

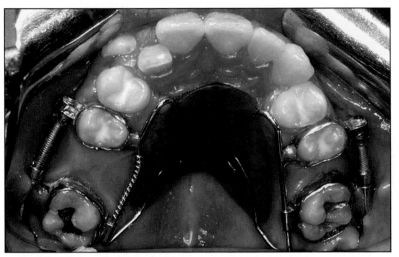

Figure 22.11 Bilateral distalization with the FCA.

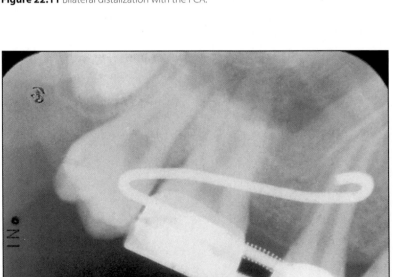

Figures 22.12, 22.13 Radiographic assessment of the molar distalization.

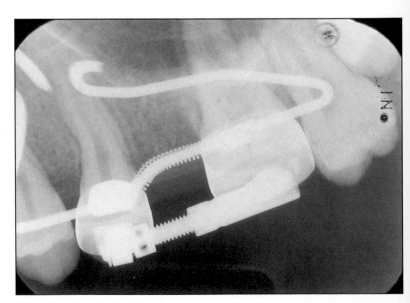

Figure 22.13

17 patients (10 males, 7 females) with Class II malocclusion. All subjects presented with bilateral full Class II molar relationship at the start of treatment and they were consecutively treated with the same treatment protocol in a single orthodontic practice. Lateral cephalograms were obtained at T1 (start of treatment with the FCA) and at T2 (end of molar distalization). All cephalograms were taken with the same X-ray device and by a single technician. Mean age at T1 was 13 years 4 months (range, 11 years 4 months to 17 years 2 months). Four patients were in the mixed dentition. In 12 out of the 13 subjects in the permanent dentition, the maxillary permanent second molars were partially or totally erupted. The mean time period between the initial T1 radiograph and the postdistalization T2 radiograph was 72 days (range 41–110 days). Gender differences were not considered a factor because of the short duration of treatment with the FCA.

Pancherz's superimposition method[44] was applied for the assessment of sagittal dental changes to avoid errors due to possible variations in the inclination of the occlusal plane after molar distalization. The cephalometric landmarks and measurements are illustrated in Figures 22.14 and 22.15.

Pre- and posttreatment cephalometric data with changes induced by the FCA at the dentoskeletal level are reported in Tables 22.1 and 22.2.

After the active phase of treatment, the maxillary first molars showed a significant distalization (ms-Ol_p) of 4.0 mm associated with a distal axial incline (mmc-ma/SN) of 4.6°. A significant mesial movement of the second premolars (anchorage loss) of 1.7 mm (ps-Ol_p) associated with a significant mesial axial incline of 2.2° (pc-pa/SN) was recorded.

The upper first molars exhibited an extrusion of 1.2 mm (mmc-SN). The second premolars (pc-SN) showed a nonsignificant tendency to extrude during treatment (1.0 mm). In the anterior region a nonsignificant mesial movement of the maxillary incisor

of 1.2 mm (is-Ol_p) was associated with a significant increment (2.6°) in the inclination of the maxillary incisor axis to the cranial base (is-ia/SN). The overjet increased significantly by 1.2 mm while the overbite showed a nonsignificant tendency to decrease (–0.8 mm).

Minimal sagittal and vertical skeletal effects (0.4° increase in SNA and 0.5° increase in the inclination of the mandibular plane to SN), although statistically significant, were not considered noteworthy from a clinical point of view. No statistically significant changes occurred in the soft tissue measurements during the distalization therapy.

Effects of Second Molar Eruption

No significant differences between subjects with unerupted second molars and subjects with partially or totally erupted second molars were found in the amount of first molar distalization (3.9 mm vs 4.0 mm) and distal inclination (–4.1° vs –4.8°) and in the amount of anchorage loss (mesial movement of the second premolars 1.5 mm vs 1.8 mm and incisor proclination 2.4° vs 2.7°). These results confirmed those reported for the Pendulum in previous studies[30–33] that the amount of distal movement and inclination of the upper first molars as well as the amount of anchorage loss were not influenced by the presence of the upper second molars. Interestingly, Bolla and coworkers[25] noted more favorable changes (less distal tipping of the first molar and less anchorage loss and extrusion) in those subjects treated with the Distal Jet after the eruption of the second molars. With the FCA no significant differences in the inclination of the mandibular plane in relation to both the cranial base and the palatal plane were found between patients who had second molars erupted and those who did not.

Despite the small sample size, these findings do not support the conclusions by Bussick & McNamara[33] who advocate starting to

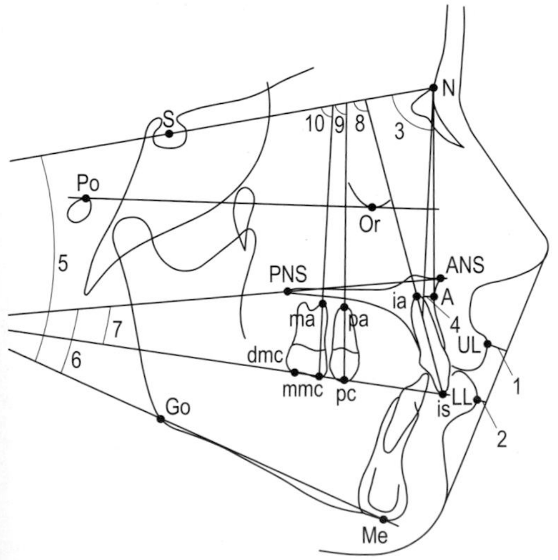

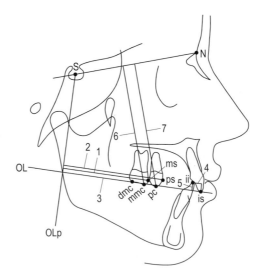

Figure 22.14 Soft tissue linear measurements: *1*, UL-E plane; *2*, LL-E plane. Skeletal measurements: *3*, SNA angle; *4*, Point A to nasion perpendicular; *5*, SN-mandibular plane angle; *6*, palatal plane-mandibular plane angle; *7*, palatal plane-occlusal line (OL) angle. Dental angular measurements: *8*, is-ia/SN; *9*, pc-pa/SN; *10*, mmc-ma/SN. (*From Fortini et al,[43] © 2004, with kind permission from the American Association of Orthodontists*)

Figure 22.15 Sagittal dental linear measurements (Pancherz's superimposition method): *1*, ms-Ol_p; *2*, ps-Ol_p; *3*, is-Ol_p; *4*, overjet (is-Ol_p minus ii-Ol_p). Vertical dental linear measurements: *5*, overbite (ii-OL); *6*, mmc-NSL; *7*, pc-NSL. (*From Fortini et al,[43] © 2004, with kind permission from the American Association of Orthodontists*)

Table 22.1. Descriptive statistics for the cephalometric skeletal and dental measurements at T1 and T2.

Measurements	Pretreatment (T1) n=17					Posttreatment (T2) n=17				
	Mean	Median	SD	Min	Max	Mean	Median	SD	Min	Max
Soft tissue (mm)										
UL-E plane	0.0	1.0	2.6	−4.5	3.5	0.3	1.0	2.4	−4.0	3.0
LL-E plane	−0.2	0.0	2.0	−4.0	2.0	0.0	0.5	2.1	−4.0	3.0
Skeletal										
SNA (°)	80.6	80.0	3.2	76.0	87.5	81.0	80.0	3.1	77.0	87.5
Pt A to nasion perp (mm)	1.5	2.0	2.1	−3.0	5.5	1.6	2.0	1.9	−1.0	6.0
SN-mand.plane (°)	31.6	31.5	6.8	18.0	42.0	32.1	33.5	6.9	19.0	42.0
Pal.plane-mand.plane (°)	23.7	23.0	6.6	12.0	38.0	24.1	25.0	7.2	10.0	40.0
Pal.plane-OL (°)	12.7	13.0	4.0	5.0	18.0	13.2	14.0	4.0	6.0	18.0
Dental angular (°)										
is-ia/SN	99.1	99.0	7.3	86.0	111.0	101.6	102.0	7.7	87.0	115.0
pc-pa/SN	74.8	73.0	5.7	67.0	85.5	77.0	75.0	6.7	67.0	89.0
mmc-ma/SN	71.3	70.0	4.9	64.0	83.5	72.4	72.5	5.6	62.0	84.5
Dental linear (mm)										
ms-OL$_p$	58.4	57.0	4.3	52.5	68.5	54.4	54.0	4.1	48.0	62.5
ps-OL$_p$	66.3	64.0	4.4	61.0	75.5	68.1	68.0	4.8	63.0	78.0
is-OL$_p$	89.6	88.0	5.6	80.5	102.0	91.0	89.5	5.3	81.0	102.0
mmc-SN	71.9	70.5	4.9	64.0	83.5	71.5	71.5	4.9	62.0	81.5
pc-SN	75.3	74.5	4.7	68.0	86.0	76.4	77.0	4.7	68.0	84.0
Overjet	6.3	6.0	2.2	3.0	11.0	7.5	7.0	1.5	5.0	11.0
Overbite	4.1	5.0	2.2	0.0	8.0	3.3	3.5	1.9	0.0	6.0

(From Fortini et al,[43] © 2004, with kind permission from the American Association of Orthodontists)

move the first molars distally with the Pendulum before the eruption of the second molars to avoid significant increases in the mandibular plane angle and in lower anterior facial height.

Distalization Rate

The FCA induced an average 4.0 mm/side distal movement of the crowns of the maxillary first molars during a period of 2.4 months (Table 22.2). It was able to produce a true "rapid" molar distalization (1.7 mm/month on average) when compared with the rate of distalization of other devices (Table 22.3). Molar distalization accounted for 70% of the change in sagittal position between the first molar and the second premolar.

Anchorage Loss: Comparison with Other Distalization Appliances

One of the unavoidable side effects when using an intraarch maxillary molar distalizer is the anchorage loss generated by the reciprocal force on the anchorage unit (first and/or second premolars and the Nance

acrylic button). The anchorage loss is expressed by the mesial movement of the premolar–incisor segment. None of the contemporary intraarch molar distalizers is able to provide completely effective anchorage control (see Table 22.3). Anchorage loss may vary from a minimum of 24% to a maximum of 55% of the spaces created between the first molars and the anchorage teeth (first or second premolars). The FCA produced 30% loss of anchorage that corresponded to 1.7 mm of premolar mesial movement with 2.2° of mesial tipping.

The FCA was quite efficient in anchorage control when compared to other distalizing devices, as the second premolars moved mesially only 0.4 mm for every millimeter of molar distalization. If we combine the information deriving from the two "efficiency indices" reported in Table 22.3, the Distal Jet, the Intraoral Bodily Molar Distalizer, and the FCA come out as the most efficient intraarch molar distalizers.

The amount of incisor flaring (2.6°) and overjet increase (1.2 mm) induced by the FCA is similar to those produced by the majority of the distalizing appliances. There is no doubt that the creation of additional overjet in a Class II case introduces an element of inefficiency into the treatment. However, if the amount of overjet increase is modest,

Table 22.2. Descriptive statistics and statistical comparisons for the changes T2–T1.

Measurements	T2–T1 changes					Wilcoxon test		
	Mean	Median	SD	Min	Max	Z	P	Significance
Soft tissue (mm)								
UL-E plane	0.3	0.0	1.1	−1.0	4.0	−0.955	0.340	NS
LL-E plane	0.2	0.0	0.5	−0.5	1.0	−1.561	0.119	NS
Skeletal								
SNA (°)	0.4	0.0	0.6	0.0	1.5	−2.232	0.026	*
Pt A to nasion perp (mm)	0.2	0.0	0.6	−1.0	2.0	−0.850	0.395	NS
SN-mand.plane (°)	0.5	0.0	0.9	−1.0	2.0	−2.549	0.011	*
Pal.plane-mand.plane (°)	0.4	0.0	1.8	−2.0	4.0	−1.922	0.055	NS
Pal.plane-OL (°)	0.5	0.0	2.7	−2.5	9.0	−0.581	0.561	NS
Dental angular (°)								
is-ia/SN	2.6	3.0	1.0	1.0	4.0	−3.659	0.000	***
pc-pa/SN	2.2	1.5	2.2	0.0	6.0	−2.673	0.008	**
mmc-ma/SN	−4.6	−5.0	2.6	−8.0	0.0	−3.066	0.002	**
Dental linear (mm)								
ms-OL$_p$	−4.0	−3.5	1.5	−7.0	−2.0	−3.187	0.001	**
ps- OL$_p$	1.7	1.5	1.5	0.0	4.5	−2.807	0.005	**
is- OL$_p$	1.3	1.0	1.3	0.0	4.0	−3.075	0.002	**
mmc-SN	1.2	1.5	2.0	−2.0	5.0	−2.212	0.027	*
pc-SN	1.0	1.0	1.7	−2.0	4.0	−1.944	0.052	NS
Overjet	1.2	1.0	1.9	−4.0	4.5	−2.341	0.019	*
Overbite	−0.8	0.0	1.6	−4.0	2.5	−1.335	0.182	NS

* = p<0.05; ** = p<0.05; *** = p<0.001; NS = not significant. *(From Fortini et al,[43] © 2004, with kind permission from the American Association of Orthodontists)*

below 2 mm according to Gianelly,[15] the use of J-hook headgear or Class II elastics to reinforce anterior anchorage control does not seem to be justified.

The End of Molar Distalization: Clinical Management

Transformation of the First Class Appliance into a Retention Device

It is mandatory to stabilize the maxillary molars once they have been moved distally as it has been clearly demonstrated that they have a strong tendency to relapse mesially towards their original position.[45]

Once the first molars have achieved a Class I occlusion, the appliance is transformed into a modified Nance holding arch by removing the bands on the second premolars together with the male screws and the palatal coil springs (Fig. 22.16). The tubes on the palatal sides of the first molar bands are crimped with a hard wire cutter to stabilize the molar in the distal position.

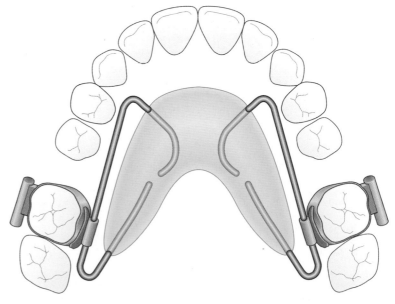

Figure 22.16 After completing molar distalization, the appliance is transformed into a modified Nance holding arch.

Table 22.3. Comparison of the effects of molar distalization appliances.

Report	Appliance	n	Treatment duration (mos)	Molar distal movement (mm)	Molar distal tipping (°)	Premolar mesial movement (mm)	Premolar tipping (°)*	Incisor vestibular movement (mm)	Incisor vestibular tipping (°)	Overjet (mm)	Distalization rate (mm/mo)	Distal tipping index (°/mm)	Anchorage loss index	Molar distalization (%)	Anchorage loss (%)
Ghosh & Nanda 1996[30]	Pendulum	41	6.2	3.4	8.4	2.5	1.3	–	2.4	1.3	0.5	2.5	0.7	57	43
Byloff & Darendeliler 1997[31]	Pendulum	13	4.1	3.4	14.5	1.6	–	0.7	1.7	–	0.8	4.3	0.5	71	29
Byloff & Darendeliler 1997[31]	Pendulum	20	6.8	4.1	6.1	2.2	–	1.0	3.2	–	0.6	1.5	0.5	64	36
Bussick & McNamara 2000[33]	Pendulum	101	7.0	5.7	10.6	1.8	1.5	1.4	3.6	0.8	0.8	1.9	0.3	76	24
Chaques-Asensi & Kalra 2001[35]	Pendulum	26	6.5	5.3	13.1	2.2	4.8	2.1	5.1	1.8	0.8	2.5	0.4	71	29
Gulati et al 1998[18]	Jones Jig	10	3.0	2.7	3.5	1.1	2.6	–	–	1.0	0.9	1.3	0.4	71	29
Runge et al 1999[19]	Jones Jig	13	6.7	2.2	4.0	2.2	9.5	–	2.0	1.5	0.3	1.8	1.0	50	50
Haydar & Uner 2000[20]	Jones Jig	20	2.5	2.8	7.8	3.3	6.0	0.2	1.0	–	1.1	2.8	1.2	46	54
Brickman et al 2000[21]	Jones Jig	72	6.3	2.5	7.5	2.0	4.8	–	2.4	-0.4	0.4	3.0	0.8	55	45
Keles & Sayinsu 2000[39]	IBMD	15	7.5	5.2	1.1	4.3	-2.7	4.8	6.7	4.1	0.7	0.2	0.8	55	45
Ngantung et al 2001[23]	Distal Jet	33	6.7	2.1	3.3	2.6	-4.3	–	12.1	1.7	0.3	1.6	1.2	45	55
Nishii et al 2002[24]	Distal Jet	15	6.4	2.6	1.8	1.5	–	2.4	4.5	–	0.4	0.7	0.6	63	37
Bolla et al 2002[25]	Distal Jet	20	5.0	3.2	3.1	1.3	-2.8	–	0.6	0.4	0.6	1.0	0.4	71	29
Fortini et al 2004[43]	First Class	17	2.4	4.0	4.6	1.7	2.2	1.2	2.6	1.2	1.7	1.1	0.4	70	30

IBMD, Intraoral Bodily Molar Distalizer; * positive value = distal tipping; negative value = mesial tipping. (From Fortini et al,[43] © 2004, with kind permission from the American Association of Orthodontists)

Alternative Retention Devices

It may happen that at the end of distalization the Nance button of the FCA cannot be used as a retention device because the bands have been damaged during the removal of the screws or because of the presence of defects in the acrylic of the Nance button. In other instances the clinician may need to use a smaller Nance button than the one incorporated in the FCA. In all these situations the FCA can be sent to the laboratory to be transformed into either a Nance holding arch or a transpalatal arch. A facebow (with or without an anterior stainless steel bite plane) can be used in conjunction with the Nance button to reinforce the anchorage during the distalization of the second premolars.

The tendency to relapse after molar distalization can be controlled by creating an overcorrection of molar relationship (a so-called "super Class I"). The maxillary molars are stabilized in the overcorrected position by placing two omega loops immediately mesial to the molar tubes.

Among the alternative retention devices, an interesting possibility is represented by the new extradental systems (microimplants, non-osseointegrated mini-screws or osseointegrated implants) that can provide absolute orthodontic anchorage.[46–50] The anchorage systems that can be used at the end of the distalization phase with the FCA are:

- Nance button of the FCA after the removal of the screws
- Nance button of the FCA modified appropriately in the laboratory
- transpalatal arch
- facebow
- overcorrection of molar relationships and omega stops on the archwire
- intermaxillary Class II elastics
- extradental anchorage on mini-implants.

There are no absolute indications for the use of any of the retention systems. The decision on which system to apply is made after evaluating the amount of distal movement of the molars produced by the FCA, the need for a short second phase of treatment with fixed appliances, and patient compliance.

Distalization of the Premolars and the Anterior Segment

After the molars have been adequately distalized, one of challenges to the clinician is to maintain molar anchorage while the premolars are retracted. A certain amount of spontaneous distal drifting of the premolars, due to the pull of the transseptal fibers between adjacent teeth ("driftodontics"), can be seen during the molar stabilization phase.[51]

Some type of retracting mechanics needs to be applied on the premolars, however, since the amount of spontaneous distal drifting cannot usually guarantee a complete distalization of the first and second premolars.

The mechanics that we utilize for retraction of the remaining maxillary teeth is based on the concept of the straight-wire technique as proposed by Bennett & McLaughlin.[52,53] According to this treatment, the premolars have to be distalized first while the upper canines will be retracted "en masse" together with the incisors during the reduction of the overjet and space closure.

One of the most frequently used systems for premolar retraction is by means of intermaxillary Class II elastics.[54] The use of intramaxillary Class I elastics for distalization of the premolars is usually contraindicated unless methods for proper anchorage control (e.g. facebow) are applied. In fact, it is a common clinical observation that application of Class I elastics can easily lead to a relapse in the position of the distalized maxillary molars that are subjected to a force in an opposite direction. With the exception of the mini-implants, there is no intraoral device (Nance button, transpalatal arch, etc.) that can provide proper anchorage control during premolar retraction with Class I intramaxillary forces. The only case in which Class I elastics can be used is when the patient (better if adult) can guarantee good cooperation with a facebow.

A typical scheme for premolar retraction is the following:

- Class II elastics, to be worn full time
- Class I elastics to be worn only during night-time hours together with the facebow.

The clinician has to be aware of the effects and side effects produced by Class II elastics. In particular, the inclination of the force vector of the elastics can influence the amount of the sagittal and vertical forces in which the vector can be decomposed. The extrusive forces on the lower posterior teeth and on the upper anterior teeth can generate either favorable or unfavorable effects in relation to the vertical dentoskeletal features of the individual patient.

In deep-bite Class II cases, while the extrusive force on the lower posterior segment can be used effectively for bite opening, the extrusive force on the upper incisors has to be adequately counteracted with intrusive forces such as those generated by a $0.019 \times 0.025''$ stainless steel archwire with accentuated curve of Spee or by J-hook headgear.

Case Studies

Patient 1

Diagnosis and Treatment Planning

GG, a female patient 12 years and 4 months old, showed bilateral Class II molar and canine relationships with increased overjet and overbite (Figs 22.17–22.23). Mild crowding was present in both arches. As for skeletal relationships, she presented with Class I skeletal pattern with a tendency to mandibular retrusion and decreased vertical skeletal relationships (Figs 22.17, 22.18 and 22.24; Table 22.4). The upper incisors were protruded and proclined while the lower incisors, though retruded, showed a normal inclination. The upper and lower lips were slightly protruded to the E-plane with a decrease in the

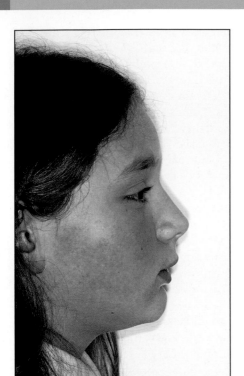

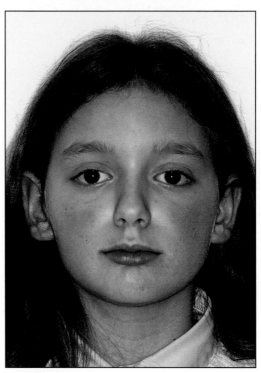

Figures 22.17, 22.18 Female patient GG. Pretreatment facial photographs.

Figure 22.18

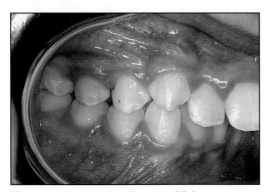

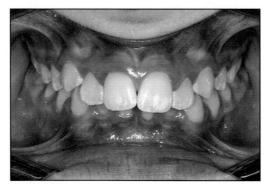

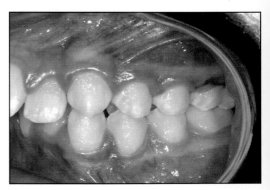

Figures 22.19–22.23 Female patient GG. Pretreatment intraoral photographs.

Figure 22.20

Figure 22.21

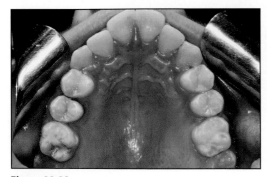

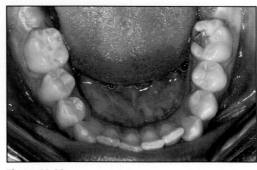

Figure 22.22

Figure 22.23

distalization revealed a bodily movement of the first molars in the absence of any unfavorable reaction on the roots of the teeth or on the periodontal structures (Figs 22.25 and 22.26).

End of Distalization
The duration of active distalization was 71 days. The appliance was then removed and sent to the laboratory to be transformed into a Nance holding arch.

Treatment Results

At the end of treatment (patient aged 13 years and 9 months), a good occlusion was achieved resulting in bilateral Class I molar and canine relationships and normal values for both overjet and overbite. Crowding was also corrected (Figs 22.27–22.33). The patient still showed a Class I skeletal relationship with a slight favorable increase in vertical relationships (Figs 22.27, 22.28 and 22.34; see Table 22.4). The position and inclination of the upper incisors were normalized while the lower incisors showed a moderate increase in protrusion and vestibular inclination. The nasolabial angle presented with normal values and the upper and lower lips exhibited a normal position in relation to the E-plane.

Patient 2

Diagnosis and Treatment Planning

AF, a female patient aged 11 years 8 months, presented with bilateral Class II molar and canine relationships and with increased overjet and overbite (Figs 22.35–22.41). Both arches exhibited moderate crowding. The lower molars were banded as the patient had worn a lip bumper. The patient showed a tendency to Class II skeletal relationship due to mandibular retrusion and normal vertical

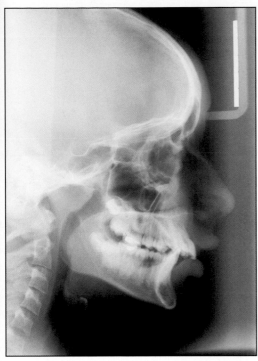

Figure 22.24 Female patient GG. Pretreatment cephalometric radiograph.

nasiolabial angle. The patient was treated with the FCA followed by comprehensive fixed appliance therapy.

Treatment Progress

Control after 35 Days of Distalization
After 35 days of activation of the FCA, 3 mm of molar distalization bilaterally had been achieved. The radiographic assessment of

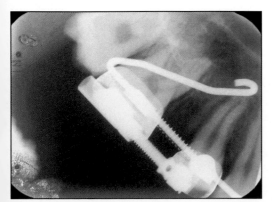

Figures 22.25, 22.26 Female patient GG. Radiographic assessment of molar distalization after 35 days of FCA activation.

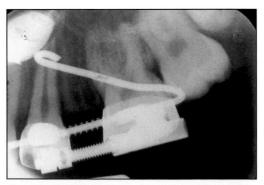

Figure 22.26

Table 22.4. Patient GG, female, 12 years 4 months. Pre- and posttreatment cephalometric measurements.

	Pretreatment		Posttreatment	
	Normal values	**GG**	**Normal values**	**GG**
OJ (mm)	2	9.8	2	2.6
OB (mm)	2	4.2	2	2.1
SNA (°)	79.7	76.4	79.9	74.6
SNB (°)	77.1	73.3	77.5	73.1
ANB (°)	2.9	3.1	2.7	1.6
A to nasion perp. (mm)	0.9	−1.5	1	−2.4
Pog to nasion perp. (mm)	−1.8	−2.7	−1	−1.8
Wits (mm)	2.1	3.8	2.2	0.3
Go-Gn to SN (°)	35	30.1	34	31.4
Mand. P. to FH (°)	26	17.1	26	18.2
Go-Me to palatal P. (°)	28.2	21.7	27.8	21.6
N-S-Ar (°)	124.7	135.4	124.9	134.1
S-Ar-Go (°)	139.9	128.5	139.9	131.5
Ar-Go-Me (°)	131.1	127.2	130.6	127.2
Sum (°)	396	391.1	395.4	392.9
Ar-Goi-Me (°)	125.6	122.2	125.2	122.7
Ar-Goi-N (°)	53.5	55.6	53.5	53.9
N-Goi-Me (°)	72.5	66.6	72.5	68.7
S-Go (mm)	65.2	70.4	66.9	71.2
Upper inc. to palatal P. (°)	110	118.7	109.4	112.3
Lower inc. to Go-Me (°)	91	92.2	90.7	100.9
Interincisal angle (°)	131.7	120.5	132.6	115.2
Upper inc. to A-Pog. (mm)	4.5	8.4	4.2	5.7
Lower inc. to A-Pog. (mm)	1.1	−1.4	1	3.3
Nasolabial angle (°)	110.2	116.9	110.4	124.5
Upper lip to E-plane (mm)	−3.2	0.8	−3.6	−0.9
Upper lip protrusion (mm)	3	5.6	3	3.7
Lower lip to E-plane (mm)	−2.2	−1.3	−2.5	0.5
Lower lip protrusion (mm)	2	1.2	2	3.4

relationships (Figs 22.35, 22.36 and 22.42; Table 22.5). The upper incisors were protruded with a normal inclination while the lower incisors were retruded with a normal inclination. Both upper and lower lips were protruded to the E-plane with a decrease in the nasolabial angle. The patient was treated with the FCA followed by comprehensive fixed appliance therapy. The second deciduous molars were used as anchorage teeth for the FCA.

Treatment Progress

Control after 68 Days of Distalization

After 68 days of treatment with the FCA, 3 mm of molar distalization were obtained bilaterally. The radiographic assessment of distalization revealed no sign of unfavorable reaction on the roots or on the periodontal structure of the molars.

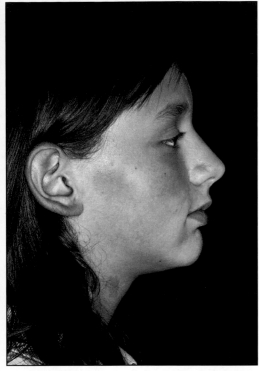

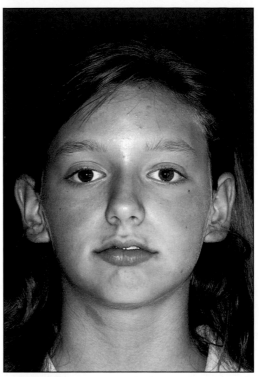

Figures 22.27, 22.28 Female patient GG. Posttreatment facial photographs.

Figure 22.28

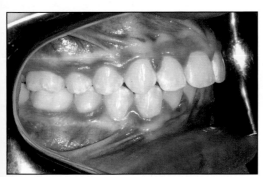

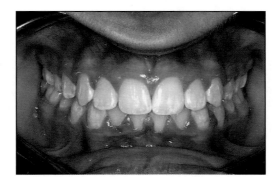

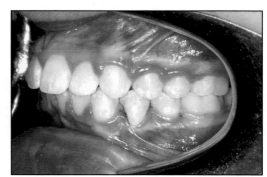

Figures 22.29–22.33 Female patient GG. Posttreatment intraoral photographs.

Figure 22.30

Figure 22.31

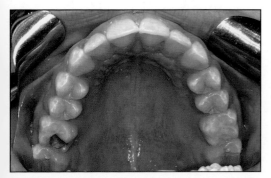

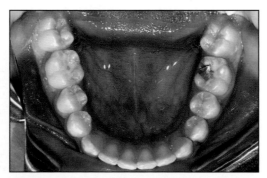

Figure 22.32

Figure 22.33

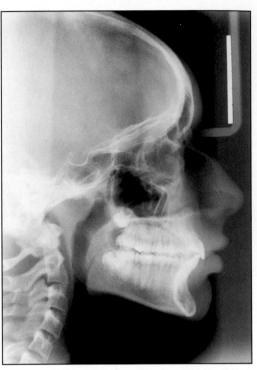

Figure 22.34 Female patient GG. Posttreatment cephalometric radiograph.

End of Distalization

Active distalization lasted 86 days (Fig. 22.43). The appliance was then removed and sent to the laboratory to be transformed into a Nance holding arch.

Treatment Results

At the end of treatment (patient aged 13 years 4 months) bilateral Class I molar and canine relationships and normal values for both overjet and overbite were obtained. Crowding was also corrected in both arches (Figs 22.44–22.50). The patient showed a Class I skeletal relationship with a favorable mandibular advancement. Vertical dimension was slightly increased (Figs 22.44, 22.45 and 22.51; see Table 22.5). The upper incisors were slightly retroclined while the lower incisors showed a moderate increase in protrusion and vestibular inclination. The nasolabial angle was slightly increased with respect to normal values while the upper and lower lips exhibited a normal position in relation to the E-plane.

Conclusion

The effectiveness of the FCA for the correction of Class II malocclusion has been evaluated by comparing the treatment effects

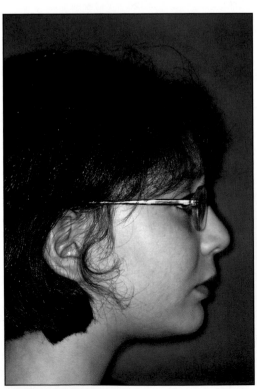

Figures 22.35, 22.36 Female patient AF. Pretreatment facial photographs.

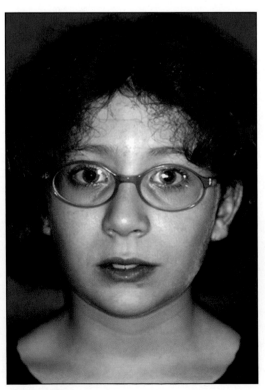

Figure 22.36

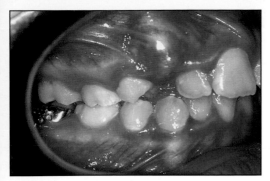

Figures 22.37–22.41 Female patient AF. Pretreatment intraoral photographs.

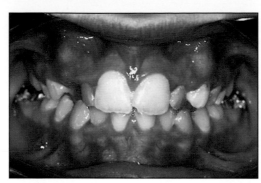

Figure 22.38

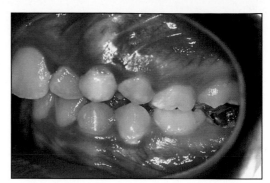

Figure 22.39

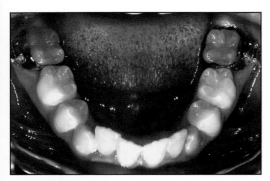

Figure 22.40

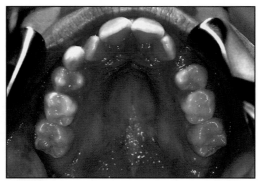

Figure 22.41

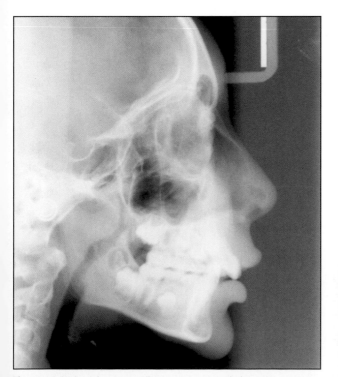

Figure 22.42 Female patient AF. Pretreatment cephalometric radiograph.

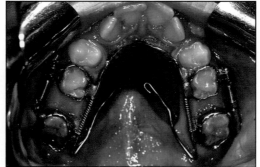

Figure 22.43 Female patient AF. Intraoral photograph at the end of molar distalization.

Table 22.5. Patient AF, female, 11 years 8 months. Pre- and posttreatment cephalometric measurements.

	Pretreatment		Posttreatment	
	Normal values	AF	Normal values	AF
OJ (mm)	2	8.9	2	2.8
OB (mm)	2	4.9	2	2.7
SNA (°)	79.4	76.7	80	77.4
SNB (°)	76.7	72.4	77.8	74.9
ANB (°)	3	4.3	2.5	3.5
A to nasion perp. (mm)	0.6	−1.2	1.1	−2.1
Pog to nasion perp. (mm)	−2.6	−12.2	−0.2	−8.7
Wits (mm)	2.1	4.9	2.1	1
Go-Gn to SN (°)	35	37.6	34	39.7
Mand. P. to FH (°)	26	25.3	26	25.2
Go-Me to palatal P. (°)	28.5	28.4	27.2	30.9
N-S-Ar (°)	124.6	123.7	124.9	124.7
S-Ar-Go (°)	140.2	152.9	140.1	157.9
Ar-Go-Me (°)	131.4	122.8	130	119.3
Sum (°)	396.2	399.4	395	401.9
Ar-Goi-Me (°)	125.8	116.6	125	114
Ar-Goi-N (°)	53.5	44.9	53.5	40.5
N-Goi-Me (°)	72.5	71.7	72.5	73.4
S-Go (mm)	63.5	64.9	68.5	71
Upper inc. to palatal P. (°)	109.8	112.2	109.5	103.8
Lower inc. to Go-Me (°)	90.8	91.1	90.1	101.6
Interincisal angle (°)	131.3	127.3	133.6	116.8
Upper inc. to A-Pog. (mm)	4.5	8.5	4.1	6.2
Lower inc. to A-Pog. (mm)	1.1	−1.4	0.9	3.5
Nasolabial angle (°)	109.4	108.8	110.5	113.6
Upper lip to E-plane (mm)	−2.8	0.8	−4	−2.1
Upper lip protrusion (mm)	3	6.2	3	4.9
Lower lip to E-plane (mm)	−1.9	−0.9	−2.9	0.8
Lower lip protrusion (mm)	2	2.3	2	5.4

produced by this appliance with those induced by other intraoral distalizing devices. It has to be emphasized, however, that the FCA cannot be considered as a completely compliance-free molar distalizing appliance. The collaboration required of the patient is minimal (one turn of a screw per day) and the screw is placed in a vestibular position that is extremely easy to reach for activation, especially when compared with other devices like the rapid maxillary expanders. However, treatment of Class II malocclusion with a nonextraction protocol using distalizing appliances can be carried out successfully only in patients who can guarantee a certain amount of collaboration. In fact, during the second phase of treatment with

fixed appliances, the patient may be asked to wear auxiliary devices (like Class II elastics or a facebow) for anchorage control.

The FCA is an efficient and reliable device for the unilateral or bilateral distalization of the maxillary permanent first molars. Both second deciduous molars and second premolars can be used as anchorage teeth.

The following treatment effects have been observed.

- The FCA produces rapid molar distalization as bilateral Class II molar relationship can be corrected in 2.4 months on average. Mean duration of treatment is shorter than that reported for other intraoral distalizing appliances and it is

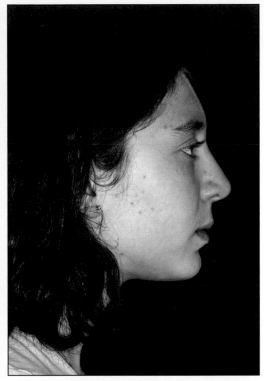

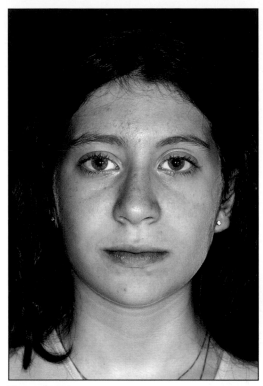

Figures 22.44, 22.45 Female patient AF. Posttreatment facial photographs.

Figure 22.45

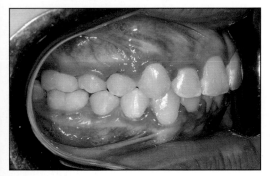

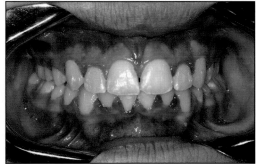

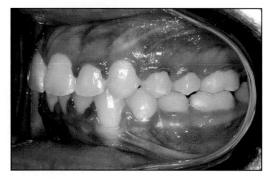

Figures 22.46–22.50 Female patient AF. Posttreatment intraoral photographs.

Figure 22.47

Figure 22.48

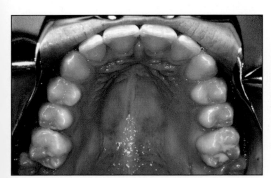

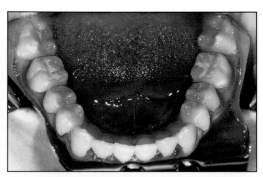

Figure 22.49

Figure 22.50

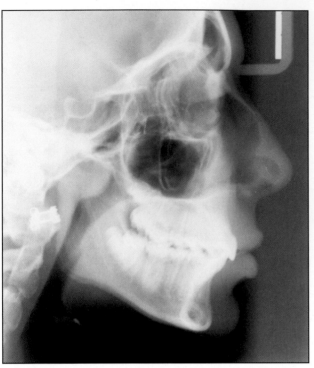

Figure 22.51 Female patient AF. Posttreatment cephalometric radiograph.

not influenced by the presence of erupted permanent second molars.

- The maxillary first molars can be moved distally an average of 4.0 mm/side with a mean distal tipping of 4.6°. These values are similar to those reported for other intraoral distalizing appliances.

- The FCA produces minimal anchorage loss. Anchorage loss measured at the second premolars is 1.7 mm on average with 2.2° of mesial tipping. The maxillary central incisors are proclined slightly during treatment (2.6°) with minimal increase in the overjet (1.2 mm). The maxillary molar distalization contributes to 70% of the space created anterior to the first molars, while 30% is due to reciprocal anchorage loss of the maxillary second premolars.

- No significant changes in either sagittal or vertical skeletal relationships can be observed.

Acknowledgements

The authors wish to thank Dr. Massimo Lupoli for his valuable help in the clinical and experimental testing of the FCA.

References

1. Kloehn SJ. Evaluation of cervical traction of the maxilla and upper first permanent molar. Angle Orthod 1961;31:91–104.

2. Hubbard GW, Nanda RS, Currier GF. A cephalometric evaluation of nonextraction cervical headgear treatment in Class II malocclusion. Angle Orthod 1994;64:359–370.

3. Haas AJ. Headgear therapy: the most efficient way to distalize molars. Semin Orthod 2000;6: 79–90.

4. Cetlin NM, Ten-Hoeve A. Nonextraction treatment. J Clin Orthod 1983;17:396–413.

5. Ferro F, Monsurro A, Perillo L. Sagittal and vertical changes after treatment of Class II division 1 malocclusion according to the Cetlin method. Am J Orthod Dentofacial Orthop 2000; 118:150–158.

6. Muse DS, Fillman MJ, Emmerson WJ, Mitchell RD. Molar and incisor changes with the Wilson rapid molar distalization. Am J Orthod Dentofacial Orthop 1993;103:556–565.

7. Rana R, Becher MK. Class II correction using the bimetric "distalizing" arch. Semin Orthod 2000;6:106–118.

8. Wilson WL, Wilson RC. Multi-directional 3D functional Class II treatment. J Clin Orthod 1987; 21:186–189.

9. Blechman AM. Magnetic force systems in orthodontics. Am J Orthod 1985;87:201–210.

10. Gianelly AA, Vaitas AS, Thomas WM. The use of magnets to move molars distally. Am J Orthod Dentofacial Orthop 1989;96:161–167.

11. Itoh T, Tokuda T, Kiyosue S, Hirose T, Matsumoto M, Chaconas SP. Molar distalization with repelling magnets. J Clin Orthod 1991;25:611–617.

12. Bondemark L, Kurol J. Distalization of maxillary first and second molars simultaneously with repelling magnets. Eur J Orthod 1992;14:264–272.

13. Bondemark L, Kurol J, Bernhold M. Repelling magnets versus superelastic nickel-titanium coils in simultaneous distal movement of maxillary first and second molars. Angle Orthod 1994;64:189–198.

14. Gianelly A, Bednar J, Dietz V. Japanese NiTi coils used to move molars distally. Am J Orthod Dentofacial Orthop 1991;99:564–566.

15. Gianelly A. A strategy for non extraction Class II treatment. Semin Orthod 1998;4:26–32.

16. Locatelli R, Bednar J, Dietz V, Giannelly A. Molar distalization with superelastic NiTi wire. J Clin Orthod 1992;26:277–279.

17. Jones R, White J. Rapid Class II molar correction with an open coil jig. J Clin Orthod 1992;26: 661–664.

18. Gulati S, Kharbanda OP, Prakash H. Dental and skeletal changes after intraoral molar distalization with sectional jig assembly. Am J Orthod Dentofacial Orthop 1998;114:319–327.

19. Runge ME, Martin JT, Bukai F. Analysis of rapid molar distal movement without patient cooperation. Am J Orthod Dentofacial Orthop 1999;115: 153–157.

20. Haydar S, Uner O. Comparison of Jones jig molar distalization appliance with extraoral traction. Am J Orthod Dentofacial Orthop 2000;117:49–53.

21. Brickman CD, Sinha PK, Nanda RS. Evaluation of the Jones jig appliance for distal molar movement. Am J Orthod Dentofacial Orthop 2000;118: 526–534.

22. Carano A, Testa M. The Distal Jet for upper molar distalization. J Clin Orthod 1996;30: 374–380.

23. Ngantung V, Nanda RS, Bowman SJ. Posttreatment evaluation of the distal jet appliance. Am J Orthod Dentofacial Orthop 2001;120:178–185.

24. Nishii Y, Hidenori K, Hideharu Y. Three-dimensional evaluation of the distal jet appliance. World J Orthod 2002;3:321–327.

25. Bolla E, Muratore F, Carano A, Bowman J. Evaluation of maxillary molar distalization with the distal jet: a comparison with other contemporary methods. Angle Orthod 2002;72:481–494.

26. Keles A. Maxillary unilateral molar distalization with sliding mechanics: a preliminary investigation. Eur J Orthod 2001;23:507–515.

27. Keles A, Pamukcu B. Bilateral maxillary molar distalization with sliding mechanics: Keles Slider. World J Orthod 2002;3:57–66.

28. Lanteri C, Beretta M, Lanteri V. Un nuovo dispositivo per la distalizzazione dei molari superiori: il Fast-back. Mondo Ortodon 2003;29:301–315.

29. Hilgers JJ. The Pendulum appliance for Class II non-compliance therapy. J Clin Orthod 1992;26: 700–703.

30. Ghosh J, Nanda RS. Evaluation of an intraoral maxillary molar distalization technique. Am J Orthod Dentofacial Orthop 1996;110:639–646.

31. Byloff FK, Darendeliler MA. Distal molar movement using the pendulum appliance. Part 1: clinical and radiological evaluation. Angle Orthod 1997;67:249–260.

32. Byloff FK, Darendeliler MA, Clar E, Darendeliler A. Distal molar movement using the pendulum appliance. Part 2: the effects of maxillary molar root uprighting bends. Angle Orthod 1997;67:261–270.

33. Bussick TJ, McNamara JA Jr. Dentoalveolar and skeletal changes associated with the pendulum appliance. Am J Orthod Dentofacial Orthop 2000;117:333–343.

34. Joseph AA, Butchart CJ. An evaluation of the pendulum "distalizing" appliance. Semin Orthod 2000;6:129–135.

35. Chaques-Asensi J, Kalra V. Effects of the pendulum appliance on the dentofacial complex. J Clin Orthod 2001;35:254–257.

36. Kinzinger G, Fuhrmann R, Gross U, Diedrich P. Modified pendulum appliance including distal screw and uprighting activation for non-compliance therapy of Class II malocclusion in children and adolescents. J Orofac Orthop 2000;61:175–190.

37. Kinzinger GSM, Fritz UB, Sander FG, Diedrich PR. Efficiency of a pendulum appliance for molar distalization related to second and third molar eruption stage. Am J Orthod Dentofacial Orthop 2004;125:8–23.

38. Kalra V. The K-loop molar distalizing appliance. J Clin Orthod 1995;24:298–301.

39. Keles A, Sayinsu K. A new approach in maxillary molar distalization: intraoral bodily molar distalizer. Am J Orthod Dentofacial Orthop 2000;117:39–48.

40. Fortini A, Lupoli M, Parri M. The First Class Appliance for rapid molar distalization. J Clin Orthod 1999;32:322–328.

41. Ricketts RM. Progressive cephalometrics: paradigm 2000. Scottsdale: American Institute for Bioprogressive Education; 1996.

42. Cisneros GJ. Molar Distalization: introduction. Semin Orthod 2000;6:77–78.

43. Fortini A, Lupoli M, Giuntoli F, Franchi L. Dentoskeletal effects induced by rapid molar distalization with the first class appliance. Am J Orthod Dentofacial Orthop 2004;125:697–705.

44. Pancherz H. The mechanism of Class II correction in Herbst appliance treatment: a cephalometric investigation. Am J Orthod 1982;82:104–113.

45. Andreasen G, Naessig C. Experimental findings on mesial relapse of maxillary first molars. Angle Orthod 1968;38:51–55.

46. Kanomi R. Mini-implant for orthodontic anchorage. J Clin Orthod 1997;31:763–767.

47. Costa A, Raffaini M, Melsen B. Miniscrews as orthodontic anchorage: a preliminary report. Int J Adult Orthod Orthogn Surg 1998;13:201–209.

48. Lee JS, Park HS, Kyung HM. Micro-implant anchorage for lingual treatment of a skeletal Class II malocclusion. J Clin Orthod 2001;35:643–647.

49. Maino BG, Mura P, Giannelly A. A retrievable palatal implant for absolute anchorage in orthodontics. World J Orthod 2002;3:125–134.

50. Lin JC, Liou EJ. A new bone screw for orthodontic anchorage. J Clin Orthod 2003;37:676–681.

51. Gianelly A. Distal movement of the maxillary molars. Am J Orthod Dentofacial Orthop 1998;114:66–72.

52. Bennett JC, McLaughlin RP. Orthodontic treatment mechanics and the preadjusted appliance. London: Wolfe Publishing; 1993.

53. Bennett JC, McLaughlin P. Orthodontic management of the dentition with the preadjusted appliance. Oxford: Isis Medical Media; 1997.

54. Philippe J. Mechanical analysis of Class II elastics. J Clin Orthod 1995;28:367–372.

CHAPTER 23

An effective and precise method for rapid molar derotation: Keles TPA

Ahmet Keles

CONTENTS

Introduction

A distal molar relationship could arise due to the mesiopalatal rotation of the maxillary molars. In some patients, an ideal Class I intercuspation can be achieved with the opposing molar and a Class II relationship can be corrected by molar derotation. The maxillary molars consist of three roots and due to the early loss of the deciduous second molars, the palatal root acts as a hinge for mesial rotation of the molars. Lemons & Holmes reported that a gain of 1–2 mm of arch length per side may be achieved following derotations.[1]

The transpalatal arch (TPA) for molar derotation was introduced to the orthodontic literature by Goshgarian.[2] Cetlin & Ten Hoeve showed that the TPA is an effective device to stabilize, rotate, and distalize the molars.[3] According to Ricketts, a line drawn from the distobuccal and mesiopalatal cusp tips of the first molars should pass through the cusp tip of the canines on the opposite side.[4] Investigators have assessed the shape of maxillary first molars and examined the arch length gain with derotation.[5–7] According to Braun et al, 2.1 mm arch length can be gained with the application of the TPA and an equivalent distal force at the level of the maxillary first molar center of resistance.[8]

The TPA can be removable or fixed, depending on the clinician's preference.

In 2003, we presented an effective method for rapid molar derotation by means of the Keles TPA.[9] Our aim in this study was to develop an easy method to rapidly and precisely rotate the maxillary molars.

TPA Construction

The maxillary first molars were banded with a Precision Lingual Hinge Cap Attachment (Ormco, Orange, CA), welded on their palatal aspect (Fig. 23.1). The hinge cap attachment is designed to accommodate 0.032 × 0.032″ wires. The TPA was constructed from the Burstone Lingual Arch System (Fig. 23.2), which was introduced to the orthodontic literature in 1988.[10–12] The wire consists of 0.032 × 0.032″ beta-titanium alloy (TMA, Ormco, Orange, CA). After the passive construction of the TPA, molar bands were cemented to the first molars (Figs 23.3 and 23.4) and the TPA was removed for activation (Fig. 23.5).

The method for activation is simple and precise. The TPA is placed on a piece of white paper and two lines are drawn along the terminal ends (rotating component) of the TPA with a black pen (Fig. 23.6). Additional lines are drawn with a 20° angle passing

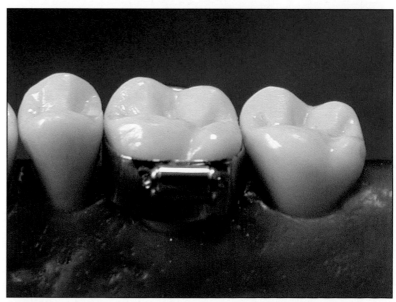

Figure 23.1 Maxillary first molars were banded with a Precision Lingual Hinge Cap Attachment welded on their palatal sides. *(From Keles & Impram,[9] with kind permission of Quintessence Publishing Co. Inc.)*

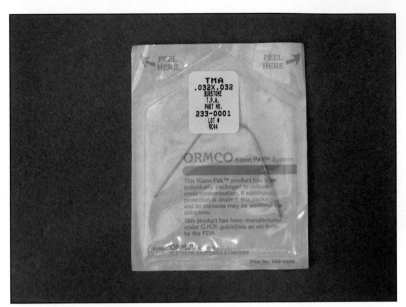

Figure 23.2 A transpalatal arch was constructed using the Burstone Lingual Arch System. *(From Keles & Impram,[9] with kind permission of Quintessence Publishing Co. Inc.)*

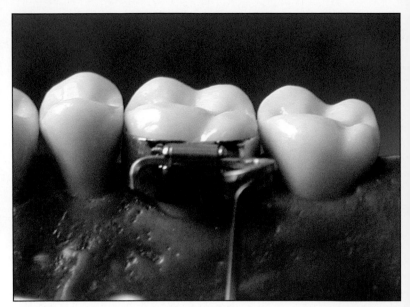

Figure 23.4 Palatal view of the TPA design. *(From Keles & Impram,[9] with kind permission of Quintessence Publishing Co. Inc.)*

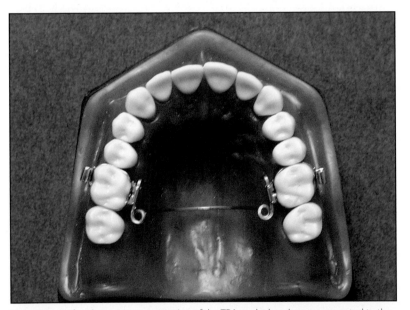

Figure 23.3 After the passive construction of the TPA, molar bands were cemented to the fist molars with the TPA. *(From Keles & Impram,[9] with kind permission of Quintessence Publishing Co. Inc.)*

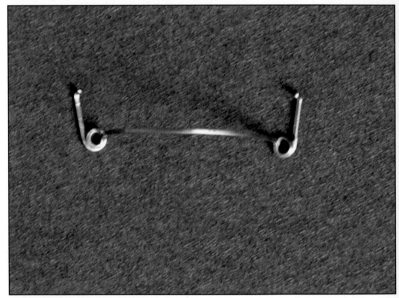

Figure 23.5 The TPA was removed for activation. *(From Keles & Impram,[9] with kind permission of Quintessence Publishing Co. Inc.)*

through the distal end of the helix of the wire. The TPA is activated on both sides with the help of a bird-beak plier (Fig. 23.7). The biomechanics of the force moment system is presented in Figure 23.8. Two equal and opposite moments are generated on both molars. Two equal and opposite forces are generated on both sides which would also help to increase the intermolar width between the mesial cusp tips of the first molars. The activation of the TPA is checked on both sides and then it is placed in the mouth (Figs 23.9 and 23.10).

Unilateral activation of a TPA, as described by Cetlin & Ten Hoeve,[3] would generate distal force on one side and rotation on the other side. After the correction of rotation of the molar on one side, Cetlin & Ten Hoeve recommend subsequent activation to rotate the molar on the other side a few months later. This would extend the treatment duration and generate unwanted distal forces. McNamara & Brudon have also indicated that the subsequent activation would generate a distal force on one side and rotation on the other side.[13]

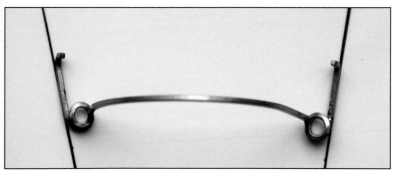

Figure 23.6 Passive stage. *(From Keles & Impram,[9] with kind permission of Quintessence Publishing Co. Inc.)*

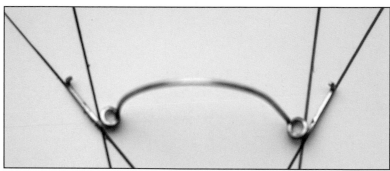

Figure 23.7 Active stage. *(From Keles & Impram,[9] with kind permission of Quintessence Publishing Co. Inc.)*

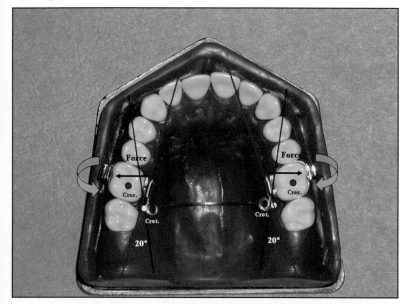

Figure 23.8 Biomechanics of the force moment system. *(From Keles & Impram,[9] with kind permission of Quintessence Publishing Co. Inc.)*

Case Study

DK was a female patient, 11 years and 3 months of age, diagnosed with edge-to-edge molar relationship. She was in the mixed dentition period and had crowding of 5.6 mm in the maxilla and 4.2 mm in the mandible. There was not adequate space for the eruption of the canines in the maxillary arch. Her maxillary first molars were severely rotated mesiopalatally. She had an 80% anterior deep bite. Her pretreatment intraoral pictures are presented in Figures 23.11–23.14.

The treatment goals were to derotate the maxillary molars, correct the deep bite, align the maxillary and mandibular arches, and achieve Class I molar and canine relationship.

The treatment was started with the engagement of the TPA and derotation of the maxillary first molars (Fig. 23.15). Twenty-degree anti-rotation bends were constructed on the TPA and 2 months later the rotations were corrected (Figs 23.16–23.18). After the

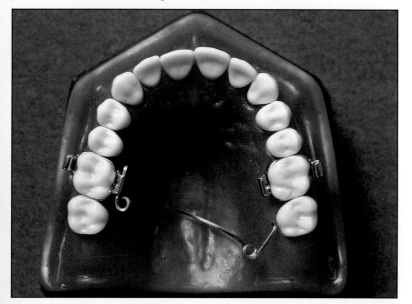

Figures 23.9, 23.10 The activation of the TPA is being checked on both sides. *(From Keles & Impram,[9] with kind permission of Quintessence Publishing Co. Inc.)*

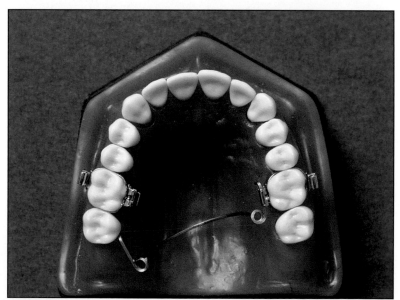

Figure 23.10

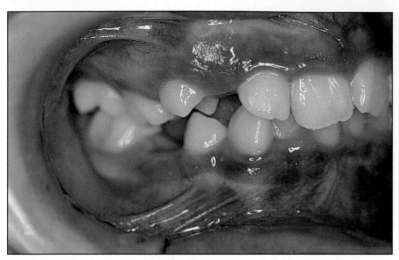

Figure 23.11 Patient 1, DK. Right intraoral photograph. *(From Keles & Impram,[9] with kind permission of Quintessence Publishing Co. Inc.)*

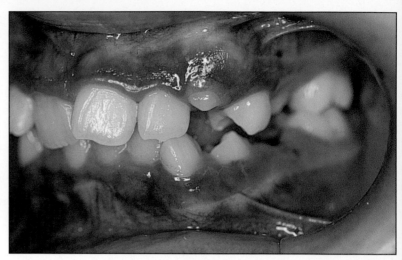

Figure 23.12 Patient 1, DK. Left intraoral photograph. *(From Keles & Impram,[9] with kind permission of Quintessence Publishing Co. Inc.)*

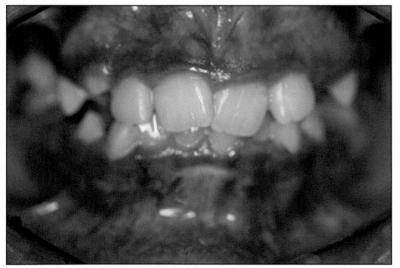

Figure 23.13 Patient 1, DK. Pretreatment anterior intraoral photograph. *(From Keles & Impram,[9] with kind permission of Quintessence Publishing Co. Inc.)*

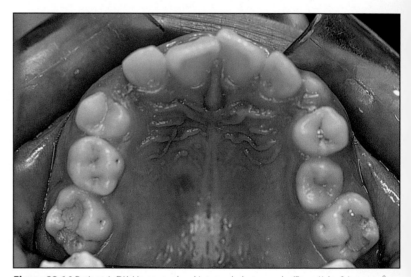

Figure 23.14 Patient 1, DK. Upper occlusal intraoral photograph. *(From Keles & Impram,[9] with kind permission of Quintessence Publishing Co. Inc.)*

placement of fixed appliances, the maxillary and mandibular arches were aligned and the deep bite was eliminated. At the end of orthodontic treatment, a Class I molar and canine relationship was achieved (Figs 23.19–23.22).

Discussion

The results showed that maxillary molars can be derotated effectively in 2–3 months. From a biomechanic point of view, the method described above has several advantages. With most techniques, due to the mesiopalatal rotation of molars, the molar width between the mesial cusp tips is decreased. The method described here increased the intermolar width between the mesial cusp tips of the molars and maintained the intermolar width on the distal (see Fig. 23.18). In fact, the subsequent use of the conventional TPA, which was described in the literature, would tend to decrease the intermolar width on the distal rather than increase intermolar width on the mesial.

With this approach, palatal hinge cup attachments were used instead of TPA sheaths. The hinge cup attachment opens and shuts easily, which makes the clinical application practical and dramatically

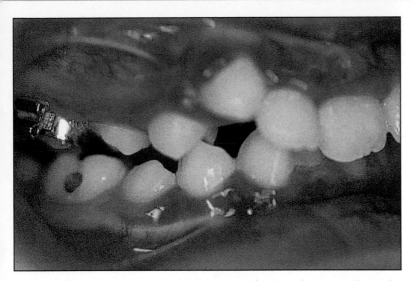

Figure 23.15 Patient 1, DK. Right intraoral photograph after the molar rotation. *(From Keles & Impram,[9] with kind permission of Quintessence Publishing Co. Inc.)*

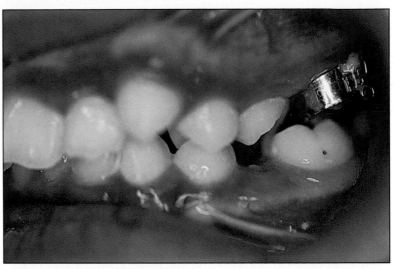

Figure 23.16 Patient 1, DK. Left intraoral photograph after the molar rotation. *(From Keles & Impram,[9] with kind permission of Quintessence Publishing Co. Inc.)*

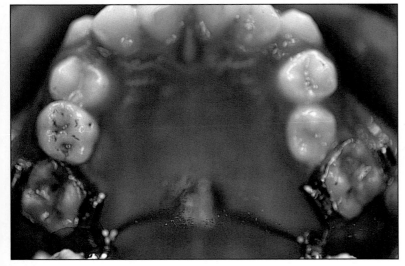

Figure 23.17 The TPA was engaged and derotation of the first molars initiated. *(From Keles & Impram,[9] with kind permission of Quintessence Publishing Co. Inc.)*

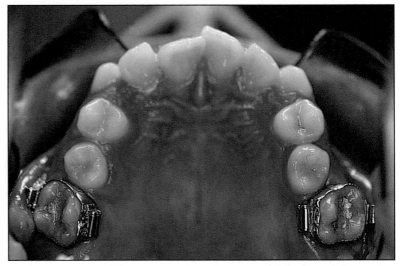

Figure 23.18 Patient 1, DK. Upper occlusal intraoral photograph after the molar rotation. *(From Keles & Impram,[9] with kind permission of Quintessence Publishing Co. Inc.)*

enhances TPA mechanics. In addition, this technique minimizes the difficulty of lingual wire insertion and removal. A secure lock over the wire eliminates the double-back bend and ligature ligation that is required in many applications of traditional TPAs. The hinge cup attachment has 12° built-in torque in its base, which makes it an equally appropriate choice for both passive and active TPA application. Some investigators prefer the soldered rather than removable TPA.[13] However, for bilateral molar rotation correction of the soldered ones, subsequent activation and repeated cementation are required in order to obtain the desired bilateral rotational result.

Square-sectioned beta-titanium alloy wire enables three-dimensional control of the molar movement. In contrast, the traditional TPA uses a round stainless steel wire. The other advantage of beta-titanium alloy wire is that it allows constant and long-lasting light force, without any plastic deformation.

In addition to rotating the molars effectively, after rapid palatal expansion this TPA can also be used to maintain and stabilize intermolar width and also to correct buccal crown tipping of molars by bilateral activation of the square-sectioned beta-titanium alloy wire for buccal root movement.

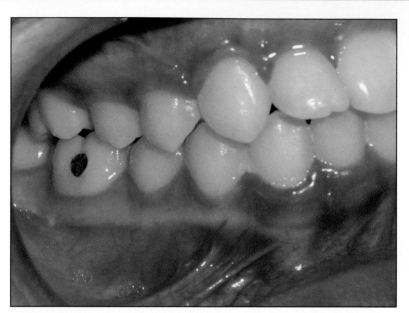

Figure 23.19 Patient 1, DK. Right intraoral photograph at the end of orthodontic treatment. *(From Keles & Impram,[9] with kind permission of Quintessence Publishing Co. Inc.)*

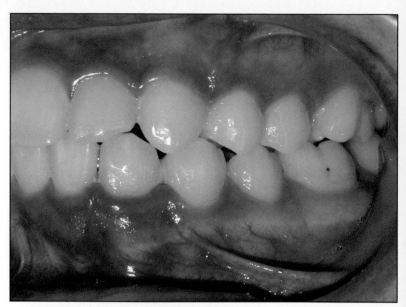

Figure 23.20 Patient 1, DK. Left intraoral photograph at the end of orthodontic treatment. *(From Keles & Impram,[9] with kind permission of Quintessence Publishing Co. Inc.)*

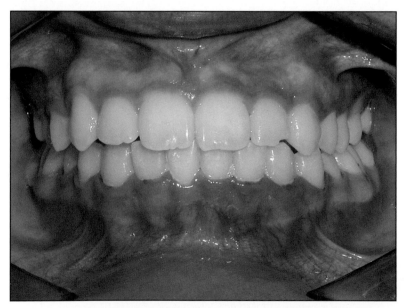

Figure 23.21 Patient 1, DK. Anterior intraoral photograph at the end of orthodontic treatment. *(From Keles & Impram,[9] with kind permission of Quintessence Publishing Co. Inc.)*

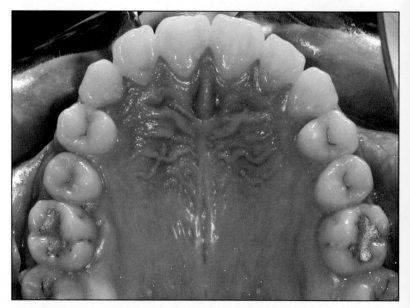

Figure 23.22 Patient 1, DK. Upper occlusal intraoral photograph at the end of orthodontic treatment. *(From Keles & Impram,[9] with kind permission of Quintessence Publishing Co. Inc.)*

Conclusion

With the Keles TPA, bilateral molar derotation can be achieved in a short period of time. From a biomechanic point of view, this method eliminated the subsequent activation process and also increased the reduced intermolar width between the mesial cusp tips of the molars.

References

1. Lemons FF, Holmes CW. The problem of the rotated maxillary first permanent molar. Am J Orthod 1961;47:246–272.

2. Goshgarian RA. Orthodontic palatal arch wires. Washington DC: United States Government Patent Office; 1972.

3. Cetlin NM, Ten Hoeve A. Nonextraction treatment. J Clin Orthod 1983;17:396–413.

4. Ricketts RM. Futures of light progressive technique. No. 5. Denver: Rocky Mountain Dental Products; 1972.

5. Cooke MS, Wreakes G. Molar derotation with a modified palatal arch: an improved technique. Br J Orthod 1978;5:201–203.

6. Orton HS. An evaluation of five methods of derotating upper molar teeth. Dent Pract Dent Rec 1966;16:279–286.

7. Rebellato J. Two-couple orthodontic appliance systems: transpalatal arches. Semin Orthod 1995; 1:44–54.

8. Braun S, Kusnoto B, Evans C. The effect of maxillary molar derotation on arch length. Am J Orthod Dentofacial Orthop 1997;112:538–544.

9. Keles A, Impram S. An effective and precise method for rapid molar derotation: Keles TPA. World J Orthod 2003;4:229–236.

10. Burstone CJ. Precision lingual arches. Active applications. J Clin Orthod 1989;23:101–109.

11. Burstone CJ. The precision lingual arch: hinge cap attachment. J Clin Orthod 1994;28:151–158.

12. Burstone CJ, Manhartsberger C. Precision lingual arches. Passive applications. J Clin Orthod 1988;22:444–451.

13. McNamara JA, Brudon W. Orthodontics and dentofacial orthopedics. Ann Arbor: Needham Press; 2002: 208.

SECTION FOUR

INTRAMAXILLARY APPLIANCES WITH ABSOLUTE ANCHORAGE USED FOR THE MANAGEMENT OF CLASS II MALOCCLUSION

This section includes chapters on the following:

Overview of the intramaxillary noncompliance appliances with absolute anchorage

Moschos A. Papadopoulos

Introduction

Stationary anchorage is often a prerequisite as well as an essential factor for the successful treatment of Class II malocclusions. Loss of stability of the anchoring teeth may lead to unfavorable occlusal relations and unsatisfactory treatment outcomes. Usually, extraoral appliances, such as headgears, or intraoral means, such as grouping of teeth or Nance appliances, can be used to reinforce anchorage. However, the use of headgears is often associated with compliance problems, while anchorage loss often occurs when intraoral modalities are used.

The continuing development of dental implants and their advantages in terms of stability have resulted in the introduction of implants for orthodontic purposes. During recent decades, many studies have shown that osseointegrated implants can resist applied forces, remaining stable after orthodontic loading.[1–18] Therefore, the use of endosseous implants for orthodontic purposes seems to be a significant alternative when maximum anchorage is required. Despite the obvious advantages of the use of implants over the other conventional methods regarding the preservation of anchorage during orthodontic treatment, the invasive technique needed for their insertion and removal remains a matter of criticism, which prevents their widespread use in everyday practice. In this respect, the introduction of new types of implants (such as mini-implants, mini-screws, and onplants), which are associated with less invasive methods than conventional implants, seems very promising to provide a stable anchorage for the treatment of Class II malocclusion in terms of posterior teeth distalization and/or anterior teeth retraction and intrusion (see Table 2.3).

In comparison to the conventional dental implants used mainly for prosthetic reasons, the application of orthodontic implants presents some differences. Orthodontic patients usually have complete dentitions and there is no available alveolar bone for the insertion of implants. Therefore, orthodontic implants need to be placed into other anatomic sites such as the palate,[19–23] the retromolar region,[3,24] or even the zygomatic region.[25] Due to the different bone characteristics in these regions, orthodontic implants have to present smaller dimensions, especially in length, but they still have to be stable in order to resist the application of orthodontic forces. Other important factors for a successful application of orthodontic implants include minimal strain on patients during insertion, active treatment and removal, the reliable fixation of orthodontic wires, and handling simplicity.[26]

Palatally Positioned Implants Used as Anchorage for Molar Distalization

Several implant systems have been used for maxillary molar distalization. These include the Graz Implant-Supported Pendulum (GISP), the Bioresorbable Implant Anchor for Orthodontics System (BIOS Implant System), the Straumann Orthosystem, the Frialit-2 Implant System, the Oric Implant System, short epithetic implants, anchorage screws, mini-screws and the Onplant System (see Table 2.3). These implants were combined with distalization appliances such as the Pendulum,[27–29] the Distal Jet Appliance,[28–30] the Keles Slider,[31] with a modified acrylic Nance button,[28] or with nickel-titanium coil springs and nickel-titanium wires.[28,29,32]

Bioresorbable Implant Anchor for Orthodontics System (BIOS Implant System)

Glatzmaier and colleagues were the first to introduce an implant-supported force system for molar distalization, the BIOS Implant System.[22,33] This consists of a biodegradable implant body and a variable metal abutment as superstructure. The implant body is fabricated from biodegradable polylactide and provides sufficient anchorage for 9–12 months until degraded. The design and dimensions of the BIOS implant originate from the ITI-Bonefit Screw Implant (Straumann, Waldenburg, Switzerland) with a fixture length of 6 mm.

Graz Implant-Supported Pendulum

Byloff et al[27] described the use of the Graz Implant-Supported Pendulum (GISP) (Mondeal Medical Systems, Tuttlingen, Germany) to distalize the maxillary first and second molars in adults. The GISP consists of two parts: the anchorage plate, which is fixed to the palatal bone via four mini-screws and incorporates two cylinders, and the removable part, which is a Pendulum-type appliance. The Nance button of the Pendulum Appliance has two cylindrical slots in the palatal surface, which correspond to the two cylinders of the anchorage plate. The system can be loaded 2 weeks after surgical placement, actively distalizes maxillary molars consecutively, serves as an active anchor unit, and provides stability against rotational movements. When the desired molar distalization has been achieved, the GISP can be used to maintain the molar position, not only passively but actively by exerting counteracting forces to the mesial forces exerted on the molars during retraction of the anterior teeth, thus providing active anchorage.[27]

Straumann Orthosystem

Giancotti et al[28,34] described the use of the Straumann Orthosystem (Straumann, Waldenburg, Switzerland) with a different stainless steel cap, for orthodontic appliance placement, from that used by Wehrbein et al.[21,26] The force necessary for molar distalization was applied either indirectly, by means of coil springs and nickel-titanium (NiTi) wires (see Figs 25.2–25.6), or directly by means of a modified Distal Jet Appliance, a modified Nance button, and a modified Pendulum Appliance (see Figs 25.7–25.10).

Frialit-2 Implant System

Keles et al[31] used the Frialit-2 Implant System (Synchro screw implants) (Friadent GmbH, Mannheim, Germany) as anchorage for molar distalization. The stepped screw titanium implant, 4.5 mm in diameter and 8 mm in length, was placed palatally, not in the mid-palatal suture but in the lateral side of the palatal suture (paramedian region). The paramedian region was selected to avoid the connective tissues of the palatine suture and because it is considered to be a suitable host site for implant placement. After 3 months of healing, the implant was osseointegrated and orthodontic treatment was initiated. Instead of a Nance button, the palatal implant was used for anchorage and a modified Keles Slider was used to distalize the maxillary molars.

Midplant System

Maino et al[29] described the use of the midplant system (HDC, Sarcedo, Italy) as absolute anchorage for maxillary molar distalization. The midplant consists of two parts: an endosseous portion, called the core, and a unit called the Orthodontic Implant Connection (Oric) that connects the core to the oral region (see Figs 25.11 and 25.12).

The core consists of a self-tapping titanium screw (3.75 mm in diameter) in five different lengths (4.5–8 mm), which is chemically treated with an acid etching process (bone lock etching) or with titanium plasma spray (TPS), and a disk (5.0 mm in diameter) as support flange. The thread is designed to be screwed into cancellous bone without damaging the insertion site. A threaded hole on the palatal surface of the core allows the attachment with the Oric.

There are two different types of orthodontic connecting system: the standard Orthodontic Implant Connection (Oric cap), which is made of titanium formed by a standard connector with a cylindrical shape fixed to a transpalatal bar (see Figs 25.14 and 25.15), and the Oric EA (easy application), which is a winged connection platform with a retaining hole providing a more flexible connection.

The implant is placed in the midpalatal region close to the maxillary first and second premolars and its length is selected according to the vertical height of the anterior part of the palate. The implant can be positioned in the palatal midline or in the paramedian area and is not orthodontically loaded for 4 months. Maino et al[29] demonstrated the use of the midplant system to distalize maxillary molars either with the indirect method, by means of Neosentalloy Coils and Sentalloy Wires, or with the direct method by means of a modified Pendulum Appliance and a Distal Jet Appliance.

Short Epithetic Implants

Bernhart et al[35] evaluated the efficacy of short epithetic implants for orthodontic anchorage positioned in the paramedian region of the palate of 21 patients, avoiding the anterior palatine suture. The flange fixture used (Branemark, Nobel Biocare, Sweden) is made of commercial pure titanium and has a diameter of 3.75 mm. The self-tapped screw-shaped endosseous part of the implant has a length of 3–4 mm. A perforated flange 5.5 mm in diameter is placed above the endosseous portion. An external hexagon is mounted on the flange to prevent rotation of the threaded abutment, on which the orthodontic construction can be screwed. After a mean period of 4 months with unloaded healing, the implants were subjected to direct or indirect orthodontic loading, aiming among other things to distalize the maxillary molars. After completion of orthodontic treatment, the implants were removed by simple counter-clockwise rotation with a defined torque using the reinserted insertion post. According to the authors, short epithetic implants are suitable for achieving maximum anchorage in the paramedian region of the hard palate during orthodontic treatment.

Anchorage Screw

Karaman et al[30] presented an implant-supported modified Distal Jet Appliance for maxillary molar distalization. The implant used was an anchorage screw (Stryker Leibinger, Freiburg, Germany) 3 mm in diameter and 14 mm long, which was placed under local anesthesia at the anterior palatal suture 2–3 mm posterior to the canalis incissivus. Stainless steel tubes of 1 mm in diameter (Dentaurum, Ispringen, Germany) were adjusted to the implant, 0.8 mm anchor wires were soldered to the tubes for occlusal rests on the first premolars, and 0.9 mm wires extended through each tube, ending in a bayonet bend, were placed into the palatal tube of the maxillary first molar bands. The connection between the implant and the tubes was secured with composite material to minimize plaque retention and to increase the stability of the modified Distal Jet. Nickel-titanium open coil springs delivered the distalization force to the first molars. When the desired distal molar movement was obtained, the implant screw was removed without anesthesia and with no discomfort for the patient.

According to Karaman et al,[30] the main advantages of the appliance include its ability to achieve adequate distal movement of the first maxillary molars without anchorage loss, its stability against rotational movements, the possibility of immediate loading, active bilateral or unilateral force application, and ease of insertion and removal.

Mini-Screws

Kyung et al[36] used mini-screws positioned in the midpalate for molar distalization. These mini-screws can be easily inserted with an engine-driven screwdriver in low speed, while their removal is also easy. In addition, orthodontic forces can be applied immediately after implant placement without waiting for osseointegration. Transpalatal arches can be attached to the mini-screws and distal molar movement takes place with the indirect method.

Onplant System

Bondemark et al[32] described the use of the Onplant System for absolute anchorage during molar distalization. The Onplant (Nobel Biocare, Gothenburg, Sweden) is a thin titanium disk 7.7 mm in diameter and 2 mm thick (see Figs 26.3 and 26.4) which is inserted subperiosteally under local anesthesia (see Fig. 26.5). The surface of the Onplant that contacts the bone is coated with a layer of hydroxyapatite 75 μm thick, which enhances osseointegration. The surface that faces the soft tissues consists of smooth titanium alloy

with an external hexagon which is protected by a cover screw and is used for abutment connection.

The matching transmucosal abutment is placed 16 weeks after onplant placement and is composed of two parts, an internal hexagon towards the implant and an internal double hexagon facing the cylinder, thus allowing attachment of a transpalatal bar. According to Bondemark et al,[32] this construction allows rotational stability in all dimensions. The stainless steel transpalatal bar 1.3 mm in diameter is welded with metal mesh on the ends to allow bonding to the palatal surfaces of the anchorage teeth (see Fig. 26.11). In addition, two stainless steel sectional arches 0.017 × 0.025″ are attached bilaterally to the brackets on the maxillary second premolars and the tubes on the first and second molars. Nickel-titanium open coil springs inserted on the sectional wires deliver the distalization force. The appliance is reactivated every 6 weeks.

When molar distalization is complete, the transpalatal bar is replaced by a new one bonded on the onplant and the maxillary first molars, which retains their position during retraction of the anterior teeth (see Fig. 26.12).

Palatally Positioned Implants Used as Posterior Anchorage for Anterior Teeth Retraction

Some of the implant systems described above, such as the Straumann Orthosystem, the Midplant System, and the short epithetic implants, are not indicated solely for maxillary molar distalization but can also serve as absolute anchorage for anterior teeth retraction.[21,26,28,29,34,35,37] For the same purpose, different types of mini-screws, onplants or mini-implants have been used by various authors.[38–42] Summaries of these applications are presented in Table 2.3.

Buccally Positioned Implants Used as Posterior Anchorage for Anterior Teeth Retraction

Implant systems, such as mini-screws positioned buccally[38,43–45] or mini-plates positioned at the zygomatic region,[25,46] have also been developed and used as absolute anchorage by some authors to distalize the posterior segments or to retract anterior teeth (see Figs 25.16–25.21). These applications are shown in summary in Table 2.3.

References

1. Roberts WE, Smith RK, Zilberman Y, Mozsary PG, Smith RS. Osseous adaptation to continuous loading of rigid endosseous implants. Am J Orthod 1984;86:95–111.
2. Roberts WE, Helm FR, Marshal KJ, Gongloff RK. Rigid endosseous implants for orthodontic and orthopedic anchorage. Angle Orthod 1989;59:247–256.
3. Roberts WE, Marshall KJ, Mossary PG. Rigid endosseous implant utilized as anchorage to protract molars and close an atrophic extraction site. Angle Orthod 1990;60:135–152.
4. Turley PK, Kean C, Sehur J, et al. Orthodontic force application to titanium endosseous implants. Angle Orthod 1988;58:151–162.
5. Shapiro P, Kokich V. Use of implants in orthodontics. Clin Oral Impl Res 1988;32:65–75.

6. Smalley WM, Shapiro PA, Hohl TH, Kokich VG, Branemark PI. Osseointegrated titanium implants for maxillofacial protraction in monkeys. Am J Orthod Dentofacial Orthop 1988;94:285–295.

7. Odman J, Lekholm U, Jemt T, Branemark PI, Thilander B. Osseointegrated titanium implants – a new approach in orthodontic treatment. Eur J Orthod 1988;10:98–105.

8. Odman J, Grondahl K, Lekholm U, Thilander B. The effect of osseointegrated implants on the dento-alveolar development. A clinical and radiographic study in growing pigs. Eur J Orthod 1991;13:279–286.

9. Odman J, Lekholm U, Jemt T, Thilander B. Osseointegrated implants as orthodontic anchorage in the treatment of partially edentulous adult patients. Eur J Orthod 1994;16:187–201.

10. Linder-Aronson S, Nordenram A, Anneroth G. Titanium implant anchorage in orthodontic treatment an experimental investigation in monkeys. Eur J Orthod 1990;12:414–419.

11. Haanaes HR, Stenvik A, Beyer Olsen ES, Tryti T, Faehn O. The efficacy of two-stage titanium implants as orthodontic anchorage in the preprosthodontic correction of third molars in adults: a report of three cases. Eur J Orthod 1991;13:287–292.

12. Thilander B, Odman J, Grondahl K, Lekholm U. Aspects on osseointegrated implants inserted in growing jaws. A biometric and radiographic study in the young pig. Eur J Orthod 1992;14:99–109.

13. Thilander B, Odman J, Grondahl K, Friberg B. Osseointegrated implants in adolescents. An alternative in replacing missing teeth? Eur J Orthod 1994;16:84–95.

14. Wehrbein H, Diedrich P. Endosseous titanium implants during and after orthodontic load. An experimental study in the dog. Clin Oral Implants Res 1993;4:76–82.

15. Sennerby L, Odman J, Lekholm U, Thilander B. Tissue reactions towards titanium implants inserted in growing jaws. A histological study in the pig. Clin Oral Impl Res 1993;4:65–75.

16. Southard TE, Buckley MJ, Spivey JD, Krizan KE, Casko JS. Intrusion anchorage potential of teeth versus rigid endosseous implants a clinical and radiographic evaluation. Am J Orthod 1995;107:115–120.

17. Chen J, Chen K, Garetto LP, Roberts WE. Mechanical response to functional and therapeutic loading of a retromolar endosseous implant used for orthodontic anchorage to mesially translate mandibular molars. Implant Dent 1995;4:246–258.

18. Melsen B, Lang NP. Biological reactions of alveolar bone to orthodontic loading of oral implants. Clin Oral Impl Res 2001;12:144–152.

19. Triaca A, Antonini M, Wintermantel E. Ein neues Titan-Flachschrauben-Implantat zur orthodontischen Verankerung am anterioren Gaumen. Inf Orthod Kieferorthop 1992;24:251–257.

20. Wehrbein H. Enossale Titanimplantate als orthodontische Verankerungselemente. Experimentelle Untersuchungen und klinische Anwendung. Fortschr Kieferorhop 1994;5:236–250.

21. Wehrbein H, Glatzmaier J, Mundwiller U, Diedrich P. The orthosystem: a new implant system for orthodontic anchorage in the palate. J Orofac Orthop 1996;57:142–153.

22. Glatzmaier J, Wehrbein H, Diedrich P. Die Entwicklung eines resorbierbaren Implantatsystems zur orthodontischen Verankerung. Fortschr Kieferorthop 1995;56:175–181.

23. Abels N, Schiel HJ, Hery-Langer G, Neugebauer J, Engel M. Bone condensing in the placement of endosteal palatal implants: a case report. Int J Oral Maxillofac Implants 1999;14:849–852.

24. Higuchi KW, Slack JM. The use of titanium fixtures for intraoral anchorage to facilitate orthodontic tooth movement. Int J Oral Maxillofac Implants 1991;6:338–344.

25. Erverdi N, Tosun T, Keles A. A new anchorage site for the treatment of anterior open bite: zygomatic anchorage. A case report. World J Orthod 2002;3:147–153.

26. Wehrbein H, Merz BR, Diedrich P, Glatzmaier J. The use of palatal implants for orthodontic anchorage. Design and clinical application of the orthosystem. Clin Oral Implants Res 1996;7:410–416.

27. Byloff FK, Karcher H, Clar E, Stoff F. An implant to eliminate anchorage loss during molar distalization: a case report involving the Graz implant-supported pendulum. Int J Adult Orthod Orthognath Surg 2000;15:129–137.

28. Giancotti A, Muzzi F, Greco M, Arcuri C. Palatal implant-supported distalizing devices: clinical application of the Straumann Orthosystem. World J Orthod 2002;3:135–139.

29. Maino BG, Mura P, Gianelly AA. A retrievable palatal implant for absolute anchorage in orthodontics. World J Orthod 2002;3:125–134.

30. Karaman AI, Basciftci FA, Polat O. Unilateral distal molar movement with an implant-supported distal jet appliance. Angle Orthod 2002;72:167–174.

31. Keles A, Erverdi N, Sezen S. Bodily distalization of molars with absolute anchorage. Angle Orthod 2003;73:471–482.

32. Bondemark L, Feldmann I, Feldmann H. Distal molar movement with an intra-arch device provided with the onplant system for absolute anchorage. World J Orthod 2002;3:117–124.

33. Glatzmaier J, Wehrbein H, Diedrich P. Biodegradable implants for orthodontic anchorage. A preliminary biomechanical study. Eur J Orthod 1996;18:465–469.

34. Giancotti A, Muzzi F, Santini F, Arcuri C. Straumann Orthosystem method for orthodontic anchorage: step-by-step procedure. World J Orthod 2002;3:140–146.

35. Bernhart T, Freudenthaler J, Dortbudak O, Bantleon HP, Watzek G. Short epithetic implants for orthodontic anchorage in the paramedian region of the palate. A clinical study. Clin Oral Implants Res 2001;12:624–631.

36. Kyung SH, Hong SG, Park YC. Distalization of maxillary molars with a midpalatal miniscrew. J Clin Orthod 2003;37:22–26.

37. Bantleon H-P, Bernhart T, Crismani AG, Zachrisson BU. Stable orthodontic anchorage with palatal osseointegrated implants. World J Orthod 2002;3:109–116.

38. Costa A, Raffainl M, Melsen B. Miniscrews as orthodontic anchorage: a preliminary report. Int J Adult Orthodon Orthognath Surg 1998;13:201–209.

39. Lee JS, Park HS, Kyung HM. Micro-implant anchorage for lingual treatment of a skeletal Class II malocclusion. J Clin Orthod 2001;35:643–647.

40. Block MS, Hoffman DR. A new device for absolute anchorage for orthodontics. Am J Orthod Dentofacial Orthop 1995;107:251–258.

41. Celenza F, Hochman MN. Absolute anchorage in orthodontics: direct and indirect implant-assisted modalities. J Clin Orthod 2000;34:397–402.

42. Fritz U, Diedrich P, Kinzinger G, Al-Said M. The anchorage quality of mini-implants towards translatory and extrusive forces. J Orofac Orthop 2003;64:293–304.

43. Kanomi R. Mini-implant for orthodontic anchorage. J Clin Orthod 1997;31:763–767.

44. Maino BG, Bednar J, Pagin P, Mura P. The spider screw for skeletal anchorage. J Clin Orthod 2003;27:90–97.

45. Park HS, Bae SM, Kyung HM, Sung JH. Micro-implant anchorage for treatment of skeletal Class I bioalveolar protrusion. J Clin Orthod 2001;35:417–422.

46. De Clerck H, Geerinckx V, Siciliano S. The zygoma anchorage system. J Clin Orthod 2002;36:455–459.

CHAPTER 25

The use of implants as absolute anchorage for Class II correction

Aldo Giancotti, Claudio Arcuri

Introduction

Osseointegration Concepts

The clinical use of endosseous implants has expanded rapidly over the last 20 years. The increasingly predictable success of implants has resulted in a wider application in dentistry.

Implants for dental use were introduced by Albrektson et al[1] who suggested that obtaining a stable implant unit necessitated creating a close connection between the implant and the bone, when the current practice was to create a connection in soft tissue. Their research focused substantially on three determining parameters: the implant shape, the surface features, and the implant features. The shape of the implant was cylindrical to better distribute the masticatory loading, the implant was made of pure titanium (from grade 2 to 4), but the critical factor seemed to be the surface features.

The implant surface can be treated in order to stimulate osseointegration. Two different methods are available: implants can be sandblasted and acid etched (SLA) or covered with plasma spray (TPS). Both methods were demonstrated to create a close connection of the implant to the bone.[2,3]

The critical determinant of endosseous implant performance is the response of the bone interface and the supporting bone to functional and therapeutic loads. The adaptive reaction to implant insertion involves a change in osseous tissue mass, architecture, and mechanical features of the supporting bone. When an implant is placed in the cortical bone, the initial healing reaction is the formation of a woven bone callus at the periosteal and endosteal surfaces. After capturing subperiosteal bone vessels in a lattice of woven bone, the primary callus then fills the paravascular space with high-quality lamellar bone by a physiologic process called lamellar compaction. This maturation of the primary bone results in rigid stabilization of the implant. Little is known about the mineralization patterns of the rapidly evolving bone which supports implants in the healing phase.[4]

After initial callus formation, bone adaptation occurs around the integrated dental implant by cancellous compaction and remodeling. Osseous adaptation is essential for the long-term stability and integrity of the bone–implant interface; remodeling replaces the nonvital bone adjacent to a recently installed implant through an accelerated response which is a regional acceleratory phenomenon. This healing reaction is called osseointegration, defined as the direct contact between a dental implant and surrounding bone without an intervening fibrous tissue layer at the interface.[5] Implant survival and success depend on maintaining the integrity of the bone–implant interface. To ensure a valid resistance to continuous loading, such as conventional orthodontic forces,[6] an osseointegration of 10% should be present between the implant surface and the nearby bone.[7,8] Osseointegrated implants preserve their stability even with continuous bone remodeling as bone turnover involves only a small part of the implant surface at any one time.[9,10]

Implants in Orthodontics

Apart from the conventional use of dental implants in providing support and retention for dental restorations, endosseous implants have assumed a new role as an alternative type of rigid osseous anchorage for orthodontic treatment. Traditionally, the successful outcome of orthodontic treatment has been dependent on a number of factors such as the availability of tooth-bone anchorage, patient compliance in wearing supplemental appliances (headgear, etc.), and the potential for further maxillofacial growth.[11,12] The anchorage planning often represents a critical and not yet clinically predictable phase of orthodontic treatment. Anchorage control systems commonly used by orthodontists are often limited by the fact that the success of the therapy relies on patient cooperation. This includes the risk of reducing the possibility of a successful clinical result. Endosseous implants can offer a direct rigid fixation to the alveolar process so there is no reciprocal movement during the treatment and no need for patient compliance.[13]

Implants used for orthodontic purposes can be divided into three different groups depending on the implant position:

- alveolar process implants
- retromolar implants
- palatal implants.

The traditional implant is positioned in the edentulous area of the alveolar process and then used as an anchorage unit. Many authors have studied the implant reaction to orthodontic loading in vitro and in vivo. The first experimental study, carried out in 1978 by Sherman, investigated the reaction of a vitreous carbon dental implant subjected to orthodontic load in dogs, when no healing period was allowed; the carbon implant was not stable and exfoliated.[14]

In 1983 Gray et al fitted two different types of implants (vitallium implant and bioglass-coated implant) in rabbits and tested their stability when subjected to orthodontic forces after 28 days of healing; no movement was noted.[15]

In 1984 Roberts et al studied bone adaptation in rabbits, after 6–10 weeks of healing, to continuous force application by means of a 100 g stainless steel coil spring placed between the implants. All implants tested remained rigid, revealing that 6 weeks' healing is an adequate time to create a rigid osseous surface around the implant.[9] The same group of researchers investigated, in 1989, the osseointegration of implants placed in dogs' mandibles and loaded with 3 N (more than 300 g) for 13 weeks; the 94% of implants with less than 10% of the endosseous interface in direct contact with bone successfully remained rigid.[13]

In 1988 Turley et al placed implants in dogs, evaluating the reaction to orthodontic and orthopedic forces; the implants remained stable under a 300 g force application for 10 weeks and provided 4 mm of movement.[16]

Wehrbein & Diedrich confirmed these series of experimental studies in dogs in 1993, achieving a rigid osseointegration after 26 weeks of force application of 2 N (more than 200 g).[17]

In 1995, Southard et al studied the adaptation of implants to orthodontic intrusive movement in the dog mandible, loading the implants with a 100 g force by means of an orthodontic arch with V-bends for a period of 16 weeks.[18] The implant remained stable while the teeth were intruded.

More recently, Saito et al assessed the different reaction to loading of two implants inserted in the dog mandible on different sides.[19] After the osseointegration period, one implant was loaded by means of an orthodontic sectional fixed appliance on the teeth with a loop exerting 200 g for a period of 32 weeks, while the other implant was not loaded. After 32 weeks, on the activated side the teeth were moved distally but at histologic examination no differences in bone volume were present around the loaded implant or the control implant.

Ohmae et al used the same criteria to test mini-implants placed in the alveolar bone of dog mandible to intrude a group of teeth, exerting 150 g for 18 weeks, while three other mini-implants were inserted but not loaded.[20] Histologic examination confirmed that calcification around the loaded mini-implants was the same as for the control group.

Further, Melsen & Costa performed a histomorphometric analysis of tissue reactions around implants subjected to a well-defined force system.[21] It was found that loading significantly influenced both the turnover and the density of the alveolar bone in the proximity of the implants. However, even unloaded implants tended to maintain the bone characteristics of the alveolar process.

Clinical studies were performed using implants inserted in the alveolar process in the edentulous area in order to achieve absolute anchorage control during traditional orthodontic movements. The first study was performed by Odman et al in 1988 using the implant anchorage to gain extrusion of a maxillary impacted canine.[22] The following year, Van Roekel used a traditional implant for orthodontic anchorage to correct a cross-bite relationship between a mandibular canine and a maxillary lateral incisor.[23]

In 1993 Stean illustrated the advantages of using implant anchorage during traditional orthodontic treatment (crowding resolution) and using the implant for fixed prosthetic reasons.[24] Odman et al in 1994 applied implants in nine edentulous patients and tested implant resistance to orthodontic movements such as tipping, torquing, rotation, intrusion, extrusion, and bodily movement.[25] Biometric and radiographic assessment confirmed that the implants remained fixed during different kinds of orthodontic loading; at the end of the orthodontic phase, the implants served as prosthetic fixtures.

Sorenson published a clinical report in 1995 describing the use of implants for Class II elastic anchorage.[26] Prosterman et al in the same year reported a case of severe open bite malocclusion due to loss of the anterior alveolar process treated with orthodontics and maxillofacial surgery by an implant-bearing prosthesis.[27] Kokich in 1996 illustrated the advantages of using implants for orthodontic anchorage in patients who do not present sufficient anchorage units.[28,29]

In 1991 Haanaes et al tested the efficacy of two-stage titanium implants as orthodontic anchorage for preprosthodontic correction of third molars in adults.[30] The same year Higuchi & Slack used implants as rigid anchorage units in the treatment of various types of malocclusion by the application of 150–400 g loading on the implant. The fixed anchorage unit remained stable.[31]

Research into implant application in orthodontics has been directed at finding an alternative site insertion in order to use the implant anchorage not only in edentulous patients but also in full dentition patients.[32] Following this tendency, Roberts et al reported in 1990 the application of an implant in the retromolar area distally to the second mandibular molar to obtain mesial translation of the second and third molars to close a first molar extraction site. Rates of unidirectional space closure for mandibular second molars were assessed with periapical radiographs. At the end of treatment, the implant remained stable and a large bone remodeling was visible close to the mandibular molar.[33,34]

The introduction of osseointegrated implants has definitely changed the use of anchorage but conventional implants as well as retromolar implants cannot always cover the spread of applications in orthodontics. The introduction of titanium mini-implants inserted in the midsagittal area of the palate has widened implant application in orthodontic anchorage. The particular histologic characteristics of the palate and its proximity to the nasal cavity required additional research to create a smaller, nonconventional implant, in respect to hard and soft tissues. The advantage of delayed loading consists of achieving osseointegration of the palatal mini-implant and absolute anchorage control as osseointegrated implants remained stable under orthodontic loading. However, a limitation of this kind of loading is that it needs a healing period of 3–4 months, during which the implants must not be loaded to guarantee the osseointegration. In order to avoid undesired effects on the implant, a removable protective appliance is normally used.

Triaca et al investigated a screw-type implant with a height (H) of 3 mm and a diameter (D) of 7.5 mm. They achieved results in relation to bone height but the implant caused invasion of soft tissue.[35]

Block & Hoffman[36] and later Bondemark et al[37] introduced a subperiostal disk (H 2 mm, D 10 mm), covered with a thick coat of hydroxyapatite (75 µm) on one side and smooth titanium on the other side with a trimming hole for implant connection.

Wehrbein and coworkers in collaboration with the Straumann Institute presented the Orthosystem, a sand-blasted and chemically treated (SLA) mini-implant that is smaller (D 3.3 mm) but longer than former types (4 or 6 mm).[17,38–43] In 2002, Giancotti et al showed first the step-by-step procedure of the Straumann Orthosystem insertion in the midpalatal area and then the application of distalizing devices supported by palatal implants.[44,45] Recently, the same authors illustrated the application of a palatal implant in extraction treatment.[46] In 2000, Bernhart et al examined dental computed tomography (CT) as a method for preimplant surgical bone volume measurement in order to avoid overestimating the amount of bone available for implants in the median hard palate and to better visualize the incisive canal.[47]

In 2002, Maino et al presented the midplant system which is composed of three parts: the core, which is a self-tapping titanium screw and a disk (D 5 mm) as support flange, chemically treated (TPS), in five lengths (4.5 mm, 5 mm, 6 mm, 7 mm, 8 mm); the Orthodontic Implant Connection (Oric), made of titanium formed by a standard connector with a cylindric shape fixed to a transpalatal bar; and the Oric EA, a winged connection platform with retaining hole for a more flexible connection.[48]

Schlegel et al indicated in 2002 the anatomic features which characterize the palatal midline region.[49] As their histologic studies showed, the palatal suture was less often ossified in the direction of the anterior nasal spine than the posterior nasal spine, and therefore the authors suggested that the distal area of the palatal suture was more suitable as an implant insertion site. Keles et al illustrated, in 2003, the characteristics of a midpalatal implant used for orthodontic anchorage in extraction cases and space-opening procedures; the surgical insertion was planned by a three-dimensional template.[50] Tosun et al illustrated the application of the Keles Appliance connected to a palatal osseointegrated implant; space opening was achieved and no anchorage loss was evident at the end of distalization.[51]

Finally, Celenza presented his clinical experience with a midpalatal endosseous implant connected to the teeth by means of a transpalatal bar; the advantage of the absolute anchorage permits en masse movements, thus shortening treatment time.[52]

Correction of Class II Molar Relationship Using Absolute Anchorage: Delayed and Immediate Loading

Several appliances with different implant methods have been proposed to gain space by means of molar distalization in the maxillary arch. For this purpose, the palatal implant offers two different options: it can be directly connected to the teeth that have to be moved by means of a distalizing device (*direct method*), so that the reaction forces are completely dissipated on the implant. Alternatively, the palatal implant can be used as a reinforcement anchorage unit, by means of a transpalatal bar connecting the first premolars and the implant; in this way the reaction forces are dissipated on the dental/implant unit (*indirect method*).

Delayed Loading Procedure

In this section two different procedures that use palatal implants for anchorage reinforcement will be described: the Straumann Orthosystem and the Midplant System. Both of these techniques require a healing period of 3–4 months, careful diagnostic planning, accurate preparation of the surgical site and no implant loading during the osseointegration period.

The Straumann Orthosystem

In 1996, Wehrbein et al presented the Orthosystem (Istitut Straumann, Waldenburg, Switzerland), a sand-blasted and chemically treated (SLA) mini-implant that is thinner (D 3.3 mm) but longer (4 or 6 mm) than conventional implants.[17,38–43] They have also investigated the midsagittal area of the palate as a valid insertion site, in spite of its bone thickness. The results suggested that vertical bone support was at least 2 mm higher than apparent on the cephalogram, so the risk of perforation of the nasal cavity was limited. Apart from the median sagittal position, the paramedian region might be a suitable host site if a relatively low vertical bone support is evident in the cephalogram.

In our clinical experience, we followed the indications given by Wehrbein et al in verifying the surgical site on a lateral cephalogram, which is a normally requested examination in orthodontic patients. However, we suggest that 6 mm implants should be used with caution, prescribing an additional dental CT. We use the following parameters for the radiologic assessment (Fig. 25.1).

- The position of the implant in relation to the section of palate. The distance between the incisive canal and posterior nasal spine (PNS) is divided into three sections; the anterior portion

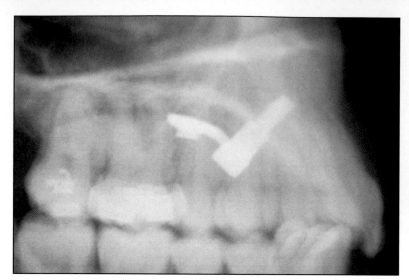

Figure 25.1 Radiologic parameters: palatal bone height assessment on a lateral cephalogram.

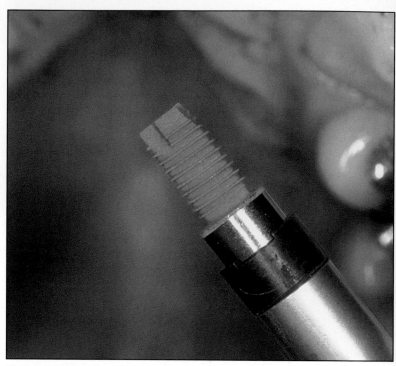

Figures 25.2, 25.3 Characteristics of the palatal mini-implant: self-thread intraosseous screw (SLA) (L. 6 mm).

is the most suitable because preimplant surgical examinations of the anterior palate have shown that the vertical bone volume decreases posteriorly. The smallest mean value, which can be explained by the direct vicinity of the incisive canal, is excluded from this trend, although Henriksen et al proved that approximately 50% of cases still had the requisite minimum 4 mm of bone inferior to the incisive canal.[53]

- The angle between the implant axis and the palatal plane and the distance between the most cranial border of the implant and the most cranial border of the palatal complex. The angulation of the implant has a considerable influence on the remaining vertical bone height. The lower the angle between the anterior and posterior nasal spine plane (ANS-PNS) and the implant axis, the wider will be the bone available. Because of this, the angulation cannot be selected freely but the implant should be inserted approximately orthogonal to the buccal surface of palate.

A reference line is constructed perpendicular to the palatal plane and passing through the point representing the most cranial border of the palatal complex (MCBPC). The distance between the most cranial border of the implant (MCBI) and the MCBPC should be the largest possible. In fact, the smaller the angle between ANS-PNS and the implant axis, the more residual bone is available above the MCBI (see Fig. 25.1).

By following these parameters of planning and choosing the right length of implant, the risk of a perforation to the nasal cavity can be minimized or even avoided. However, if a slight perforation of the bony structure occurs, the thick nasal mucosa should prevent an open connection.

In addition, the topographic position relative to the neighboring root, which represents a limiting factor for implant insertion, is evaluated on panoramic and intraoral radiographs.

Further anatomic limitations could be represented by a particular shape of bone palate and by the thickness of fibromucosa. In fact, a thick fibromucosa with marked folds can represent a contraindication to the use of midpalatal implants, while with a reduced transverse diameter of the palate and an increased concavity, it may be difficult to find the right location for the orthodontic connecting bar, which needs a minimum transverse space of 6–7 mm.

However, these limits have been partially solved by the introduction of a new steel clamping cap, which allows programming of the position of the orthodontic device distant from the palatal arch by soldering the cap directly on the bar.

Implant Features and Surgical Phase

The Straumann Orthosystem consists of a pure titanium implant, a healing cap with screw and a set of burs, and instruments for the insertion and subsequent removal of the implant.

The implant consists of an intraosseous screw (Fig. 25.2), a transmucosal smooth neck in contact with soft tissue (H 2.5 or 4.5 mm) and an exposed part of 2 mm, on which the healing cap is fixed.

The intraosseous screw is made of pure titanium (grade 4) and has a 3.3 mm diameter and two possible lengths (4 or 6 mm). It has a self-tapping thread structure sand blasted and acid etched in order to obtain good primary stability.

The surgical insertion of the implant in the middle area of palate takes place under local anesthesia (palatine and incisive nerves) and irrigation with physiologic solution. The palatal mucosa is removed with a mucosa trephine (D 4.2 mm).

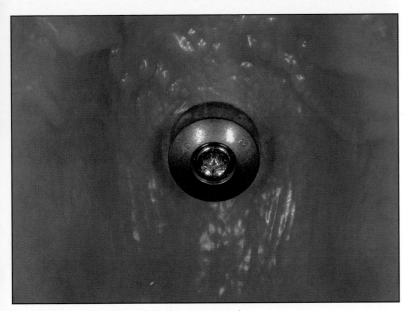

Figure 25.3 Palatal implant with healing cap inserted.

Preparation of the implant bed with a standard round bur and profile drill and intraoperative probing of the implant bed is followed by insertion of the self-threading fixture with an angle of about 60° to the occlusal plane.

The implant, taken from a sterile phial, is connected to the inserting device and placed in the surgical site by hand or using a clenching device.

The last surgical phase consists of connection of the healing cap to the implant by an occlusal screw (Fig. 25.3).

The Healing Period

In order to prevent infection after implant insertion, antibiotic therapy and dental hygiene instruction are suggested and the construction of a protective resin splint is planned in the same surgical insertion, to avoid interference by the tongue on the implant.

Postoperative checks are programmed at 7–10 days and 10 weeks from the insertion date. After the implant has been inserted, a 13-week healing period is necessary.

The principal factor which permits the dissipation of forces without the induction of any osteoclastic cell response is the absence of periodontal ligaments and/or fibrocapsula between the implant and alveolar bone (osseointegration).[54-56] Therefore, in the days immediately after surgical insertion, the implant should be protected from the tongue and only when complete osseointegration is obtained can it be finally connected to the orthodontic appliance which has been designed to produce absolute anchorage.

The Laboratory Phase

The laboratory phase starts when the osseointegration period is completed and the implant has achieved good stability (10 weeks).

The first step is the impression of the upper arch. After 10 weeks the healing cap connected to the implant is replaced by an impression cap. As with conventional implants, the purpose of the impression cap is to reproduce on the plaster cast the exact position of the implant by the transfer analog.

The first transfers were metallic with a cylindric base and exhibited loss of precision because of undesirable movements. In order to avoid this problem, Straumann introduced a new plastic transfer with a squared base, which was better covered by the impression's material (PVS).

The kit suggested by Straumann consists of:
- a healing cap (D 5 mm)
- an octagonal plastic transfer (Ortho Transfer Coping)
- a laboratory analog (Ortho Analogue, D 4.2 mm, L 14 mm)
- an octagonal steel cap (Ortho Post Cap, D 5 mm, L 3.6–5.6 mm).

The next step consists in sending the precise impression (silicon) to the laboratory where the orthodontic device is constructed following our indications.

In the indirect loading method, a transpalatal bar is constructed to connect the implant to first premolars in order to guarantee orthodontic posterior anchorage in extraction cases. Originally, the transpalatal bar was made with a round section (D 8 mm) and was connected closely to the implant by a titanium clamping cap. Nowadays, we use a squared bar (1.2 × 1.2 mm), which has better stability, and an octagonal steel cap, which allows direct soldering of the two parts. Moreover, the implant can be connected to the premolars through a transpalatal bar for anterior orthodontic anchorage or we can use devices for maxillary molar distalization directly connected to the implant.

The Orthosystem for Upper Molar Distalization

In the very first clinical experiences in maxillary molar distalization through loading of palatal mini-implants, the original Straumann Orthosystem kit was used. The first kit included a titanium clamping cap, which was designed to connect the palatal bar to the implant, while the bar was projected very close to the anterior portion of the implant.

This procedure needed an indirect loading method to connect the implant structure to the first bicuspids by the palatal bar (Figs 25.4–25.6). With an indirect loading technique such as the one described above, the dento-implant unit has to support the reaction forces itself, but when maximum anchorage is required, it does not guarantee a secure anchorage control. In fact, an undesirable coronal tipping of the first bicuspids happens during distal movement of the upper molars, even if the first circular bar has been replaced by a stronger squared one (1.2 × 1.2 mm).

In order to avoid any undesired mesial movement of the anterior dental arch, we developed a loading system directly connected to the implant, with no dental elements involved.

We considered the orthodontic devices commonly used, such as the Distal Jet, which was connected to the implant by a steel squared

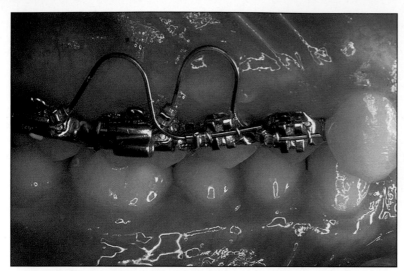

Figure 25.4 Indirect loading method: transpalatal bar connecting first premolars to implant for anterior anchorage. Right view.

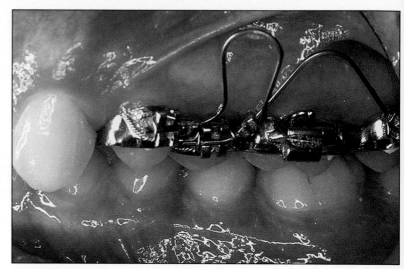

Figure 25.6 Left view.

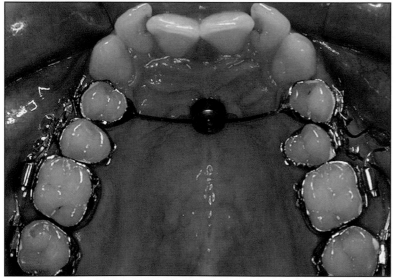

Figure 25.5 Occlusal view.

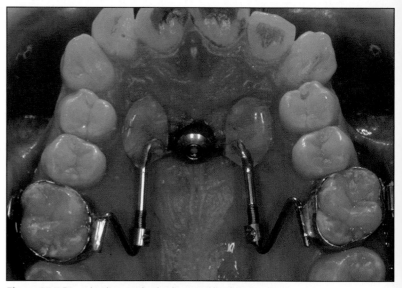

Figure 25.7 Direct loading method: telescopic distalizing system.

wire designed to pass close to the anterior portion of the implant and fixed with a titanium clamping cap (ortho-clamping). All reaction forces were released on the implant system, but this second solution showed palatal mucosa recumbency due to the presence of the clamping cap which forced the bar to stand too close to the implant, causing mucosal injury (Fig. 25.7). In order to protect the palatal mucosa, we developed a modified acrylic Nance button which was connected to the telescopic structure and included an impression cap fixed on the implant by a clamping cap.

The introduction of a new Straumann kit, including a steel connection cap, finally solved the inconvenience due to the titanium clamping cap and allowed us to use a Pendulum device connected to the palatal implant.

The current Straumann kit presents a few advantages, improving the clinical application of the Orthosystem:
- ability to laser or solder the transpalatal arch directly to the Ortho Post Cap
- simplicity of handling
- ability to treat asymmetric cases because of the cap's internal octagonal design, which avoids bar rotation
- better adaptation to different shapes of palatal arch, thanks to two possible lengths for the Ortho Post Cap.

These modifications extended the use of the Orthosystem, allowing the design and subsequent construction of distalizing devices for maxillary molars with better comfort and a more efficient clinical result.

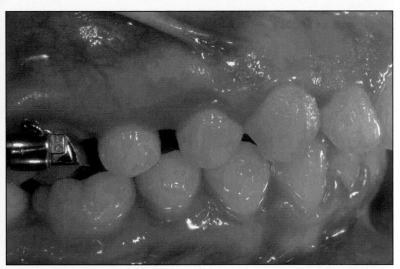

Figure 25.8 Direct loading method: implant-supported Pendulum. Right view.

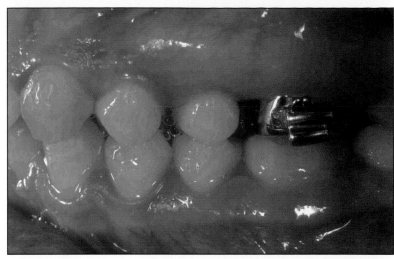

Figure 25.10 Left view.

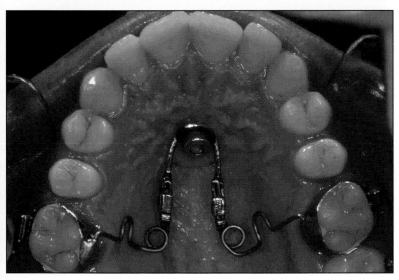

Figure 25.9 Occlusal view.

We first examined the Hilgers Pendulum,[57] which is commonly used in maxillary molar distalization with interesting results, but we finally considered a modified version of it.[58] This modified Pendulum provides better handling and permits easier activation thanks to the removable springs.

The conventional Pendulum uses a large acrylic Nance button in the palate for anchorage. Our modified Pendulum for the palatal implant uses the new octagonal cap connected to the implant with two lingual sheaths positioned on the horizontal plane and soldered on a 0.7 mm steel wire which is itself soldered to the new steel cap. Two distalizing springs are finally formed from 0.32″ TMA wire and inserted in lingual sheaths (Figs 25.8–25.10).

Clinical activation of the two distalizing springs is similar to that suggested by Hilgers: the first activation leads the springs up to 60°

from the middle plane, while the distal root inclination is controlled in a second activation phase by the inclination of the two spring ends.

Surgical Removal of the Implant

Usually when the orthodontic finishing phase is performed and maximum anchorage is no longer required, the palatal implant can be removed. Removal takes place under local anesthesia, following a standard noninvasive procedure. In this second surgical phase, the kit provided includes a profile drill with markings at 4–6 mm and an anticlockwise insertion device.

After exposing the implant screw by removing the healing cap, the removal of the bone surrounding the implant is achieved by using a proper profile drill under irrigation with physiologic solution, followed by removal of the implant itself. Finally, the surgical site is accurately cleaned and no sutures are placed.

No particular postsurgical instructions are given to the patient, except for common hygiene rules. Antibiotic therapy is not routinely used but may be indicated, depending on the individual case. Two weeks after removal, complete healing of the palatal mucosa can be seen.

The Midplant System

The Midplant System (HDC, Sarcedo, Italy) was introduced by Maino et al in 2002.[48] It consists of two components: an endosseous portion, called the core, and a unit called the orthodontic implant connection (Oric) that connects the core to the oral region (Figs 25.11 and 25.12). The core is a single unit formed by a self-tapping screw and a disk (support flange) manufactured from commercially pure titanium (grade 2). The thread is designed to be screwed into cancellous bone without damaging the insertion site. The surface of the screw that interfaces with the bone is treated with an acid-etching process (bone lock etching) or with titanium plasma spray (TPS) to increase its surface area, enhancing its retention. The diameter of the screw is

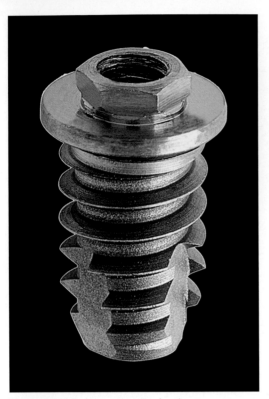

Figure 25.11 Endosseous portion (core).

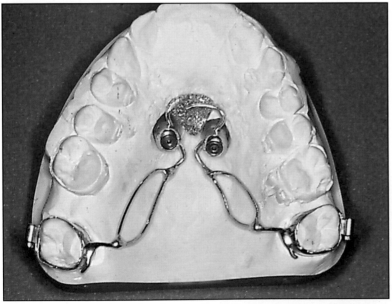

Figure 25.13 Midplant design for indirect loading method. *(Courtesy of Dr G.B. Maino)*

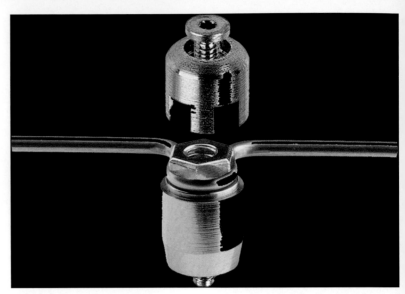

Figure 25.12 Orthodontic Implant Connection (Oric).

There are two different kinds of orthodontic implant connectors, also made of pure titanium (grade 4). Each type has specific indications: the standard connector (Oric cap) has a cylindric transmucosal portion that is 5.5 mm in diameter and is available in four lengths, depending on the thickness of the palate tissue. This component also has an internal hexagonal design on its connecting surface which connects with the hexagonal nut of the core. The use of a hexagonal design prevents rotation of the inserted connector. The transmucosal portion is secured to the core through a fixation screw; this portion has a threaded hole in its head to allow a cover cap to be attached by a screw. A transpalatal bar, made of round or rectangular wire, is used to connect the teeth to the implant and is positioned between the transmucosal portion and the fixation screw. The cover cap, which has four rectangular slots (H 1.3 mm, W 1.2 mm), is then secured to the fixation screw, enhancing the anteroposterior stability of the bar. The special design of the Oric cap ensures that the wires are locked and the reaction forces are three-dimensionally controlled. This connector is indicated when the anchorage units will not change during treatment; in this case the loading method selected is indirect, involving first the distalization by means of a traditional appliance and then the posterior anchorage by means of connection between maxillary molars and the implant (Figs 25.13–25.15).

The loading method can be selected in relation to the Orthosystem, direct or indirect, depending on whether we want to include the teeth in the anchorage unit or not.

The second version of the implant connector, called the Oric EA (easy application), is a winged connection platform with a central hole and retaining holes on the wings. It is secured to the core by a fixation screw. On the transmucosal surface, there is a hexagonal device that ensures positional stability and prevents rotation. Acrylic can be added to the platform to ensure that it is properly adapted to the palate. Transpalatal bars connecting the teeth to the Oric EA are

3.75 mm and there are five lengths available: 4.5 mm, 5 mm, 6 mm, 7 mm, and 8 mm. The disk is 5 mm in diameter and a hexagonal nut is fixed to its superior surface. On the palatal aspect of the core there is a threaded hole which permits the connection of different orthodontic connecting systems.

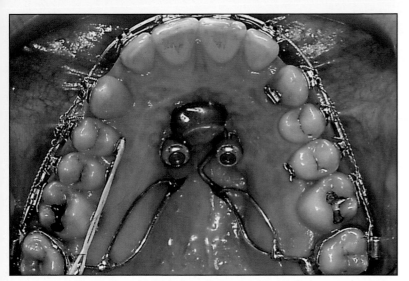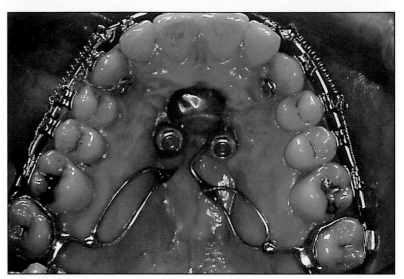

Figures 25.14, 25.15 Indirect loading method: posterior anchorage for lateral sector retraction. *(Courtesy of Dr G.B. Maino)*

Figure 25.15

fixed to the platform by light- or self-curing composites and resin. The Oric EA is more flexible because the anchorage units can be changed with minor modifications; it is indicated when more than one kind of anchorage is necessary (Class II nonextraction treatment with maxillary molars distalization).

Surgical Technique

The implants are placed in the midpalatal region proximal to the first and second premolars. This locates the implant far enough distally so that its presence will not interfere with incisor root positioning during overjet reduction. The length of the implant is selected according to the vertical height of the anterior palate noted on the radiograph. Usually the implant is inserted in the palatal midline area to use the thicker bone in that location.

After delivery of local anesthesia, an operculum of tissue is removed with a tissue punch. The implant site is opened to exposed bone by using a round bur (D 2.3 mm) at reduced speed with copious irrigation of the site with saline solution. After perforating the bone, the implant site is prepared using a 2.5 mm spiral drill with laser horizontal markings. The depth of the site is controlled by a special titanium depth-measuring gauge. Spiral drills also can be equipped with stops at the desired depth so that the preparation will be safer, avoiding direct inspection. The implant site is enlarged using a 3 mm diameter spiral drill. Finally, the area for the disk portion of the implant is created in the bone with a countersink drill.

The implant, with the preassembled mount, is screwed into the prepared site using a maximum speed of 20 turns per minute. The disk flange functions as a depth stop and the implant can be inserted without direct visual control. Once the mount has been removed, an insert, called the healing screw, is placed and works as an interim transmucosal portion of the implant during the osseointegration phase and guarantees access to the core. The length of the screw varies from 1 to 6 mm and the appropriate length is chosen according to the

thickness of the surrounding tissue; this ensures that the healing screw remains at the same level as the palatal mucosa tissues, avoiding trauma from the tongue and food, since microtrauma can jeopardize osseointegration.

After implant insertion, the patient is given antibiotic treatment for 6 days and asked to perform oral hygiene fastidiously and cleanse the area with 0.2% chlorhexidine digluconate twice a day during the 15 days following surgery.

Laboratory Phase

To accurately locate the position of the implant on a construction model after osseointegration, the healing screw is removed and a 23 mm long, two-part copying system is inserted into the implant prior to taking the impression. The copying system consists of a body with a hollow core and a long screw, placed through the hollow portion of the body and screwed securely into the implant. The hollow core presents at its end a hexagonal design in order to fit with the implant and to allow the copying system to determine precisely the implant position. An alginate impression is taken with a tray with its central part removed so that the copying system extrudes through the material. Before removing the impression, the screw of the copying system is withdrawn and then the impression is removed with the body of the system inserted in it. A replica of the osseointegrated implant is placed on the hexagonal portion of the body of the copying and the screw is reinserted into the replica of the implant to secure its position in the impression. The model is made with the replica implant in the exact position of the oral implant and it is then possible to plan the selected orthodontic implant connection system.

If a standard connector (Oric cap) is indicated, bands are placed on the teeth that will be connected to the implant by a transpalatal bar and the bar is designed properly to fit into the slot of the fixation screw. To prevent bending, the bar has to be as rigid as possible and sometimes is made of double wire.

If the Oric EA connector has been selected, it is screwed into the replica of the core and the wings are shaped to fit the palate. Acrylic is then added to the wings to form a platform. Transpalatal connection bars are fixed to the platform with resin and to the teeth with composite to stabilize the teeth that are to be used as anchorage.

Immediate Loading Procedure

The major disadvantage of dental implants is that a variable healing period is needed in order to permit osseointegration, which leads to an extension of the active treatment time compared to conventional orthodontic therapy. To overcome this, different clinical procedures with immediate loading have been investigated.

The recent introduction of titanium mini-screws has enhanced the use of skeletal anchorage because of the ability to place them in almost any area of alveolar bone by means of a simple surgical procedure.[4,59] Since osseointegration is not necessary, the mini-screws can be loaded immediately and can provide exceptional anchorage control.

Different types of mini-screw have been presented and several applications have been reported. The first and most common application of the mini-screw was the insertion in the retromolar area in order to upright and extrude impacted lower second molars after the extraction of third molars.[60] Lee et al using the lingual technique, placed micro-screws in the cortical bone of the palate to reinforce posterior anchorage in the correction of a Class II malocclusion treated with extractions.[61] Park et al applied micro-screws between the roots of maxillary and mandibular first and second molars to correct Class I malocclusion with bialveolar protrusion treated with extraction of four premolars; the upper screw provided anchorage during the retraction phase while the lower screw was used for intrusion and uprighting of the molars.[62] Recently the same authors demonstrated the use of micro-screws in nonextraction treatment for "en masse" distalization of the maxillary dentition.[63]

Kyung et al illustrated the use of a screw placed into the middle area of the palate, in the nasal crest, to distalize maxillary molars by means of an elastic chain attached from the screw, which was distal to the molars, to a transpalatal bar with a mesial loop connecting the molars.[64] The same authors then reported the use of micro-screws inserted in the cortical bone of the mandibular arch to protract the mandibular second molars by the application of a lingual arch with two vertical hooks and elastic chain between the screws and the hooks.[65]

Paik et al recently proposed a mini-screw as rigid fixation in order to reduce vertical excess in extraction treatment. The screws were placed in the midpalatal area to intrude upper molars by elastic chain attached to a transpalatal bar, and in the intraseptal area of mandibular molars to provide posterior anchorage and accomplish lower molar intrusion.[66]

Melsen & Costa placed 14 mini-screws in the zygomatic area of *Macaca fascicularis* monkeys and two in the chin area, concluding that mini-screws represent a valid alternative orthodontic anchorage unit.[21]

Freudenthaler et al inserted horizontally 12 titanium bicortical screws as anchorage for mandibular molar protraction in eight patients.[67]

Giancotti et al used mini-screws for mandibular second molar uprighting in an adult patient.[60] Mini-screws were also used by Park et al for the same purpose.[68]

The possibility provided by immediate loading is to achieve an absolute anchorage via the mechanical stability of a titanium screw inserted in the alveolar bone, rather than an osseointegration of the screw. No differences in anchorage quality are noted; if the mini-screws achieve primary stability, they remain stable during treatment. A recent study by Liou et al indicated that mini-screws remained stationary under orthodontic loading but in some cases the head of the screw can tip or extrude towards the force direction by a small amount, which is clinically insignificant.[69]

Planning for mini-screw insertion is based on a radiologic evaluation of panoramic and intraoral films in order to locate included or ectopic dental elements near to the area where the screw should be inserted, and to evaluate the space available for mini-screw insertion and the best insertion axis to support an orthodontic anchorage loading. As previously described for palatal implants, mini-screws can be loaded according to two different techniques.

- Indirect loading, in which the screws are used to maintain posterior anchorage and the force is applied from the anchorage unit, fixed with the screws, to the teeth which have to be moved (Figs 25.16 and 25.17).
- Direct loading, in which the screws are also used to maintain anchorage but the force is directly applied from the screws to the teeth that have to be moved (Figs 25.18–25.21).

The mini-screws used as immediate loading anchorage that will be described in this section are the Cizeta Modulsystem and the Spider Screw.

The Cizeta Modulsystem

The Cizeta Modulsystem 2.0™ (Cizeta Surgical, Bologna, Italy) orthodontic anchorage mini-screws are made of pure medical titanium and are provided with a partial thread which measures 2 mm on the external side. The mini-screws are 7 mm long and the emergency diameter is 2.3 mm wide. Originally, the mini-screws had a fracture loading of 550 N/mm² but this was subsequently raised to 860 N/mm² (Box 25.1). The kit also includes a drill and a screwdriver for surgical phases.

The mini-screws are always inserted under local anesthesia and two different surgical protocols are possible: direct and indirect. The direct surgical method consists of a subperiosteal flap incision and its following suture. When the marginal gingiva is thick enough, the indirect or transmucosal technique may be indicated, therefore avoiding incision or a surgical flap.

When the surgical site has been prepared using the appropriate drill, the mini-screw is inserted, screwing it down with the screwdriver provided. The mini-screw must achieve immediate stability and can then be loaded with orthodontic elastic forces.

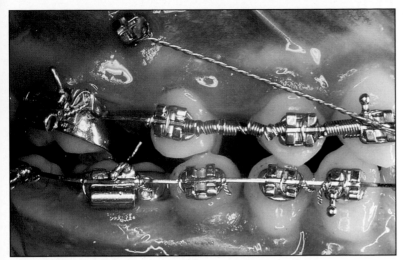

Figure 25.16 Indirect loading method: lateral sectors distalization by coil springs. Right view. *(Courtesy of Dr G.B. Maino)*

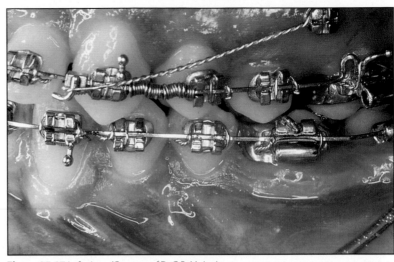

Figure 25.17 Left view. *(Courtesy of Dr G.B. Maino)*

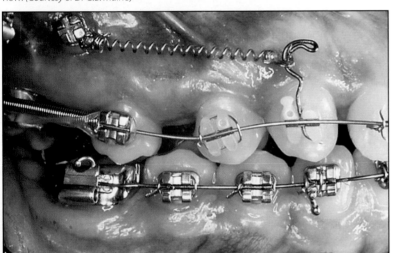

Figure 25.18 Direct loading method: canine retraction by power arm and NiTi coil springs. Right view. *(Courtesy of Dr G.B. Maino)*

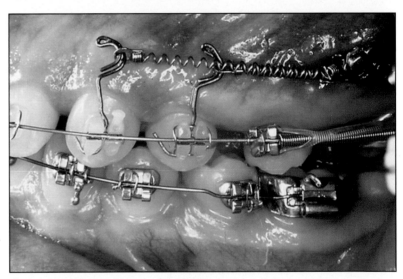

Figure 25.19 Left view. *(Courtesy of Dr G.B. Maino)*

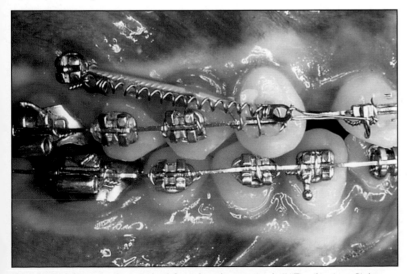

Figure 25.20 Direct loading method: frontal teeth retraction by NiTi coil springs. Right view. *(Courtesy of Dr G.B. Maino)*

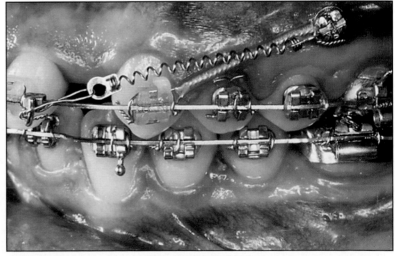

Figure 25.21 Left view. *(Courtesy of Dr G.B. Maino)*

Box 25.1 Features of Cizeta Modulsystem mini-screws

Material	pure titanium
Length	7–9 mm
Grade	5
Fracture loading	860 N/mm^2
External thread diameter	2 mm
SOS emergency	2.3 mm
Screw-head height	0.2 mm

When orthodontic therapy is concluded or when the mini-screw is no longer needed as anchorage, the screw is removed under local anesthesia in an anticlockwise manner, using the screwdriver included in the kit. Usually, the oral mucosa near the surgical site returns to normal within 10–14 days.

The Spider Screw

The Spider Screw (HDC, Sarcedo, Italy) is a self-tapping mini-screw available in three lengths (7 mm, 9 mm, and 11 mm). The screw has an internal 0.021 × 0.025″ slot, an external slot of the same dimension, and a 0.025″ round vertical slot.[70] The screw has three different heights to fit soft tissue thickness: regular with a thicker head and an intermediate length collar; low profile with a thinner head and a longer collar; and low profile flat with the same thin head and a shorter collar. All these types of Spider Screw are small enough to avoid soft tissue irritation but wide and effective for orthodontic loading.

Surgical Phase

The insertion site must be assessed on a radiograph in order to ensure that there is the correct bone depth and at least 2.5–3 mm of bone width to protect adjacent dental roots. The surgical site is prepared with a water-cooled 1.5 mm pilot drill with a corresponding screw-length stop. No separate incision is required if the area presents sufficient attached gingiva. The Spider Screw is taken from the sterile package and connected to the pick-up device; a manual screwdriver is then used for final turning until the screw collar reaches its ideal position.

Once the surgical insertion has been completed, the screw has to be immediately loaded to promote mechanical stability; because the mini-screws rely on mechanical retention rather than osseointegration, the orthodontic force exerted should be perpendicular.

The Spider Screw is easily removed after completion of treatment with a manual screwdriver without local anesthesia, and tissue healing can be expected in a few days.

References

1. Albrektsson T, Branemark PI, Hansson HA, Lindstrom J. Osseointegrated titanium implants. Requirements for ensuring a long-lasting direct bone to implant anchorage in man. Acta Orthop Scand 1981;52:255–270.
2. Hansson HA, Albrektsson T, Branemark PI. Structural aspects of the interface between tissue and titanium implants. J Prosthet Dent 1983;50:108–114.
3. Yip G, Schneider P, Roberts WE. Micro-computed tomography: high resolution imaging of bone and implants in three dimensions. Semin Orthod 2004;10:174–187.
4. Huja S, Roberts WE. Mechanism of osseointegration: characterization of supporting bone with indentation testing and backscattered imaging. Semin Orthod 2004;10:162–173.
5. Schaffler MB, Radin EL, Burr DB. Mechanical and morphological effects of strain rate on fatigue of compact bone. Bone 1989;10:207–214.
6. Gainsforth BL, Highley LB. A study of orthodontic anchorage possibilities in basal bone. Am J Orthod Oral Surg 1945;31:406–417.
7. Roberts WE. Bone tissue interface. J Dent Educ 1988;52:804–809.
8. Roberts WE, Garetto LP, Simmons KE. Endosseous implants for rigid orthodontic anchorage. In: Bell WH, ed. Surgical correction of dentofacial deformities. Philadelphia: Saunders; 1992:1230–1236.
9. Roberts WE, Smith RK, Zilberman Y, Mozsary PG, Smith RS. Osseous adaptation to continuous loading of rigid endosseous implants. Am J Orthod 1984;86:95–111.
10. Roberts WE, Turley PK, Brezniak N, Fielder PJ. Bone physiology and metabolism: implications in dental implantology. Cal Dent Ass J 1987;15:54–61.
11. Cozzani G, Gianelly A. Ortodonzia: concetti pratici. Milan, Italy: Istituto per la Comunicazione Audiovisiva; 1985.
12. Giancotti A, Gianelly AA. Three-dimensional control in extraction cases using a bi-dimensional approach. World J Orthod 2001;2:168–176.
13. Roberts WE, Helm FR, Marshall KJ, Gongloff RK. Rigid endosseous implants for orthodontic and orthopedic anchorage. Angle Orthod 1989;59:247–256.
14. Sherman AJ. Bone reaction to orthodontic forces on vitreous carbon dental implants. Am J Orthod 1978;74:79–87.
15. Gray JB, Steen ME, King GJ, Clark AE. Studies on the efficacy of implants as orthodontic anchorage. Am J Orthod 1983;83:311–317.
16. Turley PK, Kean C, Schur J, et al. Orthodontic force application to titanium endosseous implants. Angle Orthod 1988;58:151–162.
17. Wehrbein H, Diedrich P. Endosseous titanium implants during and after orthodontic load: an experimental study in the dog. Clin Oral Implants Res 1993;4:76–82.
18. Southard TE, Buckley MJ, Spivey JD, Krizan KE, Casko JS. Intrusion anchorage potential of teeth versus rigid endosseous implants a clinical and radiographic evaluation. Am J Orthod 1995;107:115–120.
19. Saito S, Sugimoto N, Morohashi T, et al. Endosseous titanium implants as anchors for mesiodistal tooth movement in the beagle dog. Am J Orthod Dentofacial Orthop 2000;118:601–607.
20. Ohmae M, Saito S, Morohashi T, et al. A clinical and histological evaluation of titanium mini-implants as anchors for orthodontic intrusion in the beagle dog. Am J Orthod Dentofacial Orthop 2001;119:489–497.
21. Melsen B, Costa A. Immediate loading of implants used for orthodontic anchorage. Clin Orthod Res 2000;3:23–28.
22. Odman J, Lekholm U, Jemt T, Branemark PI, Thilander B. Osseointegrated implants: a new approach in orthodontic treatment. Eur J Orthod 1988;10:98–105.
23. Van Roekel NB. Use of Branemark system implants for orthodontic anchorage: report of a case. Int J Oral Maxillofac Implants 1989;4:341–344.
24. Stean H. Clinical case report: an improved technique for using dental implants as orthodontic anchorage. J Oral Implantol 1993;19:336–340.
25. Odman J, Lekholm U, Jemt T, Thilander B. Osseointegrated implants as orthodontic anchorage in the treatment of partially edentulous adult patients. Eur J Orthod 1994;16:187–201.
26. Sorenson NA Jr. Use of maxillary intraosseous implants for Class II elastic anchorage. Angle Orthod 1995;65:169–173.
27. Prosterman B, Prosterman L, Fisher R, Gornitsky M. The use of implants for orthodontic correction of an open bite. Am J Orthod Dentofacial Orthop 1995;107:245–250.
28. Kokich VG. Managing complex orthodontic problems: the use of implants for anchorage. Semin Orthod 1996;2:153–160.

29. Smalley WM, Shapiro PA, Hohl TH, Kokich VG, Branemark PI. Osseointegrated titanium implants for maxillofacial protraction in monkeys. Am J Orthod Dentofacial Orthop 1988;94:285–295.

30. Haanaes HR, Stenvik A, Beyer-Olsen ES, Tryti T, Faehn O. The efficacy of two-stage titanium implants as orthodontic anchorage in the preprosthodontic correction of third molars in adults: a report of three cases. Eur J Orthod 1991;13:287–292.

31. Higuchi KW, Slack JM. The use of titanium fixtures for intraoral anchorage to facilitate orthodontic tooth movement. Int J Oral Maxillofac Implants 1991;6:338–344.

32. Chen J, Chen K, Garetto LP, Roberts WE. Mechanical response to functional and therapeutic loading of a retromolar endosseous implant used for orthodontic anchorage to mesially translate mandibular molars. Implant Dent 1995;4:246–258.

33. Roberts WE, Marshall KJ, Mozsary PG. Rigid endosseous implant utilized as anchorage to protract molars and close an atrophic extraction site. Angle Orthod 1990;60:135–152.

34. Roberts WE, Nelson CL, Goodacre CJ. Rigid implant anchorage to close a mandibular first molar extraction site. J Clin Orthod 1994;28:693–704.

35. Triaca A, Antonini M, Wintermantel E. Ein neues Titan-Flachschrauben-Implantat zur orthodontischen Verankerung am anterioren Gaumen. Inf Orthod Kieferorthop 1992;24:251–257.

36. Block MS, Hoffman DR. A new device for absolute anchorage for orthodontics. Am J Orthod Dentofacial Orthop 1995;107:251–258.

37. Bondemark L, Feldmann I, Feldmann H. Distal molar movement with an intra-arch device provided with the Onplant System for absolute anchorage. World J Orthod 2002;3:117–124.

38. Wehrbein H, Merz B. Aspects of the use of endosseous palatal implants in orthodontic therapy. J Esthet Dent 1998;10:315–324.

39. Wehrbein H, Merz B, Diedrich P, Glatzmaier J. The use of palatal implants for orthodontic anchorage. Design and clinical application of the Orthosystem. Clin Oral Implants Res 1996;7:410–416.

40. Wehrbein H, Glatzmaier J, Mundwiller U, Diedrich P. The Orthosystem: a new implant system for orthodontic anchorage in the palate. J Orofac Orthop 1996;57:142–153.

41. Wehrbein H, Merz B, Hammerle C, Lang N. Bone-to-implant contact of orthodontic implants in humans subjected to horizontal loading. Clin Oral Implants Res 1998;9:348–353.

42. Wehrbein H, Feifel H, Diedrich P. Palatal implant anchorage reinforcement of posterior teeth: a prospective study. Am J Orthod Dentofacial Orthop 1999;116:678–686.

43. Wehrbein H, Merz B, Diedrich P. Palatal bone support for orthodontic implant anchorage: a clinical and radiological study. Eur J Orthod 1999; 21:65–70.

44. Giancotti A, Muzzi F, Greco M, Arcuri C. Palatal implant-supported distalizing devices: clinical application of the Straumann Orthosystem. World J Orthod 2002;3:135–139.

45. Giancotti A, Muzzi F, Santini F, Arcuri C. Straumann Orthosystem method for orthodontic anchorage: step by step procedure. World J Orthod 2002;3:140–146.

46. Giancotti A, Greco M, Docimo R, Arcuri C. Extraction treatment using a palatal implant for anchorage. Aust Orthod J 2003;19:87–90.

47. Bernhart T, Vollgruber A, Gahleitner A, Dortbudak O, Haas R. Alternative to the median region of the palate for placement of an orthodontic implant. Clin Oral Impl Res 2000;11:595–601.

48. Maino BG, Mura P, Gianelly AA. Retrievable palatal implant for absolute anchorage in orthodontics. World J Orthod 2002;3:125–134.

49. Schlegel KA, Kinner F, Schlegel KD. The anatomic basis for palatal implants in orthodontics. Int J Adult Orthod Orthognath Surg 2002;17:133–139.

50. Keles A, Erverdi N, Sezen S. Bodily distalization of molars with absolute anchorage. Angle Orthod 2003;73:471–482.

51. Tosun T, Keles A, Erverdi N. Method for the placement of palatal implants. Int J Oral Maxillofac Implants 2002;17:95–100.

52. Celenza F. Implant-enhanced tooth movement: indirect absolute anchorage. Int J Periodontics Restorative Dent 2003;23:533–541.

53. Henriksen B, Bavitz B, Kelly B, Harn SD. Evaluation of bone thickness in the anterior hard palate relative to midsagittal orthodontic implants. Int J Oral Maxillofac Implants 2003;18:578–581.

54. Helm FR, Poon LC, Marshall KJ, Gangloff RJ, Roberts WE. Bone remodelling response to loading of rigid endosseous implants. J Dent Res 1987; 66:186–192.

55. Smith JR. Bone dynamics associated with the controlled loading of bioglass-coated aluminum oxide endosteal implants. Am J Orthod 1979;76: 618–636.

56. Turley PK, Shapiro PA, Moffett BC. The loading of bioglass-coated aluminium oxide implants to produce sutural expansion of the maxillary complex in the pigtail monkey (Macaca nemestrina). Archs Oral Biol 1980;25:459–469.

57. Hilgers JJ. The Pendulum appliance for Class II non-compliance therapy. J Clin Orthod 1992;36: 700–714.

58. Scuzzo G, Pisani F, Takemoto K. Maxillary molar distalization with a modified pendulum appliance. J Clin Orthod 1999;33:645–650.

59. Costa A, Raffaini M, Melsen B. Miniscrews as orthodontic anchorage: a preliminary report. Int J Adult Orthod Orthog Surg 1998;13:201–209.

60. Giancotti A, Muzzi F, Santini F, Arcuri C. Miniscrew treatment of ectopic mandibular molars. J Clin Orthod 2003;37:380–383.

61. Lee JS, Park HS, Kyung HM. Micro-implant anchorage for lingual treatment of a skeletal Class II malocclusion. J Clin Orthod 2001;35:643–647.

62. Park HS, Bae SM, Kyung HM, Sung JH. Micro-implant anchorage for treatment of skeletal Class I bialveolar protrusion. J Clin Orthod 2001;35: 417–422.

63. Park HS, Kwon TG, Sung JH. Nonextraction treatment with microscrew implant. Angle Orthod 2004;74:539–549.

64. Kyung SH, Hong SG, Park YC. Distalization of maxillary molars with a midpalatal miniscrew. J Clin Orthod 2003;37:22–26.

65. Kyung SH, Choi JH, Park YC. Miniscrew anchorage used to protract lower second molars into first molars extraction sites. J Clin Orthod 2003;37:575–579.

66. Paik CH, Woo YJ, Boyd RL. Treatment of an adult patient with vertical maxillary excess using miniscrew fixation. J Clin Orthod 2003;37:423–428.

67. Freudenthaler JW, Haas R, Bantleon HP. Bicortical titanium screws for critical orthodontic anchorage in the mandible: a preliminary report on clinical applications. Clin Oral Implants Res 2001;12: 358–363.

68. Park HS, Kyung HM, Sung JH. A simple method of molar uprighting with micro-implant anchorage. J Clin Orthod 2002;36:592–596.

69. Liou EJ, Pai BC, Lin JC. Do miniscrews remain stationary under orthodontic forces? Am J Orthod Dentofacial Orthop 2004;126:42–47.

70. Maino BG, Bednar J, Pagin P, Mura P. The spider screw for skeletal anchorage. J Clin Orthod 2003; 27:90–97.

CHAPTER 26

The use of onplants for maxillary molar distalization

Lars Bondemark

Introduction

When intraarch appliances are inserted to correct Class II occlusion or to create space in the maxillary arch by distal molar movement, the palatal vault together with the anterior teeth and premolars are used for anchorage. Despite the anchorage arrangement during the distal molar movement, anchorage loss still occurs, resulting in increased overjet up to 2 mm (Figs 26.1 and 26.2).[1-6]

Since loss of anchorage may lead to prolonged treatment time and less predictable treatment results, it is important for the profession to find new and better tools for its arsenal. Several experimental studies and case reports indicate that osseointegrated endosseous implants are resistant to orthodontic force application and can provide a valuable alternative for stable anchorage.[7-10] For instance, a short titanium screw-form implant in the anterior palate can serve as anchorage[11] and the use of mini-screws in various locations has been demonstrated as achieving anchorage.[12] However, endosseous implants require available bone without the presence of vital structures at the implant sites. For example, the presence of erupted or nonerupted teeth, the nasal and sinus cavities, as well as the thickness of the soft tissues may all prevent the use of an endosseous implant as an orthodontic anchor in the palatal part of the maxilla.

Research into the development of stable anchorage systems has therefore focused on some important prerequisites such as easy installation, minimum pain for the patient, and effortless removal when no longer required. For the orthodontist, the anchor system should be comfortable to handle and show a high success rate. Furthermore, it is fundamental to make a distinction between

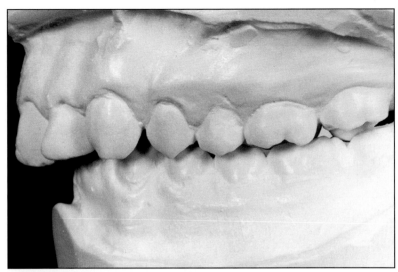

Figure 26.1 Pretreatment study cast.

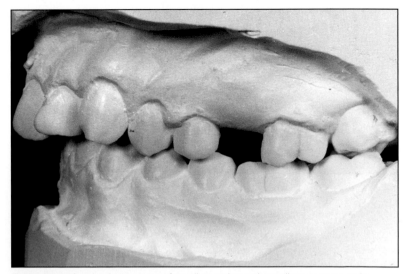

Figure 26.2 After distal movement of maxillary molars with repelling magnets and a Nance button provided as anchorage. The frequent anchorage loss associated with intraarch appliances for molar distalization has in this case resulted in increased overjet of 2 mm during the time when the molars were moved 5 mm distally.

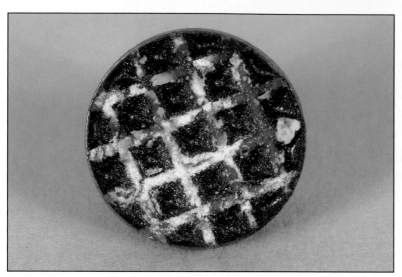

Figure 26.3 The textured and HA-coated undersurface of the titanium onplant.

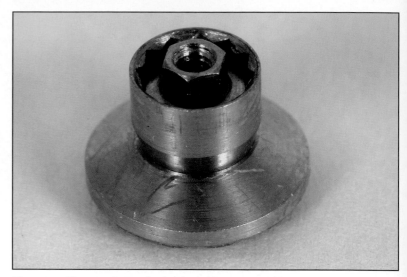

Figure 26.4 The smooth superficial surface of the onplant with the transmucosal abutment component in place.

anchoring devices that are used as abutments for prosthodontic reconstructions and those that are to be removed after commencing orthodontic treatment. In the former case, it is imperative to use systems with a well-documented long-term result, while in the latter case short-term functionality and patient tolerability are the major concerns. With this in mind and considering the criteria described above, Block & Hoffman designed and developed the onplant, a thin titanium alloy disk.[13]

The Onplant System

The term "onplant" reflects the position of the device, i.e. on the surface of the bone, not within the bone as a conventional endosseous implant. The onplant is a thin titanium alloy disk, 8 mm in diameter and 2 mm thick. The surface of the disk that lies against the bone is textured and coated with a thin layer (75 μm) of hydroxyapatite (HA) (Figs 26.3 and 26.4). This bioactive surface joins to the bone via a mechanically significant bond, termed biointegration,[14] and thus permits a favorable osseointegration/biointegration.[13] The superficial surface of the onplant that faces the soft tissue is smooth titanium alloy with an internally threaded hole and an external hexagonal head which accepts a variety of attachments. The abutment that is also the transmucosal component is secured to the onplant by a screw. Then, onto the abutment a transpalatal bar can be secured which is then soldered to bands or bonded to the lingual surfaces of the second premolar.

In a slightly modified system by Nobel Biocare, the diameter of the onplant is 7.7 mm and the abutment is a two-piece construction with an internal double hexagon with one hex facing the onplant and the other hex facing a cylinder. This arrangement makes it possible to connect a transpalatal bar and, together with the osseointegration, allows the building of a superstructure with rotational stability in all planes.

Surgical Procedure

Presurgically, the patient receives 2 g of amoxicillin as single-dose antibiotic prophylaxis. After local anesthesia of the palate, a paramarginal incision approximately 15 mm long is made in the region from the lateral incisor to the first premolar. A subperiosteal tunnel is prepared, extending across the midline in the region of the second premolar. The onplant is then inserted into the tunnel and slid into position with the HA surface directly on the bone, close to the palatal midline (Fig. 26.5). It is imperative to achieve close contact between the onplant and the underlying palatal bone, and thus a slight paramedial placement is recommended to avoid the bony ridge in the palatal midline.

After the onplant placement, the incision is closed with a few sutures and a prefabricated, relieved vacuum-form stent, lined with Viscogel tissue conditioner, is fitted (Fig. 26.6). The stent stays in place 24 hours a day during the first week, to prevent migration of the onplant and avoid hematoma formation. Throughout the first week, in addition to normal oral hygiene, the patient must also rinse the mouth twice daily with 0.1% chlorhexidine gluconate.

After 16 weeks of healing the transmucosal abutment is placed. A small amount of local anesthesia is administered to the mucosa above the onplant and the cover screw of the onplant is located with a dental probe and exposed using a tissue punch. Then, the cover screw is removed and an abutment screw with a healing cap is placed (Figs 26.7 and 26.8).

Orthodontic Procedure

When the abutment connection is completed and the soft tissue of the palate is healed, the transpalatal bar is made ready. The healing cap over the abutment is removed and an impression coping is secured on the abutment (Fig. 26.9). Then, an impression is taken

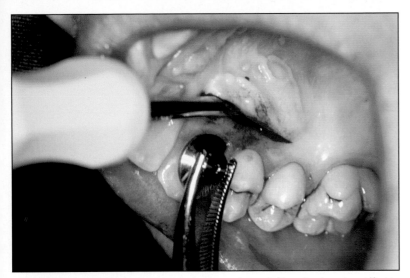

Figure 26.5 The onplant is placed via a subperiosteal tunnel. *(From Bondemark et al,[16] with kind permission of Quintessence Publishing Co. Ltd.)*

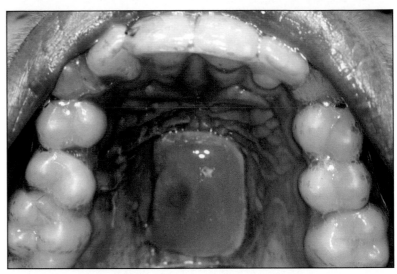

Figure 26.6 Prefabricated relieved stent with Viscogel tissue conditioner in place. *(From Bondemark et al,[16] with kind permission of Quintessence Publishing Co. Ltd.)*

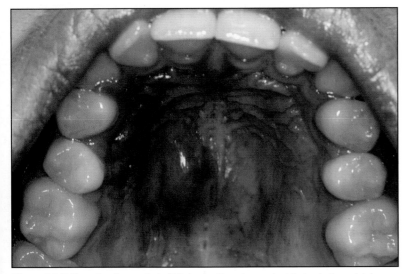

Figure 26.7 After a healing period of 16 weeks. Note the onplant bulge in the palatal mucosa. *(From Bondemark et al,[16] with kind permission of Quintessence Publishing Co. Ltd.)*

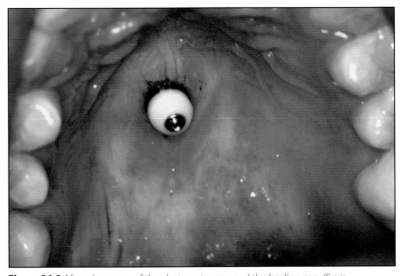

Figure 26.8 After placement of the abutment screw and the healing cap. *(From Bondemark et al,[16] with kind permission of Quintessence Publishing Co. Ltd.)*

to transfer the abutment position to a stone cast. When the impression is removed a special abutment replica is secured to the impression (Fig. 26.10). The impression with the replica is delivered to a dental technician for fabrication of the transpalatal bar. Usually, the bar has to be welded with metal mesh on both ends to allow bonding to the palatal surfaces of the anchorage teeth. As soon as the bar is inserted, two sectional arches ($0.017 \times 0.025''$ stainless steel) are attached bilaterally to brackets and tubes on the second premolars and first molars (Fig. 26.11). If the second maxillary molars have erupted, it is recommended to also engage these teeth in the sectional arches. A nickel-titanium open coil, compressed approximately 3 mm and providing a force of 150–200 g, is inserted between the first molar tube and the bracket of the second premolar.

Reactivation can be performed every 6–8 weeks and if the coil is compressed even more than 3 mm, e.g. 5–6 mm, there is no need for reactivation during the distal molar movement period.

After the molar distalization is completed, the transpalatal bar is removed. A new bar is attached to the onplant and bonded palatally to the first maxillary molars to retain the distal molar movement. Then, a multibracket mechanism is inserted to solve the crowding and retract the anterior teeth and premolars into a Class I relationship (Fig. 26.12). As soon as the orthodontic treatment is completed or it is judged that the transpalatal bar is not needed any more, the bar is removed.

When the onplant is removed, a small amount of local anesthesia is administered in the palatal mucosa close to the onplant. A small

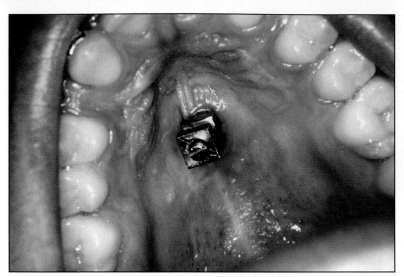

Figure 26.9 The healing cap has been removed and an impression coping is mounted to the abutment.

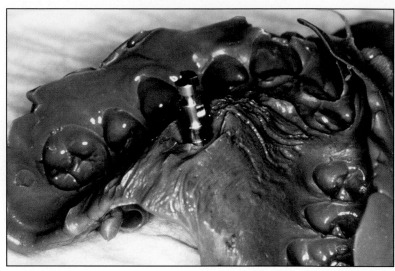

Figure 26.10 A special abutment replica is secured to the impression.

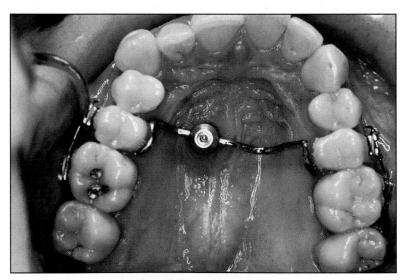

Figure 26.11 The transpalatal bar with the cylinder has been fixed to the abutment of the onplant and the ends of the bar have been bonded lingually to the anchorage teeth. The two buccal sectional arches are also shown.

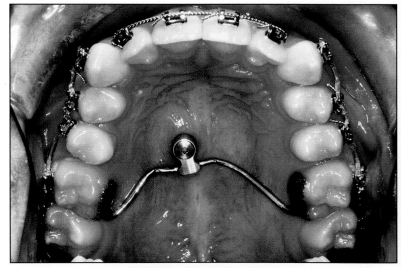

Figure 26.12 A new transpalatal bar has been attached to the onplant and bonded palatally to the first maxillary molars to retain the distal molar movement. The subsequent multibracket technique is used to solve the crowding and retract the anterior teeth and premolars into a Class I relationship.

incision is made along the edge of the onplant and the onplant is carefully elevated from the palatal bone using a periosteal elevator or an osteotome. Most often the underlying bone shows a textured pattern that mirrors the textured undersurface of the onplant.

Evaluation of the System

The Onplant System has been tested in two animal series.[13] Following a healing period of 10 weeks, the ability of the onplants to withstand orthodontic forces was tested. As expected, the onplants did not move and histologic comparison between loaded and unloaded control devices revealed no significant differences. The onplant was sufficiently anchored by the HA–bone biointegrated interface to resist a shear force of approximately 700 N. This means that orthodontic forces are well below the maximum force the onplant system is able to withstand. It was also recommended to use rigid palatal bars that can withstand the forces since deformation of the bar will result in unwanted tooth movements.

Feldmann et al have clinically documented the Onplant System in a series of 10 patients.[15] It was concluded that the Onplant System functioned well and only one of the 10 onplants failed to integrate.

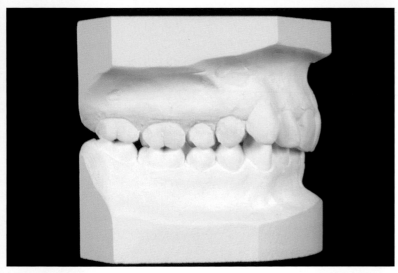 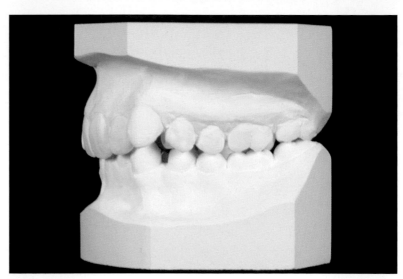

Figures 26.13, 26.14 Pretreatment study casts of a 16-year-old girl. There is an evident Class II occlusion with space deficiency of 4 mm in the maxillary arch. Both first and second maxillary molars are in occlusion and there is an overjet of 3 mm and overbite of 6 mm. *(From Bondemark et al,[16] with kind permission of Quintessence Publishing Co. Ltd.)*

Figure 26.14

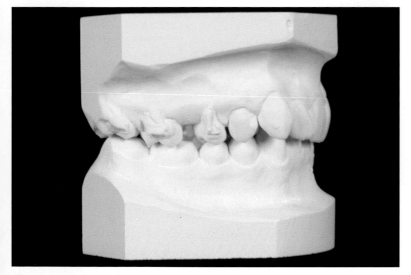 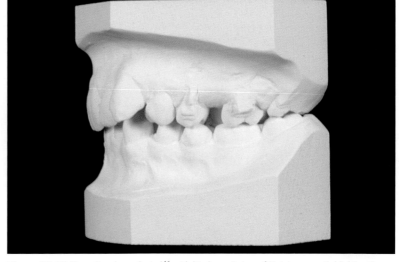

Figures 26.15, 26.16 After 4.5 months' distal molar movement. The first and second maxillary molars have been moved distally 2.5 mm and are now in a Class I relation without any anchorage loss. *(From Bondemark et al,[16] with kind permission of Quintessence Publishing Co. Ltd.)*

Figure 26.16 *(From Bondemark et al,[16] with kind permission of Quintessence Publishing Co. Ltd.)*

Moreover, the component management was straightforward and the patients' reactions were generally positive. Bondemark et al used an intraarch device provided with an Onplant System for simultaneous distal movement of maxillary first and second molars.[16] No anchorage loss, i.e. forward movement of the anterior teeth, was seen and the first and second molars were simultaneously moved distally 2.5 mm during 4.5 months (Figs 26.13–26.16). Moreover, an onplant has been used for palatal anchorage to extrude the unerupted maxillary first molars in a girl with tooth aplasia and cleft palate.[17] After a healing period of 5 months, the onplant remained stable under indirect elastic tension of approximately 160 g applied for 17 weeks, and the maxillary first molars were successfully extruded.

Advantages and Disadvantages of the Onplant System

Animal tests and case series or case reports can only be beneficial as initial reports of new techniques or ideas, and have no validity in evidence-based dentistry. As long as a paucity of controlled clinical trials exists in respect to comparisons between the Onplant System and other anchorage systems, including endosseous implants and mini-screws, the Onplant System can only be regarded as a promising method to create stable or absolute anchorage. Nevertheless, the system seems to provide sufficient absolute anchorage when intraarch appliances are used for molar distalization. The system also produces sufficient anchorage to molars to prevent anterior migration. Moreover, compared to endosseous implants, there is no need to drill in bone and the onplant is easy to insert and remove. Since drilling of bone is not required during installation or when the onplant is removed, there is no risk of tooth damage or perforating the floor of the nasal or sinus maxillary cavities.

The disadvantages are that patients have to undergo two, albeit minor, surgical procedures, the loading of the onplant cannot be started before 16 weeks of osseointegration, and the Onplant System is fairly expensive.

References

1. Bondemark L, Kurol J. Distalization of maxillary first and second molars simultaneously with repelling magnets. Eur J Orthod 1992;14:264–272.
2. Muse DS, Fillman MJ, Emmerson WJ, Mitchell RD. Molar and incisor changes with Wilson rapid molar distalization. Am J Orthod Dentofacial Orthop 1993;104:556–565.
3. Bondemark L, Kurol J, Bernhold M. Repelling magnets versus superelastic nickel-titanium coils in simultaneous distal movement of maxillary first and second molars. Angle Orthod 1994;64:189–198.
4. Ghosh J, Nanda RS. Evaluation of an intra-oral maxillary molar distalization technique. Am J Orthod Dentofacial Orthop 1996;110:639–646.
5. Byloff FK, Darendeliler MA. Distal molar movement using the pendulum appliance. Part 1: Clinical and radiological evaluation. Angle Orthod 1997;67:249–260.
6. Bondemark L. A comparative analysis of distal maxillary molar movement produced by a new lingual intra-arch Ni-Ti coil appliance and a magnetic appliance. Eur J Orthod 2000;22:683–695.
7. Roberts WE, Helm FR, Marshall KJ, Gongloff RK. Rigid endosseous implants for orthodontic and orthopedic anchorage Angle Orthod 1989;59:247–256.
8. Roberts WE, Nelson CL, Goodacre CJ. Rigid implant anchorage to close a mandibular first molar extraction site. J Clin Orthod 1994;28:693–704.
9. Wehrbein H, Diedrich P. Endosseous titanium implants during and after orthodontic load: an experimental study in the dog. Clin Oral Impl Res 1993;4:76–82.
10. Odman J, Lekholm U, Jemt T, Thilander B. Osseointegrated implants as orthodontic anchorage in the treatment of partially edentulous adult patients. Eur J Orthod 1994;16:187–201.
11. Wehrbein H, Feifel H, Diedrich P. Palatal implant anchorage reinforcement of posterior teeth: a prospective study. Am J Orthod Dentofacial Orthop 1999;116:678–686.
12. Costa A, Raffaini M, Melsen B. Miniscrews as orthodontic anchorage: a preliminary report. Int J Adult Orthod Orthognath Surg 1998;13:201–209.
13. Block MS, Hoffman DR. A new device for absolute anchorage for orthodontics. Am J Orthod Dentofacial Orthop 1995;107:251–258.
14. Block MS, Kent JN, Kay J. Evaluation of hydroxyapatite-coated titanium dental implants in dogs. J Oral Maxillofac Surg 1987;45:601–607.
15. Feldmann I, Feldmann H, Lundström F. Nobel Biocare Onplants for orthodontic anchoraging. J Parodontol d´Implantol Orale 2000;19:361–371.
16. Bondemark L, Feldmann I, Feldmann H. Distal molar movement with an intra-arch device provided with the onplant system for absolute anchorage. World J Orthod 2002;3:117–124.
17. Janssens F, Swennen G, Dujardin T, Glineur R, Malevez C. Use of an onplant as orthodontic anchorage. Am J Orthod Dentofacial Orthop 2002;122:566–570.

SECTION FIVE

CLINICAL EFFICACY OF THE NONCOMPLIANCE APPLIANCES

This section includes chapters on the following:

CHAPTER 27

Clinical efficacy of the noncompliance appliances used for Class II orthodontic correction

Moschos A. Papadopoulos

CONTENTS	

Introduction

Noncompliance approaches provide an important treatment alternative for the orthodontic management of patients with Class II malocclusion who present minimal or no cooperation, especially when nonextraction treatment protocols have to be utilized. In the past, with the use of conventional orthodontic procedures, namely headgears and functional appliances and sometimes removable appliances, patient cooperation was a significant problem to overcome in order to achieve a successful treatment outcome. Recently, a great variety of noncompliance appliances and techniques that are less dependent on patient compliance have been proposed in order to correct Class II malocclusion either by advancing the mandible in a more forward position or by distalizing the maxillary molars into a Class I relationship. The development of new wire materials, which can deliver light and continuous forces over a wide range of deactivation, as well as the better understanding of biomechanics and tissue reaction to orthodontic tooth movement have increased their efficiency and predictability. Most of the authors who introduced these appliances claim in general that they can produce more reliable and faster results in comparison to the conventional treatment approaches, while delivering more optimal forces.

Each of the noncompliant appliances advocated for Class II orthodontic correction provides clinicians with a different combination of features and characteristics, which can assist in reaching the initially defined and individual treatment goals. Consequently, depending on the individual needs of the patient, clinicians may now choose from a large number of these devices in order to achieve the best treatment outcome.

Before choosing the appropriate appliance, the clinician should be knowledgeable about its treatment and/or side effects. For example, it is known that when using intermaxillary appliances like the Herbst appliance, the lower incisors became proclined after treatment and therefore this type of therapy is not recommended in patients who have labial inclination or position of the lower incisors at the beginning of treatment. Further, when using intramaxillary distalization appliances, distal tipping of the molars and protrusion and/or proclination of the anterior teeth are considered as undesirable side effects and should be taken into consideration before initiating such a treatment procedure.

For the above reasons, investigation of the clinical efficacy of noncompliance appliances is of particular importance. Although several clinical studies documenting the dentoalveolar and skeletal effects of some of these appliances (Herbst appliance, Jasper Jumper, Pendulum Appliance, Distal Jet) have been published, some appliances (Flex Developer, Sabbagh Universal Spring, Fast Back) have only technical notes or case reports without further clinical investigations. This could be partially attributed to the fact that most of these appliances were introduced very recently and there has probably not been enough time for evaluation of their clinical efficacy.

In the following, the clinical efficacy of the noncompliance appliances used for Class II correction will be discussed based on published clinical studies and according to the classification that was presented in Chapter 2. Appliances that have been described only in technical notes or case reports and whose treatment effects have not been thoroughly studied will not be discussed. Detailed data concerning the changes observed after treatment with the intermaxillary appliances are presented in Table 27.1, while the corresponding data for the intramaxillary noncompliance distalization appliances are presented in Table 27.2.

Intermaxillary Noncompliance Appliances

Rigid Intermaxillary Appliances (RIMA)

Herbst Appliance

According to most investigators, the Herbst Appliance (Dentaurum, Ispringen, Germany) is an effective and reliable method to correct

Table 27.1. Significant changes observed after treatment with intermaxillary noncompliance appliances.

Report	Appliance	N	Tx duration	Sagittal changes — Skeletal									Sagittal changes — Dental									Vertical changes — Skeletal						Vertical changes — Dental				
				SNA angle (°)	Movement of A point (mm)	SNB angle (°)	ANB angle (°)	Wits appraisal (mm)	Co-Pg (mm)	Co-Gn (mm)	Ar-Pg (mm)	Movement of Pg point (mm)	Maxillary molar distal movement (mm)	Maxillary molar distal tipping (°)	Mandibular molar mesial movement (mm)	Molar relationship correction (mm)	Maxillary incisor distal movement (mm)	Maxillary incisor distal tipping (°)	Mandibular incisor mesial movement (mm)	Mandibular incisor mesial tipping (°)	Overjet correction (mm)	NL/NSL angle (°)	OL/NSL angle (°)	ML/NSL angle (°)	ML/NL angle (°)	Anterior lower facial height (mm)	RL/ML angle (°)	Maxillary first molar movement (mm)	Maxillary incisor movement (mm)	Mandibular incisor movement (mm)	Mandibular molar movement (mm)	Overbite (mm)
Pancherz (1979)[1]	Herbst	20	6.0	-0.7		1.2	-2.0		3.2											5.4	3.8	0.4			-0.3	1.8						-2.5
Pancherz (1982)[2]	Herbst	22	6.0	-0.5		1.4	-1.9		3.0			3.1	-2.6		1.3	6.7			1.8		5.1	0.5	1.1	0.2	-0.3							-3.0
Wieslander (1984)[27]	Headgear–Herbst	18	5.0		-0.9		-3.9			3.4					5.3	6.7	-2.4	-5.4		3.6	7.5											
Pancherz (1985)[3]	Herbst	22	6.0	-0.5	-0.4	1.4	-1.9					2.5	-2.8		1.0				1.8	6.6	5.2		1.2–5.1			1.8		-1.0		-1.8	1.3	-3.0
Pancherz & Hägg (1985)[35]	Herbst	70	7.1												1.5				2.4	8.4	5.0											
Pancherz & Hansen (1986)[4]	Herbst	40	7.0	-0.5		1.0	-1.5	-2.4				2.5	-2.0		2.1	6.4	-2.3		2.4		6.9		1.2	0.4								
Pancherz & Hansen (1988)[5]	Herbst	65	7.0	-0.5		1.2	-1.7	-2.7							1.9				2.5	9.4	8.0			0.4								
Panchertz et al (1989)[6]	Herbst	36	6.0			1.2	-1.8					1.9	-2.7		1.9	6.4	-3.0	-6.2	3.1	8.8	7.9		5.0									
Valant & Sinclair (1989)[7]	Herbst	32	10.0		-0.7	1.3	-2.0						-1.5	-6.4	1.6				2.4					0.5				0.2				
Panchertz & Fackel (1990)[8]	Herbst	17	7.0				-1.5				4.3											0.8					2.0				
McNamara et al (1990)[30]	Herbst	21	12.0	0.4		1.7	-1.9			4.4			-1.3		1.4		-0.6		1.6			2.8				1.7		0.5	1.9	-1.0	1.4	
Panchertz (1991)[19]	Herbst[1]	14	6.0	0.4		1.6	-1.2									6.3		-5.1		7.8	7.4	0.9	1.8		-0.6							-3.8
	Herbst[2]	15	6.0	0.2		1.3	-1.1									6.2		-8.2		8.2	7.6	0.5	2.1		0.7							-4.5
Hansen et al (1991)[9]	Herbst[3]	19	12.7	-0.5	0.7	1.0	-1.6					2.9	-0.6		1.8	4.6	-1.2	-2.9	0.8	2.7	4.2	0.8		-0.2	-0.9	1.0						
	Herbst[4]	15	13.1	-0.1	1.7	1.2	-1.3					3.8	-1.5		1.5	5.1	-3.5	-6.6	1.7	1.7	5.8	0.8		-0.1	-0.9	0.6						
	Herbst[5]	6	13.8	0.1	1.9	1.4	-1.2					4.5	-1.9		1.9	5.2	-2.7	-6.0		4.2	5.6	-0.4		-1.5	-1.1	-0.4						
Schiavoni et al (1992)[38]	Herbst[6]	11	9.0																							0.9						
	Herbst[7]	8	9.0																							0.4						

Table 27.1. Significant changes observed after treatment with intermaxillary noncompliance appliances (cont'd).

Report	Appliance	N	Tx duration	SNA angle (°)	Movement of A point (mm)	SNB angle (°)	ANB angle (°)	Wits appraisal (mm)	Co-Pg (mm)	Co-Gn (mm)	Ar-Pg (mm)	Movement of Pg point (mm)	Maxillary molar distal movement (mm)	Maxillary molar distal tipping (°)	Mandibular molar mesial movement (mm)	Molar relationship correction (mm)	Maxillary incisor distal movement (mm)	Maxillary incisor distal tipping (°)	Mandibular incisor mesial movement (mm)	Mandibular incisor mesial tipping (°)	Overjet correction (mm)	NL/NSL angle (°)	OL/NSL angle (°)	ML/NSL angle (°)	ML/NL angle (°)	Anterior lower facial height (mm)	RL/ML angle (°)	Maxillary first molar movement (mm)	Maxillary incisor movement (mm)	Mandibular incisor movement (mm)	Mandibular molar movement (mm)	Overbite (mm)
Hansen & Pancherz (1992)[10]	Herbst	32	7.0	-0.4	1.1	1.1	-1.6					3.5	-1.2		1.4	5.0	-2.8	-6.6	0.4	2.5	5.7	0.8			-0.9		0.7					-3.5
Pancherz & Anehus-Pancherz (1993)[28]	Herbst	45	7.0										-2.1										2.0					-0.7				
Windmiller (1993)[11]	Herbst	46	11.6	-0.9		1.1	-1.9	-3.0		5.7		2.5	-2.0		1.5		-0.9	-3.7	1.6	5.6	5.6	0.4	1.8			2.4						
Sidhu et al (1995)[31]	Herbst	8	8.0			3.1	-2.1		4.0			3.7		-6.5	5.5			-5.5			6.3					4.1				-0.9		-0.4
Hansen et al (1995)[36]	Herbst	53	6.0																	6.8							-3.4					-3.4
Ruf & Pancherz (1996)[37]	Herbst	80	7.0																						-0.5							
Wong et al (1997)[15]	Herbst[8]	14	6–8			1.8	-1.8				5.0	3.4	-1.9		2.1	7.2		-9.3	4.0	11	9.2		2.5	0.1	0.1							
	Herbst[9]	14	6–8			0.9	-1.3				3.8	2.3	-2.6		2.1	6.7	-2.4	-6.8	2.8	9.5	7.2	0.5	2.3	0.7	0.2							
Hansen et al (1997)[12]	Herbst	24	7.0	-0.6	0.1	1.3	-1.8					3.1						-6.6		10.8		0.6			-0.2							
Ruf & Pancherz (1997)[21]	Herbst[10]	16	7.0		0.2						2.7	3.0	-1.5		2.1	6.4	-1.8		3.0		7.6											
	Herbst[11]	15	7.0		0.5						2.0	1.9	-2.4		1.9	5.7	-1.9		2.2		5.5											
Konik et al (1997)[20]	Herbst[12]	21	7.7		0.1								-2.0		1.8	6.1	-2.6		3.5		8.4											
	Herbst[13]	22	6.2		0.3								-2.6		1.3	6.7	-0.5		1.8		5.1											
Obijou & Pancherz (1997)[13]	Herbst[14]	14	7.5	-0.6	0.8	1.3	-2.9	-5.1				3.5	-1.6		1.6	5.9	3.0				3.1		2.6									
	Herbst[15]	40	7.0	-0.5	0.3	1.0	-1.5	-2.4				2.5	-2.0		2.1	6.4	-2.3				6.9		1.2	0.4								
Omlus et al (1997)[14]	Herbst	18	6.0	-0.6	0.1	1.2	-1.8					1.9	-2.7		1.9	6.4	-3.0	-6.2	3.1	8.8	7.9	0.6	5.0	0.5								
Pancherz et al (1998)[96]	Herbst	98	6.0												2.2																	

Table 27.1. Significant changes observed after treatment with intermaxillary noncompliance appliances (cont'd).

Report	Appliance	N	Tx duration	Sagittal changes — Skeletal									Sagittal changes — Dental									Vertical changes — Skeletal						Vertical changes — Dental				
				SNA angle (°)	Movement of A point (mm)	SNB angle (°)	ANB angle (°)	Wits appraisal (mm)	Co-Pg (mm)	Co-Gn (mm)	Ar-Pg (mm)	Movement of Pg point (mm)	Maxillary molar distal movement (mm)	Maxillary molar distal tipping (°)	Mandibular molar mesial movement (mm)	Molar relationship correction (mm)	Maxillary incisor distal movement (mm)	Maxillary incisor distal tipping (°)	Mandibular incisor mesial movement (mm)	Mandibular incisor mesial tipping (°)	Overjet correction (mm)	NL/NSL angle (°)	OL/NSL angle (°)	ML/NSL angle (°)	ML/NL angle (°)	Anterior lower facial height (mm)	RL/ML angle (°)	Maxillary first molar movement (mm)	Maxillary incisor movement (mm)	Mandibular incisor movement (mm)	Mandibular molar movement (mm)	Overbite (mm)
Eberhard & Herbst Hirschfelder (1998)[32]	Herbst	22	6.4	2.6		-2.4	-2.4						-2.2				2.4		0.2				1.1	2.0	2.6							
Ruf & Pancherz (1999)[22]	Herbst[16]	14	8.5		0.2						1.5	2.3	-2.7		3.8	8.6	-3.6		3.8		9.5											
	Herbst[17]	25	7.1		0.5						4.0	4.3	-3.0		2.5	9.3	-3.3		2.7		9.8											
Franchi et al (1999)[23]	Herbst	55	12.0		0.6				4.8			3.1	-1.4		1.4	5.3			1.3		4.1											
Croft et al (1999)[16]	Herbst[18]	40	17.0	-0.8	0.6	0.5	-1.4		7.5		6.5	2.3	0.6		3.7	3.4	0.8		3.4		3.3											
Nelson et al (2000)[24]	Herbst[19]	18	6.0	0.3								2.6				3.5	-2.2				4.6				-0.3	3.2						-2.4
Schweitzer & Pancherz (2001)[33]	Herbst[18]	19	22.0					-3.0										15.3		9.6								1.5	-0.4	-0.4	2.2	-5.6
Baltromejus Herbst et al (2002)[34]	Herbst	98	7.2									2.2																				
Hagg et al (2002)[17]	Headgear-Herbst	22	12.0	-0.6								5.0	-2.8		2.5	10.9	-1.8		3.2	12.5	10.6			-0.6		2.7		-1.1	2.2	-2.3	2.0	
Du et al (2002)[25]	Headgear-Herbst[20]	21	12.0	-0.5								4.9	-2.8		2.6	10.8	-2.0		3.0		10.4			-0.7		2.7		-1.0	2.2	-2.4	2.0	
	Herbst[21]	24	10.0	1.0								3.5	-1.7		2.1	6.3	-2.6		3.6		8.7			0.4		3.1		1.4		-1.4	1.5	
Burkhardt et al (2003)[18,22]	Herbst[22]	30	29.5	-0.6	-1.0	0.9	-1.6			6.4		0.9	0.2	-0.0	1.4	3.6	-0.9	-3.2	1.0	3.4	4.0			-0.4		4.0		1.4	1.4	1.4	2.8	-1.9
	Herbst[23]	30	28.0	-1.2	-0.9	0.2	-1.4			6.4		0.9	0.6	2.2	2.6	3.7	-0.9	1.0	1.7	5.2	3.9			-0.3		3.2		1.4	0.2	0.1	1.9	-3.5
O'Brien et al (2003)[26]	Herbst	82	5.8			1.2			3.4			3.7	0.5		1.1	3.0	-2.4		0.9		5.8					5.8						
Pangrazio-Kulbersh et al (2003)[51]	MARA[24]	30	10.7	1.1		-1.4				4.8		2.3	-1.1		1.2	5.8			0.6	3.9	3.9		0.4			2.5		-1.1				
Cope et al (1994)[57]	Jasper Jumper[25]	31	6.0-9.0									-4.3	-4.3		2.7		-4.7			5.3								-1.0	2.5	-1.7	1.4	

Table 27.1. Significant changes observed after treatment with intermaxillary noncompliance appliances (cont'd).

Report	Appliance	N	Tx duration	SNA angle (°)	Movement of A point (mm)	SNB angle (°)	ANB angle (°)	Wits appraisal (mm)	Co-Pg (mm)	Co-Gn (mm)	Ar-Pg (mm)	Movement of Pg point (mm)	Maxillary molar distal movement (mm)	Maxillary molar distal tipping (°)	Mandibular molar mesial movement (mm)	Molar relationship correction (mm)	Maxillary incisor distal movement (mm)	Maxillary incisor distal tipping (°)	Mandibular incisor mesial movement (mm)	Mandibular incisor mesial tipping (°)	Overjet correction (mm)	NL/NSL angle (°)	OL/NSL angle (°)	ML/NSL angle (°)	ML/NL angle (°)	Anterior lower facial height (mm)	RL/ML angle (°)	Maxillary first molar movement (mm)	Maxillary incisor movement (mm)	Mandibular incisor movement (mm)	Mandibular molar movement (mm)	Overbite (mm)
Weiland & Bantleon (1995)[56]	Jasper Jumper	17	6.0			1.2	-2.0				1.7	3.1	-1.4		1.6	5.0	-2.4	-5.8		4.2	5.2		3.2									
Weiland et al (1997)[52]	Jasper Jumper	25	6.0	-0.6	0.4		-1.0				2.2		-1.1		3.7	4.7			3.1	4.3	4.0	0.5	1.3							-1.7	1.0	-3.1
Stucki & Ingervall (1998)[53]	Jasper Jumper	26	5.0	-0.6		0.7	-1.0				1.4		-0.9		2.6	3.4	-1.6	-2.7	2.9	6.4	4.7			-1.2	-1.5	-1.7		-0.6	0.6	-1.7	0.7	-1.1
Covell et al (1999)[54]	Jasper Jumper	12	5.0	-0.8	0.0		-1.0						-2.1	-4.3	1.1		-2.6	-6.5	1.9	8.6			2.4			-0.2		-0.7	0.9	-1.2	0.9	
Sari et al (2003)[55]	Jasper Jumper	20	8.5	-1.1		0.8	-1.9						-1.7		4.5		-1.7	-6.8	1.2	2.5						-3.4		-0.5		0.1	1.9	
Heinig & Goz (2001)[58]	Forsus Spring	13	4.0			0.5						1.4	-0.8		3.1	3.9	-1.4	-5.3	3.3	9.6	4.7		4.2									-1.2
Stromeyer et al (2002)[59]	Eureka Spring	37	4.0										-1.2		1.5	2.7	-1.5	-2.9	3.4		2.1							0.8		2.1		

[+ indicates mesial or extrusive movement; –, distal or intrusive.] [Measurements corresponding to the 1: stable group, 2: relapsed group, 3: pre-peak group and performed at the end of the settling period, 4: peak group and performed at the end of the settling period, 5: post-peak group and performed at the end of settling period, 6: banded group, 7: splinted group, 8: Chinese group, 9: Swedish group, 10: hyperdivergent group, 11: hypodivergent group, 12: late treatment group, 13: early treatment group, 14: Class II, division 2 group, 15: Class II, division 1 group, 16: young adult group, 17: adolescent group, 18: at the end of the overall treatment, 19: 6 months after appliance removal, 20: HHSSA group, 21: HMJ group, 22: acrylic Herbst group performed at the end of the overall treatment, 23: crown Herbst group at the end of the overall treatment, 24: 6 weeks after MARA removal, 25: annualized figures.]

Table 27.2. Significant changes observed after treatment with intramaxillary noncompliance distalization appliances.

Report	Appliance	N	Tx duration (months)	Sagittal changes												Vertical changes					
				Molar distal movement (mm)	Molar distal tipping (°)	Premolar mesial movement (mm)	Premolar tipping (°)	Incisor mesial movement (mm)	Incisor mesial tipping (°)	Overjet (mm)	Distalization rate (mm/mo)	Distal tipping index (°/mm)	Anchorage loss index	Molar distalization (%)	Anchorage loss (%)	Maxillary molar movement (mm)	Maxillary premolar movement (mm)	Maxillary incisor movement (mm)	Mandibular first molar movement (mm)	Overbite correction (mm)	Lower anterior facial height increase (mm)
Ghosh & Nanda (1996)[64]	Pendulum	41	6.2	3.4	8.4	2.5	1.3	1.3	2.4	1.3	0.55	2.5	0.7	58	42	-0.1	1.7			1.4	2.8
Bussick & McNamara (2000)[60]	Pendulum	101	7.0	5.7	10.6	1.8	1.5	1.4	3.6	0.8	0.81	1.9	0.3	76	24	-0.1	1.1	0.9	-1.0	1.1	2.2
Chaques-Asensi & Kalra (2001)[63]	Pendulum	26	6.5	5.3	13.1	2.2	4.8	2.1	5.1	0.8	0.8	1.9	0.3	76	24	-1.2					
Toroglu et al (2001)[1,61]	Pendulum[1]	30	5.0	4.1	13.4	6.6	5.9	4.1	8.7	1.4	0.82	3.3	1.6	38	62				-0.8		
	Pendulum[2]	30	5.7	5.9	14.9	4.8	3.9	2.1	3.6	1.2	1.03	2.5	0.8	55	45				1.3		
Burkhardt et al (2003)[18]	Pendulum[3]	30	31.6	0.8	3.7			1.1	4.1	1.5		4.6		42	58	-1.7		1.0	2.8	1.6	
Byloff & Darendeliler (1997)[74]	Pendex	13	4.0	3.4	14.5	1.6		0.7	1.7		0.85	4.3	0.5	68	32	-1.2	0.8				
Byloff et al (1997)[75]	Pendex	20	6.8	4.1	6.1	2.2			3.2		0.6	1.5	0.5	65	35	-1.4	1.4	0.5			
Kinzinger et al (2000)[76]	K-Pendulum	50	5.2	2.9	3.1			1.1	4.1		0.67	1.1	1.1	72.5	27.5	0.4	3.3		1.5		
Kinzinger et al (2003)[77]	K-Pendulum	20			5.73														2.6		
Kinzinger et al (2004)[72]	K-Pendulum	36	5.1	3.1	3.3			1.3	4.5		0.61	1.1	1.1	70	30						
Keles & Sayinsu (2000)[78]	BMD	15	7.5	5.2	1.1	4.3	-2.7	4.8	6.7	4.1	0.69	0.2	0.8	55	45						
Ngantung et al (2001)[79]	Distal Jet	33	6.7	2.1	3.3	2.6	-4.3		12.2	1.7	0.31	1.6	1.2	45	55	-1.0	1.6			3.9	2.4
Bolla et al (2002)[81]	Distal Jet	20	5.0	3.2	3.1	1.3	-2.8	1.3			0.64	1.0	0.4	71	29	0.5	1.1			0.3	0.9
Nishii et al (2002)[80]	Distal Jet	15	6.4	2.4	1.8	1.4		1.5	4.5		0.37	0.7	0.6	63	37						
Keles (2001)[82]	Keles Slider[4]	15	6.1	4.9	0.9	1.3		1.8	3.2	2.1	0.8	0.2	0.3	79	21			0.9		3.1	
Bondemark (2000)[83]	Nance Appliance with NiTi coils	21	6.5	2.5	2.2	1.2	2.1	1.5	4.7	1.2	0.38	0.9	0.5	67	33					1.5	1.3
Gulati et al (1998)[84]	Jones Jig	10	3.0	2.8	3.5	1.1	2.6			1.0	0.93	1.2	0.4	72	28	1.6					1.0

Table 27.2. Significant changes observed after treatment with intramaxillary noncompliance distalization appliances (cont'd).

Report	Appliance	N	Tx duration (months)	Molar distal movement (mm)	Molar distal tipping (°)	Premolar mesial movement (mm)	Premolar tipping (°)	Incisor mesial movement (mm)	Incisor mesial tipping (°)	Overjet (mm)	Distalization rate (mm/mo)	Distal tipping index (°/mm)	Anchorage loss index	Molar distalization (%)	Anchorage loss (%)	Maxillary molar movement (mm)	Maxillary premolar movement (mm)	Maxillary incisor movement (mm)	Mandibular first molar movement (mm)	Overbite correction (mm)	Lower anterior facial height increase (mm)
						Sagittal changes											Vertical changes				
Runge et al (1999)[85]	Jones Jig	13	6.3	2.2	4.0	2.2	9.5		2.0	1.5	0.35	1.8	1.0	50	50	2.1	3.2	3.1		0.2	1.0
Brickman et al (2000)[86]	Jones Jig	72	6.4	2.5	7.5	2.0	4.8				0.86	3.0	0.8	55	45	0.1	1.9				
Haydar & Uner (2000)[87]	Jones Jig	20	2.5	2.8	7.8	3.3	6.0	0.55			0.39	2.8	1.2	46	54		-1.8	-0.9			
Papadopoulos et al (2004)[89]	Sectional jig assembly	14	3.8	1.4	6.8	2.6	8.1	2.3	4.8	0.9	0.37	4.9	1.9	35	65					1.0	
Mavropoulos et al (2005)[90]	Sectional jig assembly	10	4.1	2.8	6.8	3.3	7.5	1.8	5.2		0.68	2.4	1.2	46	54						
Erverdi et al (1997)[91]	NiTi coil springs	15	3.0	3.8	9.9	-0.8					1.27	2.6	-0.2								
Itoh et al (1991)[93]	Magnets	10	1.9	2.1	7.4			1.2	3.8		1.11	3.5		64	36						
Bondemark & Kurol (1992)[92]	Magnets	10	3.9	4.2	8.0						1.07	1.9									
Bondemark et al (1994)[71]	Magnets	18	6.0	2.2	1.0			1.2	4.4	1.5	0.37	0.4		65	35	0.8				3.6	
Bondemark (2000)[83]	Magnets	21	5.8	2.6	8.8	1.8	6.7	1.9	5.5	1.7	0.45	3.4	0.7	59	41					1.6	1.1
Fortini et al (2004)[94]	First Class	17	2.4	4.0	4.6	1.7	2.2	1.3	2.6	1.2	1.67	1.1	0.4	70	30	1.2					

[Measurements corresponding 1: to low angle cases, 2: to high angle cases, 3: at the end of the overall treatment, and 4: 2 months after appliance removal.]

Class II malocclusion without relying on patient compliance. Herbst treatment affects not only the dentition but also the craniofacial skeleton, the associated soft tissues, and the temporomandibular joint. The following discussion covers the effects of the Herbst appliance during treatment, as well as in the long-term observation period (more than 6–12 months post treatment). A more detailed discussion of the effects of the appliance is presented in Chapter 4.

Sagittal Changes

The use of the Herbst appliance in Class II patients appears to have a restraining effect on the maxillary growth, as shown by the 0.4–1.2° decrease in the SNA angle seen during treatment.[1–18] In the long-term post-treatment period the SNA angle was increased between 0.2° and 4°,[9,10,19] whereas other investigators observed a decrease of 0.6–0.8° for the same period.[12,14]

The restraining effect on the maxilla was also evident by the reduction in the forward movement of the maxillary base (A point). In particular, the maxillary base moved forward 0.1–1.2 mm during treatment,[3,10,12–14,16,20–26] which was 0.2–1.2 mm less than the forward movement observed in the normal population or in the control group. However, in some studies it moved backward 0.5–1 mm.[3,17,18,25,27] The restraining effect on the maxilla was diminished in the long-term posttreatment period as the maxillary base moved forward 1.3–5.1 mm,[8–10,12,14,28,29] thus showing that maxillary growth inhibition by the Herbst appliance was of a temporary nature.

The increase in sagittal mandibular growth was evident by the increase in the SNB angle which was between 0.2° and 3.1° during Herbst treatment.[1–7,10–16,18,19,30–32] During the long-term posttreatment period the SNB angle remained approximately unchanged,[12,14] whereas in some studies an increase between 0.3° and 2.6° was evident.[9,10,14,19]

The sagittal intermaxillary jaw relationships were also improved after Herbst appliance treatment. In particular, the ANB angle was decreased between 1.1° and 3.9° as a result of the changes observed in the SNA and SNB angles, which could be attributed to the skeletal changes produced by the treatment.[1–16,18,19,27,30–32] In addition, a further decrease between 0.4° and 4° was observed during the long-term posttreatment period[9,12,14,29] while Pancherz[19] found an increase between 0.2° and 1°. The Wits appraisal was also affected during Herbst treatment, and a decrease between 2.4 and 5.1 mm was found.[4,5,11,13,32,33]

The increase in mandibular length produced by the Herbst appliance during treatment was also confirmed by various variables. The Co-Pg distance increased between 3 and 7.5 mm during treatment,[1,2,16,23,26,31] the Co-Gn distance increased between 3.4 and 6.4 mm,[11,18,27,30] the Ar-Pg distance was increased between 1.5 and 5 mm,[8,15,21,22] and finally, the S-Pg distance was also increased by 4.2 mm.[8] On a long-term posttreatment basis, the mandibular length was also increased significantly as shown by the 5.6 mm increase in the S-Pg and the 5.7 mm increase in the Ar-Pg distance.[8] In addition, a 0.9–5 mm forward movement of the mandibular jaw base (as measured by Pg-point) was found.[2–4,6,9–18,20–27,31,34,35]

The dental changes observed in both the maxilla and the mandible can be attributed to the fact that the Herbst appliance exerts a posteriorly directed force on the maxillary dentition and an anteriorly directed force on the mandibular dentition,[1,2,6,13,19,20,36] which results in distalization of the maxillary molars, retroclination of the maxillary incisors, mesial movement of the mandibular molars, and proclination of the mandibular incisors.[2,6,30,31,36] The latter is undesirable, especially in patients with initial incisor proclination, and can be considered as anchorage loss along with the spaces between maxillary canines and first premolars, which are often observed after Herbst treatment.[2] However, the mandibular incisors showed a tendency to return to their former position after Herbst removal, without causing anterior maxillary crowding.[4,5] According to Pancherz,[2] dental changes during Herbst treatment are generally undesirable, with the exception of cases presenting anterior crowding, in which distal movement of the posterior teeth is favorable.

The overjet was corrected as a result of the dental and skeletal changes produced by Herbst treatment. In particular, a reduction between 3.1 and 9.8 mm was evident at the end of Herbst treatment.[1–6,9,10,13–16,18–24,26,27,31,36,37] This reduction was even more pronounced (approx. 10.5 mm) when the headgear Herbst and a step-by-step mandibular advancement was used.[17,25] On a long-term posttreatment basis, a relapse in the overjet between 0.3 and 2.4 mm was observed,[9,10,14,19,29] while an additional correction of 0.8 mm was also evident.[19] In total, the Herbst appliance caused an overjet correction between 3.3 and 5.7 mm from the pretreatment to long-term posttreatment period.[9,10,14,19,37]

Vertical Changes

Regarding the effect of the Herbst appliance on the maxilla, it was found that the palatal plane inclination (NL/NSL angle) was changed during the treatment and posttreatment period, showing a rotational effect of the Herbst telescopic mechanism on the maxillary skeleton. In particular, the palatal plane tipped downwards 0.2–1°,[1,2,7–12,14,15,19,28] while a decrease of 0.4° was also observed.[9]

The occlusal plane also tipped clockwise during treatment (as was shown by the increase of the OL/NSL angle) between 1.1° and 5.1°, which was significantly different from the control group mainly because of the distalization and intrusion of the maxillary first molars.[2–4,6,11,13–15,19,28,30,32] However, it tipped counterclockwise during the long-term posttreatment period.[14,19,28]

Regarding the effect of the Herbst appliance on the mandibular plane (ML/NSL) angle, the majority of the investigators found an increase of 0.2–0.8° during Herbst treatment.[2,4–7,12–15,19,25,32,38] In contrast, others observed that the ML/NSL angle was decreased 0.3–1.5°,[9,17,18,25,38] whereas some investigators found that it remained unaffected.[1,10,24] During the long-term posttreatment period the mandibular plane angle further decreased 1.6–5.8°,[8–10,12,14,19,38] which can be attributed to the marked forward rotation of the mandible[14] or to normal growth.[37]

In relation to vertical jaw relationships, the maxillomandibular plane (ML/NL) angle was decreased by 0.2–1.1° at the end of

.

Herbst treatment,[1,2,9,10,19,23,24] while other investigators found an increase of 0.1–2.6°.[15,32] The same angle was further decreased during the long-term posttreatment period.[2,9,12,19]

The anterior lower facial height (ANS-Me) was increased 0.4–4.1 mm[1,3,11,17,18,24,25,30,31,39] but according to Pancherz,[3] no difference was evident between the treatment and the control groups in the 12-month posttreatment period.

The Herbst appliance also affected the dental components of both maxilla and mandible. Regarding the maxillary dental changes, it was observed that the maxillary first molars were intruded between 0.5 and 1 mm during the treatment period.[3,17,28,30,33] In contrast, an extrusion of 1.4–1.5 mm was evident in other studies.[18,33] The maxillary second premolars also extruded during Herbst treatment.[3] Regarding the maxillary incisors, an extrusion between 0.2 and 2.2 mm was observed at the end of Herbst treatment,[17,18,25] while no significant changes were found during the retention period.[17] With regard to the mandibular dental changes, the incisors were intruded by 0.4–2.4 mm and the molars extruded 1.3–2.8 mm.[3,17,25,30,31,33] However, Burkhardt et al[18] observed an incisor extrusion of 0.1–1.4 mm. Finally, the mandibular second premolars were extruded after treatment.[3]

After Herbst treatment the overbite was reduced between 1.9 and 5.6 mm,[1–3,10,18,19,24,31,33,37] while an increase of 0.5–1.1 mm was observed during the long-term follow-up.[10,19,37] Thus, the total overbite reduction during the total observation period was between 1 and 2.6 mm.[19,37]

Transverse Changes
During Herbst treatment, maxillary arch length, intercanine width, and intermolar width were increased significantly, while the mandibular arch displayed minimal changes.[7] Similarly, Hansen et al[37] found after Herbst treatment an increase of the upper and lower arch perimeters, which relapsed during the short-term observation period.

Soft Tissue Changes
At the end of Herbst treatment, the soft tissue profile was improved.[1,40,41] The upper lip was retruded during treatment,[18,41] while the lower lip remained unchanged[41] or retruded less than the upper lip.[18] Regarding the long-term posttreatment effects on the soft tissues, a retrusion of 4.4–4.5 mm of the upper lip was observed, while the lower lip showed a retrusion of 2.9–3.4 mm.[41] The soft tissue profile changes and the upper and lower lip retrusion can be at least partially attributed to the increase in nasal growth, which affected the position of the lips in relation to the E-line,[41] and to the tendency of the lower incisors to relapse.[4,41]

Effects on Temporomandibular Joint
The placement of the Herbst appliance caused an anterior and downward movement of the condyle which induced the remodeling of the condyle, the glenoid fossa, and the articular tubercle. The articular disk, which retruded at the start of treatment as an adaptive response to the incisal edge-to-edge position, returned to approximately its initial position after appliance removal while only in some cases a slightly retruded position remained.[42]

Some undesirable functional disturbances could be observed during Herbst treatment, such as temporomandibular joint (TMJ) sounds,[43] masticatory muscle tenderness,[3,43] and TMJ tenderness on palpation, which can be attributed to the lack of occlusal buffer during the first months of the treatment.[3,44] The frequency of condylar displacement, TMJ sound findings or temporomandibular disorders (TMDs) in patients treated with the Herbst appliance was not significantly greater than in the normal population, both for the short-term and long-term periods.[45,46] In addition, anamnestic, clinical, and radiographic findings were similar to those observed in untreated groups.[43]

Thus, the functional disturbances observed were of a temporary nature and Herbst treatment did not seem to have any adverse effects on TMJ function or to cause TMDs or unfavorable structural changes on a short- or long-term basis.[3,43,45–47]

Effects on Muscles
Regarding the effects of the Herbst appliance on the masticatory muscles, the incisal edge-to-edge relationship caused a noticeable reduction in the electromyographic (EMG) activity of both the masseter and temporal muscles during maximal biting in the intercuspal position, which recovered noticeably almost to pretreatment values 3–6 months after placement of the Herbst appliance.[44,48,49] Regarding the lateral pterygoid muscle activity, an increase in the EMG pattern was observed after wearing the appliance which was reduced remarkably in a 6-month period, which led to the conclusion that muscular adaptation takes place soon after Herbst placement and before the appearance of morphologic changes due to functional treatment.[50]

When the Herbst appliance was removed, the EMG activity of the masseter and temporal muscles was increased in comparison to pretreatment values,[48] while this increase was greater for the masseter than for the temporal muscle. Twelve months post treatment, when the occlusion was stabilized, the contraction pattern in the two muscles was similar to that observed in subjects with normal occlusion.[3]

In addition, following treatment with the Herbst appliance, the moment arms of the masseter muscle increased, mainly due to the mandibular protrusion which caused changes in the muscle and jaw geometry.[51] In contrast, the moment arms of the temporal muscle presented no significant changes, possibly because the temporal muscle application vector is far from the area where the geometric changes occurred. Moreover, the mechanical advantages of masseter and temporal muscles related to the occlusal bite force on the mandibular and occlusal planes as well as the number and intensity of occlusal contacts were reduced after treatment.[51]

Mandibular Anterior Repositioning Appliance (MARA™)
According to Pangrazio-Kulbersh et al,[52] the MARA (AOA/Pro Orthodontic Appliances, Sturtevant, WI) is effective in correcting

Class II malocclusions by producing skeletal and dental changes, which were measured in annualized values.

Sagittal Changes

Pangrazio-Kulbersh et al[52] did not observe a significant change in the maxillary skeletal parameters and concluded that the appliance did not exert a restraining effect on maxillary forward growth. However, the MARA had an effect on mandibular growth, which was increased in comparison to the growth observed in the control group, as shown by the 4.8 mm increase in the Co-Gn distance, which was 2.7 mm more than that observed in the control group, the 2.3 mm increase in the Pog/N perpendicular distance, which was 2 mm greater than that of the control group, and the 1.1° increase in the SNB angle. The sagittal intermaxillary relationship was also improved as demonstrated by the 1.4° decrease of the ANB angle.

In relation to the maxillary dentition, the maxillary molars moved 1.1 mm in a distal direction in comparison with the 1.3 mm mesial movement observed in the control group.[52] The mandibular molars moved mesially 1.2 mm, 0.7 mm greater than the movement observed in the control group, and the incisors also moved mesially 0.6 mm, in contrast to the 0.4 mm distal movement observed in the control group, and proclined 3.9°, 3° greater than that of the control group.

Vertical Changes

The MARA had a significant effect on the anterior face height (ANS-Me) which was increased by 2.5 mm, 1.5 mm greater than the increase in the control group, and on the posterior facial height (Co-Go), which was increased 4 mm, 2.7 mm greater than the increase observed in the control group. The latter can be attributed to the use of molar crowns, which caused an inferior displacement of the condyle in the fossa and an increase in the condylar growth in a posterior and superior direction.[52] According to the same investigators, the occlusal plane increased 0.4°, while in the control group a decrease of 0.9° was observed. The MARA did not have a significant effect on the mandibular plane, SN-Go-Gn, and FMA angles.

Comparison with Other Appliances

When comparing the MARA with the Herbst and Frankel appliances, it was found that the MARA had similar effects to the Herbst appliance and greater dentoalveolar effects than the Frankel appliance. However, some differences between the MARA and the Herbst were noticed, such as the greater restriction in maxillary growth in the Herbst group, the lack of headgear effect in the MARA group, the greater intrusion of the maxillary molars and the intrusion and mesial movement of the mandibular incisors observed in the Herbst group.[52]

Flexible Intermaxillary Appliances (FIMA)

Jasper Jumper™

According to most investigators, the Jasper Jumper (American Orthodontics, Sheboygan, WI) is an effective appliance to correct Class II malocclusion by producing skeletal and dental changes, especially in patients in the early permanent dentition. These changes, observed after active treatment as well as after a short-term posttreatment period of 7 months, will be further discussed below.

Sagittal Changes

The use of the Jasper Jumper seems to restrain maxillary growth, as indicated by the 0.6–1.1° decrease of the SNA angle during treatment.[53–56] However, Weiland & Bantleon[57] did not observe a significant change in the SNA angle. According to Covell et al,[55] the sagittal forward movement of the A point was unchanged, showing a restriction in maxillary growth during treatment, whereas Weiland et al[53] found a 0.5 mm forward movement. Regarding the effect of the appliance on the mandibular skeleton, an increase in forward growth was found during treatment, as demonstrated by the 0.7–1.2° increase in the SNB angle.[54,57] Further, the mandibular base was moved anteriorly between 1.4 and 3.1 mm during treatment as demonstrated by the forward movement of point Pg, and the mandibular length (Pg-Ar) was also increased 1.7 mm.[53,54,56] The sagittal intermaxillary relationship was also improved after treatment with the Jasper Jumper, as shown by the 1–2° decrease of the ANB angle, and can be attributed to the changes observed in the SNA and SNB angles.[53–57]

The dental changes observed during treatment in both the maxilla and the mandible could be attributed to the distally directed forces applied on the maxillary dentition and the mesially directed forces delivered to the mandibular dentition.[55] More specifically, treatment with the Jasper Jumper had an effect on the maxillary molars, which were distalized between 0.9 and 2.1 mm and tipped distally 4.3° at the end of treatment.[53–58] The mandibular molars were also affected during treatment with the appliance, as shown by the 1.1–4.5 mm mesial movement and the 2.9–4.2° mesial tipping.[53–58] As a result of both the skeletal and dental changes observed during treatment, the molar relationship was corrected between 3.4 and 5 mm.[53–55,57] Regarding the effect of the appliance on the maxillary incisors during treatment, they were moved distally between 1.6 and 2.6 mm and retroclined between 2.7° and 6.8°,[54–58] whereas in the short-term posttreatment period, a forward movement of 0.8 mm and a proclination of 1.8° were observed which can be considered as relapse.[54] The mandibular incisors were also influenced by the Jasper Jumper treatment due to the mesial forces delivered on the mandibular dentition, which produced a mesial movement between 1.2 and 3.1 mm and a proclination of 2.5–8.6°.[53–58] During the short-term posttreatment period, a retroclination of 4.4° was observed.[54] Finally, the overjet was corrected between 4 and 5.2 mm as an effect of the skeletal and dental changes produced by the Jasper Jumper treatment.[53,54,57]

In comparison with other treatment options, such as the Herren Activator and the activator-headgear combination, the Jasper Jumper seems to achieve better treatment results. In particular, it showed a greater correction of the overjet and the molar relationship in comparison with the Herren Activator and the activator-headgear combination.[53] When comparing the group treated with removable Jasper Jumpers with the activator-headgear combination group, Sari et al[56] found that the ANB angle was significantly decreased in both treatment groups compared with the controls. The total facial height was increased more in the activator-headgear group than in the Jasper Jumper group, while the vertical growth inhibition of the lower incisors was greater in the Jasper Jumper group. The activator-headgear appliance was more effective on the mandible, whereas the Jasper Jumper was mainly active on the maxilla. The authors suggested that ideal patients for the Jasper Jumper splinted appliance would be high-angle cases, particularly with maxillary excess and some mandibular deficiency.

Vertical Changes

The Jasper Jumper affected the mandibular and maxillary skeletal and dentoalveolar structures in the vertical plane. More specifically, the vertical effect of the appliance on the maxillary skeletal structures was evident from the 0.5° increase in the NL/NSL angle during treatment.[53] Regarding the mandibular skeletal changes, a 1.2° decrease in the ML/NSL angle was observed during treatment, which could be attributed to normal growth.[54] However, Weiland et al[53] found this angle to be stable after treatment. Further, the vertical jaw relationship (NL/ML) was also affected by the Jasper Jumper, as shown by the 1.5° decrease found at the end of the treatment.[54] Regarding the effect of the appliance on the occlusal plane (OL/NSL), a clockwise rotation between 1.3° and 3.2° was observed during treatment, mainly due to direction of the force vector of the Jasper Jumper.[55-57] The lower anterior facial height (ANS-Me) was decreased between 0.2 and 3.4 mm.[55,56] Stucki & Ingervall[54] also found this distance decreased 1.7 mm after treatment with the Jasper Jumper, while it relapsed to approximately pretreatment values during the short-term posttreatment period. Further, the same authors also observed a decrease in the total anterior facial height (N-Me) of about 1.1 mm during treatment, which again relapsed to the pretreatment values during the short-term posttreatment period.

With regard to the maxillary dental changes in the vertical plane, it was found that the maxillary molars were intruded 0.5–1 mm during treatment, whereas an extrusion to almost pretreatment values was observed during the posttreatment period.[54-56,58] The maxillary incisors were also extruded between 0.6 and 2.5 mm during treatment.[54,55,58] The mandibular dentition was also affected by the Jasper Jumper treatment, as the mandibular incisors were intruded between 1.2 and 1.7 mm,[53-56,58] while Sari et al[55] found an extrusion of 0.1 mm. The mandibular molars extruded between 0.7 and 1.9 mm.[53,54,56,58] The overbite was corrected between 1.1 and 3.1 mm during treatment, mainly due to the mandibular incisors' intrusion and changes in the mandibular and maxillary incisors' inclination,[53,54] but at the end of the short-term posttreatment period no significant change was evident in comparison to the pretreatment values, indicating an almost equal relapse.[54]

Soft Tissue Changes

Significant decreases of the soft A point to sella vertical (A'-SV) distance of 0.3 mm and the upper lip to sella vertical (UL-SV) distance of 0.9 mm were evident after treatment in comparison to the control group, which can be attributed to the inhibition of forward movement of the lip due to the restraining effect on the A point and the maxillary incisor retrusion.[56]

Forsus™ Nitinol Flat Spring

Sagittal Changes

The skeletal effect of the Forsus Nitinol Flat Spring (3M Unitek, Monrovia, CA) on the mandible was evident from the 0.5° increase in the SNB angle and the 1.4 mm forward movement of the pogonion, while the maxilla presented only an insignificant forward growth.[59]

Regarding the maxillary dental changes, the Forsus Nitinol Flat Spring caused a 1.4 mm absolute maxillary incisors distal movement and a 0.8 mm absolute distal molar movement.[59] According to the same investigators, the appliance confirmed the headgear effect which was evident in other Class II appliance systems like the Herbst and the Jasper Jumper. Regarding the effect of the Forsus Spring on the mandibular dentition, the mandibular first molars were moved mesially 3.1 mm and the mandibular incisors moved mesially 3.3 mm and proclined 9.6°.

The overjet was corrected by 4.7 mm and the molar relationship by 3.9 mm, as a result of the skeletal and dental changes during treatment with the Forsus Spring.[59]

Vertical Changes

The Forsus Spring had an effect on the occlusion plane, which was rotated 4.2° in terms of bite opening, and on the overbite, which was decreased by 1.2 mm.[59]

Transverse Changes

The dental cast analysis showed an increase of the maxillary dental arch width, 2.2 mm anteriorly and 2.5 mm posteriorly, while the corresponding values of the mandibular arch width increase were 0.6 mm and 1.2 mm, respectively.[59]

Hybrid Appliances (Combination of RIMA and FIMA)

Eureka Spring™

According to Stromeyer et al,[60] the Eureka Spring (Eureka Orthodontics, San Luis Obispo, CA) is an effective and reliable method to correct Class II malocclusions in noncompliant patients, producing mainly dentoalveolar changes in both arches.

Sagittal Changes

After treatment with the Eureka Spring, a distal maxillary molar movement of 1.2 mm was observed, whereas the mandibular molars were moved mesially 1.5 mm. The maxillary incisors retroclined 3° and moved distally 1 mm, whereas the mandibular incisors proclined 3° and moved mesially 1 mm. Stromeyer et al noticed that the mandibular molars moved mesially more than the mandibular incisors, thereby reducing the mandibular arch length. Finally, the overjet correction was 2.1 mm and the molar correction 2.7 mm, mainly as a result of dental changes.[60]

Vertical Changes

Regarding the effect of the Eureka Spring on the dentition, the maxillary molars were intruded 1 mm and the mandibular incisors 2 mm, but no other change was evident in the vertical dimension.[60]

Twin Force Bite Corrector (TFBC)

Except for the short- and long-term effects of the Twin Force Bite Corrector (Ortho Organizers Inc., San Marcos, CA), derived from a prospective study that has been part of two thesis projects at the Department of Orthodontics at the University of Connecticut, which are thoroughly described in Chapter 13, no other papers regarding the clinical efficacy of this appliance have been published.

Appliances Acting as Substitute for Elastics

No clinical studies concerning the clinical efficacy of the noncompliance distalization appliances of this category (Calibrated Force Module, Alpern Class II Closers, Saif Springs) have been published yet.

Intramaxillary Noncompliance Distalization Appliances

Appliances with a Flexible Distalization Force System Palatally Positioned

Pendulum Appliance

According to most investigators, the Pendulum Appliance is an effective and reliable method for distalizing maxillary molars at the expense of moderate anchorage loss without, however, relying on patient compliance. Further, Pendulum treatment affects primarily the maxillary dentition, while less pronounced effects on the craniofacial skeleton and associated soft tissues also occur.

Sagittal Changes

Bussick & McNamara[61] found after treatment with the Pendulum Appliance a mean first molar distalization of 5.7 mm, a change that contributed substantially to the Class II correction. This distalization was similar in patients with various vertical growth patterns, a result which was in contrast to the findings of Toroglu et al[62] who found that the molars were distalized 5.9 mm in the high-angle group and 4.1 mm in the low-angle group. Burkhardt et al[18] also found that the maxillary molars were distalized 5.9 mm; however, 87% of the molar distalization was lost during the stabilization phase of treatment. A similar amount of 5.1 mm of molar distalization was also observed by Joseph & Butchart[63] and Chaques-Asensi & Kalra,[64] whereas Ghosh & Nanda[65] found a mean maxillary first molar distalization of only 3.4 mm. However, distal tipping almost always accompanies the distalization of the maxillary first molars as an undesirable effect. Bussick & McNamara[61] reported that the mean molar distal tipping during Pendulum treatment was 10.6°. Ghosh & Nanda[65] observed a similar distal tipping of 8.4°, whereas greater tipping of the upper first molars of 13.1° and 15.7° was reported by Chaques-Asensi & Kalra[64] and Joseph & Butchart,[63] respectively.

The maxillary second and third molars can also be influenced through the distal movement of first molars. After Pendulum treatment, the second molars were distalized almost 2.3 mm and tipped distally 12–14.2°,[64,65] while the third molars were distalized 0.2 mm and tipped distally 2.5°. During the treatment period the mandibular molars also moved mesially by an amount from 0.2 to 1.4 mm,[18,61,65] a fact that also contributed to the correction of Class II molar relationship to Class I.

The anchor unit is unable to completely resist the reciprocal mesial forces of the Pendulum Appliance. Anterior anchorage loss, expressed as mesial movement of premolars and incisors, was therefore a constant finding in several studies following distalization with the Pendulum Appliance. Consequently, Bussick & McNamara[61] found that the first premolars moved mesially 1.8 mm and tipped 1.5°, while Ghosh & Nanda[65] observed a mesial movement of 2.6 mm and tipping of 1.3°. Further, Chaques-Asensi & Kalra[64] observed a mesial movement of 2.2 mm and tipping of 4.8°. The second premolars experienced even more anchorage loss, as was found by Toroglu et al.[62] They moved mesially between 4.8 and 6.6 mm and tipped between 3.9° and 5.9° in their low- and high-angle groups, respectively. Thus, for every millimeter of distal molar movement, the premolars moved mesially 0.8 mm in the sample of Ghosh & Nanda,[65] while Bussick & McNamara[61] reported that the premolar or deciduous first molar moved mesially only 0.3 mm for every 1 mm of molar distalization. In other words, the maxillary molar distalization contributed to 76% of the total space opening anterior to the maxillary first molar, whereas 24% was due to reciprocal anchorage loss of the maxillary premolars.[61]

Following treatment with the Pendulum Appliance, anterior movement and proclination of the incisors were also observed. In the various studies, it was found that the incisors moved mesially from 1.1 to 4.1 mm and tipped up to 4.9°.[18,61–65] Thus, the overjet was also increased between 0.8 and 1.5 mm.[18,61,62,64,65] In order to minimize anchorage loss, Ghosh & Nanda[65] recommended reinforcement of the anchor unit so that the anterior framework includes all anterior teeth and complete coverage of the palate.

The presence of second permanent molars still remains a matter of discussion regarding the effectiveness of distalization. Hilgers[66] suggested that the appliance would be more efficient if the second molars were not erupted. On the other hand, Bussick & McNamara[61] and Ghosh & Nanda[65] found no significant mean differences in the amount of distal movement of the maxillary first molars and sagittal anchorage loss between patients who had second molars erupted and those who did not. However, there are other authors who believe that distalization of the first molars depends on the stage of eruption of the second molars.[67–69] More specifically, it has been reported that the presence of second molars increases the treatment time,[70,71] produces more tipping[72] and more anchorage loss, and that tipping of the second molar is greater when a third molar bud is present.[73]

Regarding the skeletal changes in the sagittal plane, Bussick & McNamara[61] found that these were only minimal, expressed as a slight forward movement of the maxilla and a backward and downward movement of the mandible, while the mandible length was increased.

Vertical Changes

Distalization and tipping of the maxillary first molars following treatment with the Pendulum Appliance can result in molar intrusion. Bussick & McNamara[61] observed an intrusion of 0.7 mm of the upper first molars, which was more pronounced in the group of patients with erupted second maxillary molars, and Chaques-Asensi & Kalra[64] an intrusion of 1.2 mm. In addition, Ghosh & Nanda[65] reported a nonsignificant maxillary molar intrusion of 0.1 mm for the first molar and 0.5 mm for the second molar. In contrast, Toroglu et al[62] found an extrusion of the maxillary molars, although this was not significant.

Bussick & McNamara,[61] Ghosh & Nanda,[65] and Chaques-Asensi & Kalra[64] observed an extrusion of upper first premolars or deciduous molars of 1 mm and 1.7 mm, respectively. The upper incisors were also found to be extruded by 0.8–0.9 mm.[61,64] However, Toroglu et al[62] found this extrusion to be insignificant for both the second premolars and incisors.

The overbite is also influenced after treatment with the Pendulum Appliance. More specifically, it was decreased between 1.4 and 1.8 mm.[61,65] This reduction in overbite was more pronounced in the group of patients with second maxillary molars erupted as well as in the group in whom the second premolars were used for anterior anchorage of the appliance instead of the second deciduous molars.

In contrast to these findings, Toroglu et al[62] found no significant changes in overbite after treatment.

It was found that mandibular first molars were extruded by an amount ranging between 0.5 and 2.8 mm,[18,61,62,65] which can probably be considered a result of normal growth during the treatment period.[74] Further, this could also be an effect of the occlusal rests and the bonding on the upper first and second premolars or deciduous molars.[61] The bonded occlusal rests could have acted as a bite plate, allowing extrusion of the molars as well as a slight clockwise rotation of the mandible.

Regarding the skeletal changes in the vertical plane, Bussick & McNamara[61] and Chaques-Asensi & Kalra[64] found that the lower anterior facial height was increased 2.2–2.8 mm after treatment with the Pendulum Appliance. Further, no significant differences in lower anterior facial height increase between patients with high, neutral or low mandibular plane angles were observed. These findings are in agreement with those of Toroglu et al,[62] who also observed an increase in lower facial height which did not differ significantly between their low- and high-angle patients. However, Bussick & McNamara[61] found that in patients with erupted maxillary second molars, there was a slightly greater increase in lower anterior face height and in the mandibular plane angle in comparison to patients with unerupted second molars, as well as in patients with second premolar anchorage versus those with second deciduous molar anchorage. According to the authors, the increase in lower anterior facial height can be attributed to a 0.7 mm extrusion of the mandibular molars, as well as to the fact that the maxillary molars are moving distally into the arc of closure. Similar to the above results Ghosh & Nanda[65] found that the lower anterior face height increased by 2.8 mm. This increase was, however, greater in patients with higher Frankfort-mandibular plane angle. In addition, the mandibular plane angle was increased by 1.1° with treatment.

Transverse Changes

Regarding the transverse changes after treatment, Ghosh & Nanda[65] observed an increase of 1.4 mm of the width between the mesiobuccal cusps of the right and left first maxillary molars, whereas the width between the distobuccal cusps showed no increase. In addition, the same authors also found that the width between the mesiobuccal cusps of the second maxillary molars was increased by 2.3 mm, while that of the second maxillary premolars was increased by 2 mm.

Soft Tissue Changes

As a result of incisor proclination due to anchorage loss, Bussick & McNamara[61] and Ghosh & Nanda[65] found that the upper lip was protruded by 0.6 mm and 0.3 mm, respectively. According to Bussick & McNamara,[61] this slight protrusion may have also resulted from the bracket placement on the incisors in some of their patients. In addition, it was observed that the lower lip was also protruded after treatment by almost 1 mm.[61,65] Finally, Bussick & McNamara[61] found the nasolabial angle to be decreased by 2.5°, which was in contrast to the findings of Toroglu et al.[62]

Pendex Appliance

Bussick & McNamara[61] evaluated the Pendex and Pendulum appliances in a sample of patients without differentiating between the two groups. For this reason, the results from their study have been presented and discussed in the previous section regarding the standard Pendulum Appliance. The clinical efficacy of the Pendex Appliance was evaluated by Byloff & Darendeliler[75] and Byloff et al,[76] who however modified the original Pendex design of Hilgers,[66] as was described in Chapters 15 and 16.

Sagittal Changes

The Pendex Appliance is effective in obtaining distal movement of the first maxillary molars. The mean molar distalization observed by Byloff & Darendeliler[75] was 3.4 mm and by Byloff et al[76] 4.1 mm. The first maxillary molars were also tipped distally by 14.5°.[75] However, when uprighting bends were incorporated into the distalizing springs this tipping effect was significantly reduced to 6.1°.[76] The rate of distal molar movement varied from 0.7 mm[76] to 1 mm[75] per month.

Regarding the anchorage unit, the maxillary second premolars moved mesially 1.6 mm and the central incisors moved anteriorly 0.9 mm and tipped labially 1.7°.[75] However, when uprighting bends were incorporated into the distalizing springs, the anchorage loss was more pronounced; the maxillary second premolars moved mesially 2.2 mm and the central incisors moved anteriorly 1.5 mm and tipped labially 3.2°.[76] Nevertheless, this anchorage loss was found to be nonsignificant between the patients with and without expansion.[76]

The space opened between the maxillary first molars and the maxillary second premolars was found to be 5.5 mm by Byloff & Darendeliler[75] and 7.3 mm by Byloff et al.[76] However, the molar distalization represented 71% and 64% of this space in the first and second studies, respectively. The difference between the two studies may be attributed to the incorporation of the uprighting bends, which caused increased distalization and less tipping of the molars at the cost of increased anchorage loss in terms of increased mesialization and extrusion of the premolars and proclination of the incisors.[76]

In addition, both of the above studies found that the eruption stage of second molars did not influence the amount of distal molar movement and incisor anchorage loss. However, it must be mentioned that the number of patients in the three different eruption stages were small in both studies.

Regarding skeletal changes, the SNA angle presented no significant differences between the studies, which may lead to the conclusion that the A point was not affected by the anteriorly directed forces within a relative short period of time.

Vertical Changes

The first maxillary molars were significantly intruded almost 1.5 mm after treatment.[75,76] Byloff & Darendeliler[75] observed a small but significant amount of second premolar extrusion of 0.8 mm, while this extrusion was found to be increased (1.4 mm) after incorporating the uprighting bends.[76] Although the central incisors demonstrated a nonsignificant extrusion of 0.5 mm,[75] after the incorporation of the uprighting bends this extrusion was found to be slightly increased (0.5 mm) and significant.[76]

Regarding skeletal effects in the vertical dimension, no significant changes were observed in the y-axis and NL/ML angle, probably due to maxillary molar intrusion, although bite opening is normally expected after distal movement and tipping of the maxillary molars.[75] However, the vertical skeletal dimensions were increased significantly by 0.8° for the y-axis and by 0.9° for the NL/ML angle when uprighting bends were incorporated into the distalizing springs.[76]

K-Pendulum Appliance

Sagittal Changes

After treatment with the K-Pendulum, the first maxillary molars were distalized approximately 3 mm (or 0.6 mm per month, which represents 70.3% of the total movement in the sagittal plane), while they also tipped distally up to 5.9° in relation to the palatal plane.[73,77,78] However, the distal tipping of the first molars in patients with erupted second molars was less (0.9°), while in patients with incompletely erupted maxillary second molars, this tipping was found to be significantly greater (5.9°).[73] In addition, when the third molar was in the eruption phase, the distal tipping of the second molar was also greater.

The second molars were distalized 2.6 mm and also tipped distally. This distal tipping was moderate when the second molars were in the budding stage (4.1°), greater in patients with fully erupted second molars (7.9°) and smaller in patients in whom germectomy of the third molars was undertaken (2°).[73]

After treatment, the maxillary incisors demonstrated a mean protrusion of 1–1.3 mm, which represents 27.5–29.8% of the total sagittal movement.[73,77] The labial tipping of the central incisors was 4.4°. Moreover, the incisor protrusion was significantly smaller in patients with incompletely erupted second molars (3.3°) than in patients with erupted second molars (5.5°), regardless of whether germectomy of the third molars had been performed or not.[73]

Regarding skeletal changes, no significant differences were observed after treatment.[73,77]

Vertical Changes

Following treatment with the K-Pendulum, the first molars extruded between 0.4 and 0.6 mm, while no significant skeletal changes were observed.[73,77]

Transverse Changes

Although a tendency to expansion (ranging from 0.7 to 2.6 mm) was observed after treatment, this was not significant for the total sample or for the different groups of patients. In addition, the first and second molars experienced mesiobuccal rotations (ranging from 2.2° to 5.2°), which were also not significant.

Intraoral Bodily Molar Distalizer (IBMD)

Sagittal Changes

Keles & Sayinsu investigated the effects of the IBMD in 15 patients and found that after treatment, the maxillary first molars were distalized 5.2 mm with a minimal and nonsignificant distal tipping of 1.2°.[79]

Regarding anchorage loss, the maxillary incisors protruded 4.8 mm and also tipped labially 6.7°, while the overjet was increased 4.1 mm. However, after the removal of the appliance and the distal drift of the premolars, both incisor proclination and overjet were reduced. The first premolars also moved mesially 4.3 mm and tipped distally 2.7° during treatment. For every 1 mm of molar distalization, 0.8 mm of anchorage loss of the first premolars occurred. No statistical difference has been observed concerning anchorage loss between patients with erupted and nonerupted maxillary second molars.

Regarding skeletal effects of the appliance, the SNA angle was found to be increased by 1.6°, which can be attributed to the proclination of the maxillary incisors and the remodeling of the A point. The ANB angle was also increased by 1.7° while the SNB angle did not change after maxillary first molar distalization.

Vertical Changes

No significant extrusion of the maxillary first molars was observed after treatment with the appliance. In contrast, the maxillary first premolars were extruded 3.3 mm and the overbite was reduced by 2.6 mm. In addition, the first mandibular molars extruded 1.5 mm.

Regarding skeletal effects, a significant increase in the vertical dimension was observed. The anterior lower face height to total face height ratio was increased by 1 mm and the ML/NSL angle was increased by 1.7°. Further, the OL/NSL angle and the NL/NSL angle were also increased by 1° and 0.3°, respectively. According to Keles & Sayinsu, the reduction of overbite, the increase of the ML/NSL angle, and the increase of the lower face height to total face height ratio could be related to the mandibular molar extrusion and cuspal interference.[79]

Transverse Changes

Model cast analysis has demonstrated that the intermolar distance was increased by 0.5 mm and that the first maxillary molars were rotated by 0.8° after treatment with the IBMD. However, neither measurement was statistically significant.

Distal Jet™

According to most authors, the Distal Jet Appliance (American Orthodontics, Sheboygan, WI) is effective in distalizing the maxillary first molars with no reliance in patient compliance, although some anchorage loss may occur. The Distal Jet mainly affects the maxillary dentition, although less marked effects can be observed on the hard and soft tissues.

Sagittal Changes

Following distalization with the Distal Jet, the maxillary first molars were distalized between 2.1 and 3.2 mm.[80–82] However, the distal molar movement in most cases was associated with undesirable distal tipping which varied between 1.8° and 3.3°. Tipping of maxillary first molars was less when second molars were in eruption (2.3°) than when unerupted (4.3°).[82] The maxillary second molars were also affected through the first molar distal movement, being distalized 2.6–2.7 mm and tipped distally 4.9–11.8°.[80,82]

The anchor unit was not able to resist the reciprocal mesial forces of the Distal Jet and anterior anchorage loss was a constant finding in the studies evaluating the efficacy of the appliance. According to Bolla et al[82] the first premolars, which supported the appliance, moved mesially 1.3 mm and tipped distally 2.8°. The second premolars, when they were used as supporting teeth, moved mesially from 1.4 mm[81] to 2.6 mm[80] and tipped distally 4.3°.[80] The space created mesial of the first molars was 4.5 mm, of which 71% was due to the molar distalization and 29% to the anchorage loss.[82] Nishii et al found that for every millimeter of maxillary first molar distalization, the second premolars moved mesially 0.6 mm.[81] Further, anterior movement and proclination of the maxillary incisors were also found after molar distalization. Nishii et al[81] observed that the maxillary incisors moved mesially 2.4 mm and proclined up to 4.5°, while Ngantung et al[80] found this mesial tipping more increased (12.2°), probably due to the simultaneous use of full-fixed appliances during distalization. In contrast, Bolla et al found no significant incisor proclination or mesial movement.[82] Further, no significant differences were observed in the maxillary incisor angulation among patients with high, medium, and low Frankfort-mandibular plane angles (FMA).[80]

Regarding changes in overjet, Ngantung et al[80] found an increase of 1.7 mm, while Bolla et al[82] found this to be unchanged during the distalization phase. In general, less anchorage loss was observed when the distal jet was used alone than with fixed appliances.[80]

The presence of the second permanent molars is an issue of debate regarding the effectiveness of the appliance. Bolla et al found that maxillary first molar tipping was less pronounced when second molars were erupted (2.3°) than unerupted (4.3°).[82]

Vertical Changes

The first molars were extruded 0.5 mm after treatment with the appliance.[81,82] The first maxillary premolars also presented some extrusion (1.1 mm)[82] while the second premolars were found to be extruded 0.5 mm by Nishii et al[81] and 1.6 mm by Ngantung et al.[80] Further, the maxillary incisors were also found to be extruded by 0.3 mm,[81] while in contrast Ngantung et al found an incisor intrusion of 1 mm and an overbite decrease of 3.9 mm during the distalization phase.[80]

Some skeletal changes, in terms of an increase in the vertical dimensions, were also observed during the distalization phase with the Distal Jet. The lower anterior facial height was increased from an insignificant 0.9 mm[82] to a significant 2.4 mm.[80] The percentage of lower anterior face height was also increased by 0.5%. However, this increase did not differ significantly among subjects with high, neutral or low pretreatment mandibular plane angles.[80] The palatal plane angle was found to be slightly increased (0.6°)[80] or remained unchanged,[82] while distalization with the Distal Jet did not cause significant changes in the mandibular plane angle.[80,82]

Transverse Changes

Bolla et al found that distalization with the Distal Jet Appliance produced 2.9 mm of intermolar width expansion, which was accompanied by a mild distal rotation of the palatal cusps of the first maxillary molars.[82] In addition, Nishii et al also observed a 1.2 mm increase in the intermolar width.[81] This increase in width is necessary to maintain a proper transverse relationship of the maxillary to mandibular molars during distalization.[82] The increase in maxillary width was also observed in the regions of second maxillary molars and first and second premolars, although less than in the first molar region.[81,82]

Soft Tissue Changes

Ngantung et al found that the distance of the upper and lower lip to Rickett's E-plane was increased 0.8 mm and 2.1 mm, respectively.[80] In contrast, Bolla et al found these distances to be decreased, 0.4 mm for the upper lip and 0.3 mm for the lower lip.[82]

Keles Slider

The Keles Slider (patent pending) seems to be an effective device for bodily distalization of the maxillary first molars with minimal reliance on patient compliance, although some anchorage loss may occur. Keles used the appliance for maxillary unilateral molar distalization in 15 patients and evaluated its effects by means of initial and final lateral cephalograms.[83] However, the fact that the final cephalograms were taken 2 months after distalization (after completion of the stabilization period) and not immediately after appliance removal could have possibly positively influenced the results of this investigation.

Sagittal Changes

After treatment with the Keles Slider, the unilateral Class II molar relationship was corrected in all patients in a period of 6.1 months and the first maxillary molars were moved distally 4.9 mm on average, almost in a bodily fashion. A 0.9° distal tipping of the first molar was also present, but this was not statistically significant.

The anchor unit could not resist the reciprocal mesial forces of the appliance and anterior anchorage loss was evident. The maxillary first premolars presented a mesial movement of 1.3 mm. For every 1 mm of molar distal movement, 0.3 mm of anchorage loss was observed on the first premolars. The appliance also caused 1.8 mm upper incisor protrusion and 3.2° incisor proclination. Furthermore, the overjet was also increased by 2.1 mm. However, during the stabilization period, the anteriorly protruded incisors and the mesially migrated first premolars relapsed distally.

Vertical Changes

No extrusion of the maxillary molars was observed. The first premolars and incisors extruded nonsignificantly 1.9 and 0.9 mm, respectively. In addition, the overbite was reduced by 3.1 mm, probably due to the use of the anterior bite plane incorporated in the Nance button.

Transverse Changes

A slight distobuccal rotation of the maxillary first molars was found at the end of the distalization phase. According to Keles, this was due to the interplay between the 1.1 mm tube and 0.9 mm wire or due to the point of force application which was located more palatally.[83]

Nance Appliance with NiTi Coil Springs

Sagittal Changes

Bondemark found that after bilateral simultaneous distalization of first and second molars with the intraarch NiTi coil appliance, the maxillary first molars were distalized into a Class I relationship in 6.5 months.[84] In this period, they moved distally 2.5 mm and tipped 2.2°. The second molars were also affected by the distalization of the first molars and they tipped distally 5.9°.

Regarding anchorage loss, the maxillary second premolars moved mesially 1.2 mm, thus causing 1.5 mm mesial movement of the maxillary incisors, 4.7° incisor proclination, and 1.2 mm increase in overjet.[84]

Vertical Changes

Bondemark found that the lower anterior facial height was increased by 1.3 mm and the mandibular plane angle increased by 0.6° after molar distalization with the intraarch NiTi coil appliance. A small backward rotation of the mandible of 0.6° was also evident, which caused a decrease in overbite of 1.5 mm.[84]

Appliances with a Flexible Distalization Force System Buccally Positioned

Jones Jig™

According to most investigators, the Jones Jig (American Orthodontics, Sheboygan, WI) was effective in distalizing the maxillary first molars with no dependence on patient cooperation, although some anchorage loss occurred at the same time.

Sagittal Changes
Following distalization with the Jones Jig, the maxillary first molars were distalized between 1.2 and 2.8 mm[85–89] with a monthly rate of 0.8 mm.[85] However, the distal movement of the first molars was in most cases accompanied with unfavorable distal tipping that varied between 3.5° and 7.9°.[85–89] The maxillary second molars were also influenced by the first molar distal movement, being distalized from 1.5 to 2.7 mm[85–87] and tipped distally from 3.3°[85] up to 7.9°.[87]

The anchor unit could not resist the reciprocal mesial forces of the Jones Jig and anterior anchorage loss was found in most of the studies. The maxillary first premolars moved mesially 1.1 mm and tipped also mesially 2.6°.[85] The second premolars, when used as anchor teeth, moved mesially about 2 to 3 mm and tipped mesially between 2.6° and 9.4°.[86–88]

In addition, anterior movement and proclination of the maxillary incisors were also found during the distalization phase with the appliance. The maxillary incisors were found to move mesially 0.6 mm and to procline between 1° and 2°.[86,88] The overjet was found to be increased between 1 and 1.5 mm.[85,86]

Vertical Changes
The first molars were influenced during the distalization phase. Some investigators observed an extrusion between 0.9 and 2.1 mm[85,86,88] while others found an nonsignificant extrusion of 0.1 mm.[87] The maxillary second molars were also extruded by 2 mm.[86]

Further, the maxillary first premolars presented a 3.2 mm extrusion.[86] The second premolars were extruded 1.9 mm according to Brickman et al,[87] while in contrast Haydar & Uner found 1.9 mm of intrusion.[88]

The maxillary incisors also presented a 3.1 mm extrusion[86] while in contrast Haydar & Uner observed an intrusion of 1.0 mm.[88] Further, the overbite was decreased between 0.2 and 1.3 mm.[85–87]

Skeletal changes concerning the vertical dimension were also found after distalization with the Jones Jig. The lower anterior facial height was increased from 1 to 1.5 mm.[86,87] The mandibular plane angle was also increased by 1.3°,[85] whereas Runge et al found this angle almost unchanged after treatment.[86]

Soft Tissue Changes
The soft tissues were also affected by the anchorage loss of the anterior teeth. Runge et al observed a 0.4 mm protrusion of the upper lip and a 1.1 mm protrusion of the lower lip, as measured from their distances to the E-plane.[86] Brickman et al observed similar changes for the upper and lower lip.[87]

Modified Sectional Jig Assembly
The modified sectional jig assembly is an effective and reliable method for distalizing simultaneously the maxillary first and second

molars at the cost of anchorage loss, without depending on patient cooperation. The appliance mainly affects the maxillary dentition, with less marked effects on the craniofacial skeleton and the soft tissues.

Sagittal Changes
The modified sectional jig assembly has been shown to produce effective simultaneous distalization of maxillary first and second molars.[90] A Class II molar relationship was corrected into a Class I on both sides, in all cases in a mean treatment period of 16.5 weeks. Following distalization with the appliance, the maxillary first molars were distalized 1.4–2.8 mm and tipped distally 6.8°.[90,91] The rate of first molar distal movement was 0.4 mm per month.[90] The maxillary second molars were also distalized by 1.2 mm and tipped distally 8.3°. The effect of distalization on the maxillary third molars was extremely varied. In general, no distal movement was observed but distal tipping occurred by a mean 4° but this was not statistically significant.

The anchorage unit was unable to completely resist the reciprocal mesial forces of the activated coil springs. Anchorage loss was expressed as mesial tipping of the second premolars and as an increase in overjet. According to Papadopoulos et al,[90] the maxillary second premolars were moved mesially by a mean 2.6 mm and tipped by a mean 8.1° without significant extrusion. Mavropoulos et al observed that the space created between the first molars and the second premolars averaged 6.1 mm.[91] However, only 46% of this space was due to the distalization of the first molars. Furthermore, the maxillary incisors were moved forward 1.8–2.3 mm and proclined 4.8–5.2°,[90,91] while the overjet was increased by 0.9 mm.[90]

In relation to skeletal changes, the SNA angle showed no statistically significant difference before and after treatment with the distalization appliance, confirming previous findings using similar noncompliance approaches with NiTi coil springs.[85,87,88] However, the distance from the A point to PtV plane was significantly increased by a mean 1.4 mm. In addition, the SNB angle showed a statistically significant increase during the same period, most probably due to normal mandibular growth. For this reason it seems relevant to consider that the correction to a Class I molar relationship resulted not only from the distal movement of the upper first molars but also from the mesial repositioning of the lower first molars as the mandible grew forward.

Vertical Changes
During the distalization phase with the modified sectional jig assembly, the overbite was significantly decreased by 1 mm, while no significant changes were observed in lower anterior facial height (ANS-Me) and in the inclination of the palatal, mandibular, and functional occlusal planes in relation to the anterior cranial base (SN).[90]

Transverse Changes
The distal movement of the first maxillary molars was found to be accompanied by a distal rotation of 7.9° and a slight mesial rotation

of the second premolars of 3.7°.[91] The most interesting finding was the asymmetric effect which amounted to more than 1.5 mm. This observation could be attributed to the different states of leveling and alignment between the two sides of the dental arch.

Soft Tissue Changes

The evaluation of the soft tissue changes revealed that the upper lip protruded by a mean of 0.7 mm relative to the esthetic line; this was, however, not statistically significant. This tendency can be probably attributed to the proclination of the maxillary incisors and the forward movement of the A point. Surprisingly, the lower lip also protruded by a mean 1.3 mm, probably as a consequence of mandibular growth.[90]

NiTi Coil Springs Used for Molar Distalization

Sagittal Changes

Erverdi et al found that following distalization with the use of NiTi coil springs, the first molars were moved to a Class I relationship in a period of 3 months.[92] The first maxillary molars were distalized by an average of 3.8 mm and their crowns were tipped distally by 9.9°. The maxillary second premolars were also affected by the maxillary first molar distalization, and a distal movement of 0.8 mm was observed. Erverdi et al did not investigate the possible loss of anchorage on first premolars or incisors.[92]

Transverse Changes

According to Erverdi et al, a first molar distopalatal rotation of 8.6° was evident at the end of the distalization phase.[92]

Magnets used for molar distalization

Sagittal Changes

Following distalization with magnets, the maxillary first molars were distalized between 2.1 and 4.2 mm.[72,84,93,94] Nevertheless, the distal movement of the first molars was in most cases associated with undesirable distal tipping, which varied between 1° and 8.8°. The maxillary second molars were also affected by the first molar distal movement and they tipped distally between 3.8° and 8.9°.

The anchor unit could not resist the reciprocal mesial forces of the appliance and some anterior anchorage loss was found in most of the studies. The second premolars moved mesially 1.8 mm and tipped mesially 6.7°.[83] Further, anterior movement and proclination of the maxillary incisors were also evident after treatment. The incisors moved anteriorly between 1.2 and 1.9 mm and proclined between 3.8° and 5.5°.[72,84,93,94] The overjet was also influenced during the distalization phase, being increased between 1.5 and 1.7 mm.[72,84,93,94]

Some minor skeletal changes were also observed during the distalization phase of the treatment. In particular, the ANB angle was increased by 0.4°.[72]

Vertical Changes

The maxillary first molars were influenced during the distalization period and an extrusion of 0.8 mm was observed, while the overbite was decreased between 1.6 and 3.6 mm.[72,84]

Skeletal changes were also observed regarding the vertical dimension. The lower anterior facial height was increased 1.1 mm[84] while the mandibular plane angle was also increased by 1.1°.[72]

Transverse Changes

The maxillary first molars rotated distobuccally between 2° and 8.5° and the maxillary second molars between 5.9° and 7°.[72,93,94]

Appliances with a Double Flexible Distalization Force System Positioned Both Palatally and Buccally

No clinical studies have been published yet concerning the clinical efficacy of the noncompliance distalization appliances in this category (Piston Appliance, Nance Appliance with NiTi Coil Springs).

Appliances with a Rigid Distalization Force System Palatally Positioned

No clinical studies concerning the treatment effects of the distalization appliances in this category (Veltri's Distalizer, New Distalizer, P-Rax Molar Distalizer) have been reported in the literature to date.

Hybrid Appliances

First Class Appliance

According to the authors who evaluated the First Class Appliance (FCA) (Leone SpA, Firenze, Italy), it is an efficient and reliable device for the distalization of the maxillary first molars.[95]

Sagittal Changes

Following distalization with the FCA, the maxillary first molars were moved distally 4 mm. However, this was accompanied with undesirable distal tipping of 4.6°.

The anchorage unit could not resist the reciprocal mesial forces and anterior anchorage loss was observed. The maxillary second premolars moved mesially 1.7 mm and tipped mesially 2.2°, which corresponds to a 30% loss of anchorage. The maxillary incisors moved also mesially 1.3 mm and proclined 2.6°, while the overjet was increased 1.2 mm after distalization with the appliance.

Minimal skeletal changes occurred in the sagittal plane. In particular, the SNA angle was found increased by 0.4°.

Vertical Changes

The maxillary first molars extruded 1.2 mm and the second premolars extruded by a nonsignificant amount of 1 mm, while the overbite decreased also nonsignificantly by 0.8 mm.

Minimal skeletal changes were also found in the vertical dimension. The inclination of the mandibular pane to SN was increased by 0.5°.

Transpalatal Arches for Molar Rotation and/or Distalization

The transpalatal arches (TPA) have been found to be effective in rotating the maxillary molars. Dahlquist et al investigated the effects of a prefabricated transpalatal arch manufactured by GAC (GAC International Inc., Islandia, NY) used for the correction of first molar rotation in 50 children and compared the molar positions with those in 34 individuals with normal occlusion.[96] Following the use of the TPA for 60–198 days, the first molars were effectively derotated. In about two-thirds of the cases, the mesiobuccal cusp of the molar moved distally during derotation. In the remaining patients, it moved mesially or remained unchanged. The median distal movement was 0.3 mm on the right and 0.5 mm on the left side. Because many molars moved mesially, there was no gain in space on average in the dental arch from the derotation. Finally, in most cases the derotation resulted in a small, unintended expansion.

References

1. Pancherz H. Treatment of Class II malocclusions by jumping the bite with the Herbst appliance. A cephalometric investigation. Am J Orthod 1979;76:423–442.

2. Pancherz H. The mechanism of Class II correction in Herbst appliance treatment. A cephalometric investigation. Am J Orthod 1982;82:104–113.

3. Pancherz H. The Herbst appliance – its biologic effects and clinical use. Am J Orthod 1985; 87:1–20.

4. Pancherz H, Hansen K. Occlusal changes during and after Herbst treatment: a cephalometric investigation. Eur J Orthod 1986;8:215–228.

5. Pancherz H, Hansen K. Mandibular anchorage in Herbst treatment. Eur J Orthod 1988;10:149–164.

6. Pancherz H, Malmgren O, Hagg U, Omblus J, Hansen K. Class II correction in Herbst and Bass therapy. Eur J Orthod 1989;11:17–30.

7. Valant JR, Sinclair PM. Treatment effects of the Herbst appliance. Am J Orthod Dentofacial Orthop 1989;95:138–147.

8. Pancherz H, Fackel U. The skeletofacial growth pattern pre- and post-dentofacial orthopaedics. A long-term study of Class II malocclusions treated with the Herbst appliance. Eur J Orthod 1990;12:209–218.

9. Hansen K, Pancherz H, Hagg U. Long-term effects of the Herbst appliance in relation to the treatment growth period: a cephalometric study. Eur J Orthod 1991;13:471–481.

10. Hansen K, Pancherz H. Long-term effects of Herbst treatment in relation to normal growth development: a cephalometric study. Eur J Orthod 1992;14:285–295.

11. Windmiller EC. The acrylic-splint Herbst appliance: a cephalometric evaluation. Am J Orthod Dentofacial Orthop 1993;104:73–84.

12. Hansen K, Koutsonas TG, Pancherz H. Long-term effects of Herbst treatment on the mandibular incisor segment: a cephalometric and biometric investigation. Am J Orthod Dentofacial Orthop 1997;112:92–103.

13. Obijou C, Pancherz H. Herbst appliance treatment of Class II, division 2 malocclusions. Am J Orthod Dentofacial Orthop 1997;112:287–291.

14. Omblus J, Malmgren O, Pancherz H, Hagg U, Hansen K. Long-term effects of Class II correction in Herbst and Bass therapy. Eur J Orthod 1997;19:185–193.

15. Wong GW, So LL, Hagg U. A comparative study of sagittal correction with the Herbst appliance in two different ethnic groups. Eur J Orthod 1997;19: 195–204.

16. Croft RS, Buschang PH, English JD, Meyer R. A cephalometric and tomographic evaluation of Herbst treatment in the mixed dentition. Am J Orthod Dentofacial Orthop 1999;116:435–443.

17. Hagg U, Du X, Rabie AB. Initial and late treatment effects of headgear-Herbst appliance with mandibular step-by-step advancement. Am J Orthod Dentofacial Orthop 2002;122:477–485.

18. Burkhardt DR, McNamara JA Jr, Baccetti T. Maxillary molar distalization or mandibular enhancement: a cephalometric comparison of comprehensive orthodontic treatment including the pendulum and the Herbst appliances. Am J Orthod Dentofacial Orthop 2003;123:108–116.

19. Pancherz H. The nature of Class II relapse after Herbst appliance treatment: a cephalometric long-term investigation. Am J Orthod Dentofacial Orthop 1991;100:220–233.

20. Konik M, Pancherz H, Hansen K. The mechanism of Class II correction in late Herbst treatment. Am J Orthod Dentofacial Orthop 1997;112:87–91.

21. Ruf S, Pancherz H. The mechanism of Class II correction during Herbst therapy in relation to the vertical jaw base relationship: a cephalometric roentgenographic study. Angle Orthod 1997;67: 271–276.

22. Ruf S, Pancherz H. Dentoskeletal effects and facial profile changes in young adults treated with the Herbst appliance. Angle Orthod 1999;69:239–246.

23. Franchi L, Baccetti T, McNamara JA Jr. Treatment and post-treatment effects of acrylic splint Herbst appliance therapy. Am J Orthod Dentofacial Orthop 1999;115:429–438.

24. Nelson B, Hansen K, Hagg U. Class II correction in patients treated with class II elastics and with fixed functional appliances: a comparative study. Am J Orthod Dentofacial Orthop 2000;118:142–149.

25. Du X, Hagg U, Rabie AB. Effects of headgear Herbst and mandibular step-by-step advancement versus conventional Herbst appliance and maximal jumping of the mandible. Eur J Orthod 2002;24: 167–174.

26. O'Brien K, Wright J, Conboy F, et al. Effectiveness of treatment for Class II malocclusion with the Herbst or twin-block appliances: a randomized, controlled trial. Am J Orthod Dentofacial Orthop 2003;124:128–137.

27. Wieslander L. Intensive treatment of severe Class II malocclusions with a headgear-Herbst appliance in the early mixed dentition. Am J Orthod 1984;86:1–13.

28. Pancherz H, Anehus-Pancherz M. The headgear effect of the Herbst appliance: a cephalometric long-term study. Am J Orthod Dentofacial Orthop 1993;103:510–520.

29. Wieslander L. Long-term effect of treatment with the headgear-Herbst appliance in the early mixed dentition. Stability or relapse? Am J Orthod Dentofacial Orthop 1993;104:319–329.

30. McNamara JA Jr, Howe RP, Dischinger TG. A comparison of the Herbst and Frankel appliances in the treatment of Class II malocclusion. Am J Orthod Dentofacial Orthop 1990;98:134–144.

31. Sidhu MS, Kharbanda OP, Sidhu SS. Cephalometric analysis of changes produced by a modified Herbst appliance in the treatment of Class II division 1 malocclusion. Br J Orthod 1995;22:1–12.

32. Eberhard H, Hirschfelder U. Treatment of Class II, Division 2 in the late growth period. J Orofac Orthop 1998;59:352–361.

33. Schweitzer M, Pancherz H. The incisor-lip relationship in Herbst/multibracket appliance treatment of Class II, Division 2 malocclusions. Angle Orthod 2001;71:358–363.

34. Baltromejus S, Ruf S, Pancherz H. Effective temporomandibular joint growth and chin position changes: Activator versus Herbst treatment. A cephalometric roentgenographic study. Eur J Orthod 2002;24:627–637.

35. Pancherz H, Ruf S, Kohlhas P. Effective condylar growth and chin position changes in Herbst treatment: a cephalometric roentgenographic long-term study. Am J Orthod Dentofacial Orthop 1998;114:437–446.

36. Pancherz H, Hagg U. Dentofacial orthopedics in relation to somatic maturation. An analysis of 70 consecutive cases treated with the Herbst appliance. Am J Orthod 1985;88:273–287.

37. Hansen K, Iemamnueisuk P, Pancherz H. Long-term effects of the Herbst appliance on the dental arches and arch relationships: a biometric study. Br J Orthod 1995;22:123–134.

38. Ruf S, Pancherz H. The effect of Herbst appliance treatment on the mandibular plane angle: a cephalometric roentgenographic study. Am J Orthod Dentofacial Orthop 1996;110:225–229.

39. Schiavoni R, Grenga V, Macri V. Treatment of Class II high angle malocclusions with the Herbst appliance: a cephalometric investigation. Am J Orthod Dentofacial Orthop 1992;102:393–409.

40. Eicke C, Wieslander L. [Soft-tissue profile changes through therapy with the Herbst hinge appliance.] Schweiz Monatsschr Zahnmed 1990;100:149–153.

41. Pancherz H, Anehus-Pancherz M. Facial profile changes during and after Herbst appliance treatment. Eur J Orthod 1994;16:275–286.

42. Pancherz H, Ruf S, Thomalske-Faubert C. Mandibular articular disk position changes during Herbst treatment: a prospective longitudinal MRI study. Am J Orthod Dentofacial Orthop 1999;116: 207–214.

43. Hansen K, Pancherz H, Petersson A. Long-term effects of the Herbst appliance on the craniomandibular system with special reference to the TMJ. Eur J Orthod 1990;12:244–253.

44. Pancherz H, Anehus-Pancherz M. The effect of continuous bite jumping with the Herbst appliance on the masticatory system: a functional analysis of treated Class II malocclusions. Eur J Orthod 1982; 4:37–44.

45. Hansen K. Post-treatment effects of the Herbst appliance. A radiographic, clinical and biometric investigation. Swed Dent J Suppl 1992;88:1–49.

46. Ruf S, Pancherz H. Long-term TMJ effects of Herbst treatment: a clinical and MRI study. Am J Orthod Dentofacial Orthop 1998;114:475–483.

47. Ruf S, Pancherz H. Does bite-jumping damage the TMJ? A prospective longitudinal clinical and MRI study of Herbst patients. Angle Orthod 2000;70: 183–199.

48. Pancherz H, Anehus-Pancherz M. Muscle activity in Class II, division 1 malocclusions treated by bite jumping with the Herbst appliance. An electromyographic study. Am J Orthod 1980;78: 321–329.

49. Leung DK, Hagg U. An electromyographic investigation of the first six months of progressive mandibular advancement of the Herbst appliance in adolescents. Angle Orthod 2001;71:177–184.

50. Hiyama S, Ono PT, Ishiwata Y, Kuroda T, McNamara JA Jr. Neuromuscular and skeletal adaptations following mandibular forward positioning induced by the Herbst appliance. Angle Orthod 2000;70:442–453.

51. Athanasiou AE, Papadopoulos MA, Nasiopoulos AT, Ioannidou I, Kolokithas G. Changes in the mechanical advantages of the masseter and temporal muscles and the number and intensity of occlusal contacts following Herbst appliance treatment of Class II, division 1 malocclusion: an early evaluation. J Marmara Univ Dental Faculty 2004; 5:435–444.

52. Pangrazio-Kulbersh V, Berger JL, Chermak DS, Kaczynski R, Simon ES, Haerian A. Treatment effects of the mandibular anterior repositioning appliance on patients with Class II malocclusion. Am J Orthod Dentofacial Orthop 2003;123:286–295.

53. Weiland FJ, Ingervall B, Bantleon HP, Droschl H. Initial effects of treatment of Class II malocclusion with the Herren activator, activator-headgear combination, and Jasper Jumper. Am J Orthod Dentofacial Orthop 1997;112:19–27.

54. Stucki N, Ingervall B. The use of the Jasper Jumper for the correction of Class II malocclusion in the young permanent dentition. Eur J Orthod 1998; 20:271–281.

55. Covell DA Jr, Trammell DW, Boero RP, West R. A cephalometric study of class II Division 1 malocclusions treated with the Jasper Jumper appliance. Angle Orthod 1999;69:311–320.

56. Sari Z, Goyenc Y, Doruk C, Usumez S. Comparative evaluation of a new removable Jasper Jumper functional appliance vs an activator-headgear combination. Angle Orthod 2003;73:286–293.

57. Weiland FJ, Bantleon HP. Treatment of Class II malocclusions with the Jasper Jumper appliance. A preliminary report. Am J Orthod Dentofacial Orthop 1995;108:341–350.

58. Cope JB, Buschang PH, Cope DD, Parker J, Blackwood HO 3rd. Quantitative evaluation of craniofacial changes with Jasper Jumper therapy. Angle Orthod 1994;64:113–122.

59. Heinig N, Goz G. Clinical application and effects of the Forsus spring. A study of a new Herbst hybrid. J Orofac Orthop 2001;62:436–450.

60. Stromeyer EL, Caruso JM, DeVincenzo JP. A cephalometric study of the Class II correction effects of the Eureka Spring. Angle Orthod 2002;72:203–210.

61. Bussick TJ, McNamara JA Jr. Dentoalveolar and skeletal changes associated with the pendulum appliance. Am J Orthod Dentofacial Orthop 2000;117:333–343.

62. Toroglu MS, Uzel I, Cam OY, Hancioglu ZB. Cephalometric evaluation of the effects of pendulum appliance on various vertical growth patterns and of the changes during short-term stabilization. Clin Orthod Res 2001;4:15–27.

63. Joseph AA, Butchart CJ. An evaluation of the pendulum distalizing appliance. Semin Orthod 2000;6:129–135.

64. Chaques-Asensi J, Kalra V. Effects of the pendulum appliance on the dentofacial complex. J Clin Orthod 2001;35:254–257.

65. Ghosh J, Nanda RS. Evaluation of an intraoral maxillary molar distalization technique. Am J Orthod Dentofacial Orthop 1996;110:639–646.

66. Hilgers JJ. The pendulum appliance for Class II noncompliance therapy. J Clin Orthod 1992; 26:706–714.

67. Ten Hoeve A. Palatal bar and lip bumper in nonextraction treatment. J Clin Orthod 1985;19: 272–291.

68. Gianelly AA, Vaitas AS, Thomas WM, Berger OG. Distalization of molars with repelling magnets, case report. J Clin Orthod 1988;22:40–44.

69. Jeckel N, Rakosi T. Molar distalization by intra-oral force application. Eur J Orthod 1991;3:43–46.

70. Gianelly AA, Vaitas AS, Thomas WM. The use of magnets to move molars distally. Am J Orthod Dentofacial Orthop 1989;96:161–167.

71. Gianelly AA, Bednar J, Dietz VS. Japanese NiTi coils used to move molars distally. Am J Orthod Dentofacial Orthop 1991;99:564–566.

72. Bondemark L, Kurol J, Bernhold M. Repelling magnets versus superelastic nickel-titanium coils in simultaneous distal movement of maxillary first and second molars. Angle Orthod 1994;64:189–198.

73. Kinzinger GS, Fritz UB, Sander FG, Diedrich PR. Efficiency of a pendulum appliance for molar distalization related to second and third molar eruption stage. Am J Orthod Dentofacial Orthop 2004;125:8–23.

74. Riolo ML, Moyers RE, McNamara JA Jr, Hunter WS. An atlas of craniofacial growth: cephalometric standards from the University School Growth Study, The University of Michigan. Craniofacial Growth Monograph Series, Vol. 2. Ann Arbor: Center for Human Growth and Development, University of Michigan; 1974.

75. Byloff FK, Darendeliler MA. Distal molar movement using the pendulum appliance. Part 1: Clinical and radiological evaluation. Angle Orthod 1997;67:249–260.

76. Byloff FK, Darendeliler MA, Clar E, Darendeliler A. Distal molar movement using the pendulum appliance. Part 2: The effects of maxillary molar root uprighting bands. Angle Orthod 1997;67: 261–270.

77. Kinzinger G, Fuhrmann R, Gross U, Diedrich P. Modified pendulum appliance including distal screw and uprighting activation for noncompliance therapy of Class II malocclusion in children and adolescents. J Orofac Orthop 2000;61:175–190.

78. Kinzinger G, Fritz U, Diedrich P. Combined therapy with pendulum and lingual arch appliances in the early mixed dentition. J Orofac Orthop 2003;64:201–213.

79. Keles A, Sayinsu K. A new approach in maxillary molar distalization: intraoral bodily molar distalizer. Am J Orthod Dentofacial Orthop 2000;117: 39–48.

80. Ngantung V, Nanda RS, Bowman, SJ. Posttreatment evaluation of the distal jet appliance. Am J Orthod Dentofacial Orthop 2001;120:178–185.

81. Nishii Y, Katada H, Yamaguchi H. Three-dimensional evaluation of the distal jet appliance. World J Orthod 2002;3:321–327.

82. Bolla E, Muratore F, Carano A, Bowman SJ. Evaluation of maxillary molar distalization with the distal jet: a comparison with other contemporary methods. Angle Orthod 2002;72:481–494.

83. Keles A. Maxillary unilateral molar distalization with sliding mechanics: a preliminary investigation. Eur J Orthod 2001;23:507–515.

84. Bondemark L. A comparative analysis of distal maxillary molar movement produced by a new lingual intra-arch NiTi coil appliance and a magnetic appliance. Eur J Orthod 2000;22: 683–695.

85. Gulati S, Kharbanda OP, Parkash H. Dental and skeletal changes after intraoral molar distalization with sectional jig assembly. Am J Orthod Dentofacial Orthop 1998;114:319–327.

86. Runge ME, Martin JT, Bukai F. Analysis of rapid maxillary molar distal movement without patient cooperation. Am J Orthod Dentofacial Orthop 1999;115:153–157.

87. Brickman CD, Sinha PK, Nanda RS. Evaluation of the Jones jig appliance for distal molar movement. Am J Orthod Dentofacial Orthop 2000;118: 526–534.

88. Haydar S, Uner O. Comparison of Jones jig molar distalization appliance with extraoral traction. Am J Orthod Dentofacial Orthop 2000;117:49–53.

89. Paul LD, O'Brien KD, Mandall NA. Upper removable appliance or Jones jig for distalizing first molars? A randomized clinical trial. Orthod Craniofac Res 2002;5:238–242.

90. Papadopoulos MA, Mavropoulos A, Karamouzos A. Cephalometric changes following simultaneous first and second maxillary molar distalization using a noncompliance intraoral appliance. J Orofac Orthop 2004;65:123–136.

91. Mavropoulos A, Karamouzos A, Kiliaridis S, Papadopoulos MA. Efficiency of noncompliance simultaneous first and second upper molar distalization: a 3D tooth movement analysis. Angle Orthod 2005;75:468–475.

92. Erverdi N, Koyuturk O, Kucukkeles N. Nickel-titanium coil springs and repelling magnets: a comparison of two different intra-oral molar distalization techniques. Br J Orthod 1997;24: 47–53.

93. Bondemark L, Kurol J. Distalization of maxillary first and second molars simultaneously with repelling magnets. Eur J Orthod 1992;14: 264–272.

94. Itoh T, Tokuda T, Kiyosue S, Hirose T, Matsumoto M, Chaconas SJ. Molar distalization with repelling magnets. J Clin Orthod 1991;25:611–617.

95. Fortini A, Lupoli M, Giuntoli F, Franchi L. Dentoskeletal effects induced by rapid molar distalization with the first class appliance. Am J Orthod Dentofacial Orthop 2004;125:697–705.

96. Dahlquist A, Gebauer U, Ingervall B. The effect of a transpalatal arch for the correction of first molar rotation. Eur J Orthod 1996;18:257–267.

Index